handbook of
OBSTETRICS
& GYNECOLOGY

Bony Pelvis 17

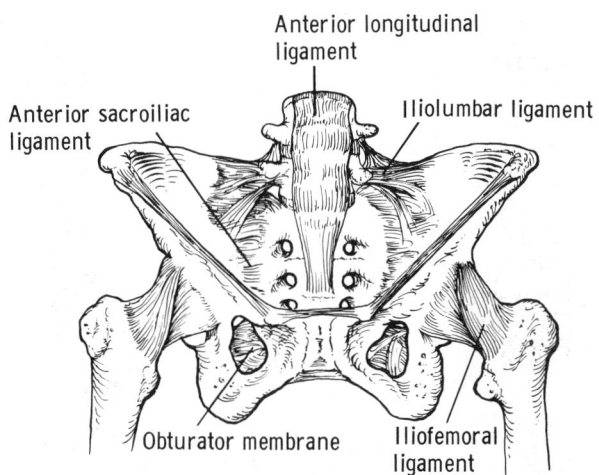

Fig 1-6. The bony pelvis (anterior view).

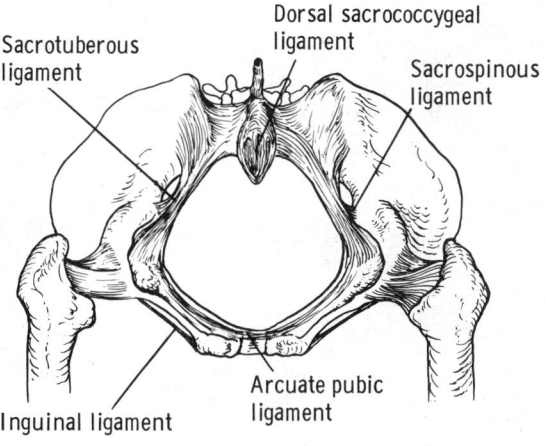

Fig 1-7. The bony pelvis (inferior view).

18 Bony Pelvis

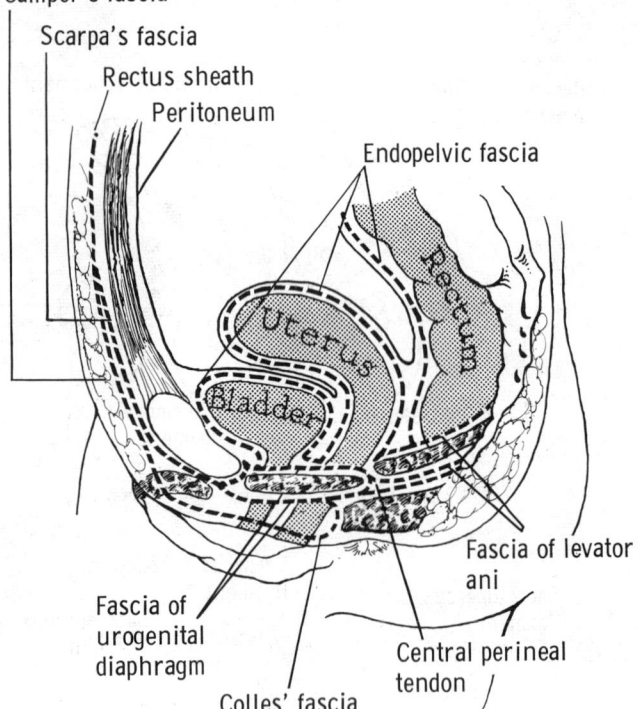

Fig 1-8. Fascial planes of the pelvis. (Modified after Netter.)

The true pelvis is bounded by the sacrum and coccyx posteriorly, by the innominate bones laterally, and by the pubes anteriorly. The posterior portion of the true pelvis is 3 times deeper than its anterior segment. The shape of the pelvic cavity along its axis suggests a bent tube with a considerably shortened anterior curve.

The upper limit of the true pelvis is the slightly heart-shaped brim, superior strait, or inlet. The lower limit, which forms an anterior-posterior ellipse, is the inferior strait or outlet (see Fig 1-7).

No 2 pelves are identical. Size and shape vary according to individual, familial, and racial characteristics. Disease may further modify the features of the bony pelvis.

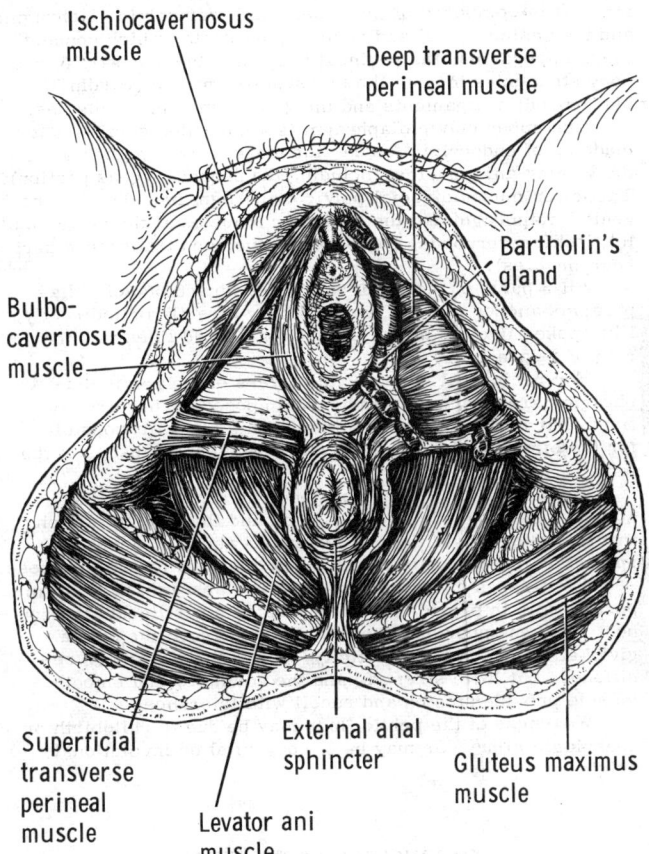

Fig 1-9. Pelvic musculature (inferior view).

THE PELVIC FLOOR

The pelvic floor consists of muscle, ligaments, and fascia arranged in such a manner as to (1) support the pelvic viscera; (2) provide sphincter-like action for the urethra, vagina, and rectum; and (3) permit the passage of a term infant. It is composed of the upper and lower pelvic diaphragms and the vesicovaginal and rectovaginal septa, which connect the 2 diaphragms, the perineal body, and the coccyx. Accessory structures include the transverse cervical (cardinal, Mackenrodt's) ligaments and the gluteus maximus muscles.

The upper pelvic diaphragm is a musculofascial structure made up of endopelvic fascia, the uterosacral ligaments, and the levator ani muscles (including the pubococcygeus portion). The lower musculofascial pelvic diaphragm includes the urogenital diaphragm and the sphincter muscles at the vulvar outlet (ischiocavernosus, bulbocavernosus, and transverse perineal muscles).

All 5 parts of the upper and lower musculofascial diaphragms anchor into the perineal body directly or indirectly, like spokes into the hub of a wheel or shroud lines into the ring of a parachute.

For reciprocal support, the layers of the pelvic diaphragms are interwoven and superimposed. They are not fixed, but move upon one another. This makes it possible for the birth canal to dilate to capacity during passage of the fetus.

The pelvic floor is perforated centrally by 3 tubular structures: the urethra, the vagina, and the rectum. Each traverses the pelvic floor at an angle, which enhances the sphincter-like action of the muscles designed for this purpose.

The tissues of the musculofascial diaphragm play an important role in providing both support and resilience: the connective tissue provides support, but no recoil; the fascia gives strength, but no elasticity; the elastic tissue has resilience, but little strength; and the voluntary and smooth muscle provide stretch and recoil with tolerance.

Weakness of the pelvic floor may be due to childbirth or neurologic injury, or may be of congenital or involutional origin.

EMBRYOLOGY OF THE FEMALE UROGENITAL TRACT

FORMATION & EARLY DEVELOPMENT OF THE CLOACA

As early as the first week following implantation of the fertilized ovum, the hindgut evaginates to form the allantois, or forerunner of the bladder. After the second week, the gut caudal to the allantois widens to form the cloaca. This incompletely developed urogenital ostium extends from the umbilical stalk to the rudimentary tail—virtually the extent of

SECOND EDITION

handbook of
OBSTETRICS & GYNECOLOGY

RALPH C. BENSON, MD
Professor of Obstetrics and Gynecology
and Chairman, Department of Obstetrics
and Gynecology, University of Oregon
Medical School, Hospitals and Clinic
Portland, Oregon

Lange Medical Publications
Los Altos, California

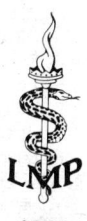

1966

Copyright © 1964, 1966

All Rights Reserved

by

Lange Medical Publications

Copyright in Canada

Library of Congress Catalog Card No. 66-16731

A Concise Medical Library for Practitioner and Student

Physician's Handbook, 14th edition, 1966 M. A. Krupp, N. J. Sweet, E. Jawetz, E. G. Biglieri	$5.00
Handbook of Medical Treatment, 10th edition, 1966 M. J. Chatton, S. Margen, H. Brainerd, Editors	$5.50
Handbook of Pediatrics, 6th edition, 1965 H. K. Silver, C. H. Kempe, H. B. Bruyn	$5.00
Handbook of Poisoning: Diagnosis & Treatment, 5th edition, 1966 R. H. Dreisbach	$5.00
Current Medical References, 4th edition, 1965 M. J. Chatton, P. J. Sanazaro, Editors	$6.50
Handbook of Surgery, 3rd edition, 1966 J. L. Wilson, J. J. McDonald, Editors	$5.50
Handbook of Obstetrics & Gynecology, 2nd edition, 1966 R. C. Benson	$5.50
Correlative Neuroanatomy and Functional Neurology, 12th edition, 1964 J. G. Chusid, J. J. McDonald	$6.00
Review of Physiological Chemistry, 10th edition, 1965 H. A. Harper	$6.50
Review of Medical Microbiology, 7th edition, 1966 E. Jawetz, J. L. Melnick, E. A. Adelberg	$6.50
Principles of Clinical Electrocardiography, 5th edition, 1964 M. J. Goldman	$5.50
General Urology, 5th edition, 1966 D. R. Smith	$6.50
General Ophthalmology, 4th edition, 1965 D. Vaughan, R. Cook, T. Asbury	$6.00
Current Diagnosis & Treatment 1966 H. Brainerd, S. Margen, M. J. Chatton, Editors	$9.50
Review of Medical Physiology, 2nd edition, 1965 W. F. Ganong	$7.00

Lithographed in U. S. A.

Preface

This Handbook is presented as a compact, ready reference for the student, house officer, and practitioner and as an abbreviated but reasonably comprehensive companion to the large, "standard" textbooks of obstetrics and gynecology. Although no effort has been made to provide definitive and complete discussions of either basic subject, we have attempted to provide a concise digest of important clinical concepts within this specialty. We trust that this book will enable the nonspecialist physician to properly diagnose and treat many of the disorders encountered in practice and to avoid certain common pitfalls. Outlines of anatomy, physiology, pathology, differential diagnosis, and complications have been included both for review and to provide a logical background to treatment.

For the Second Edition, substantial additions have been made to the Gynecology section, and a new chapter on gynecologic procedures has been provided.

The author is pleased to be able to report that a Spanish language edition of this Handbook has been brought out under the imprint of El Manual Moderno in Mexico City.

I wish to express my gratitude to many colleagues who offered suggestions for additions and revisions in this edition. In particular, I wish to thank Dr. Jack M. Futoran for systematically reviewing the entire text and suggesting several important revisions. Laurel V. Gilliland substantially increased her contribution to the success of the Handbook by providing many excellent new illustrations. I am most grateful also to Grace Brophy for editorial counsel and to Maureen Amlong and Merrie Gagnet for secretarial assistance.

Ralph C. Benson

Portland, Oregon
August, 1966

1...
Anatomy & Physiology of the Female Reproductive System

The female reproductive system may be divided into the external and internal genitalia and their supporting structures.

The **external genitalia**, collectively termed the pudendum or vulva, comprise the following structures, all easily visible on external examination: mons veneris (mons pubis), labia majora, labia minora, clitoris, vestibule and external urethral meatus, Skene's glands (paraurethral glands), Bartholin's glands (vulvovaginal glands), hymen, fourchet, perineal body, and fossa navicularis. They present varying contours around the urogenital cleft, which lies anteroposteriorly between the vaginal and urethral openings. The contours of the external genitalia are determined by the bony configuration of the antero-inferior pelvic girdle as well as by the subcutaneous fat, muscle, and fascial arrangement.

The **internal genitalia** comprise the vagina, cervix, uterus, fallopian tubes, and ovaries. They require special instruments for inspection; the intra-abdominal group can be examined visually only by means of celiotomy, peritoneoscopy, or culdoscopy.

The anatomy of the bony pelvis and the pelvic floor is discussed on pp. 15 and 19.

EXTERNAL GENITALIA

MONS VENERIS
(Mons Pubis)

Gross Appearance.

The mons veneris is a rounded pad of fatty tissue overlying the symphysis pubis; it is not an organ, but a region or landmark. Coarse, dark hair normally appears over the mons early in puberty.

During reproductive life the pubic hair is abundant, but after the menopause it becomes sparse. The normal female escutcheon is typically a "triangle with the base up," in contrast with the "triangle with the base down" male pattern.

2 Mons Veneris

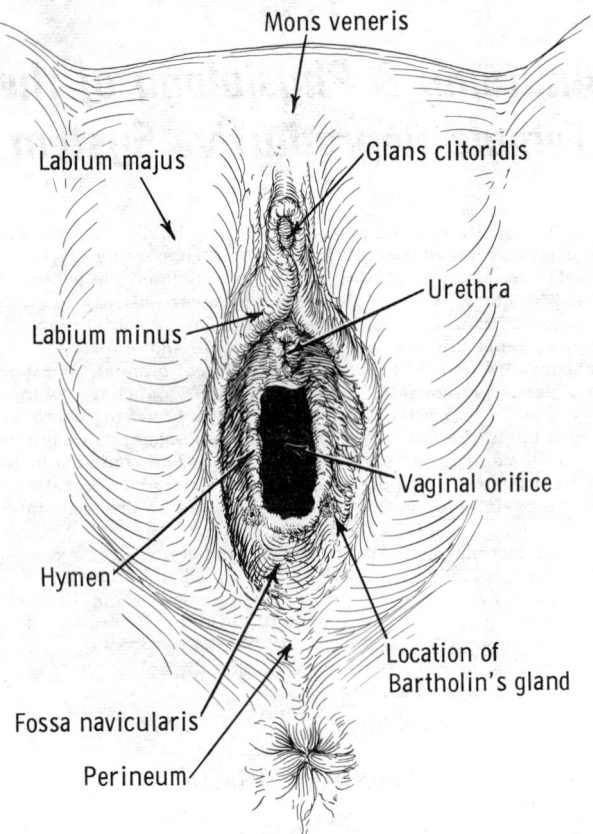

Fig 1-1. External female genitalia.

Histology.
The skin of the mons contains sudoriferous and sebaceous glands. The amount of subcutaneous fat is determined by nutritional and possibly by steroid hormonal factors.

Innervation.
The sensory nerves of the mons are the ilioinguinal and genitofemoral nerves.

Blood & Lymph Supply.

The mons is supplied by the external pudendal artery and vein. The lymphatics merge with those from other parts of the vulva and from the superficial abdomen. The crossed lymphatic circulation from the labia within the mons is of clinical interest since it permits carcinoma metastases from one side of the vulva to appear in the inguinal glands of the opposite, as well as the affected, side.

Clinical Importance.

Dermatitis is common in the pubic area. Edema may occur secondary to vulvar varicosities or to carcinomatous infiltration of the lymphatics. Cancer elsewhere in the vulva may also involve the mons.

LABIA MAJORA

Gross Appearance.

In the adult female, these 2 raised, rounded, longitudinal folds of skin are the most prominent features of the external genitalia. Arising from the perineal body, they extend anteriorly around the labia minora to merge with the mons. The labia are normally closed in nulliparous women but usually gape widely after childbirth and become thin, with sparse hair in old age.

The skin of the lateral surfaces of the labia is thick and often pigmented; it is covered with coarse hair similar to that of the mons. The skin of the inner labia majora is thin and fine and contains no hairs.

Histology.

The labia majora are made up of connective and areolar tissue, with many sebaceous glands. They are homologous to the scrotum. A thin fascial layer similar to the tunica dartos of the scrotum is found within the labia just below the surface. The round ligaments of the uterus pass through the canal of Nuck to end in a fibrous insertion in the anterior portion of the labia majora.

Innervation.

Anteriorly, the labia majora are supplied by the ilioinguinal and pudendal nerves. Laterally and posteriorly they are innervated by the posterior femoral cutaneous nerve.

Blood Supply.

The labia majora are supplied by the internal pudendal artery, derived from the anterior parietal division of the internal iliac (hypogastric) artery; and by the external pudendal artery (from the femoral artery). Drainage is via the internal and external pudendal veins.

Clinical Importance.

No special function is performed by the labia majora. A cyst of the canal of Nuck is often mistaken for an indirect inguinal hernia. Adherence of the labia may indicate vulvitis. External force or the complications of labor may cause vulvar hematoma.

LABIA MINORA

Gross Appearance.

The labia minora are small, narrow, elongated folds of skin between the labia majora and the vaginal introitus. Normally the labia minora are in apposition, concealing the introitus. Posteriorly, the labia minora merge at the fourchet. The labia are separate from the hymen, which is an individual structure marking the vaginal entrance or introitus. Anteriorly, each labium merges into a median ridge which fuses with its mate to form the frenulum of the clitoris; and an anterior fold, which becomes the prepuce of the clitoris.

The lateral and anterior surfaces of the labia minora are usually pigmented; their inner aspect is pink and moist, resembling the vaginal mucosa.

Histology.

Neither hair follicles nor sweat glands are found in the labia minora. They are rich in sebaceous glands, however.

Innervation & Blood Supply.

The innervation of the labia minora is via the ilioinguinal, pudendal, and hemorrhoidal nerves.

The labia minora are not truly erectile, but a rich vasculature permits marked turgescence with emotional or physical stimulation. They are supplied by the external and internal pudendal arteries.

Clinical Importance.

The labia minora increase in size as the result of ovarian hormonal stimulation. After the menopause they all but disappear unless estrogens are administered. Squamous cell carcinoma of the vulva often originates in the labia minora; sebaceous cysts also develop in these structures. Fused labia minora in the infant may indicate sexual maldifferentiation.

CLITORIS

Gross Appearance & Histology.

This 2-3 cm long homologue of the penis is found in the midline slightly anterior to the urethral meatus. It is composed of 2 small, erectile corpora, each attached to the periosteum of the symphysis, and a diminutive structure (glans clitoridis) which is generously supplied with sensory nerve endings. The glans is partially hooded by the labia minora.

Innervation & Blood Supply.
The clitoris is supplied by the hypogastric and pudendal nerves and pelvic sympathetics, and by the internal pudendal artery and vein.

Clinical Importance.
Cancer of the clitoris is rare, but it is extremely serious because of early metastases. The inguinal and femoral nodes are usually first involved.

VESTIBULE & URETHRAL MEATUS

Gross Appearance & Histology.
The area between the labia minora anteriorly is the vestibule. It contains the urethral, vaginal, and gland orifices. It is covered by delicate stratified squamous epithelium.

The urinary meatus is visible as an anteroposterior slit or an inverted V. Like the urethra, it is lined with transitional epithelium. The vascular mucosa of the meatus often pouts or everts. This makes it appear more red than the neighboring vaginal mucosa.

Innervation & Blood Supply.
The vestibule and terminal urethra are supplied by the pudendal nerve and by the internal pudendal artery and vein.

Clinical Importance.
Caruncles, as well as squamous cell or transitional cell carcinoma, may develop in the urethrovestibular area.

SKENE'S GLANDS
(Paraurethral Glands)

Gross Appearance & Histology.
Immediately within the urethra on its posterolateral aspect are 2 small orifices leading to the shallow tubular ducts or glands of Skene. The glands are lined by transitional cells, and are the sparse equivalent of the numerous male prostatic glands.

Blood Supply.
Like the vestibule and urethral meatus, Skene's glands are supplied by the internal pudendal artery and vein.

Clinical Importance.

Skene's glands are especially susceptible to gonococcal infection; infection is often first evident here. Following successful antigonorrheal therapy, nonspecific infection with other purulent organisms is common.

BARTHOLIN'S GLANDS & DUCTS
(Paravaginal or Vulvovaginal Glands & Ducts)

Gross Appearance & Histology.

Just inside the lower vagina, on either side, are 2 tiny apertures. Each is connected by a narrow duct, 1-2 cm long, with a small flattened mucus-producing gland which lies between the labia minora and vaginal wall. These are Bartholin's glands (paravaginal or vulvovaginal glands), the counterpart of Cowper's glands in the male. The ducts are lined with transitional epithelium.

Innervation & Blood Supply.

The internal pudendal nerve, artery, and vein serve Bartholin's glands.

Clinical Importance.

Gonorrhea frequently causes Bartholin's ducts to become abscessed and cystic, although the glands themselves are usually not affected. Nonvenereal bacterial infections uncommonly result in this complication. Primary adenocarcinoma is a rare neoplasm in the external genitalia, but it may originate in Bartholin's glands. Transitional cell epidermoid carcinoma of Bartholin's duct may also occur.

HYMEN

Gross Appearance & Histology.

A circular or crescent-shaped membrane just inside but separate from the labia minora marks the entrance to the vagina. This moderately elastic barrier partially or, in rare instances, completely occludes the vaginal canal. It is a double-faced epithelial plate covering a vascular, fibrous tissue matrix.

Innervation & Blood Supply.

The hymen is supplied by the pudendal and inferior hemorrhoidal nerves, arteries, and veins.

Clinical Importance.

A tight hymen may result in symptomatic gynatresia, in which case hymenotomy or dilatation will be required. The remnants of the lacerated hymen following intercourse or delivery are called carunculae hymenales (myrtiformes).

PERINEAL BODY, FOURCHET, & FOSSA NAVICULARIS

Gross Appearance.
   The perineal body includes the skin and underlying tissues between the anal orifice and the vaginal entrance. It is supported by the transverse perineal muscle and the lower portions of the bulbocavernosus muscle.
   The labia minora and majora converge posteriorly to form a low ridge called the fourchet. Just beyond this fold, extending about 1 cm anteriorly to the hymen, is a shallow depression, the fossa navicularis.

Innervation & Blood Supply.
   These structures are supplied by the pudendal and inferior hemorrhoidal nerves, arteries, and veins.

Clinical Importance.
   These structures are often lacerated during childbirth and may require repair. Because of their vascularity, an early episiotomy can result in the loss of several hundred ml of blood; faulty repair may be followed by dyspareunia or by pelvic relaxation in later years.

INTERNAL GENITALIA

VAGINA

Gross Appearance.
   The vagina is a thin, muscular, partially collapsed rugose canal 8-10 cm long and about 4 cm in diameter. It extends from the urogenital cleft to the cervix and curves upward and posteriorly from the vulva. The cervix protrudes several cm into the upper vagina to form the fornices. Since the posterior lip of the cervix is longer than its anterior lip, the posterior fornix is deeper than the anterior fornix.
   The vagina lies between the bladder and the rectum and is supported principally by the transverse cervical ligaments (cardinal ligaments, Mackenrodt's ligaments) and the levator ani muscles.
   The peritoneum of the posterior cul-de-sac (pouch of Douglas) and the posterior vaginal fornix are close together at the vaginal vault (a detail of surgical importance).

8 Vagina

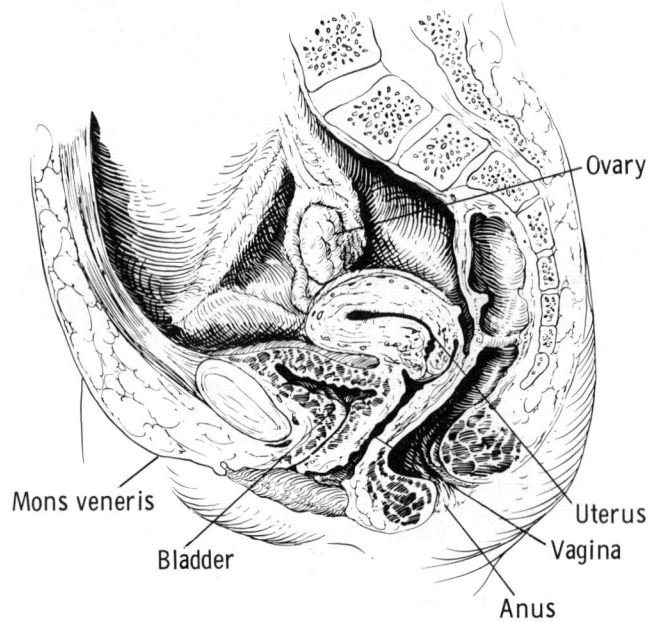

Fig 1-2. Midsagittal view of the female pelvic organs.

Histology.

The vagina is lined by mucous membrane, which is thick and folded transversely in the nulliparous woman. Many of these rugae are lost with repeated vaginal delivery and after the menopause. Normally, no glands are found in the vagina.

Innervation & Blood Supply.

The nerve supply to the vagina is via the pudendal and hemorrhoidal nerves and the pelvic sympathetic chain. The blood supply is from the vaginal artery, which is derived from a descending branch of the uterine artery, and from the middle hemorrhoidal and internal pudendal arteries. It is drained by the pudendal, external hemorrhoidal, and uterine veins.

The lymphatic drainage of the lower vagina is directed toward the superficial inguinal nodes; that of the upper vagina is to the presacral, external iliac, and hypogastric nodes. This is important in vulvovaginal infections and cancer spread.

Vagina 9

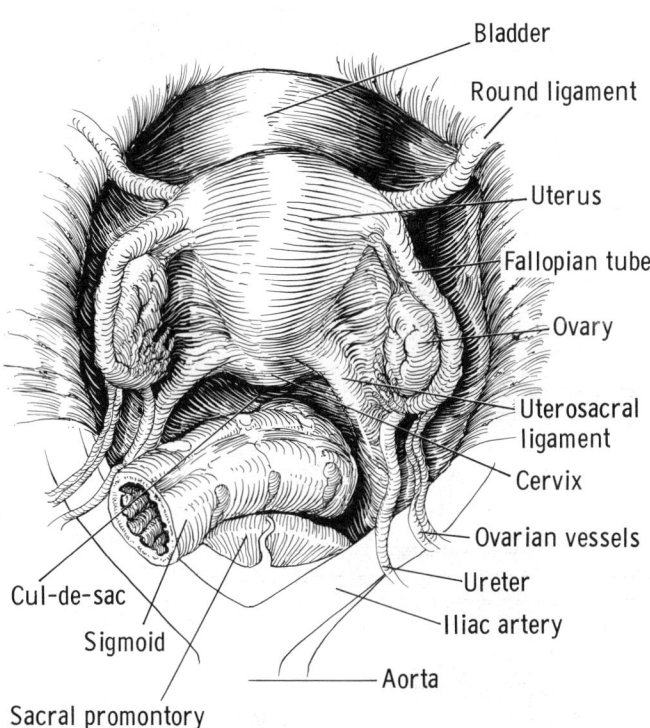

Fig 1-3. Pelvic organs (superior view).

Clinical Importance.
Vaginal discharge (leukorrhea) is common and may be due to local or systemic disorders. Infections of the lower reproductive tract are the most common cause of leukorrhea; estrogen depletion (senile or atrophic vaginitis) and estrogen or psychic stimulation are other causes.

Primary cancer of the vagina is exceedingly rare, but secondary carcinoma of the vagina, most frequently from extension of cervical cancer, is not uncommon.

CERVIX

Gross Appearance.
　　The cervix of the nonpregnant uterus is a conical, moderately firm organ about 2-4 cm long and about 2.5 cm in outside diameter. A central spindle-shaped canal communicates with the uterus above and the vagina below. About half the length of the cervix is supravaginal and is in close relation anteriorly to the bladder.
　　Childbirth lacerations account for most cervical distortions. The external os, which is initially round and only a fraction of a cm in diameter, may gape as a result of these tears. Even in the absence of distortions, however, it is customary to refer to the cervix as having anterior and posterior lips.
　　The cervix is supported by the uterosacral ligaments and transverse cervical ligaments (cardinal ligaments, Mackenrodt's ligaments).

Histology.
　　The intravaginal portion of the cervix is covered by stratified squamous cells, which usually extend to just inside the external os. The countless crevices, which give the cervix a honeycombed appearance on transection, were once believed to be glands. It is now known that they are infoldings of a mucus-secreting membrane. Peripherally, the cervix contains circular muscle fibers, which connect with the uterine myometrium above.

Innervation & Blood Supply.
　　Innervation of the cervix is via the second, third, and 4th sacral nerves and the pelvic sympathetic plexus. The cervical artery and vein, major branches of the uterine circulation, carry most of the blood to and from the cervix.

Clinical Importance.
　　Cervical cancer is the second most common female malignancy. Infection is a major cause of infertility; leukorrhea is often due to overactivity of the mucus-secreting membrane.

BODY & FUNDUS OF THE UTERUS

Gross Appearance.
　　The uterus is a muscular organ with a narrow central cavity situated deep in the true pelvis between the bladder and the rectum. It is shaped like an inverted pear. The adult nonpregnant uterus is approximately 7-8 cm long and is about 4 cm in its widest diameter. The fallopian tubes join the uterus, one on either side, about two-thirds of the distance to the

top of the uterus. That portion of the uterus above the tubal insertion is called the fundus; below the insertion is the body or corpus of the uterus, which is continuous with the supravaginal segment of the cervix. In the nulliparous woman the uterus and cervix are usually directed forward at almost a right angle with the long axis of the vagina, but 25-35% of women will have a retroverted or retroflexed uterus.

Except for the antero-inferior portion of the corpus, which is in close relation to the bladder, the uterus is covered by peritoneum.

The uterus is supported by (1) the muscular round ligaments (ligamentum teres), each of which originates in the fundus laterally and ends in a labium majus; (2) the broad ligaments, wide peritoneal folds sweeping laterally from either side of the corpus to the lateral pelvic walls; (3) the uterosacral ligaments, fibrous strands which originate in the cervico-uterine junction and insert into the periosteum of the sacrum; (4) the transverse cervical ligaments (cardinal ligaments, Mackenrodt's ligaments); and (5) the levator ani muscles.

Histology.

The uterine wall is composed of interwoven smooth muscle fibers, which are especially thick in the fundal portion. The cavity is small and is lined by endometrium, which thickens, bleeds, desquamates, and regenerates periodically during reproductive life.

Innervation.

Efferent impulses leave the uterus via S2-S4. The afferent impulses reach the central nervous system via the posterior roots of T10-T12, L1, and S2-S4 and carry sympathetic stimuli.

Blood Supply.

The uterine circulation is derived from the uterine and ovarian arteries and veins. During pregnancy especially, these channels anastomose freely within the uterus and a much greater vasculature develops to supply not only the hyperplastic, hypertrophic uterus itself but also the growing placenta and fetus.

Lymphatics.

Embryologically, the uterine lymphatic system is derived from venous channels. Lymph drainage from the uterus is directed to the (1) iliac, (2) aortic, (3) sacral, and (4) inguinal lymph glands. Nevertheless, the lymphatics of the uterus and neighboring organs intermingle, permitting progressive and retrogressive flow.

12 Fallopian Tubes

Clinical Importance.

The uterus is capable of enormous expansion to accommodate the products of conception. During pregnancy it increases in weight from about 30-40 gm to about 1 kg and its capacity is multiplied more than 4000 times. Normally, the fertilized ovum implants in the uterine endometrium, where it develops through the embryonal and fetal stages. Delivery prior to viability (28 weeks) constitutes abortion and, almost invariably, death of the fetus. After viability, the likelihood of survival of the newborn increases in direct proportion to the duration of pregnancy.

Uterine developmental anomalies and tumors cause gynecologic problems such as abnormal uterine bleeding and pelvic pain. These result in obstetric complications also—particularly dystocia.

Cancer of the uterine corpus is the second most common female genital malignancy, exceeded only by cervical carcinoma.

FALLOPIAN TUBES

Gross Appearance.

The fallopian (uterine) tubes are a pair of delicate, peristaltic ducts 10-12 cm in length. Each extends posterolaterally from the cornu of the uterus and opens into the peritoneal cavity just below and medial to the ovary on the same side. The diameter of the canal varies from 1-2 mm at either end to more than twice that in the midportion. The distal tube is connected with the ovary by a single elongated fimbria which retains the ovary and tubal extremity in close proximity.

Histology.

The fallopian tubes are composed of thin, superficial longitudinal and deep circular smooth muscle layers. They are lined by cuboidal epithelium (endosalpinx), which is similar to endometrium but has a sparse stroma. Many filmy transverse plicae or folds characterize the endosalpinx, especially in the distal half of the tube. The fallopian tubes are encased in a peritoneal fold, the mesosalpinx, a portion of the broad ligament of the uterus.

Structurally, the fallopian tubes vary in different segments. The distal end of the tube, which communicates with the peritoneal cavity through a minute opening (abdominal ostium), is fimbriated and almost erectile when turgid. The cavity of the distal 2-3 cm of the tube is termed the infundibulum because of its cornucopia-like shape. Continuous with this segment and about 6-8 cm long is the ampulla, which is somewhat dilated. The narrower isthmus, 1-2 cm in length, extends from the ampulla to the uterine wall. The portion of the tube within the uterus proper (the interstitial segment) is about 1 cm long. The lumen of the tube is narrowest at this end.

Innervation & Blood Supply.

The nerve supply to the tubes is similar to that of the uterus. The blood supply to the proximal portions of the tubes is via the uterine artery; to the distal portions, via both the uterine and ovarian arteries. Drainage is via the uterine and ovarian veins. The ampulla drains laterally through the mesosalpinx and broad ligaments to the hypogastric and iliac nodes. The isthmus and infundibulum drain toward lymph nodes supplying the uterus and ovaries.

Clinical Importance.

The ovum is fertilized in the fallopian tube and, after 3-4 days of movement down the tube, implants in the uterine endometrium. If both tubes are completely occluded, conception cannot occur. With partial occlusion, retention of the fertilized ovum within the tube may result in a tubal pregnancy. Infection of the tube (salpingitis) with resultant scarring, occlusion, and infertility is a common sequel to septic abortion or gonorrhea.

OVARIES

Gross Appearance.

The ovaries, or female gonads, are a pair of whitish, ovoid, flattened, solid organs, about $1.5 \times 3 \times 3.5$ cm, found in the true pelvis. In the nullipara, each ovary usually rests almost vertically against the peritoneum of the lateral pelvic wall in a shallow depression, the ovarian fossa. This space is bounded by (1) the obliterated umbilical artery medially; (2) the ureter and uterine vessels laterally; and (3) the obturator nerve and its accompanying artery and vein inferiorly. The fimbriated end of the tube usually curls up and over the superior medial aspect of the ovary.

The ovary is suspended between the lateral pelvic wall and the uterus by the mesovarium, which is part of the posterior segment of the broad ligament of the uterus. The mesovarium does not surround or cover the ovary but fuses with its superficial epithelial layer. It is also loosely attached to the uterus by a band-like ovarian ligament, which traverses the broad ligament.

Histology.

The ovary is composed mainly of fibroareolar tissue. The cortex, or outer one-third to one-half of the ovary, is covered by a single layer of cuboidal cells, the so-called germinal epithelium. The cortical stroma is composed of characteristic spindle- or oat-shaped cells. The inner one-half to two-thirds of the ovary is the medulla.

The cortex of the newborn ovary contains thousands of ova in various stages of development. Before puberty each ovum is surrounded by a single layer of epithelial cells and is termed a primordial follicle. These follicles, each measuring about 0.25 mm in diameter, contain a single, eccentrically placed, large, well developed sex cell with a granular hyperchromatic nucleus. The epithelial layer is composed of small, flattened, darkly-staining cells, the granulosa cells. Immediately surrounding the ovum is a cavity filled with clear serous fluid.

After puberty the primordial follicles may become graafian follicles under gonadotropic hormone stimulation. Gonadotropic hormones stimulate certain follicles cyclically, so that crops of ova begin maturing approximately once each month. The original flattened cells become cuboidal and more numerous. As they multiply, they separate into 2 layers: the tunica interna, which is the inner vesicular layer; and the tunica externa, which is composed of columnar cells. Immediately surrounding the eccentrically placed ovum and lining the entire cavity are granulosa cells, or the granulosa membrane. The fluid within the cavity is called the liquor folliculi. It contains a high concentration of estrogens, which are produced by follicular cells.

About once each month 1-2 graafian follicles reach full development and rupture to extrude the ova. The empty follicle, now termed a corpus luteum, produces both estrogens and progesterone. Partially matured follicles, still containing their ova, regress and finally disappear (atresia). If pregnancy ensues, the corpus luteum becomes even larger and more productive of steroid sex hormones. If pregnancy fails to occur, the corpus luteum degenerates, menstruation occurs, and after a number of months it becomes a hyalinized remnant called a corpus albicans. An extensive circulation within the ovary is apparent during adult life, so that each maturing follicle is well vascularized. During the climacteric, the ovary becomes less vascular and more dense in appearance.

Innervation & Blood Supply.

The nerves and blood vessels of the ovary traverse its suspensory ligament and enter and leave the hilus within the mesovarium. The ovarian arteries, which arise from the aorta just below the renal arteries, anastomose freely with branches from the uterine artery. A venous network within the mesovarium (pampiniform plexus) directs blood into the uterine and ovarian veins. The right ovarian vein empties into the inferior vena cava, whereas the left ovarian vein drains into the left renal vein.

Nerves from the dorsal roots of T10 and L1 and fibers from the pelvic and lumbar sympathetics accompany the arteries and veins.

The lymphatics of the ovary join those of the uterus to drain to the iliac and aortic nodes.

Clinical Importance.
 The ovary performs numerous functions. It is a repository for primordial sex cells, the woman's chromosomal endowment for procreation. In ovarian dysgenesis (ovarian agenesis of Turner), no primordial ova are present and the individual is sterile.
 The ovary is the organ for the production, "ripening," and monthly release of mature ova during reproductive life. Infertility follows failure of proper maturation of the ova, as in phase defects of the menstrual cycle, and retention of a fully developed ovum within a primary follicle which should have ruptured but could not because of adhesions of the ovary to a neighboring organ or a thickened ovarian tunica following perioophoritis.
 The production of steroid sex hormones (estrogens, progestogens, and androgens) in proper amounts by the ovary is required for normal female growth, development, and function. For example, hypoestrinism results in dwarfism in childhood, failure of appearance of the secondary sex characteristics and menstruation at puberty, and infertility as well as the symptomatology of the climacteric in adulthood.

BONY PELVIS

 The pelvis is a basin-shaped structure composed of 4 bones: the right and left innominates anteriorly and laterally and the sacrum and coccyx posteriorly. It rests on the femurs and supports the spinal column.
 The sacrum articulates with L5 above by an arthrodial joint; the innominate bones articulate with the femurs below by enarthroses. Within the pelvis itself are 2 types of joints: a synchondrosis uniting the 2 pubic bones, and diarthroses between the sacrum and ilium and between the sacrum and coccyx. When the sacrococcygeal joint is not ankylosed, a forward and backward movement of the coccyx is possible.
 The arrangement of the pelvic bones forms 2 cavities: the upper, larger, shallower **false pelvis** and the lower, smaller, deeper **true pelvis**. They are demarcated from one another by the ileopectineal line (linea terminalis), an oblique ridge on the inner surface of the ilium which is continued onto the pubes (see Figs 1-5 and 1-7).
 The false pelvis is bounded anteriorly by the abdominal muscles and posteriorly by the vertebral column. The flat, funnel-like false pelvis aids in supporting the intestines, but the uterus is within the true pelvis when the woman is erect. Abdominal constriction, obesity, tumors, and pregnancy also force the uterus into the true pelvis.

16 Bony Pelvis

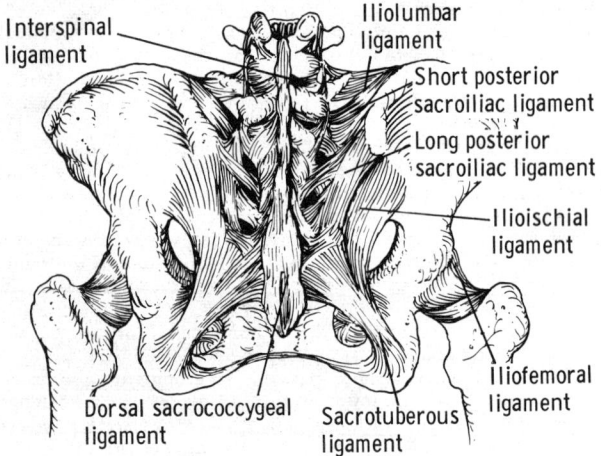

Fig 1-4. The bony pelvis (posterior view).

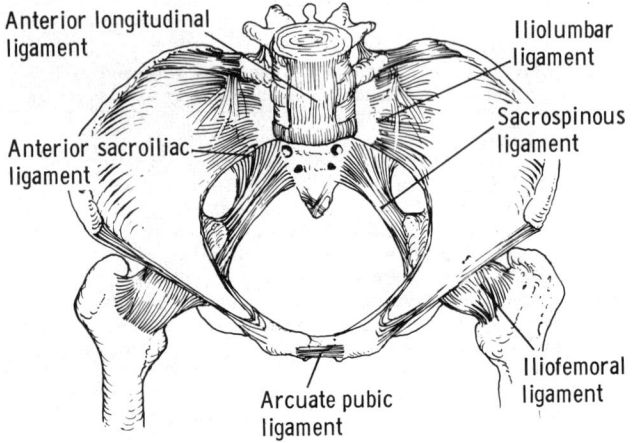

Fig 1-5. The bony pelvis (superior view).

the inferior ventral aspect of the embryo. This prevails until as late as the 6th week.

Initially, the gut does not open into the cloaca but ends abruptly in a thin partition, the cloacal membrane or proctodeum, which is found behind a slight depression just anterior to the short tail segment. Normally the membrane soon disintegrates, providing a communication between the bowel and cloaca.

During formation of the proctodeum, the cloaca divides into a dorsal portion (the hindgut) and a ventral portion (the urogenital sinus). The tissue separation between these 2 structures is called the urogenital fold. It inserts at the juncture of the allantois and the gut.

The lower hindgut becomes the rectum; its exit is the anus. The external opening of the ventral cloaca is the urogenital ostium.

When the proctodeum fails to open, an imperforate anus is the result. In the female, a rectovaginal fistula will often be present as well. (In males, a rectovesical fistula generally develops.)

DEVELOPMENT OF THE RENAL EXCRETORY APPARATUS

The pronephros (primordial kidney) is transitory and does not function in the human embryo. Its main duct persists, however, and continues to develop longitudinally. It is recognizable lateral to the mesodermal somites in the thoracolumbar region on each side as early as the second week. This passage becomes the excretory conduit of the mesonephros (wolffian body), which appears at about the third week but performs no true excretory function. After the second month of life the channel, now termed the wolffian duct, extends to the cloaca.

The metanephros (hind or true kidney) and its ureter appear about the 4th week on the right and left as a dorsolateral bud from the wolffian duct near the cloaca. These permanent kidneys develop rapidly. The ureter becomes independent of the wolffian ducts, and separate ureteral openings into the cloaca are formed promptly.

At about the 5th-6th week, the ureter divides within the metanephric mass to form calyces. Collecting and secretory tubules promptly begin to radiate into the renal mesenchyme from the calyces to connect with glomeruli which appear in the kidney cortex at about the same time. As the metanephric excretory units develop, those of mesonephric origin atrophy. Nevertheless, the wolffian ducts remain, at least until sexual differentiation has occurred. The metanephros gradually migrates from the medial to the lateral aspect of both the wolffian and the müllerian ducts. Meanwhile, because of elongation of the embryo, due mainly to growth of the body segments, the kidney is ultimately found in the dorsolumbar region. A long ureter is thus required.

The allantois, the remnant of the yolk stalk, normally inserts into the anterior portion of the cloaca. Just below this juncture, the urogenital canal enlarges the cloaca by incorporation of the terminal wolffian ducts. Between the second and third months, the lower ends of the wolffian ducts progressively widen, the allantoic stoma opens appreciably, and the upper part of the cloaca becomes partially separated from the lower or rectal portion. Thus, the bladder is formed by entodermal and mesodermal elements. Extreme maldevelopment results in exstrophy of the bladder.

The allantoic extension in the umbilical ligament and cord becomes the urachus, which may fail to obliterate late in fetal life. Urine may drain from an umbilical urachal fistula after delivery.

The prostatic urethra develops from the terminal portion of the wolffian ducts; the membranous urethra from a subdivision of the urogenital sinus; and the penile urethra (in part ectodermal) forms from the closure of a groove beneath the phallus. In the female, the origins are similar but there is, of course, no penile urethra.

ORIGIN OF THE FEMALE GENERATIVE DUCTS

An embryo 6 weeks of age reveals the beginnings of the müllerian ducts, which are destined to become the fallopian tubes, uterus, cervix, and part of the vagina. On each side, just lateral to the mesonephric structures in the lumbodorsal mesenchyme, these new channels develop parallel to the wolffian duct. The müllerian system develops caudally and ventrally to converge and end near the cloaca. The cephalad portions of the müllerian ducts become the fallopian tubes, which open to the peritoneal cavity. The upper end of the müllerian duct is often marked by a small persistent cyst (hydatid cyst of Morgagni) attached to one of the tubal fimbriæ. At the caudad end the ducts fuse in the midline and a central canal forms from which develop the uterus, the cervix, and the upper two-thirds of the vagina. Concomitantly, an invagination of the inferior part of the cloaca (urogenital sinus) is converted into the lower third of the vagina.

The mesonephric ducts disappear except for the vestigial epoophoron and paroophoron within the mesovarium.

The uterus, cervix, and upper vagina are at first solid and then become septate. The cervix is the first part of the müllerian system to lose its longitudinal septum; then the vagina; the uterus at 4-5 months. Partial or total failure of disappearance of these septa results in abnormal septa which are found in later life.

The wolffian ducts continue distally from below the ovary and pass just lateral to the uterus within the folds of the broad ligament; they traverse the peripheral tissues of the cervix and proceed down the anterolateral vaginal wall to the introitus. Parovarian cysts and Gartner's vaginal cysts are benign neoplasms of wolffian duct origin which may require excision. Atrophy of the wolffian ducts proceeds in accordance with the genetic heritage determined at fertilization. Normally, most of the unessential wolffian structures are obliterated. Carcinoma or cysts of wolffian origin are uncommonly discovered in the female after birth.

ORIGIN OF THE GONADS

Primitive Stage.

At about the 5th-6th week of embryonic existence, the genital ridges form in the right and left dorsolumbar regions within the celomic cavity. These developments involve the medial aspect of the mesonephric mesenchyme on each side. The cephalad portions of these ridges become the gonads. Finally, the genital ridges separate from the mesonephros. A few mesonephric tubules may remain as vestiges in the epoophoron. Low cells of mesodermal origin line the celomic cavity and cover the genital ridge. Concomitantly, primordial sex cells migrate across the gut mesentery into the cortex of the gonads from the yolk stalk. Meanwhile, broken columns of partially differentiated cells (Waldeyer's cords), which later become canalized (Pfleuger's tubules), appear within the substance of the early gonad, apparently as a downgrowth of superficial cells.

Indifferent or Neuter Stage.

Before the 6th-7th week after nidation the gonads are sexually indistinct. Soon thereafter, chromosomal inheritance determines whether the structures of the neuter stage will become male or female. Sex hormones of endogenous or exogenous origin stimulate or retard the full development of genitalia of the embryo or fetus.

Stage of Ovarian Development.

By the 8th week, if the conceptus is destined to become a female, the sex cells seem to organize the mesenchymal elements of the gonad. Primordial clusters of ova develop as islands of cells which contain one large primitive ovum surrounded by smaller, moderately differentiated cells which will become granulosa cells. Less well differentiated stromal cells become theca cells, and completely nondescript elements remain in the connective tissue series. Waldeyer's columns and the subsequent Pfleuger's tubules, helpful in testicular development, are not required by the ovary. Hence they disappear in the female. A few vestiges may remain, and these account for unusual cell patterns or even rare ovarian tumors such as Pick's adenoma.

ORIGIN OF THE EXTERNAL GENITALIA

The external genitalia of the male and female are similarly derived from the ectodermal cloaca. The genital or cloacal tubercle and the coccygeal tubercle mark the anterior and posterior extensions of the proctodeum. The genital tubercle becomes the clitoris in the female and the penis in the male. The anus forms just forward of the coccygeal tubercle. Labioscrotal folds develop on each side of the urogenital cleft. In the female, these ridges become the labia. In the male, scrotal pouches develop as fingerlike projections of the peritoneum. The testes descend into these recesses through the inguinal canals after the 36th week.

In the female, fatty infiltrations soon fill the labia. Although peritoneal downgrowths do form, as in the male, they are imperfect and are rapidly obliterated. In rare individuals cysts of the canal of Nuck persist as vestiges of the peritoneal attenuations. The distal end of the vagina is at first closed off from the urogenital septum by a membrane. If this barrier does not disintegrate properly, an imperforate or abnormally thick hymen results. The genital tubercle is transformed into the clitoris and the urogenital cleft remains patent, providing access to the vaginal introitus and the urethral meatus.

In the male, the scrotal folds fuse in the midline. This causes partial closure of the urogenital cleft and displaces forward the small remaining opening which is the incompletely formed urethra. The cloacal eminence rapidly becomes the penis. The remaining urogenital cleft defect closes completely when the edges of the ventral tract between the corpora cavernosa adhere to complete the terminal urethra. Because of these changes and the small size of the parts, the sex of the fetus cannot be determined grossly with confidence until after the 28th week.

MENSTRUATION

Menstruation, or normal periodic uterine bleeding, is a physiologic function which occurs only in female primates. It is basically a catabolic process and is under the influence of pituitary and ovarian hormones. Its onset, the **menarche**, occurs usually between the ages of 11 and 14 years; its termination, the **menopause**, normally occurs at 45-55 years, although medical or surgical intervention may cause an artificial menopause at an earlier age.

The interval between menstrual periods varies according to age, physical and emotional well-being, and environment. The normal menstrual cycle is commonly stated to be 28 days, but intervals of 24-32 days are still considered normal unless grossly irregular. At both poles of reproductive life the cycle is likely to be irregular and unpredictable due to failure of ovulation. Upon reaching maturity, approximately two-thirds of women maintain a reasonably regular periodicity, barring pregnancy, stress, or illness.

The average duration of menstrual bleeding is 3-7 days, but this also may vary.

The amount of blood lost in menstruation is usually about 50 ml, but many presumably normal women lose considerably more than this each month. Unless an actual hemorrhagic flow occurs, the blood passed through the cervix will not clot. This is because it has already coagulated and been hemolyzed, and is then passed with serum and tissue fragments in a reliquefied, defibrinated state.

The physiology of menstrual bleeding is not clearly understood. Many investigators believe that it represents the abortion of an unfertilized or unimplanted ovum. However, ovulation is not indispensable to regular uterine bleeding, and women can bleed from virtually any type of endometrium. Most gynecologists therefore make a distinction between **ovulatory** and **anovulatory menstruation**.

The following factors are believed to influence menstrual bleeding: (1) fluctuations in ovarian and pituitary hormone levels; (2) characteristics of the endometrium (phase, receptivity to hormones); (3) activity of the autonomic nervous system; (4) vascular changes (stasis, spasm-dilatation); (5) enzymes ("menstrual toxin" or "bleeding factor"); and (6) other factors, such as nutrition and psychologic states.

Hormonal Factors in Menstruation.

The ovarian cycle is initiated by the anterior pituitary follicle-stimulating hormone (FSH), which in turn causes the estrogen level to rise. Anterior pituitary luteinizing hormone (LH) and luteotropic hormone (LTH) later cause a rise in progesterone level. The rising titer of progesterone inhibits FSH production, and the estrogen level drops sharply. Uterine bleeding follows shortly thereafter. Although progesterone is important, it is not essential to the bleeding phenomenon; bleeding is initiated by a critical drop in the blood estrogen level.

26 Menstruation

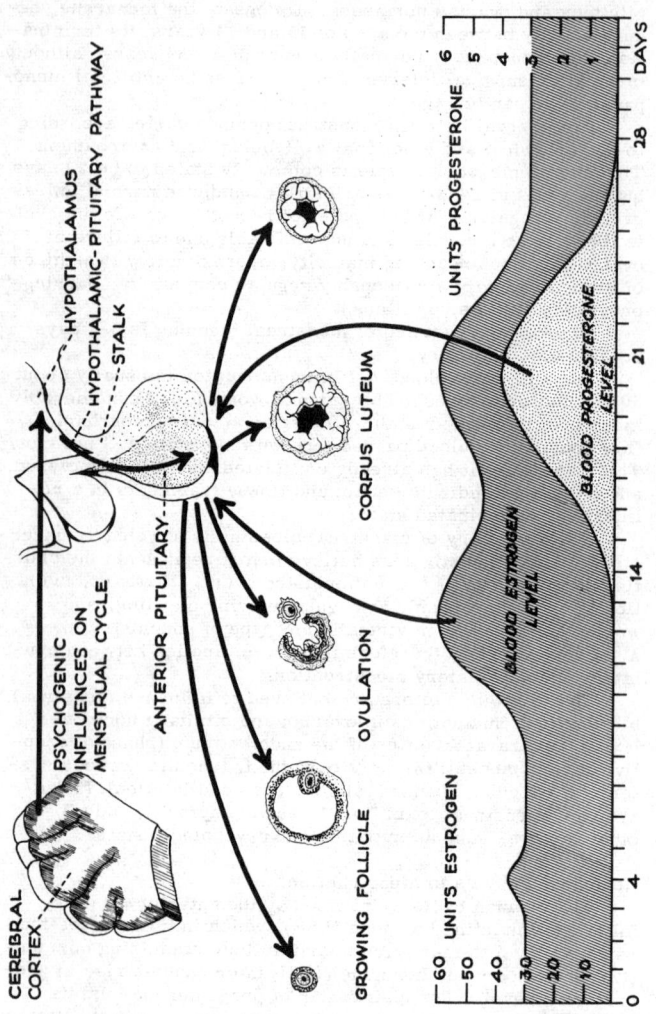

Fig 1-10. Menstrual cycle (hormones, histologic changes, BBT).

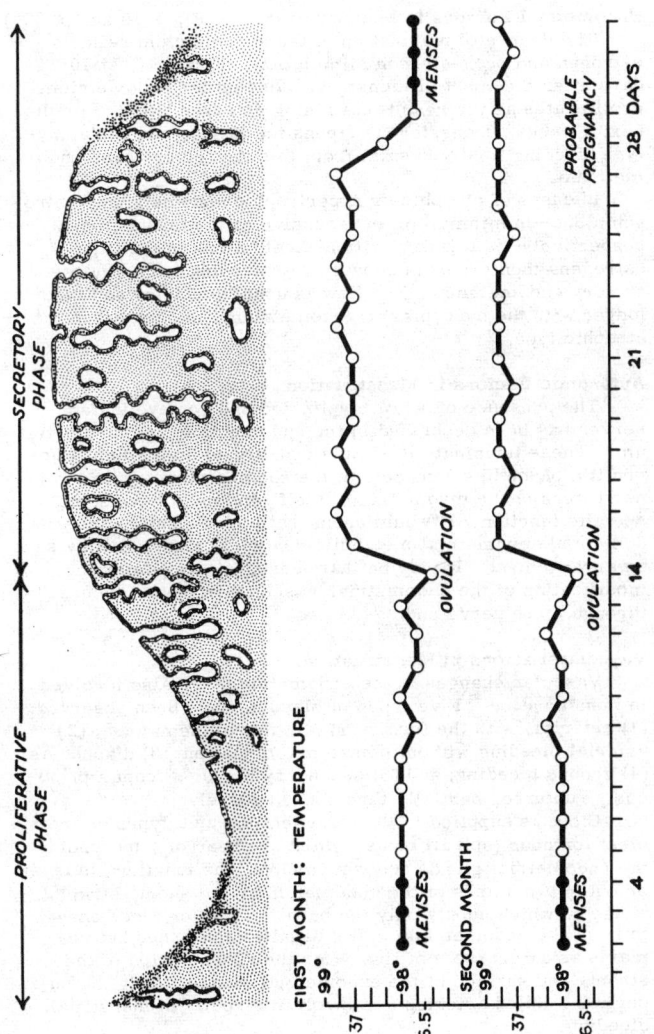

Fig 1-10. Menstrual cycle (hormones, histologic changes, BBT). (Cont'd.)

28 Menstruation

Endometrial Factors in Menstruation. (See Fig 1-10 and p. 30.)

The degree of maturation of the endometrium reflects estrogen and progesterone stimulation. For the first 10-14 days after the onset of menstrual bleeding the endometrium proliferates as the result of a rising estrogen titer. For the next 2 weeks, progesterone ripens the lining, and ovulatory-type bleeding finally results from this secretory phase endometrium.

In cases of atrophic or hypertrophic endometrium, estrogen alone—in minimal or in excessive or continued amounts, respectively—is found. Critical fluctuations in the titer of estrogens then result in anovulatory bleeding from a nonsecretory endometrium. The flow is usually heavier and lasts longer with the hyperplastic endometrium, in contrast to the atrophic type.

Autonomic Factors in Menstruation.

The presence of a few myelinated and nonmyelinated nerves has been described in the endometrium and myometrium. These terminate in simple end-organs in the tunica adventitia of the blood vessels of the endometrium and in the inner layers of the myometrium itself, and must have some specific function. It would seem that both sensation and endometrial-myometrial metabolic control are mediated by such an arrangement. It may be that neurogenic regulation or modification of the endometrial-vascular response occurs through these nerve endings.

Vascular Factors in Menstruation.

Vascular changes in the endometrium are also involved in menstruation. Five types of bleeding have been observed: (1) arterial, with the formation of a minute hematoma; (2) arterial bleeding without hematoma formation; (3) diapedesis; (4) venous bleeding; and (5) secondary bleeding from a previously ruptured, partially thrombosed vessel.

Blood is supplied to the endometrium by 2 types of arterioles: tortuous (spiral) types, which are near or surrounding the endometrial glands and which supply the functionalis layer or outer two-thirds of the endometrium; and short, straight vessels, which supply only the basalis layer or inner one-third of the endometrium. The basalis is not shed but remains as a reservoir of tissue for the regeneration of the stroma and surface of the endometrial glands. Only the superficial coiled arteries are involved directly in menstrual bleeding.

For the first week after the onset of menstrual bleeding, the spiral arterioles are short and relatively straight. During the period of thickening of the endometrium they lengthen as each day passes. The vessels grow more rapidly than the endometrium, however, so that they become coiled, particularly in the midportion of the functionalis.

In the monkey, just before menstrual bleeding begins, a rapid endometrial regression due to marked estrogen-progesterone depletion results in (1) buckling of the coiled arterioles in the functionalis; (2) stasis of the blood within the arteriovenous channels; (3) necrosis of the terminal arteriolar walls; (4) constriction of these arterioles within the basalis (outer one-third of the endometrium); and (5) periodic relaxation and hemorrhage from these peripheral branches.

Four to 24 hours before the onset of menstruation, periodic (every 60-90 seconds) vasoconstriction of the coiled arterioles apparently causes a type of "blanch and blush" phenomenon due to relaxation and contraction of the vessel musculature. At this time there seems to be considerable dehydration of the endometrium. Bleeding soon follows from various areas in the endometrium.

Enzymatic Factors in Menstruation.

The presence of a noxious substance in menstrual blood has been suspected for centuries. Menstrual toxin or "bleeding factor" has since been identified as a euglobulin-like material similar to the necrosin which has been extracted from tissues following crushing injuries. This substance is toxic to laboratory animals and causes intense arterial spasm when injected into endometrial transplants. It has been postulated that it is the cause of the vasoconstriction in the endometrium which precedes dilatation and menstrual bleeding.

Other Factors in Menstruation.

Numerous other factors can profoundly affect the menstrual cycle and flow. Undernutrition or avitaminosis (particularly deficiency of vitamin B complex, since the B vitamins aid the liver in inactivation of estrogen), obesity and other metabolic disturbances, inadequate rest, and emotional tension may each have an effect upon the cycle.

One of the most labile mechanisms in the body is the synergistic relationship between ovaries and pituitary. It is often the first to be disturbed in systemic or psychic illness, and menstrual aberrations frequently result.

THE TYPICAL MENSTRUAL CYCLE

During the first week after cessation of menstrual bleeding, FSH stimulates the development of immature or primordial follicles in the ovary. For unknown reasons, one follicle (rarely 2) is destined to complete the development of an ovum. On about the 10th or 11th day, this follicle outstrips its contemporaries and becomes the major producer of both estrogens and progesterone during that cycle.

By about midcycle, the fully-developed graafian follicle contains a mature ovum. Just prior to extrusion of the egg, the anterior pituitary gland begins production of luteinizing hormone (LH). Following actual ovulation, luteotropic hormone (LTH) is also released by the pituitary. The ovary, which is producing estrogen now, begins the production of progesterone also. Both estrogen and progesterone are operative for the next two weeks; the progesterone titer is further maintained while the corpus luteum is functional. It may be that ovarian theca cells cause this effect by releasing small bursts of estrogens and progesterone.

FSH and LH are probably required for actual ovulation, but luteotropic hormone (LTH) is necessary for the continued function of the corpus luteum itself following extrusion of the ovum. Immediately following ovulation, the blood estrogen titer falls slightly. This would seem to be one reason for the slight macroscopic bleeding from the endometrium which occurs in about 12% of women at midcycle.

Unless fertilization and nidation occur, the corpus luteum regresses in approximately 14 days. This is accompanied by a sharp decline in the output of both progesterone and estrogens. A marked reduction in the blood level of estrogens is invariably followed by increased production of FSH, with the result that a new follicle is stimulated for the next cycle.

Endometrial Changes. (See Fig 1-10.)

During reproductive life the endometrium undergoes continuous cyclic change. For each cycle, it is generally considered to have 4 phases, which correspond to ovarian hormone activity and which can be identified by endometrial biopsy.

A. Proliferative Phase: The proliferative (estrogenic) phase varies in length, but is about 14 days in a 28-day cycle.

The early proliferative phase lasts 2-3 days. The end of this phase coincides with about the 7th day of the classic cycle. Surface epithelium is repaired, but is thin or defective; its thickness depends upon the loss of tissue during menstrual bleeding. Glands are straight. Nuclei of epithelial cells are pseudostratified and mitoses are frequent. Stromal cells show relatively large nuclei and little cytoplasm. There are few phagocytic cells.

The midproliferative phase coincides with about the 10th day of the cycle. It differs from the foregoing only in degree. The surface is more regular, the glands more tortuous, and glandular cells are pseudostratified. Thickness of the endometrium is increased.

The late proliferative phase is about the 14th day of the average cycle. The surface is undulating; stromal cells are closely packed; and variable amounts of extracellular fluid are lost. Thickness is about as before, but with greater cellular concentration. The glands are in-

creasingly tortuous and contain minimal secretion. There is no glycogen in the fluid.
B. Ovulatory Phase: Ovulation occurs on about the 14th day of a 28-day cycle. Because there is no appreciable change in the endometrium within the 24-36 hours following ovulation, one cannot distinguish between the 14th- and 15th-day endometrium. Distinctive changes appear in gland cells on the 16th day and thereafter, indicating corpus luteum activity and presumably ovulation.
C. Secretory (Progestational) Phase: On the 16th day there is increased tortuosity of the glands, many mitotic figures, and the appearance of glycogen-laden basal vacuoles. On the 17th day the most pronounced vacuolization of cells occurs. Almost two-thirds of the basal portion of such glands contain glycogen-laden fluid. Slight edema is noted. Mitoses are rare. On the 18th day secretion of fluid within the glands is apparent. (This corresponds to the time when the ovum is free within the uterine cavity and must derive nourishment from uterine secretion.) On the 22nd day, the glands are more tortuous but there is less secretory activity. Considerable inspissated secretion is seen in their lumens. Stromal edema is now at the peak. (This may facilitate implantation of the ovum.) The high points of secretory activity and stromal edema coincide with the period of greatest corpus luteum activity. From the 24th to the 27th day edema regresses and the stromal cells are metamorphosed into elements suggestive of decidua cells. The first change is noted in cells around the spiral arterioles with the appearance of mitotic figures in the perivascular stroma. The glands become more and more tortuous, with serrations of their walls. Secretion of gland cells diminishes. There is infiltration by polymorphonuclear neutrophils and monocytes. Finally, necrosis and slough occur.
D. Pregnant Phase: If gestation occurs, active secretion and edema persist. Glands become more feathery and serrated. The predecidua is not immediately accentuated except around the ovum. The presence of all 3 (secretion, edema, and predecidua) strongly suggests early pregnancy, even though the patient has not yet missed a menstrual period.

After a menstrual period of from 4-7 days, bleeding gradually diminishes. Regional ooze is reduced by constriction and thrombosis of the remaining undamaged coiled arterioles, so that the spotting finally ceases.

Shedding of tissue fragments usually begins in a patchy fashion about 12 hours after bleeding starts in ovulatory cycles, although an entire cast of the endometrial cavity is separated in the so-called membranous dysmenorrhea. This painful condition results from the sudden separation of the entire secretory endometrial lining, presumably due to an abnormally rapid and complete sequence of events as noted previously.

About two-thirds of the endometrium is presumed to be lost with each ovulatory menstruation. By the time brisk flow ceases, tissue separation has occurred over the greater portion of the surface of the uterine cavity.

The interval between ovulation and menstruation is normally almost exactly 14 days. In contrast, the preovulatory period, the interval from the first day of menstruation to the day of ovulation, may vary from 7 or 8 days to over a month. This accounts for the variability of the interval between menstrual periods previously discussed.

Changes in Cervical Mucus.

Vaginal cytology reflects estrogen and progesterone variations. During reproductive life, the 4 phases corresponding to the endometrium (proliferative, ovulatory, secretory, and pregnant) can also be noted in suitably stained vaginal spreads.

The amount and consistency of the cervical mucus varies during the menstrual cycle. If a smear of the cervical mucus is allowed to dry in air without fixation and examined under a microscope, characteristic patterns of crystallization can be identified at various stages. At the time of ovulation the mucus dries to a striking fern-like pattern (fern test). Before and after ovulation and during pregnancy, other characteristic granular patterns can be observed.

At about the time of ovulation, the cervical mucus becomes extremely clear and liquid in contrast to the yellowish, viscid mucus normally observed during the extreme pre- and postovulatory phases of the cycle. Just before ovulation, a drop of endocervical mucus can be stretched into a thin cobweb-like strand 6 or more cm long. This quality ("spinnbarkeit") is related to a high estrogen level and low saline content.

Systemic Changes.

During the preovulatory phase of the cycle, resting temperatures taken each morning will usually be low (< 98° F). (Slightly elevated individual daily variations can be ascribed to activity, infections, late hours, and alcoholic beverages.) On the day of ovulation the temperature rises sharply almost one degree (C or F) and remains elevated until just before the menstrual period, when the temperature begins to fall toward the low preovulatory levels (see Fig 1-10). This occurs only in ovulating women.

Other changes associated with uterine bleeding after ovulation are as follows: (1) Extracellular edema, which is the cause of premenstrual weight gain, sometimes amounting to 10 lb or more. (2) Muscle sensitivity or hypertonicity. (Such patients are irritable and agitated.) (3) Vascular alterations, including pelvic hyperemia and increased capillary fragility or a tendency toward bruising. (4) Mastalgia due to increased breast size and turgescence. (5) Emotional tensions and headache which are related to faulty conditioning or psychoneurosis.

ANOVULATORY CYCLES

In anovulatory cycles, the maturation and differentiation of the endometrium by progesterone does not occur, and the sequence of events is therefore abbreviated. The period is qualitatively similar to an ovulatory one, but minimal coiling of the spiral arterioles probably can cause only small fissures and no propagating hematomas. The peeling away of the functionalis layer thus takes place only imperfectly in the proliferative or hyperplastic endometrium.. Bleeding from terminal arteriolar loops must occur, but tissue loss is minimal. The endometrium continues to proliferate from month to month, with the result that hemorrhage finally ensues in subsequent periods from this grossly thickened tissue.

THE MENARCHE

Because menstruation is the objective manifestation of optimal ovarian function in nonpregnant women, its onset constitutes important evidence that the rhythm and amplitude of hormone production are developing normally. During early childhood, both sexes secrete small, rather constant amounts of estrogens. Between 8 and 11 years of age, however, there is a marked increase in estrogen excretion, particularly in girls. It has been noted that for a little over a year before the onset of puberty estrogen production and excretion become cyclic. Estrogen production continues in increasing amounts to the menarche. The average age at onset of menses is 13 years.

Presumably because the degree of ovarian stimulation is insufficient to induce complete maturation and release of an ovum, the first menstrual periods are nearly always anovulatory. Several years often pass before ovulation occurs. In young girls the average interval is longer and irregularity is much more common than in adult women. After about age 20, more or less regular episodes of ovulation can be expected in the majority of women, although frequent anovulatory cycles are noted in about 30% of mature individuals.

It is no longer believed that women in colder climates begin to menstruate later and cease to menstruate earlier than women in temperate or tropical latitudes. However, race, nutrition, and perhaps social mores may play a part in determining the age at which menarche and menopause occur.

For some months after menarche and before the menopause, only estrogen is produced; this causes the endometrium to thicken, and endometrial hyperplasia may develop. Although periodic bleeding does occur, it is usually not regular and may be quite unpredictable, with excessive bleeding upon occasion. These are anovulatory cycles in which the differentiation of the endometrium and the brake-like effect of progesterone do not play a role. Unopposed or unduly prolonged estrogen stimulation therefore results in a thick, overgrown, nonsecretory endometrium from which marked bleeding may result.

THE MENOPAUSE AND CLIMACTERIC
(See also Chapter 26.)

Menopause is the time when menstruation ceases. It may occur at any time between 45 and 55 years of age (usually 49-50), and marks the end of reproductive life. Menopause may be natural or artificial (ovarian resection or irradiation), and is the result of estrogen depletion.

The **climacteric** is that era in a woman's life when the body undergoes involution or decline. This is in part due to pituitary, ovarian, and adrenal insufficiency, but it is also evidence that anabolism and repair have not kept pace with catabolism. Involution begins at about age 35 and is complete at age 65, after which time senile changes develop rapidly.

The term "change of life" is probably best understood as referring to the climacteric, which is highlighted by the menopause but which may present physical and emotional problems only vaguely related to menstrual function.

HORMONAL CHANGES DURING PREGNANCY

Metabolic studies indicate that in pregnancy estrogens are produced and excreted at about the same level as during the postovulatory phase of the menstrual cycle. During the third month of pregnancy, however, the estrogen titer slowly rises, beginning apparently with the first placental contribution to hormone production. From the third month to term the estrogen level continues to rise.

Because it is difficult to identify progesterone specifically in the blood or urine, determinations are usually based upon estimates of its catabolite, pregnanediol. Such an appraisal correlates well with progesterone production. Following implantation, pregnanediol excretion persists at approximately the same level as during the secretory phase of the cycle. Beginning at about the third month of pregnancy, pregnanediol excretion increases gradually to reach a rather high level at the 6th month. This is followed by a slight decrease, with another peak noted several weeks before delivery. Immediately before parturition, both estrogen and progesterone levels decline rapidly.

A rapid rise in chorionic gonadotropin occurs almost immediately following nidation; at about the 6th week of gestation the urine chorionic gonadotropin level is approximately 3 times that noted very early in pregnancy. As the weeks go by, this hormone further declines to a lower level between the 5th and 6th months of pregnancy and then to another lower level between the 7th and 8th months. From this point on, a gradual decline occurs until term and delivery. Chorionic gonadotropin substitutes for pituitary LH hormone, thereby ensuring a continuation and persistent functioning of the corpus luteum. It is believed that amenorrhea during pregnancy can be explained in this manner.

2...
Diagnosis of Pregnancy & the Duration of Pregnancy

DIAGNOSIS OF PREGNANCY

Although most women appear for prenatal care knowing they are pregnant, in about one-third of cases it is difficult to make a definite diagnosis of pregnancy before the second missed period. This is due largely to the variability of the physical changes, the possibility of tumors, and because obesity and poor patient relaxation often interfere with examination. Consequently, even an experienced physician may make a false-positive or false-negative diagnosis of pregnancy. The grave emotional and perhaps legal consequences of misdiagnosis should make the physician cautious; if there is any doubt, a re-examination should be done in 3-4 weeks. If the patient demands earlier confirmation, one of the pregnancy tests may be ordered, but even these are not 100% accurate. A record of the time and frequency of coitus may be of considerable importance in the diagnosis of pregnancy.

Pregnancy causes both obvious and subtle changes which involve many organ systems but are most pronounced in the generative system. Because these subjective and objective alterations vary so widely, the diagnostic criteria of pregnancy are classified as (1) presumptive, (2) probable, and (3) positive.

Presumptive Manifestations of Pregnancy.

The following signs and symptoms are presumptive evidence of pregnancy, but even 2 or more are not diagnostic.

A. Symptoms:
  1. Amenorrhea - In the majority of cases, conception is followed by immediate cessation of menses due to the rising titer of chorionic gonadotropin. About 25% of pregnant women experience slight painless bleeding at some time during the first few months, either at the time of implantation or near the time of the expected period. The cause of this bleeding is not known.
  2. Nausea and vomiting - Distaste for food, queasiness, other digestive disturbances, and nausea and vomiting are reported by almost half of pregnant women during the first 3 months. Because it is most often noted

upon arising, this reaction is called morning sickness; in some patients, however, it may occur only in the evening. Pungent smells or cooking odors frequently will precipitate a gastric upset even if the recommended light dry diet has been adhered to. Psychic tensions may be responsible.
3. Breast tenderness and tingling - Engorgement of the breasts after the first few weeks of pregnancy is caused by estrogens, which stimulate the mammary duct system; and by progesterone, which stimulates the alveolar components.
4. Urinary frequency and urgency - Estrogens and progesterone increase the turgescence of the bladder and urethra. During the first trimester, bladder irritability, urinary frequency, and nocturia are common. These symptoms decrease during the second trimester, but during the third trimester the pressure of the presenting part reduces the capacity of the bladder and the urinary symptoms become more severe.
5. Constipation - Early in pregnancy, constipation may occur—possibly as a result of a change in food habits or bowel motility; later, it is caused by uterine enlargement, which displaces the intestines and compresses the colon.
6. Fatigue - Lassitude and easy fatigability are noted by many pregnant women even a few weeks after the missed period. This slowed behavior pattern, observed also in lower forms of animal life, has not been explained.
7. Quickening - The perception of fetal movements is described by many primiparas at about the 16th week; multiparas report such sensations as early as the 14th week.
8. Weight gain - During pregnancy there is usually a steady gain in weight. A sense of well-being in some, anxiety and compensatory overeating in others, or the mistaken impression that a pregnant woman should "eat for two" is usually responsible for excessive gain. It should be noted whether weight has been average and stable in recent months.

B. Signs:
1. Skin pigmentation - Facial chloasma and darkening of the skin over the forehead, the bridge of the nose, and the malar prominences ("mask of pregnancy") occur to a variable degree in most pregnant women after the 16th week. Pigmentation of the nipples and areolas appears at about the same time. The linea nigra (pigmented linea alba) is noted after the third month and is particularly marked in brunets. In primigravidas it follows the uterine fundus to the umbilicus; in multigravidas the linea nigra reappears in its entirety early

in the second trimester. Pigmentation is caused by adrenal and placental corticoids and ketosteroids, which stimulate the melanophores in these areas particularly.

2. Epulis - Hypertrophic gingival papillae are often seen after the first trimester of pregnancy. Unidentified hormones are probably responsible.
3. Leukorrhea - Increased cervical mucus and pronounced exfoliation of vaginal epithelial cells are caused by augmented estrogen-progesterone levels during pregnancy. The whitish, mucoid, nonpruritic discharge increases to the point where a perineal pad may be needed in late pregnancy.
4. Breast changes -
   a. Enlargement and vascular engorgement of the breasts begin at about the 6th or 8th week after conception.
   b. Secondary areola, a pink periareolar pigmentation, and enlargement of the circumlacteal sebaceous glands (Montgomery's tubercles) may be noted at approximately 6-8 weeks and are presumed to be due to steroid sex hormone stimulation.
   c. Colostrum ("pre-milk" secretion) is produced by lactogenic hormone and progesterone and may be expressed after the 16th week.
5. Abdominal enlargement - Protuberance of the lower abdomen is usually evident after the 14th week.
6. Pelvic organ changes - See Figs 2-2 to 2-5.
   a. Cyanosis of the vagina (Chadwick's sign, Jacquemier's sign) occurs by about the 6th week.
   b. Softening of the cervix at the tip is occasionally noted as early as the 4th or 5th week of pregnancy; however, fibrosis, infection, or scarring may prevent softening until late in pregnancy.
   c. Softening of the cervico-uterine junction occurs often as early as the 5th or 6th week. It is first noted as a soft spot anteriorly in the midline of the uterus near the junction of the body and the cervix (Ladin's sign). A wider zone of softness and compressibility at the lower uterine segment (Hegar's sign) is the most valuable sign of early pregnancy and can usually be noted by the 6th week. Ease in flexing the fundus on the cervix (McDonald's sign) generally appears by the 7th or 8th week.
   d. Irregular softening and slight enlargement of the fundus at the site of or on the side of implantation (Von Fernwald's sign) occurs by about the 5th week. When implantation is in the region of a uterine cornu, a more pronounced softening and almost tumor-like enlargement may occur (Piskacek's sign).

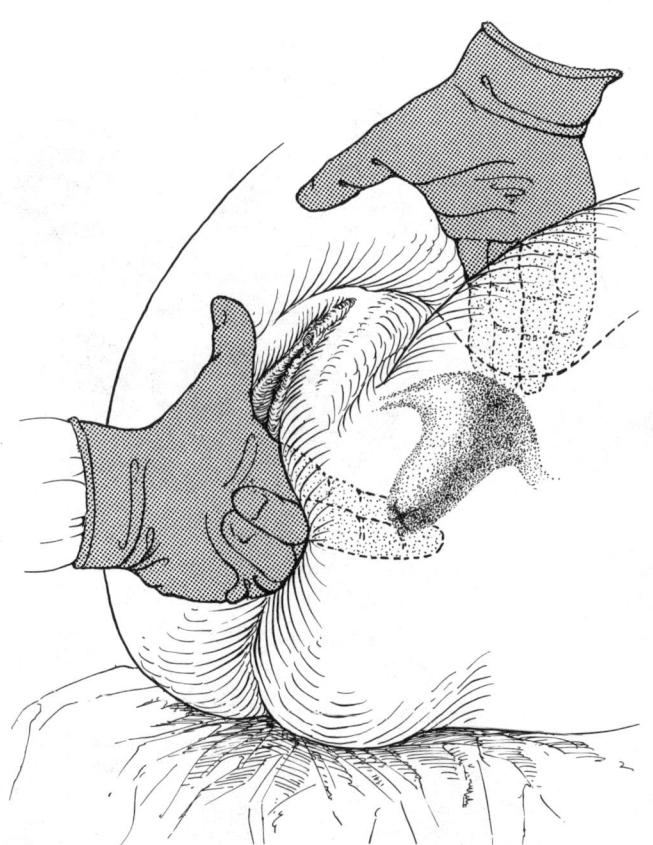

Fig 2-1. Bimanual pelvic examination.

    e. Generalized enlargement and diffuse softening of the corpus of the uterus are usually present after the 8th week of pregnancy.

Probable Manifestations of Pregnancy.*
A. Symptoms: Same as presumptive symptoms, above.
B. Signs:
  1. Uterine enlargement - Correlation of uterine size with the duration of amenorrhea or the date of conception is significant from the 6th to the 28th week. After 28

---

*See also Tables 2-1 and 2-2, p. 44.

40 Diagnosis of Pregnancy

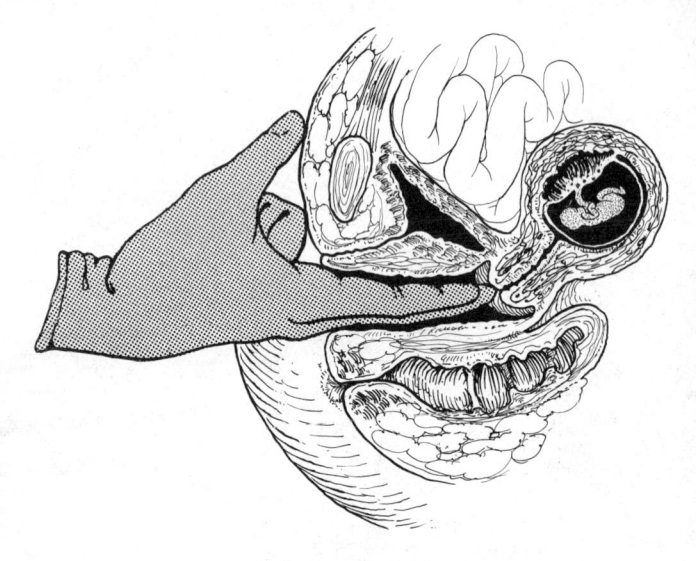

Fig 2-2. Softening of the cervix.

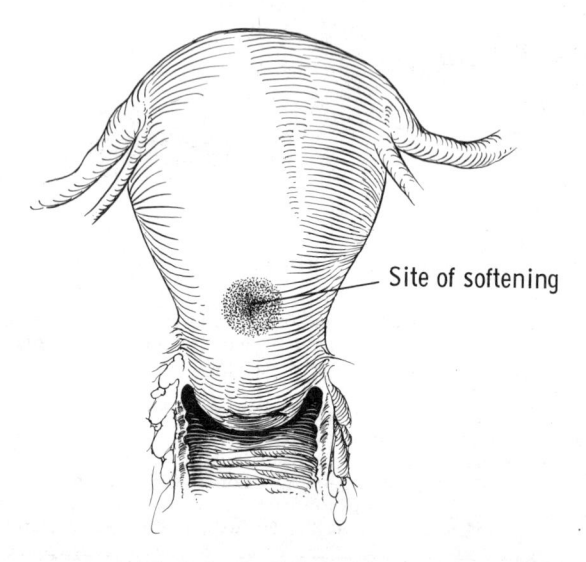

Site of softening

Fig 2-3. Ladin's sign.

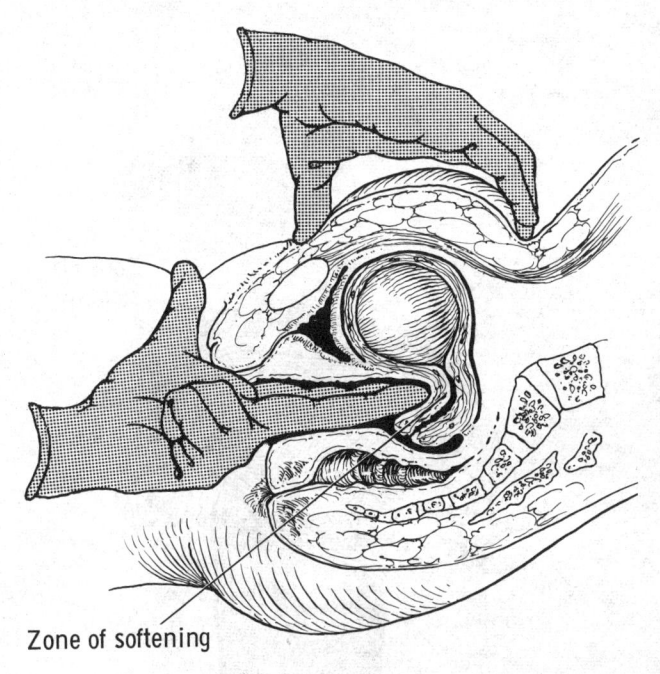

Fig 2-4. Hegar's sign.

Zone of softening

weeks, changes in the shape of the fundus, the varying positions of the fetus, and the increasing quantity of amniotic fluid may make such a relation invalid.
2. Uterine souffle (bruit) - After the 16th week a rushing sound synchronous with the mother's pulse can sometimes be heard bilaterally just above the symphysis. This sound is due to increased blood flow to the uterus, and usually indicates pregnancy. The funic or cord souffle (synchronous with the fetal heart sounds) can rarely be identified.
3. Uterine contractions (Braxton Hicks sign, Hicks's sign) - Upon bimanual examination, irregular uterine contractions may be felt after the 28th week, especially in asthenic women. These are not painful, as distinct from the contractions of premature labor.

42 Diagnosis of Pregnancy

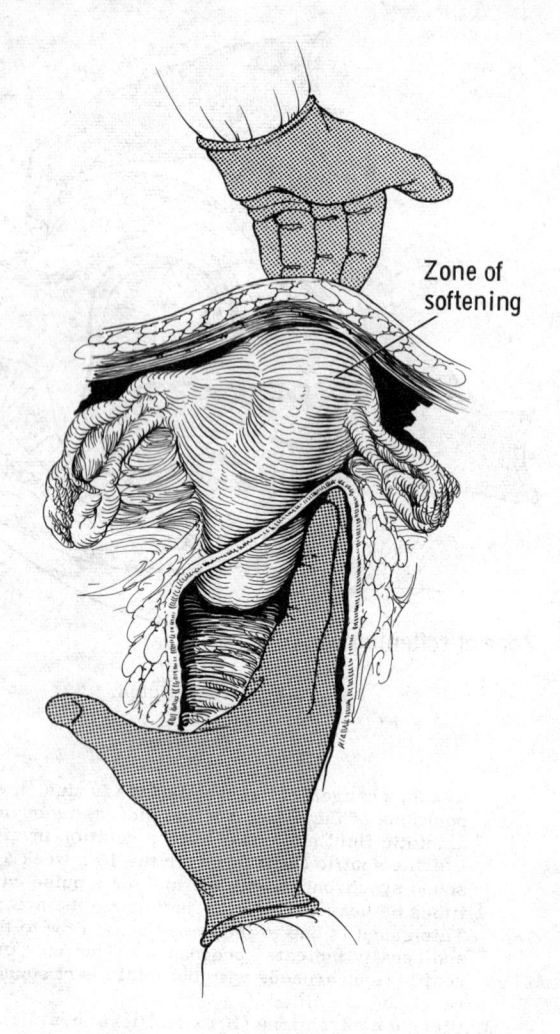

Fig 2-5. Von Fernwald's sign.

Positive Manifestations of Pregnancy.
A. Symptoms: There is no subjective evidence of pregnancy which can be accepted as diagnostic.
B. Signs: Any one of the following signs is medical and legal proof of pregnancy. They are usually not present until after the 4th month.
   1. Auscultation of fetal heartbeat - One must be able to hear distinctly **and count** the fetal heartbeat. It is faster than the mother's and resembles the tick of a watch under a pillow. Auscultation is generally possible in slender women after the 17th-18th week.
   2. Palpation of fetal outline - After the 24th week the fetal outline may be identified in many pregnant women.
   3. Recognition of fetal movements -
      a. Active movements are usually palpable after the 18th week.
      b. By the 16th-18th week passive movements of the fetus can often be elicited by abdominal and vaginal palpation. A firm tap on the uterine wall or vaginal fornix displaces the fetus as a "floating body," which can then be felt as a thrust as it moves back to its accustomed position (ballottement). Ascites and tumors must be excluded.
   4. X-ray demonstration of fetal skeleton - An oblique view of the abdomen may reveal fetal bones as early as the 12th week. An anteroposterior film may not disclose a definite skeleton until the 16th week because of the interference of bowel shadows and the variable density of the sacrum. X-ray films should be avoided whenever possible during pregnancy to protect against gonadal damage and the possibility of genetic abnormalities.

DIFFERENTIAL DIAGNOSIS OF PREGNANCY

All of the presumptive and probable symptoms and signs of pregnancy, as well as positive clinical and laboratory test results indicative of pregnancy, can be caused by other conditions.

Differential Diagnosis of Symptoms.
A. Amenorrhea:
   1. Psychic factors - Emotional shock, fear of pregnancy or venereal disease, intense desire for pregnancy (pseudocyesis).
   2. Endocrine factors - Early menopause, lactation; pituitary, thyroid, adrenal, or ovarian dysfunction.
   3. Metabolic factors - Anemia, malnutrition, climatic changes, diabetes mellitus, degenerative disorders.

44 Differential Diagnosis of Pregnancy

Table 2-1. Laboratory pregnancy tests.

Name	Test Animal*	Procedure	Time, Accuracy	Pregnancy Indicated By	Remarks
Aschheim-Zondek	5 mice (3 weeks old)	0.4 ml patient's first morning urine (acidified), injected 6× during 2 days.	96 hrs (98%)	Ovulation (corpus luteum)	Moderately expensive. Need mouse colony, multiple injections.
Friedman-Hoffman	Rabbit (10-12 weeks old)	2.5 ml patient's serum injected into rabbit's ear vein.	24 hrs (96%)	Ovulation (corpus luteum)	Moderate cost. Relatively simple test.

Name	Procedure	Accuracy	Interpretation & Remarks
Hemagglutination inhibition test (Prognosticon®)	Red cells sensitized to human chorionic gonadotropin (HCG) + urine (?HCG) + anti-HCG serum.	80-95% with increasing reliability from 40th day after first day of LMP.	Immunodiagnostic test depends upon: (1) HCG injected into a rabbit which develops anti-HCG serum. (2) Sheep red cells are tanned, formalized, and sensitized to HCG. (3) When antibodies are bound or "coated" to red cells, hemagglutination results; but addition of urine from a pregnant woman blocks the reaction between antibody and red cells. Therefore, clumping (ring formation in bottom of test tube) indicates that the patient is not pregnant; no clumping, patient is pregnant.
Agglutination	Anti-HCG serum + urine + HCG antigen (latex particles). Interpret in 3 minutes.	Similar to above.	Similar to above but latex particles with adsorbed HCG used instead of red cells.

*If the animal dies, the test should be repeated. Be certain the patient is not taking any medication which might interfere with the test, e.g., aspirin in large doses, or phenothiazines.

Table 2-2. Clinical pregnancy tests.

Name	Procedure	Accuracy	Interpretation & Remarks
Estrogen-progesterone	Progesterone, 20 mg, and estradiol benzoate, 2 mg I.M.	98%	If bleeding does not occur within 10 days after administration of estrogen-progesterone or 7 days after administration of progesterone, norethindrone, or norethynodrel, and if other causes of amenorrhea have been ruled out, pregnancy is probable. **Note:** If bleeding occurs, the test is inconclusive.
Progesterone	Delalutin® , 250 mg (2 ml) I.M.	96%	
Norethindrone or norethynodrel	Give 20 mg orally	98%	

Differential Diagnosis of Pregnancy 45

    4. Systemic disease (acute or chronic) - Infections such as tuberculosis or brucellosis; malignancy.
- B. Nausea and Vomiting:
    1. Emotional disorders - Pseudocyesis, anorexia nervosa.
    2. Gastrointestinal disorders - Enteritis, peptic ulcer, hiatus hernia, appendicitis, intestinal obstruction, "food poisoning" (bacterial contamination of foods, toxins, allergens).
    3. Acute infections - Influenza, poliomyelitis.
- C. Breast Tenderness: Premenstrual tension, hyperestrinism (due to hormone therapy or anovulatory cycles), chronic cystic mastitis, pseudocyesis.
- D. Urinary Frequency: Urinary tract infection, cystocele, urethral diverticula, pelvic tumors, emotional tension.
- E. Quickening: Increased peristalsis, "gas" (especially in women preoccupied with thoughts of pregnancy), abdominal muscle contractions, shifting abdominal contents.

Differential Diagnosis of Signs.
- A. Epulis: Local infection, dental calculus, vitamin C deficiency.
- B. "Milk" Secretion: Persistent manual breast stimulation, residual fluid from a previous pregnancy.
- C. Abdominal Enlargement: Obesity of rapid onset, relaxation of abdominal muscles (as often in pseudocyesis), pelvo-abdominal tumors, tympanites, ascites, ventral hernia.
- D. Leukorrhea: Infections and tumors of the vagina and cervix, psychically-induced excessive cervical mucus.
- E. Vaginal and Cervical Color Changes: Premenstrual turgescence, "pelvic congestion syndrome" of psychosomatic origin, venous obstruction due to pelvic tumor or infection.
- F. Changes in Consistency, Size, and Shape of Cervix and Uterus: Premenstrual engorgement, notable in multiparas with uterine hypertrophy; uterine tumors, usually myomas; tubo-ovarian cysts closely adherent to the uterus; cervical stenosis and hemato-, muco-, or pyometra.

Differential Diagnosis of Clinical & Laboratory Tests.*
- A. Elevation of Basal Body Temperature (BBT) for Longer Than 2 Weeks: Corpus luteum cyst; chorionic gonadotropin or progesterone therapy; faulty thermometer, incorrect temperature-taking or recording.
- B. Vaginal Bleeding Following Estrogen or Progesterone Therapy: (**Note:** Such bleeding is evidence against pregnancy, but it may actually be coincidental abnormal bleeding in a pregnant woman.) Threatened abortion of

---
*See Tables 2-1 and 2-2.

uterine or ectopic pregnancy; cervical or vaginal infections, tumors, or a bleeding varix.

C. Laboratory Tests: Laboratory animal tests which are based upon elevation of gonadotropins are not usually positive until the 4th-6th week, and at best are only about 98% accurate.
  1. False-positive results - Inadequate safeguards against sexual stimulation or exposure of the test animal.
  2. False-negative results - Animals too young or too old; insufficient gonadotropin in patient's specimen (too early in pregnancy or urine sample too dilute).
  3. Incorrect interpretation of results - Inexperience of observer; injection of wrong specimen; failure to inject all of specimen; failure to keep accurate records; death of test animal (if animal dies, the test should be repeated).
  4. Recently introduced serologic tests for pregnancy appear to be promising since the results to date indicate that they are convenient, accurate, and positive earlier in pregnancy than the animal tests.

DURATION OF PREGNANCY & EXPECTED DATE OF CONFINEMENT (EDC)

Pregnancy in women lasts about 10 lunar months (9 calendar months). (See Fig 2-6.) The average length of pregnancy is 266 days. (The median duration of pregnancy initiated by a known single sexual exposure is 269 days.) An authenticated case of a pregnancy of 360 days duration is on record.

In the absence of medical or obstetric complications, the physician's prediction regarding the duration of pregnancy is influenced by the length of gestation in previous pregnancies (often prolonged in certain families) and by parity (generally longer in subsequent pregnancies).

Nägele's Rule. (See also inside of back cover.)

The expected date of confinement (EDC), or estimated date of delivery, cannot be precisely stated.

It has become traditional to calculate the EDC from Nägele's rule: Add 7 days to the first day of the last menstrual period (LMP); subtract 3 months; add 1 year (EDC = [LMP + 7 days] − 3 months + 1 year). For example, if the first day of the LMP was June 4, 1964, the EDC will be March 11, 1965.

Nägele's rule is based on a 28-day menstrual cycle, with the expectation that ovulation occurred on the 14th day; in calculating the EDC, an adjustment should be made if the patient's cycle is shorter or longer than 28 days.

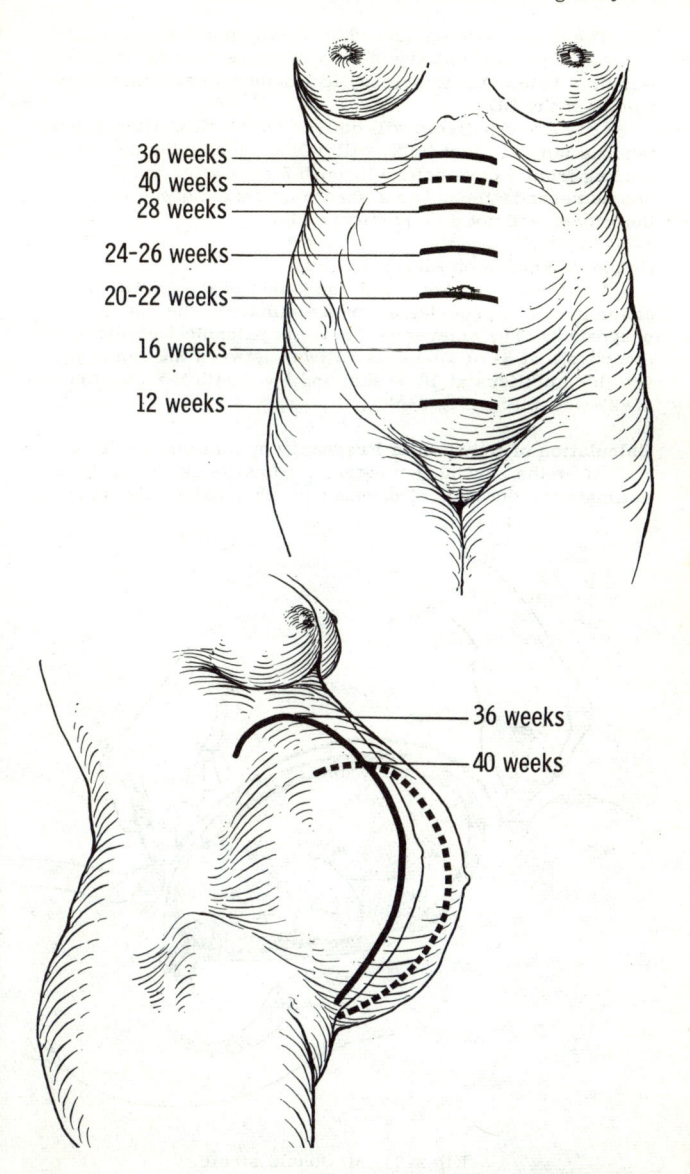

Fig 2-6. Height of fundus at various weeks during pregnancy.

48 Duration of Pregnancy

The discrepancies caused by 31-day months and the 29-day variation in February of leap year are not correctible by Nägele's rule. Nevertheless, it provides an acceptable estimate of the EDC.

Only 4% of patients will deliver on the EDC after a spontaneous labor. Most (60%) will deliver during the period extending from 5 days before through 5 days after the EDC. One should regard "term" as a season or period of maturity, therefore, and not as a particular day.

Height of Fundus on Abdominal Wall.

Until about the 6th month the height of the fundus on the abdominal wall provides a rough estimate of the duration of pregnancy. The anteverted fundus is palpable just above the symphysis at 8-10 weeks; is halfway between the symphysis and the umbilicus at 16 weeks; and level with the umbilicus at 20-22 weeks (see Fig 2-6).

Calculation of Duration of Pregnancy by McDonald's Rule.

After the second trimester, landmarks cannot be used to estimate the duration of pregnancy; other calculations are re-

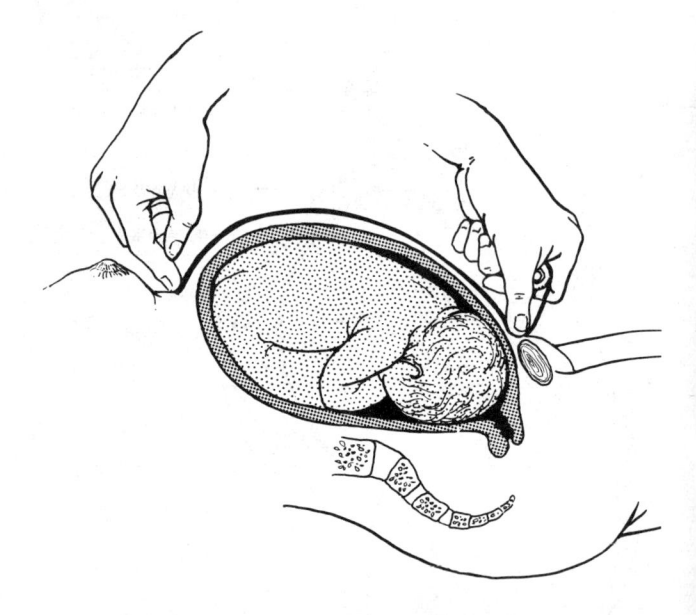

Fig 2-7. McDonald's rule.

quired. The height of the fundus above the symphysis (measured with a flexible tape, Fig 2-7) allows the following approximations (McDonald's rule):

(1) Height of the fundus (cm) × 2/7 = duration of pregnancy (lunar months); or -

(2) Height of the fundus (cm) × 8/7 = duration of pregnancy (weeks).

Although not exact, such periodic estimates do record the progress of pregnancy. Unexpectedly large measurements suggest either that the date of conception is incorrect or that the patient has a tumor, multiple pregnancy, or polyhydramnios. Unusually slow enlargement of the uterus suggests fetal abnormality or oligohydramnios, perhaps associated with placental dysmaturity. Failure of the uterus to enlarge is associated with missed abortion and fetal death in utero.

Wide variations must be expected in the weights of fetuses during the last trimester because of (1) the age-weight patterns of previous offspring, (2) the slight increase in infant weight with progressive parity, and (3) hereditary traits and acquired disorders affecting infant size (race, nutrition, diabetes mellitus, toxemia of pregnancy).

Johnson's Calculation of Fetal Weight.

A formula for calculating the weight of the fetus presenting by the vertex has been devised by R.W. Johnson:

Fundal measurement (cm) − n × 155 = fetal weight (gm), where "n" refers to the station of the head and 155 is a constant. When the head is at minus station (vertex at or above the level of the ischial spines), n = 12; at plus station (vertex below the level of the ischial spines), n = 11.

If the patient weighs 200 lb or more, subtract 1 from the fundal measurement before proceeding with the calculation.

Table 2-3. Duration of pregnancy according to fundal height and fetal weight.

Weight of Fetus (gm)	(lb)	Height of Fundus* (cm)	Station†	Duration of Pregnancy (weeks)
2100	4.6	27	minus	34
2500	5.5	29	minus	36
2800	6.2	30	minus	37
3000	6.6	31	minus	38
3150	7.0	32	minus	39
3300	7.3	33	zero	40
3450	7.6	35	zero to plus	43

*Symphysis to top of fundus. See Fig 2-7.
†Vertex presentations only.

Example:
   Height of the fundus = 35 cm
   Head engaged (vertex at zero station)
   Weight of the patient = 210 lb
   (1) 35 − 12 = 23 (height of the fundus minus n)
   (2) 23 − 1 = 22 (correction for the mother's obesity)
   (3) 22 × 155 = 3410 gm (weight of the fetus)

Approximately 70% of newborns will be within about 375 gm of the estimated birth weight as calculated by Johnson's method; at least 50% will be within about 240 gm.

TERM PREGNANCY

The diagnosis of term pregnancy is based on the estimated period of gestation and fetal measurements. Term is reached when the pregnancy has persisted for at least 36 weeks or the infant weighs 2500 gm or more (Caucasians) or the crown-rump measurement is 32 cm or more. (Other criteria: crown-heel length 47 cm or more; occipitofrontal diameter 11.5 cm or more; head circumference 33 cm or more; thorax circumference 30 cm or more.) Under the best circumstances such an infant has a 95% chance of surviving the first 28 days (neonatal period). Full term (ideal maturity) is reached at 40 weeks of gestation, with the infant weighing at least 3300 gm. The prognosis for survival at full term is raised to 99%.

When discrepancies in the dates or confusion regarding the weight of the infant arise, other observations (see below) will be required to diagnose term or full-term states.

Engagement.

In nulliparas, a zero or plus station suggests a term pregnancy. In multiparas it is strong evidence that term has been reached.

Status of the Cervix.

At full term the cervix is soft, partially effaced, and slightly patulous, and has moved from a posterior situation to the apex of the vaginal vault. Complete effacement and partial dilatation of the cervix are unequivocal evidence that the pregnancy is at term.

X-Ray Visualization of Fetal Ossification Centers.

A lateral film of the abdomen with the patient lying on the side opposite that to which the infant's back is directed will bring the fetal small parts nearer the film for delineation of the distal femoral and proximal tibial ossification centers. Precautions should be taken to protect the ovaries to avoid possible genetic abnormalities. The following possibilities exist, assuming good penetration and no subject motion:

A. If no ossification centers are visualized, the patient is probably not at term.
B. If only the distal femoral epiphysis is visualized, the patient is 36-38 weeks.
C. If the distal femoral and the proximal tibial epiphyses are visualized, the patient is at least at full term (40 weeks or more).
D. If the femoral and tibial centers and the sacral, ankle, or wrist centers are recognized, the patient is beyond full term. However, x-ray films for fetal ossification centers usually fail to reveal bone age in excess of that expected at full term.

PROLONGED PREGNANCY
(Postdate or Extended Pregnancy)

Although human pregnancy has extended to 360 days with delivery of a normal infant, prolonged pregnancy is defined as one which extends 2 or more weeks beyond the EDC as calculated from the LMP (280 + 14 = 294 days or 42 weeks). Living anencephalic monsters have been retained for as long as 389 days before spontaneous labor and delivery.

Although some women consistently carry normal pregnancies beyond the EDC, concern regarding the overdue gravida may be serious because (1) an accurate determination of the end point of pregnancy is not yet available, and (2) a perinatal mortality 2-3 times that reported at term has been recorded for offspring delivered after prolonged pregnancy. Nevertheless, the hazards of postmaturity largely relate either to (1) primiparas, especially those over 35 years of age; or (2) obstetric patients with complications such as malposition, isoimmunization, hypertension, etc.

Postmaturity presents more difficulty in diagnosis than in treatment. The major problems caused by prolonged pregnancy are the following:

(1) **Fetopelvic disproportion (large babies)**: The fetus continues to grow after 280 days; a disproportionate presenting part and lack of engagement often delays the onset of labor; prolonged labor and the need for operative delivery are more common.

(2) **Malpresentation**, i.e., face, breech, or malposition (mentum-posterior, etc.) often complicate postdate pregnancy.

(3) **Placental dysfunction**: Theoretically, aging and reduced reserve or capacity, or the inability of the placenta (a poorly compensated organ) to maintain an ever-growing fetus may cause the fetus to be smaller than expected.

Management of Prolonged Pregnancy.
A. Recheck the EDC: Estimates from the history and time of quickening should agree with the date determined from fundal height—e.g., at 28 weeks. If all agree, the EDC is more certain. The patient is rarely overdue if the cervix is not soft, slightly dilated, and somewhat effaced ("ripe"). Even so, examination of the cervix does not indicate when the fetus should be delivered.

B. Examination at Term: Reevaluate primigravidas especially at term and frequently thereafter. The following possibilities must be assessed:
  1. Dystocia - Estimate the size of the fetus. Consider x-ray and repeat standard pelvimetry.
  2. Fetal distress - FHT abnormality, amniocentesis for turbid or meconium-stained fluid.
  3. Placental incompetency - This is suggested by a high eosinophilic (acidophilic) index (>1), an increased karyopyknotic index (>10), lack of navicular (pregnancy) cells, dispersion of clumps of cells, absence of lactobacilli with a mixed flora, and a markedly reduced urinary estriol level (<10 mg/24 hours is cause for concern; 4 mg/24 hours or less is alarmingly low).
  4. Medical problems which might compromise the fetus (toxemia, diabetes mellitus, erythroblastosis).

C. Induction and Delivery: Cesarean section in uncomplicated cases of postmaturity is not warranted. Moreover, routine induction of all overdue patients would increase rather than decrease perinatal mortality. Nevertheless, if induction is decided upon, amniotomy is the preferred method. (The hypoxic or otherwise compromised fetus may not withstand unintentional uterine overstimulation by oxytocin.) If uncomplicated and reasonably rapid progress and uneventful vaginal delivery appear unlikely after a brief trial of labor, or if fetal distress develops, cesarean section should be performed at once.

3...
The Placenta & Fetus

THE PLACENTA & ITS STRUCTURES

Fertilization.

Beginning on about the 14th day of the average ovulatory menstrual cycle, the uterine glands develop the feathery contour characteristic of pregnancy endometrium and the stromal cells assume the polygonal shape of decidua cells. This preparation for implantation of the fertilized ovum is influenced by progesterone (elaborated by the corpus luteum) and, to a lesser extent, by estrogens.

Following fertilization, which usually occurs in the distal third of the fallopian tube, the ovum develops into the embryonic blastocyst. About 3-4 days are required for the blastocyst to reach the uterus, and implantation ensues 5-6 days after this. During the entire period prior to implantation the embryo depends upon adherent granulosa cells and perhaps nutrient fluids within the tube and uterus for sustenance (histotrophic phase of embryo).

Implantation.

The outermost layer of the fertilized ovum, or zygote, is termed the chorion. It serves for nutrition and protection of the embryo, and consists of an inner mesodermal layer and an outer ectodermal layer, the trophoblast. Initially the trophoblast is a poorly-defined syncytium, but it soon develops into 2 tissue types: an inner, distinctly cellular cytotrophoblast (Langhans' stria) and an outer, confluent but differentiated plasmotrophoblast (syntrophoblast).

The trophoblast produces proteolytic enzymes capable of rapid destruction of endometrium and even myometrium. They enable the embryo to erode deeply and without delay into the functionalis layer of the endometrium (but usually not beyond the compacta). Deeper invasion is prevented by formation of Nitabuch's stria, a layer of hyalinized fibrin just beyond the advancing trophoblast.

Normally, the blastocyst implants on the 5th or 6th day after entry into the uterus, most commonly in the decidua lining the anterior or posterior wall of the fundus. The site of nidation immediately heals over. Three decidual areas

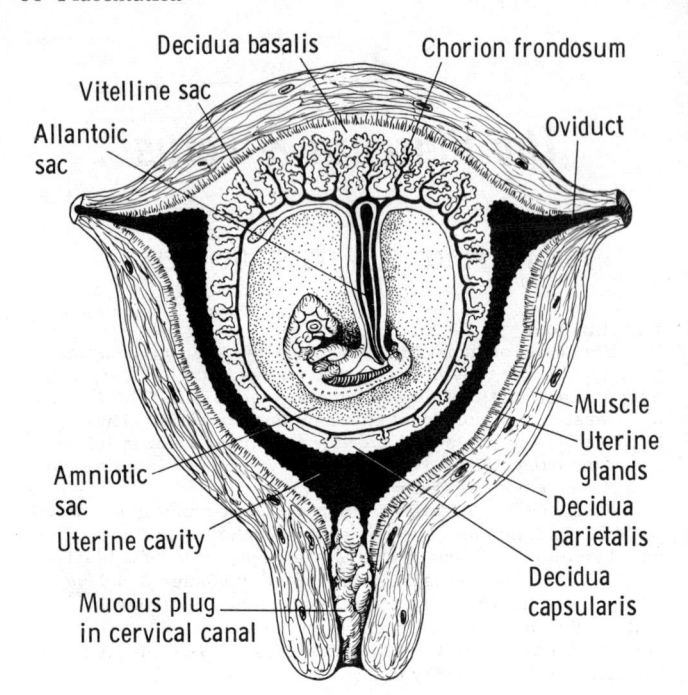

Fig 3-1. Relationships of structures in the uterus at the end of the 7th week of pregnancy.

may now be recognized: (1) decidua capsularis (reflexa), or that portion of the uterine mucosa immediately overlying the embryo; (2) decidua basalis, beneath the embryo; and (3) decidua parietalis, the remainder of the uterine lining. The decidua capsularis disappears as the embryo increases in size to fill the uterine cavity. The decidua basalis is the site of future development of the placenta.

PLACENTATION

Fetoplacental Circulation.

Following implantation, small lacunae, which later become confluent, develop in the plasmotrophoblast. These lacunae (future intervillous spaces) fill with maternal blood by reflux from previously tapped veins. An occasional maternal artery then opens and a sluggish circulation is established (hematotrophic phase of embryo).

The lacunar system is separated by trabeculae, many of which develop buds or extensions. Within these branching projections the cytotrophoblast forms a mesenchymal core. Later the core is canalized and connections are established with other potential blood vessels. The vascularized tufts are now referred to as villi.

The most extensive ramification of the villous tree occurs on that part of the chorion which is closest to the maternal blood supply (chorion frondosum). This is the site of the future placenta. Scattered villi also form over the remainder of the chorion (chorion reflexa) but soon atrophy, leaving a smooth surface (chorion laeve).

The villous system compares with an inverted fir tree (rather than an inverted chandelier). The branches pass obliquely downward and outward within the intervillous spaces. This arrangement probably permits preferential currents or gradients of blood, as in the liver. Nevertheless, such an arrangement undoubtedly encourages intervillous fibrin deposition, commonly seen in the mature placenta.

Cotyledons (subdivisions of the placenta) can be identified early in placentation. They are separated by columns of fibrous tissue, the placental septa. As the placenta develops, the maternal tissue in these septa is autolyzed by pressure and replaced by fetal tissue. The septa contain no vessels.

Communication within each cotyledon is provided by fenestrations. In contrast, intercotyledinous septa contain few openings. Fair communication between cotyledons does exist, however, via the subchorionic lake in the roof of the intervillous spaces.

Fetal blood flow between villi probably does not occur. Hence, the concept of the placenta being a sponge is not accurate anatomically.

The old theory that the trophoblast sends out finger-like projections which become invaded by proliferating mesoderm as a prelude to vascularization has also been discarded. Moreover, although a core of maternal decidua and fibrous tissue acts as the initial framework, the fibrous intercotyledinous septa are largely of fetal, not maternal, origin.

Uteroplacental Circulation.
A. Veins: Many randomly placed venous orifices can be identified over the entire decidua basalis (basal plate of placenta). They remain numerous throughout gestation. These veins have no sphincters, and there is no arteriolization of the veins to suggest comparison of the placenta to an arteriovenous fistula.

The human placenta has no peripheral venous collecting system, a function frequently ascribed to a marginal sinus. Less than one-third of the blood drains from the placenta at its margin. A marginal sinus is not seen even in the early placenta, and subchorionic marginal lakes are not commonly found in the mature placenta. Occasionally, dilated maternal vessels are found beneath the periphery of the placenta; these have been described as wreath veins, or venous lakes. They may or may not communicate with the intervillous spaces and their significance is still debated. Nonetheless, one of these thin-walled veins may be torn during premature marginal separation of the placenta, resulting in the bleeding problem erroneously called "marginal sinus rupture."

B. Arteries: In contrast to the veins, the arteries are grouped closer to the decidual attachments of the intercotyledinous septa. As the placenta matures, thrombosis decreases the number of arterial openings into the basal plate. At term, the ratio of veins to arteries is 2:1, approximately that found in other mature organs.

Even in an area beneath a well-formed placenta, some spiral arterioles empty into the intervillous spaces, but many remain coiled and compressed. Arterioles supplying the intervillous spaces appear circuitous and angulated because of fixation of the vessels and growth of the placenta. The tortuosity creates baffles or points of deflection which tend to slow the afferent blood stream.

Near their entry into the intervillous spaces, the terminal maternal arterioles lose their elastic reticulum. Since the distal portions of these vessels are lost with the placenta, bleeding from this source can be controlled only by uterine contraction.

THE MATURE PLACENTA

The mature placenta (Fig 3-2) is a blue-red, rounded, flattened, meaty organ about 15-20 cm in diameter and 3 cm thick. It weighs 400-600 gm, or about one-sixth the normal weight of the newborn. The umbilical cord (funis) extends from the fetal surface of the placenta to the umbilicus of the fetus; the fetal membranes arise from the placenta at its margin. In multiple pregnancy, one or more placentas may be present depending upon the number of ova implanted and the type of segmentation which occurs. The placenta is derived from both maternal and fetal tissue. At term, about four-fifths are of fetal origin.

The maternal portion of the placenta amounts to less than one-fifth of the total placenta by weight. It is composed of compressed sheets of decidua basalis, remnants of blood vessels, and, at the margin, spongy decidua. Irregular grooves or clefts divide the placenta into cotyledons. The maternal surface is torn from the uterine wall at birth and as a result is rough, red, and spongy.

Mature Placenta 57

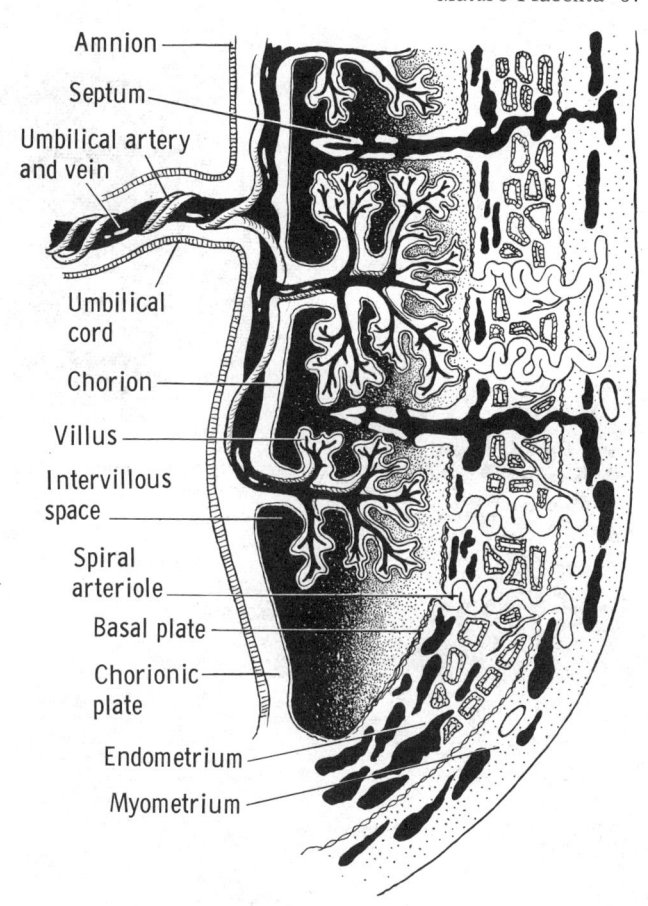

Fig 3-2. Cross-section of the mature placenta. (Considerably modified after Netter.)

The fetal portion of the placenta is composed of numerous functional units called villi. These are branched terminals of the fetal circulation, and provide for transfer of metabolic products. The villous surface, which is exposed to maternal blood, may be as much as 160 feet square. The fetal capillary system within the villi is almost 30 miles long. Most villi are free within the intervillous spaces, but an oc-

58 Mature Placenta

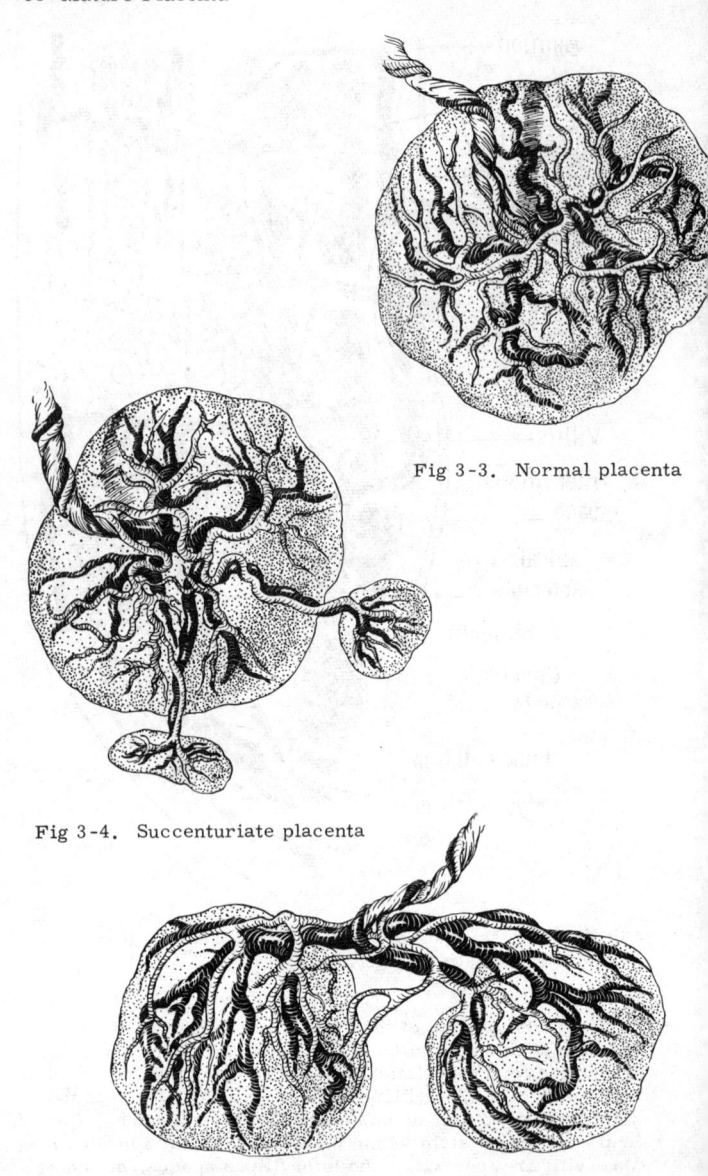

Fig 3-3. Normal placenta

Fig 3-4. Succenturiate placenta

Fig 3-5. Bipartite placenta

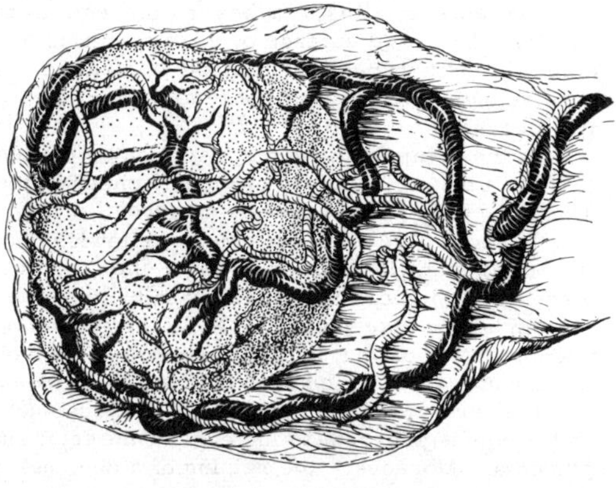

Mature Placenta 59

Fig 3-6. Velamentous insertion of cord.

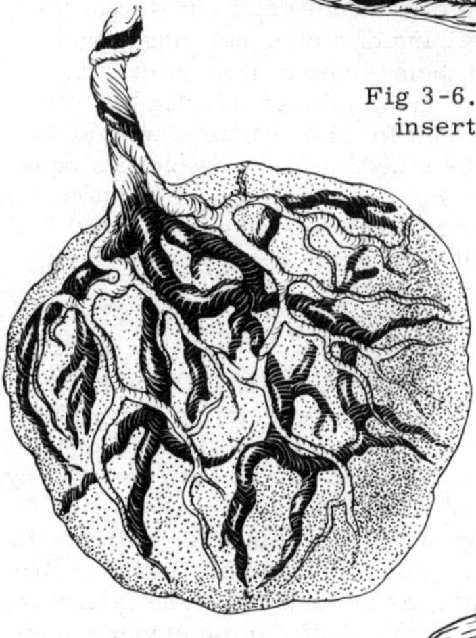

Fig 3-7. Marginal insertion or battledore placenta.

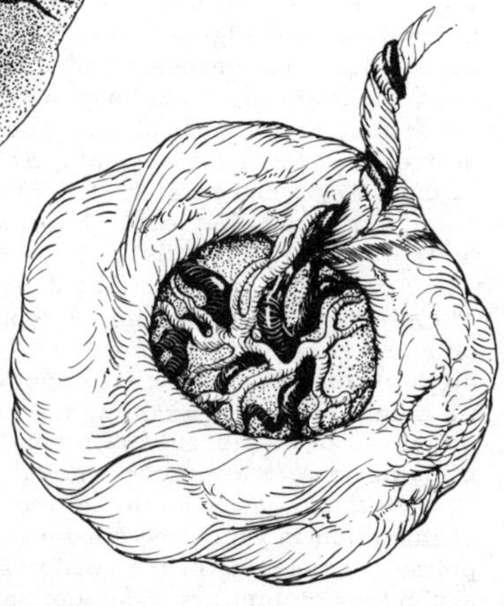

Fig 3-8. Marked circumvallate placenta.

casional anchor villus attaches the placenta to the decidua basalis. The fetal surface of the placenta is covered by amniotic membrane and is smooth and shiny. The umbilical cord vessels course over the fetal surface before entering the placenta.

In the common marginal insertion or **battledore placenta** (Fig 3-7) the cord inserts at the periphery of the placenta. The battledore placenta poses no special problems.

In about 0.5% of deliveries, a yellowish opaque band of fibrous tissue will be seen to cover the fetal surface of the placenta at the periphery. Early in the development of such **circumvallate placentas** (Fig 3-8), the growth of villi at the margin outstrips that of the membranous part of the chorion frondosum. The peripheral villi tend to grow obliquely outward under these circumstances. The decidua is undermined and becomes adherent to the edge of the fetal surface of the placenta. Moreover, the raising of a decidual ridge causes the membranes to fold upon themselves at this point. Eventual fibrinoid degeneration of the displaced decidua and a double layer of membranes account for the opaque placental edge. The "reinforced" edge of the placenta may restrict its growth and function. Late abortion and premature (usually marginal) separation of the placenta are sometimes associated with circumvallate placenta, which for some reason is often repetitious in sequential pregnancies.

Placental Types.

The normal placenta is shown in Fig 3-3. Occasionally, the placenta may have one or more succenturiate or satellite lobes (Fig 3-4). These are attached to the main body of the placenta by a bridging major fetal artery and vein covered by intervening membranes. Succenturiate lobes may fail to separate from the main body of the placenta after delivery of the fetus. Subsequent bleeding or infection may result. After delivery, inspect the placenta for evidence of vessels severed at the margin and retained fragments of the membranes suggestive of a missing lobe. Express or remove the succenturiate portion promptly.

A bipartite placenta (Fig 3-5) is an uncommon variety. The placenta is divided into 2 separate lobes but united by primary vessels and membranes. Retention of one lobe after birth of the infant will cause postpartal hemorrhagic and septic complications. Examine the vasculature and note the completeness of membranes of a small placenta for evidence of a missing lobe, and recover the adherent portion without delay.

Velamentous insertion of the cord (Fig 3-6) is a rare type of insertion in which the cord ends at the membranes where primary branching of the cord vessels occurs. Delicate secondary or tertiary vascular radicals supported only by the membranes pass to the placenta. Prepartal trauma to the membranes or traction on the cord during the birth process may lacerate placental arteries or veins, and fetal blood loss may be critical. Although ante- or intrapartal vaginal bleeding and fetal distress may be observed, there is no simple means of diagnosing membranous insertion of the cord prior to inspection of the cord and placenta. Undue traction on the cord during the third stage may sever the cord at its membranous insertion. Manual removal of the placenta may then be necessary.

The Umbilical Cord (Funis).

The umbilical cord is a gray, soft, coiled, easily compressible structure which connects the fetus with its placenta. It averages 50 cm in length and 2 cm in diameter and is covered by a thin layer of stratified squamous epithelium which is comparable to fetal skin. The cord contains a framework of loose fibrous connective tissue and is filled with a mucoid proteinaceous material (Wharton's jelly). Normally, the cord contains 2 arteries which carry deoxygenated blood from the fetus, and one vein, which supplies the fetus with oxygenated blood. The cord usually has an eccentric insertion into the placenta. The absence of one umbilical artery is noted in 1% of singletons and over 3% of twins. A two-vessel cord is associated with other anomalies in about 10% of neonates.

Fetal Membranes.

The chorion and amnion arise from the placenta at its margin to envelop the fetus. They strip easily from the fetal surface of the placenta and can be separated from one another by careful dissection.

The amnion is a double-layered translucent membrane; its outer layer is mesodermal connective tissue and its inner layer is ectoderm. The amnion may be considered an extension of the skin of the fetus. Although it consists generally of a few layers of stratified squamous cells, patches of low cuboidal cells are also seen. Thickened squamous areas are occasionally observed, especially near the umbilical cord.

(Note: A check for completeness of the membranes at delivery is essential. Large portions of the membranes may remain adherent to the decidua parietalis high in the fundus of the uterus and give rise to endometritis. It is important also to note the point of rupture of the membranes. This site will usually correspond with that portion of membranes which was over the cervical os or beneath the incision at cesarean section. By reference to the point of rupture, the area of implantation of the placenta may be determined—an important detail in proof of low-lying placenta.)

The Amniotic Fluid.

At term, the fetus is submerged in about 1 liter of clear watery fluid (though up to 2 liters may be normally present) of low specific gravity (about 1.008) and mild alkalinity (about pH 7.2). The amniotic fluid protects the fetus from direct injury, aids in maintaining its temperature, allows free movement of the fetus, and minimizes the likelihood of adherence of the fetus to the amniotic membrane. It contains fetal squamous debris, flecks of vernix, a few leukocytes, and small quantities of albumin, urates, and other organic and inorganic salts. The calcium content of amniotic fluid is low (5.5 mg/100 ml), but the electrolyte concentration is otherwise equivalent to that of maternal plasma.

The fluid is variously considered to be a secretion of the amnion, a vascular transudate, or fetal urine. Probably all 3 contribute, but the first is the most important. Approximately 350-375 ml of amniotic fluid are replaced each hour, a very rapid turnover considering the morphologic simplicity of the amnion. It is curious that the quality and the constituents of the amniotic fluid do not vary grossly with the total amount of fluid present. Nevertheless, a retention deficit of only a few ml/hour will soon result in polyhydramnios (> 2 liters of amniotic fluid); an undue clearance will cause oligohydramnios (< 300 ml at term).

PHYSIOLOGY OF THE PLACENTA

The placenta has 2 principal functions: It acts as a transfer organ for metabolic products, and it produces the hormones and enzymes necessary for the maintenance of pregnancy. It thus acts as a lung, a gastrointestinal tract, a kidney, and a complex of ductless glands for the conceptus.

Like any other organ, the placenta lives and "breathes." It derives most, if not all, of its nourishment from maternal blood. The metabolic activity of the placenta may be measured by its oxygen consumption. Continued growth of the placenta is feasible only to a point, however, and its functional capacity and oxygen consumption decline with age.

Hemodynamics.

Prior to labor, placental filling occurs whenever the uterus contracts (Braxton Hicks contractions). At these times, the maternal venous exits are closed, but the thicker-walled arteries are only slightly narrowed. When the uterus relaxes, blood drains out by the maternal veins. Hence, blood is not squeezed out of the placenta with each contraction, nor does it enter in appreciably greater amounts during relaxation.

The quantity and relative arterial pressure of the blood within different parts of the placenta vary from time to time. Nevertheless, there is little short-circuiting of blood from an arterial opening to an adjacent venous outlet because the arterial pressure of the maternal blood (60-70 mm Hg) actually causes it to be squirted into the low pressure (20 mm Hg) intervillous space. The direction of flow depends mainly upon the relative pressures in each circulation. Maternal arterial blood is directed toward the chorionic plate, whereas venous blood in the placenta tends to flow along the basal plate and out. This establishes circulation currents.

Maternal blood flow through the placenta at term approximates 500 ml/minute, whereas only about 400 ml of fetal blood circulate through the placenta each minute.

The slow rate of circulation within the placenta is offset by the capacity of the placenta, which exceeds that of the vessels supplying and draining it, as well as by the excess of maternal over fetal blood. Changes in maternal blood pressure therefore have only a gradual effect on the intervillous blood pressure in the placenta. Mechanisms to improve placental transfer are few, however. An increased rate of rhythmic uterine contractions is helpful; but strong, prolonged labor contractions are detrimental to the placental and fetal circulation. An increased fetal heart rate tends to expand the villi during systole, and this is a minor aid in circulatory transfer.

The pressure gradient within the fetal circulation changes slowly with the mother's posture, fetal movements, and physical stress. The pressure within the placental intervillous space is about 10 mm Hg when the pregnant woman is lying down. After standing for a few minutes, this pressure exceeds 30 mm Hg. In comparison, the fetal capillary pressure remains at about 20 mm Hg.

The Placental Barrier.

The human placental barrier is represented initially by 2 layers of trophoblastic cells which separate the maternal and fetal blood streams. The outer layer is the syntrophoblast or plasmotrophoblast; the inner is the cytotrophoblast or Langhans' stria. After the third month the cytotrophoblast normally loses its continuity and the cells become less numerous. Hence, in late pregnancy the only separation between maternal blood and the fetal vascular endothelium is the syntrophoblast, a single cell layer.

Placental Transfer.

Transfer across the placental barrier is accomplished by at least 4 different processes: (1) diffusion, (2) selection by means of enzyme carriers, (3) pinocytosis (engulfment of particles by cells), and (4) leakage through defects.
  A. Diffusion: Substances required for the maintenance of fetal life and the elimination of its waste products are handled largely by diffusion across the placental barrier. Included in this group are oxygen, CO_2, water, electrolytes, and urea. Fetal and maternal blood have similar

diffusion constants, so that passage of these substances is rapid in either direction. Large quantities of certain substances are involved; near term, almost 4 liters of water clear the placenta each hour.

Fortunately, the fetal oxygen requirements are less than those of the newborn. Oxygen tension in the intervillous space is only about half that in the maternal pulmonary veins. The fetus is compensated to a degree, at least, because fetal hemoglobin carries slightly more oxygen than adult hemoglobin. Moreover, fetal blood also eliminates CO_2 better than the blood of the child.

Substances of low molecular weight (< 1000) diffuse across the placenta with ease. Thyroxin, thiamine, and many drugs, including alcohol and morphine, are in this group. Large molecules (with molecular weights > 1000) such as blood proteins and chorionic gonadotropin will not pass the placental barrier by diffusion.

B. Selective Transfer: Enzymatic processes, often involving slight energy exchange, supply many fetal nutritional needs. Glucose, amino acids, calcium, phosphorus, iron, and probably some of the vitamins cross the placental barrier by this means. Specificity through selection is thus possible despite the capacity for diffusion of many of these substances. For example, because the fetus manufactures its own protein, essential amino acids are transferred more rapidly than polypeptides.

C. Pinocytosis: Ultramicroscopy has shown moving pseudopodical projections of the plasmotrophoblastic layer which reach out, as it were, to surround minute amounts of maternal plasma. These particles are carried across the cell intact to be released on the other side, whereupon they promptly gain access to the fetal circulation. This process may work both to and from the fetus, but how selective it is has not been determined. Complex proteins, small amounts of fat, and perhaps immune bodies may traverse the placenta in this way.

D. Leakage Through Defects: Trophoblastic endothelial junctions may "leak" small amounts of plasma and blood cells. Maternal and fetal blood may mix as a result of any of the following processes:
  1. Degenerative changes, e.g., subchorionic fibrin accumulation ("fibrinoid" degeneration), which may cause necrosis within the area; intervillous fibrin deposition with ischemic necrosis of the villi; infarction of a small portion of the placenta or even of entire cotyledons following the occlusion of the umbilical artery or any of its tributaries; and syncytial degeneration or incomplete loss of investment of villi (partially "naked" villi).
  2. Functional stresses, e.g., stretching of the villous tree during increased fetal intracapillary pressure or

relaxation of the villous tree after fetal capillary contraction.
3. Infection, e.g., tuberculous placentitis, granulomatous lesions of coccidiomycosis, or pyogenic abscess of the placenta.
4. Trauma, e.g., premature separation of the placenta (especially abruptio placentae) or manipulation of the uterus.
5. Abnormal development of the placenta, e.g., hydatidiform mole or chorio-epithelioma with local necrosis.

Production of Hormones.

Placental hormones can theoretically supply most of the endocrine needs of a pregnant woman who has been deprived of the anterior and posterior pituitary glands, the adrenal cortices, and the ovaries. At delivery, however, her condition would become critical.

Tissue culture studies show that the cytotrophoblast produces chorionic gonadotropin (CGT). The plasmotrophoblast is the source of the sex steroid hormones (estrogens and progesterone), corticoids, and even adrenocorticotropic hormone (ACTH).

CGT is produced from the first week after implantation, and is secreted into the maternal (but not the fetal) circulation. Maximal blood and urine levels are reached by the end of the 10th week. After this time, and concomitantly with the diminution in the number of Langhans' cells, the CGT titer falls, but it is maintained at easily detectable levels until 1-2 weeks after delivery. CGT aids in the maintenance of the corpus luteum of pregnancy and is the basis for the Aschheim-Zondek and Friedman pregnancy tests.

Estrogens are bound to serum albumin in the maternal circulation and are therefore metabolized slowly. Progesterone, on the other hand, is unbound and is metabolized rapidly. Thyroxin is bound to alpha globulin and prealbumin. Corticoids are held in relatively inactive form by a plasma protein, transcortin. Thus, although the titer of hydroxycorticosteroids is high during pregnancy, frank hypercortisonism is uncommon.

Placental Insufficiency.

Placental insufficiency is the relative inability of the placenta to sustain a normal rate of fetal growth and development. It may be present in the embryonic stage as trophoblastic deficiency. Later, maternal complications such as toxemia of pregnancy, chronic nephritis, hypertensive cardiovascular disease, or postmaturity may cause placental insufficiency.

Clinically, the uterus fails to enlarge at the normal rate, and oligohydramnios is common. The infant may be small or malnourished. The placenta is frequently quite small. Pathologic examination of placental tissue shows microinfarcts,

Table 3-1. Embryonic and fetal growth and development.

Fertilization Age (weeks)	Crown-Rump Length (approx.)	Crown-Heel Length (approx.)	Weight (approx.)	Gross Appearance	Internal Development
Embryonic Stage					
1	0.5 mm	0.5 mm	?	Minute clone free in uterus.	Early morula. No organ differentiation.
2	2 mm	2 mm	?	Ovoid vesicle superficially buried in endometrium.	External trophoblast. Flat embryonic disk forming 2 inner vesicles (amnio-ecto-mesodermal and entodermal).
3	3 mm	3 mm	?	Early dorsal concavity changes to convexity; head, tail folds form; neural grooves close partially.	Optic vesicles appear. Double heart recognized. Fourteen mesodermal somites present.
4	4 mm	4 mm	0.4 gm	Head is at right angle to body; limb rudiments obvious, tail prominent.	Vitelline duct only communication between umbilical vesicle and intestines. Initial stage of most organs has begun.
8	3 cm	3.5 cm	2 gm	Eyes, ears, nose, mouth recognizable; digits formed, tail almost gone.	Sensory organ development well along. Ossification beginning in occiput, mandible, and humerus (diaphysis). Small intestines coil within umbilical cord. Pleural, pericardial cavities forming. Gonadal development advanced without differentiation.
Fetal Stage					
12	8 cm	11.5 cm	19 gm	Skin pink, delicate; resembles a human being, but head is disproportionately large.	Brain configuration roughly complete. Internal sex organs now specific. Uterus no longer bicornuate. Blood forming in marrow. Upper cervical to lower sacral arches and bodies ossify.

Physiology of Placenta 67

16	13.5 cm	19 cm	100 gm	Scalp hair appears. Fetus active. Arm-leg ratio now proportionate. Sex determination possible.	Sex organs grossly formed. Myelenization recognized. Heart muscle well developed. Lobulated kidneys in final situation. Meconium first appears in bowel. Vagina and anus open. Ischium (descending ramus) ossified.
20	18.5 cm	22 cm	300 gm	Legs lengthen appreciably. Distance from umbilicus to pubis increases.	Sternum ossifies.
24	23 cm	32 cm	600 gm	Skin is reddish and wrinkled. Slight newly deposited subcuticular fat. Vernix appears. Primitive respiratory-like movements begin.	Os pubis (horizontal ramus) ossifies.
28	27 cm	36 cm	1100 gm	Skin less wrinkled; more fat present. Nails first appear. If delivered, breathes, cries, moves poorly. A rare child survives with optimal care.	Testes at internal inguinal ring or below. Astragalus ossifies.
32	31 cm	41 cm	1800 gm	Fetal weight increased proportionately more than length.	Middle 4th phalanges ossify.
36	35 cm	46 cm	2200 gm	Skin pale, body rounded. Generalized lanugo disappearing. Umbilicus now in center of ventral portion of body.	Distal femoral ossification centers present.
40	40 cm	52 cm	3200+ gm	Skin is smooth and pink. Copious vernix often present. Moderate to profuse dark, heavy hair on head. Lanugo hair on shoulders and upper back only. Nasal and alar cartilages apparent. Nails extend over tips of digits. Testes in scrotum or labia majora well developed.	Proximal tibial ossification centers present. Cuboid, tibia (proximal epiphysis) ossify.

diffuse perivillous fibrin deposition, and occlusion of vessels of the villous system, all of which imply reduced function.

Extended fetal deprivation in utero probably accounts for the high perinatal mortality rate. Further study and follow-up will be required to determine whether placental insufficiency is associated with persistent central nervous system deficits or other developmental defects in the infants who survive.

FETAL NUTRITION

There are 3 stages of fetal nutrition: (1) Absorption. Minimal quantities of tubal and uterine fluid are taken in by the fertilized ovum during the 3-4 days prior to nidation. (2) Histotrophic transfer. Strategic and waste materials are passed between the early embryo and decidua for about 3 months before the establishment of an effective fetal circulation. (3) Hematotrophic transfer. Anabolic and catabolic products traverse the placental barrier between the fetal and maternal circulations by both active and passive processes.

HEMATOPOIESIS

Unmistakable hematopoiesis begins in the liver, spleen, and mesonephros about the second month, although clumps or "islands" of blood cells may be seen in the yolk sac during the first 1-2 months of fetal life. All the circulating red cells are nucleated very early in human development. By the third month, however, only about 10% of the red cells still retain their nuclei; at term, only 5-8% are nucleated.

Premature as well as mature infants are polycythemic by adult standards, having red cell counts of 4-6 million/cu mm. The fetus also presents a relative leukocytosis, the white count being 15-20 thousand/cu mm at term. Macrocytic erythrocytes are typical of the entire fetal period. The span of life of the fetal and adult red cell is the same, approximately 120 days.

A gradual, relative increase in hemoglobin occurs in the developing fetus. Normally, the hemoglobin totals about 20 gm and the hematocrit 40-60% at term. Fetal hemoglobin (hemoglobin F) is the type present from the 13th week until about the 24th week, when adult hemoglobin (hemoglobin A) appears. At term, 15-45% of the hemoglobin is type A. After delivery, the proportion of hemoglobin A in the infant's blood increases rapidly; less than 2% hemoglobin F is detected at one year in most instances.

Ferritin, the iron form essential to the production of hemoglobin, is present in the placenta as early as the first month and increases in amount through the 6th month. Ferritin appears in the fetal liver during the second and third month and may be recovered from the spleen after the 4th month. In contrast with the newborn and the adult, it is absent from the intestines. The relative amount of ferritin in the fetus does not vary significantly during gestation.

Fetal blood is slightly more saturated with oxygen than maternal blood. This heightened affinity for oxygen is due probably to increased permeability of the fetal erythrocyte membrane rather than to the type of hemoglobin contained.

FETAL CIRCULATION

Environmental changes occurring in the abrupt transition from intrauterine life to an independent existence necessitate certain circulatory adaptations in the newborn. These include diversion of blood flow through the lungs, closure of the ductus arteriosus and foramen ovale, and obliteration of the ductus venosus and umbilical vessels.

Infant circulation has 3 phases (Figs 3-9 to 3-11): (1) the predelivery phase, in which the fetus depends upon the placenta; (2) the intermediate phase, which begins immediately after delivery with the infant's first breath; and (3) the adult phase, which is normally completed during the first few months of life.

Predelivery Phase.

The umbilical vein carries oxygenated blood from the placenta to the fetus. At the umbilicus the vein branches and enters the liver; a small branch bypasses the liver as the ductus venosus to enter the inferior vena cava directly.

Blood from the inferior vena cava enters the right heart, and most of it is immediately shunted through the widely patent foramen ovale into the left atrium. A smaller quantity enters the pulmonary artery. From the left atrium the oxygenated blood passes quickly into the left ventricle and thence into the ascending aorta. The head, coronary arteries, and upper extremities are thus well supplied with oxygenated blood. Only a small amount of blood from the left ventricle flows into the descending aorta.

Blood returning from the head enters the right atrium via the superior vena cava. From here it flows into the right ventricle and thence into the pulmonary artery. A small amount of the pulmonary arterial blood is directed to the lungs; the major portion flows directly into the descending aorta via the ductus arteriosus.

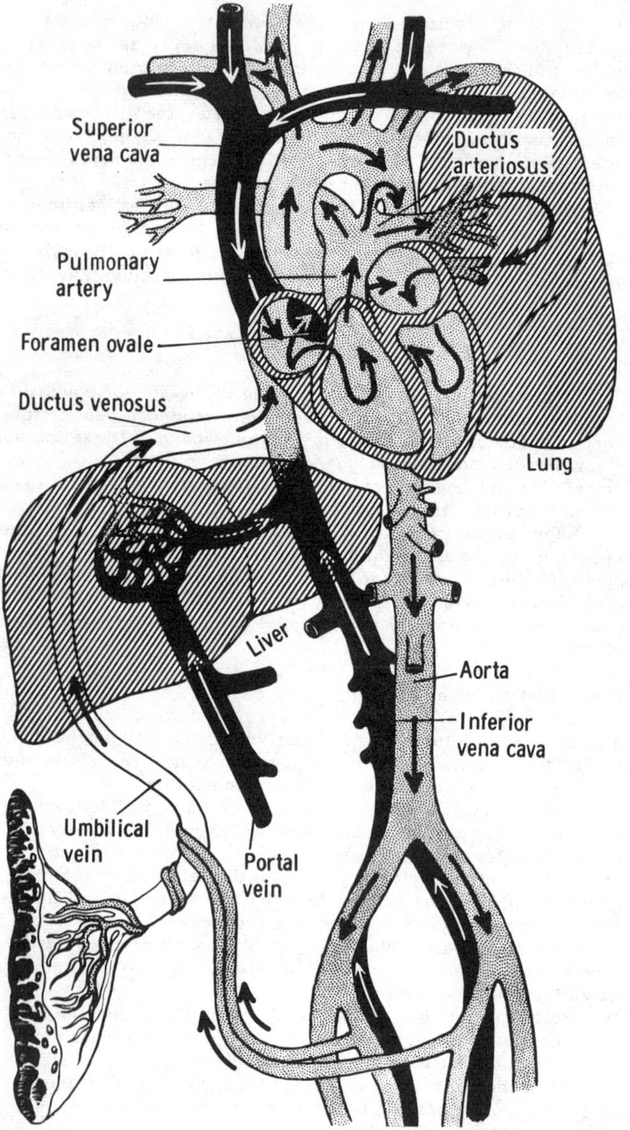

70 Fetal Circulation

Fig 3-9. Fetal circulation.

Fetal Circulation 71

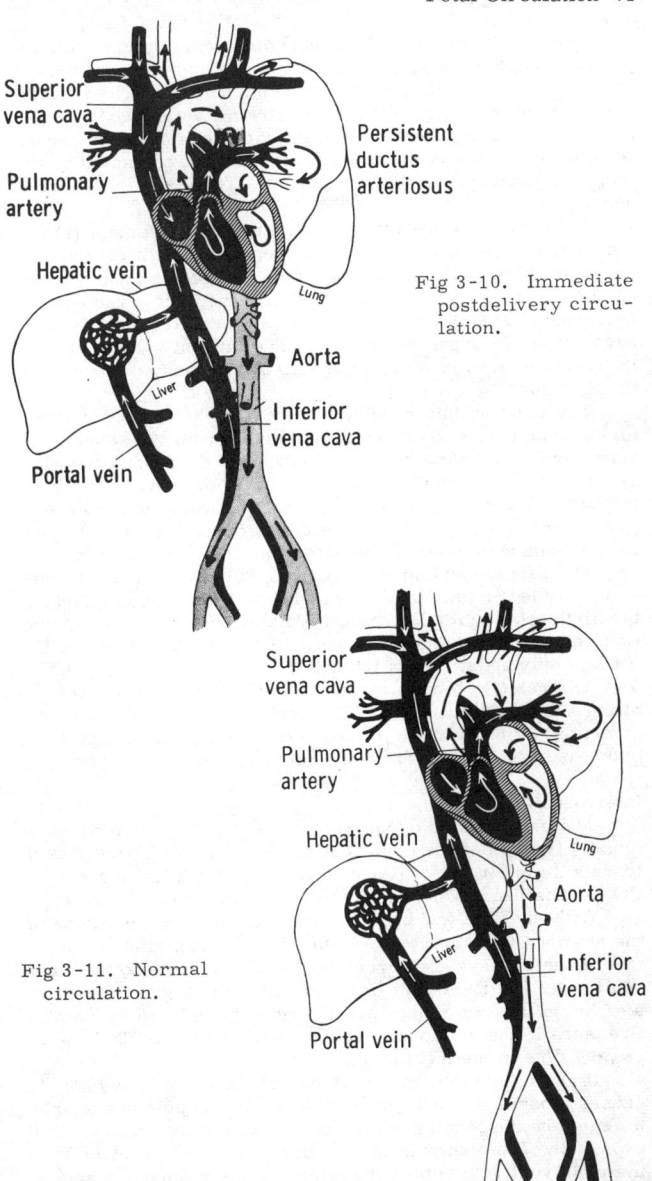

Fig 3-10. Immediate postdelivery circulation.

Fig 3-11. Normal circulation.

Most of the blood in the descending aorta returns to the placenta via the hypogastric arteries (which become the umbilical arteries as they leave at the umbilicus). The remainder circulates through the lower extremities and abdominal pelvic viscera and then into the inferior vena cava, whence it is returned, along with the large volume of oxygenated blood from the placenta, to the right heart. The cycle is then repeated.

Blood reaches the inferior vena cava by 4 routes: (1) from the liver via the hepatic veins (oxygenated blood); (2) from the liver via the hepatic and portal veins (oxygenated and deoxygenated blood); (3) around the liver via the ductus venosus (oxygenated blood); and (4) from the lower extremities via the iliac veins (deoxygenated blood). The largest volume of blood in the inferior vena cava, however, is oxygenated blood from the placenta.

The right atrium receives oxygenated blood from the inferior vena cava and deoxygenated blood from the superior vena cava. The structure and position of the foramen ovale between the right and left atria is such, however, that the stream of blood is split; most of the inferior vena cava blood passes through the foramen ovale into the left atrium; the superior vena cava blood is directed into the right ventricle.

The oxygen tension of blood in the umbilical vein is considerably lower than that of arterial or even venous blood after birth. In the fetal circulation itself, blood oxygen saturation varies widely (umbilical vein, 80%; left ventricle, 60%). This is only about 30% of the normal adult P_{O_2}.

The relative blood flow in the fetus also differs from that of the adult. Fifty to 60% of the cardiac output traverses the placenta, which offers a low resistance; only 10-15% of the output passes through the more resistant pulmonary bed.

Intermediate Phase.

At birth 2 events occur which alter the fetal hemodynamics: (1) ligation of the umbilical cord causes an abrupt though transient rise in arterial pressure; and (2) a rise in plasma CO_2 and fall in blood P_{O_2} usually initiate regular breathing.

With the first few breaths, the intrathoracic pressure of the newborn remains low (−40 to −50 mm Hg); after distention of the airways, however, the pressure rises to the normal adult level (−7 to −8 mm Hg). The initially high vascular resistance of the pulmonary bed is probably reduced by 75-80%. Pressure in the pulmonary artery falls by at least 60%, whereas pressure in the left atrium doubles.

In the fetus the high resistance of the pulmonary bed causes most of the deoxygenated blood in the pulmonary artery to enter the descending aorta via the ductus arteriosus. With expansion of the lungs in the newborn, most of the blood from the right ventricle enters the lungs via the pulmonary artery.

Further, the increased arterial pressure reverses the flow of blood through the ductus arteriosus: blood flows from the high-pressure aorta to the low-pressure pulmonary artery.

The increased pressure in the left atrium would normally result in backflow into the right heart through a patent foramen ovale. However, the anatomic configuration of the foramen is such that the increased pressure causes closure of the foramen by a valve-like fold situated in the wall of the left atrium.

The neonatal circulation is complete with closure of the ductus arteriosus and foramen ovale, but adjustments continue for 1-2 months, when the adult phase begins.

Adult Phase.

The ductus arteriosus usually is obliterated in the early postnatal period, probably by reflex action secondary to an elevated oxygen tension and the action of epinephrine-like metabolites. If the ductus remains open, a systolic crescendo murmur which diminishes during diastole ("machinery murmur") is often heard over the second left interspace.

Obliteration of the foramen ovale is usually complete in 6-8 weeks, with fusion of its valve to the left interatrial septum. The foramen may remain patent in some individuals, however, with few or no symptoms. The obliterated ductus venosus from the liver to the vena cava becomes the ligamentum venosum. The occluded umbilical vein becomes the ligamentum teres of the liver.

The hemodynamics of the normal adult differ from those of the fetus in the following respects: (1) venous and arterial blood are no longer mixed in the atria; (2) the vena cava carries only deoxygenated blood into the right atrium, whence it is pumped into the pulmonary arteries and thence to the pulmonary capillary bed; and (3) the aorta carries only oxygenated blood from the left heart via the pulmonary veins for distribution to the rest of the body.

4...
Prenatal Care

HISTORY & PHYSICAL EXAMINATION

A thorough medical history and physical examination early in pregnancy provide the groundwork for the diagnosis and treatment of disorders which may compromise the pregnancy. Knowing his patient's general health problems permits the obstetrician to interpret developing symptomatology correctly and treat complications promptly. Good antenatal care is preventive medicine of a high order.

In obstetric practice the history and physical findings are usually recorded on an outline form of the checklist type. However, many commercially available forms do not provide sufficient detail or adequate space for notes and comments.

Vital Statistics.

The following information should be recorded by the physician for each patient:

A. Date of first examination, and unit number (hospital number).
B. Patient's full name, address, home telephone number, husband's first name.
C. Patient's occupation. This information may be helpful in interpreting symptoms due to fatigue, exposure to industrial hazards, or occupational tensions. It must be considered in recommending exercise and rest periods and in determining how long the patient can continue outside employment during pregnancy and how soon she can return to work after delivery.
D. The date of marriage, especially of a primigravida, may alert the physician to possible problems regarding the patient's attitude toward the pregnancy. If the patient is unmarried, the question of adoption is often best raised at this time. Knowledge of the patient's racial customs and religious views will aid in the management of the pregnancy and may suggest the possibility of hereditary disorders which may be more frequent among certain races or ethnic groups.
E. Husband's age, height, weight, race, country of origin, and occupation. The physical inheritance of the father is of significance in anticipating hereditary disorders.

History of Present Pregnancy.

The patient is more concerned with the present pregnancy than with those which have occurred in the past. By taking a sincere interest in her current status, the physician can establish good rapport at the outset.

A. Symptoms, Signs, Infections, Injuries: At the initial visit the patient's complaints will probably include breast tenderness, nausea, headache, constipation, and other minor problems. She must be questioned specifically about drug ingestion and about infections and injuries in early pregnancy, as these may enable the physician to anticipate complications.

B. Menstrual History: The patient's menstrual history includes the date of onset and character of the last menstrual period (LMP), the date of the previous menstrual period (PMP), the date of quickening, if present, in relation to the LMP; calculation of the expected date of confinement (EDC); age at the menarche, average interval between periods, duration and amount of flow, pain and relation to flow, presence or absence of intermenstrual bleeding (note day of cycle), and existence of significant leukorrhea or other abnormalities. Pregnant women occasionally experience one or more episodes of painless, quasiperiodic bleeding during the months following conception. In such instances, the date of the PMP may be necessary to determine the EDC.

History of Previous Pregnancies.

For each previous pregnancy, whether completed successfully or not, the following information should be recorded:

A. Date (month and year) of termination; name of hospital and name of physician.

B. Labor:
1. Note whether spontaneous or induced and the reason for induction.
2. Note the duration of each pregnancy in comparison with its EDC. A consistent pattern of early or late delivery may be noted.
3. Length of labor - The length of previous labors is helpful in anticipating and preparing for problems of dystocia or precipitate delivery. Judgment is necessary in evaluating the patient's estimate of the actual duration of labor. Although patients' estimates are rarely accurate, one should attempt to determine the duration of "strong labor" rather than the interval between onset of contractions or admission to the hospital and delivery. Long labors may indicate dystocia (due to fetal disproportion or inadequate, uncoordinated contractions). Dystocia may recur if similar problems are present again. If previous labors have been brief or precipitate at term (3 hours or less), induction may

be indicated; this is particularly true when the patient lives far from the hospital.

C. Delivery:
1. Note method of delivery (vaginal, cesarean), presentation (vertex, breech), and whether assisted or not (forceps, version, extraction).
2. Complications of previous deliveries can often be inferred from the patient's statements regarding the perineum. "A few stitches" usually indicates a routine episiotomy or minor lacerations, and "no stitches" indicates a relaxed perineum. "Many stitches" may indicate tears which required extensive repair.
3. Anesthesia - Type used and any complications or difficulties which occurred.

D. Child at Birth:
1. The birth weights of each of the patient's children are important in determining the weight pattern, maturity, and maternal disease (e.g., diabetes). In the case of multiparas, or if the infant was delivered at home, the reported birth weight may be inaccurate.
2. Condition - A damaged ("marked") child usually implies a difficult delivery. Developmental abnormalities (especially cardiopulmonary anomalies) should be suspected if the infant's color was unusual ("blue baby").
3. Sex - If sex-linked disorders exist in previous children, the same possibility will exist for the expected infant if it is the same sex.

E. Nursing: Note whether the patient nursed any of her previous infants and for how long. Re-evaluation of previous failures may indicate whether or not the mother will nurse the expected infant.

F. Present Health of Child: Note whether the child is living and well. A stillbirth or death of a child under one year of age is significant obstetrically.

G. Note whether complications were antepartal, intrapartal, or postpartal. The occurrence of toxemia, infection, or hemorrhage should be determined and described fully. Suspect serious complications if the patient was hospitalized before the onset of labor or for more than 5 days after deliveries.

Past Medical History.

Record all important illnesses and **all** medications, allergies, drug sensitivities, and blood transfusions. Describe briefly when necessary. Fertility studies and contraceptive methods should also be noted.

Past Surgical History.

List and give the dates of all operations and serious injuries. Of particular importance are surgery or injury to the pelvis and its contents, the spine, or the abdominal wall.

If the patient has had one or more cesarean deliveries, note the type, indications, whether or not the patient had a trial of labor, and special surgical problems or postoperative complications. Such information is necessary in determining how the present fetus will be delivered.

Family History.

List medical, hereditary, psychiatric, and obstetric disorders which may affect the patient or her offspring, especially diabetes mellitus, malignancy, and cardiovascular renal disease.

History by Systems.

A careful system review often provides clues to the existence of significant diseases omitted from the past history. Symptoms or signs should be recorded in the following categories: general, dermal, head, cardiorespiratory, gastrointestinal, genitourinary, and neuromuscular.

Patient's Attitudes.

A. Nursing: If the mother has previously tried breast feeding, inquire casually about its success or failure. However, defer until the last trimester any decision about nursing the new infant. This gives the physician time to correct any misconceptions the patient may have about nursing, and if abortion should occur the emotional trauma may be minimized.

B. Anesthesia and Analgesia: Note any fear the patient may have of anesthesia in general or of specific anesthetic procedures. Attempt also to assess her pain threshold, i.e., how soon in labor she will require analgesics.

C. Emotional Balance: Estimate the patient's general emotional stability. Is she fearful or confident? Does she appear to want the baby? Note any alterations of mood at subsequent visits.

Antepartal Notes.

From the time of the initial office visit until delivery, a continuing record of the progress of the pregnancy should be maintained. Include symptoms, habits, contacts or exposures to illnesses, medications, fetal progress, laboratory studies, urinalyses, cervical and fundal changes, and initial signs, including pulse, temperature, weight, and blood pressure.

Physical Examination.

The general examination is conducted much as any other routine physical examination. It should be done carefully and thoroughly, however, since for many apparently healthy young women pregnancy represents the only occasion for a complete physical examination. Serious diseases are often first noted as a result of the physical examination during pregnancy (e.g., lymphoma, tuberculosis, breast tumors).

Pay particular attention to the following:

A. General Examination: Record the blood pressure, both systolic and diastolic, at each antenatal visit. A significantly elevated blood pressure together with excessive weight gain and proteinuria indicate the onset of toxemia. Note body build and state of nutrition. Palpate the breasts and axillas, examine the nipples, auscultate the heart and lungs, and look for hemorrhoids. The following must not be overlooked:

1. Skin and hair - Metabolic disorders such as hypothyroidism are often first manifested by dermatologic changes.
2. Teeth - Treat caries and maintain good dental hygiene throughout pregnancy.
3. Thyroid - Slight physiologic enlargement of the thyroid gland occurs in 60% of pregnant patients.
4. Abdomen - Consider especially the following:
    a. Uterine size, shape, and consistency. The height of the fundus above the symphysis should be measured carefully.
    b. Hernias - Umbilical, inguinal, femoral (and lumbar) hernias often become larger during pregnancy.
    c. Masses - Organs and tumors must be identified and described.
5. Extremities - Note development, deformity, and restriction of movement of legs, arms, and back. Varicosities and edema must be explained and treated.
6. Note posture and body mechanics.

B. Pelvic Examination: A thorough, stepwise pelvic examination can be performed at any time before term, and is most important for each new obstetric patient. Gloves and instruments must be clean but need not be sterile unless bleeding or gross infection is present or the patient is in labor.

Pay particular attention to the following:

1. Vulvar and vaginal varicosities which may bleed at delivery.
2. Cervix and uterus - Examine as described on p. 108. Near term it is essential to note the degree of effacement and dilatation of the cervix. Record the site and extent of previous lacerations of the cervix; tears may recur at these sites at delivery.
3. Pelvic masses - Distinguish between ovarian and other pelvic tumors and other retroperitoneal neoplasms and uterine bosselations. Suspected or actual cancer, severe pain, or dystocia at previous deliveries are indications for removal of certain pelvic tumors before term.

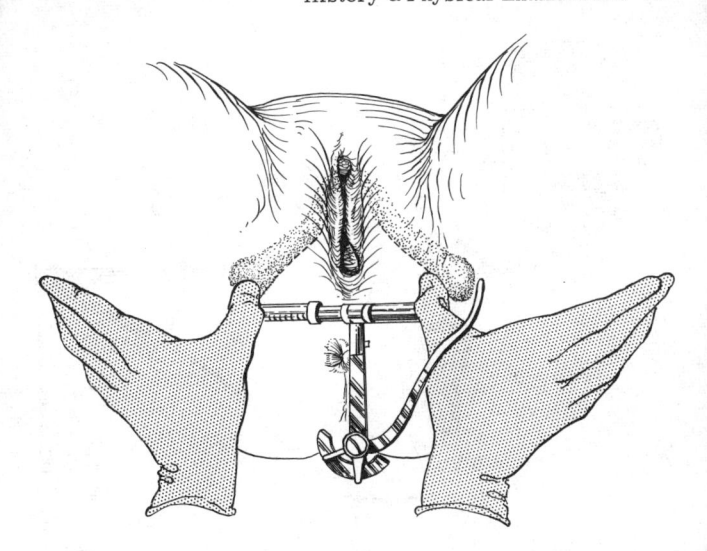

Fig 4-1. Measurement of biischial or intertuberous diameter with Thoms's pelvimeter.

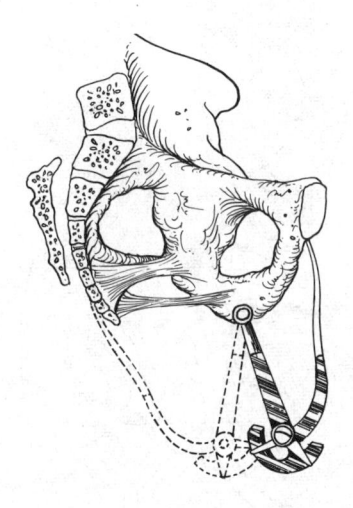

Fig 4-2. Anterior and posterior sagittal measurements with Thoms's pelvimeter.

80 History & Physical Examination

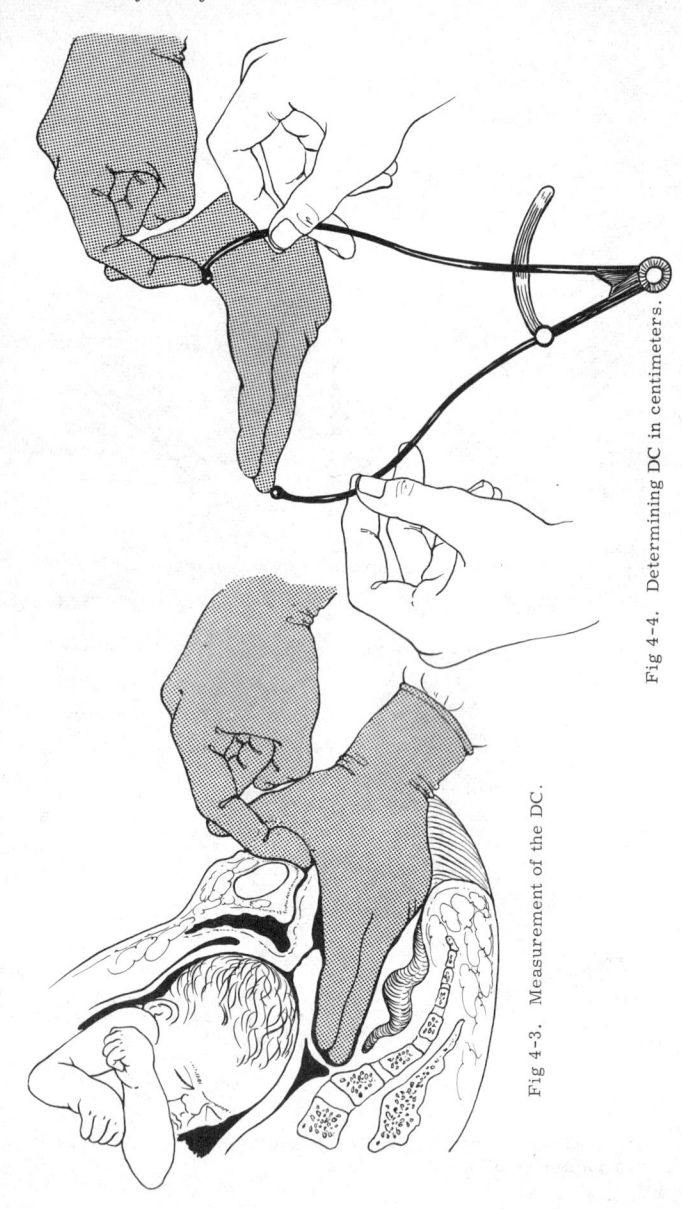

Fig 4-3. Measurement of the DC.

Fig 4-4. Determining DC in centimeters.

4. Pelvic measurements - Indirect (external) dimensions, such as the interspinal or intercristal and between the trochanters of the ilium, and Baudelocque's measurement are now regarded as misleading or of little value. Those clinical measurements which are likely to afford a reasonably good estimate of the pelvic outlet and inlet diameters are as follows:
   a. Biischial diameter (BI) or tuberischial diameter (TI) (normal: 8 cm or more) - This is measured between the tuberosities of the ischium. Thoms's and Williams' outlet pelvimeters are useful for measuring the BI with accuracy (Fig 4-1). A rough estimate of this diameter may be obtained by pressing the closed fist against the pudendum beneath the arch and comparing the known width of the fist across the knuckles with the BI.
   b. Posterior sagittal diameter of the pelvic outlet (PS) (normal: see Thoms's rule, below) - This is the distance from the midpoint of the line between the ischial tuberosities and the external surface of the tip of the sacrum. Thoms's pelvimeter measures this indirectly (Fig 4-2).

   Thoms's rule: Outlet dystocia with an average-sized baby is unlikely when the sum of the BI and the PS is more than 15 cm. The smaller the measurement, the greater the difficulty in delivery.
   c. Anteroposterior diameter of the pelvic outlet (AP) (normal: 11.9 cm or more) - This is the distance from the inferior border of the symphysis to the posterior aspect of the tip of the sacrum. A Martin or Breisky pelvimeter is generally used. This is virtually as accurate as x-ray measurement even in the moderately obese patient.

   A metal ring 8.5 cm in diameter (equivalent to the biparietal diameter of the average term infant's head) can also be fitted beneath the pelvic arch between the pelvic rami as an estimate of the available space at the pelvic outlet.
   d. Diagonal conjugate of the pelvic inlet (DC—also called the conjugata diagonalis, CD) (normal: over 11.5 cm), probably the most important single measurement of the pelvis, is a dimension measured from the inner inferior border of the symphysis to the sacral promontory (or false promontory, whichever is shorter). (Figs 4-3 and 4-4.) The true conjugate (conjugata vera, CV) is the distance from the sacral or false promontory to the inner surface of the symphysis, and is calculated to be 1.5 cm shorter than the DC; this represents the actual available anteroposterior space at the inlet. (See

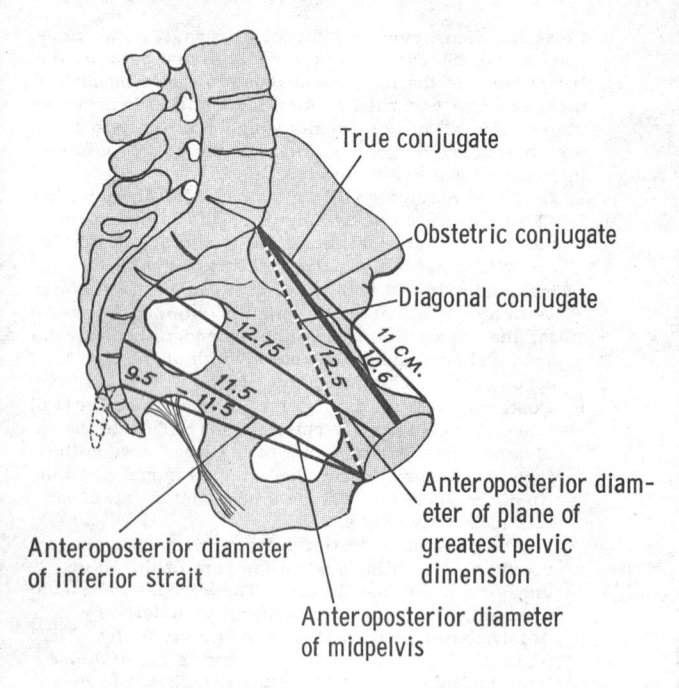

Fig 4-5. Pelvic measurements.

Fig 4-3.) Measurements of 11.5 cm or less indicate contracture of the pelvic inlet or superior strait; the likelihood of dystocia, assuming an average-sized infant, is inversely proportional to this measurement (see p. 330).
5. Palpation -
   a. Pubic arch - Trace the pubic arch with the examining fingers. Estimate the angle of the rami at the pubis: "narrow" (< 90°), "medium" (about 90°), or "wide" (> 90°).
   b. Spines of the ischium - Consider the degree of prominence, sharpness, and extent of encroachment of the spines into the birth canal.
   c. Sacrum - The contour, depth, and irregularities (e.g., bosses of rickets, false promontory) are important. Record the curvature as "hollow" (deep), "average" (normally capacious), and "flat" (shallow).

d. Coccyx - By grasping the coccyx between the fingers of the examining hand with the other hand placed in the cleft between the buttocks, the direction of the coccyx, its degree of movement at the sacrococcygeal articulation, and local tenderness may be determined.
   e. Sacrosciatic notch - The width of this space should be estimated in cm, not "fingerbreadths."
C. X-Ray Pelvimetry: (Contraindicated except in anticipation of cephalopelvic disproportion.) The measurements with average dimensions for comparison are entered. The inlet, midpelvis, and pelvic outlet are thus evaluated. The type of pelvis as well as fetal skull size, presentation, position, and relative size of the fetus are determined.

Laboratory Examinations.

The following basic laboratory tests are required for all obstetric patients as early as possible in pregnancy:
A. A serologic test for syphilis is required by all states in the USA. If positive, adequate early treatment of the mother will prevent congenital syphilis in the fetus. The traditional complement fixation (e.g., Kolmer) or precipitin (e.g., VDRL) tests are usually employed.
B. Urinalysis: A voided, first morning specimen of urine and a two-hour postprandial specimen should be tested at the second visit and every visit thereafter for protein and glucose. Instruct the patient to cleanse the urethral meatus with damp cotton and request that she obtain a "clean catch" ("midstream") specimen promptly while the urine is being passed. This prevents contamination with vaginal mucus and blood and gives almost the equivalent of a catheterized specimen.

   Should more than the faintest trace of protein or glucose be revealed, special tests for renal disease and diabetes mellitus may be required.
C. Papanicolaou Smears: See p. 495.
D. Hematologic Tests:
   1. A hematocrit, packed cell volume (PCV), or the less accurate hemoglobin (Hgb) determination is routine for the diagnosis of maternal anemia early in pregnancy. It should be repeated at about the 32nd week.
   2. White cell and differential counts are done when infection or blood dyscrasia is suspected.
   3. Blood grouping (ABO) and Rh typing of the patient and her husband are necessary in case transfusion is needed and as an indication of the possibility of erythroblastosis in the fetus.
   4. Screening tests for antibodies - See Hemantigen® Test, p. 172.

Diagnosis.

The duration of pregnancy, normal or abnormal, is entered.

Prognosis.

Record an initial prediction of the outcome of the pregnancy (vaginal or cesarean delivery) and the likelihood of medical or surgical complications (e.g., diabetes mellitus, inguinal hernia). The prognosis may have to be altered if obstetric problems develop later.

Anticipate disproportion, toxemia, and other problems which seem likely.

MANAGEMENT OF NORMAL PREGNANCY

Visits & Examinations.

Plan to see the patient in the office or clinic once a month until the 32nd week; every 2 weeks until the 36th week; and weekly thereafter until delivery, and more often if complications arise. Essential procedures at each visit are as follows:

A. Ask the patient about her general health and any complaints she may have.

B. Weigh the patient and record her weight on the prenatal chart. Evaluate weight changes in comparison with the average curve and your plan for her total gain or loss during the pregnancy.

C. Examine a urine sample for protein and glucose.

D. Record the patient's blood pressure.

E. Palpate the abdomen; measure and record the height of the rounded uterus above the symphysis and any abnormal observations.
  1. After the 20th week, estimate the presentation of the fetus and auscultate the fetal heartbeat.
  2. From the 32nd week on, record, in addition to the above, the position of the fetus, engagement of the presenting part, and the probable weight of the fetus.

F. Rectal or vaginal examinations may be done at virtually any time (in the absence of bleeding) to (1) confirm the identity of the presenting part, (2) establish its station, and (3) determine the status of the cervix. These data are most important if labor is imminent or if induction is contemplated.

G. Repeat the PCV or Hgb at about the 32nd week of pregnancy; treat anemia vigorously before term. Repeat Hemantigen® test (see p. 172) at 32-36 weeks if isoimmunization seems likely.

MINOR DISCOMFORTS OF NORMAL PREGNANCY

Backache.

Virtually all pregnant women suffer from at least minor degrees of lumbar backache during gestation. Fatigue, muscle spasm, and postural and other types of back strain, especially during the last trimester, are most often responsible. Relaxation of the pelvic joints due to the steroid sex hormones and perhaps relaxin are also responsible. Treatment is as follows:

A. Improved posture. Stress the "tall" posture, with abdomen flattened as much as possible, the pelvis tilted forward, and the buttocks "tucked under" to straighten the back.

B. Moderately vigorous daily exercises to "tone" and maintain muscle strength.

C. Heels for general wear should be of medium height to further straighten the back, particularly when flat footwear has been worn extensively.

D. A firm mattress. A sagging mattress may cause painful, prolonged flexion of the back (after exaggerated extension while erect). Bedboards between the springs and mattress often provide welcome support.

E. Local heat and light massage relax tense, taut back muscles.

F. A maternity girdle for back support may be indicated for patients with backache due to extreme lordosis or kyphoscoliosis or associated with obesity or multiple pregnancy.

G. Analgesics: Acetylsalicylic acid, 0.3-0.6 gm orally every 4 hours, will be adequate for mild distress.

H. Orthopedic evaluation is necessary when disability results from backache. Note neurologic signs and symptoms indicative of intervertebral disk syndrome or other nerve compression problems, radiculitis, and similar disorders.

Syncope & Faintness.

Syncope and faintness are most common in early pregnancy. Vasomotor instability, often associated with postural hypotension, results in transient cerebral hypoxia with pooling of blood in the legs and in the splanchnic and pelvic areas, especially after prolonged sitting or standing in a warm room. Hypoglycemia before or between meals, more common during pregnancy, may result in "lightheadedness" or even fainting.

These attacks can be prevented by avoiding inactivity and utilizing deep breathing (unless the patient shows evidence of anxiety with hyperventilation syndrome), vigorous leg motions, elastic stockings, and slow change of motion. Encourage the patient to eat 6 small meals a day rather than 3 large ones.

Stimulants (spirits of ammonia, coffee, tea, or amphetamines) are indicated for attacks due to hypotension; food for hypoglycemia.

Morning Sickness.

About half of all pregnant women complain of nausea and sometimes vomiting, often upon arising, at some time during gestation. This is most common during the first 10 weeks. About 5% of women with "morning sickness" develop intractable rejection of food and fluids (hyperemesis gravidarum; pernicious vomiting of pregnancy). Psychologic morning sickness may be due to anxieties, uncertainties, conflicts, ambivalence, or subconscious rejection of the pregnancy. Reduced gastric motility or gastroesophageal reflux are contributory factors in most cases. The roles of altered endocrine function, "metabolic shifts," and varied nutritional requirements have not been convincingly elucidated.

Explanation, sympathetic reassurance, and symptomatic relief are usually sufficient. Encourage an active, satisfying routine of life, emphasizing the advantages and happy features of pregnancy and minimizing minor vexations. Psychotherapy, often involving hypnotherapy, may be required in severe cases. Almost any form of therapy may have a favorable result on a purely psychic basis depending upon the skill and personality of the physician and the emotional status and suggestibility of the patient.

A. Diet and Vitamins: Prescribe 6 small meals a day. Nausea is more common when the stomach is empty. Advise eating dry foods which are not easily vomited. Hot cereal, bread, toast, crackers, and other foods high in carbohydrates are better tolerated. Eliminate greasy, odorous, and spiced dishes and those not ordinarily preferred by the patient. Urge the patient to drink water or other fluids between meals to avoid dehydration and acidosis, which predispose to nausea. Increase the general vitamin supplement if food intake is restricted. Vitamins are of speculative value, however, unless deficiencies have developed. Intravenous or intramuscular administration of any substance has a powerful psychologic effect.

B. Drugs: **Note:** The possibility of teratogenicity of many drugs (especially in the first trimester of pregnancy), including some antinauseants, cannot be overlooked in selecting patients for medical treatment of nausea of pregnancy and in deciding which drugs to use and in what dosages. In general, it is probably best to give medical treatment only when urgently required; to avoid new and experimental drugs and all drugs which have been suggested as potential teratogens; and to give the lowest dosage which is consistent with clinical efficacy.

   1. Antinauseants - Relief of nausea may follow administration of pyridoxine hydrochloride, 100 mg I.V. 2-3

times per week. If nausea is prolonged and severe and constitutes a serious threat to the health of the patient, promethazine (Phenergan®), meclizine (Bonine®), or a combination of meclizine with pyridoxine (Bonadoxin®), 25 mg 3 times daily before meals, may be effective. Many others are also available.
2. Sedatives - Phenobarbital, 15 mg ($1/4$ gr) orally 1-3 times during the day and 30 mg ($1/2$ gr) at bedtime, is helpful, although the patient may become so drowsy that the drug must be discontinued.
3. Stimulants such as amphetamine (e.g., Desoxyn Gradumet®) tablets, 5-10 mg orally before breakfast, often give the patient more energy and a more optimistic attitude; such preparations are particularly beneficial for mildly depressed patients with nausea.

Leukorrhea. (See also p. 451.)

A gradual increase in the amount of vaginal discharge must be expected throughout pregnancy. Augmented estrogen production increases the secretion of cervical mucus. The milky color is due to the epithelial desquamation which accompanies hypertrophy and hyperplasia of the vaginal and cervical surfaces.

Vaginal fluid is thin and nonirritating to the mucous surfaces unless infection occurs. Persistent external moisture due to mucus may cause mild pruritus, but itching is rarely severe unless trichomoniasis or fungal infection is present.

The long bacillus of Döderlein (B. vaginalis, Lactobacillus acidophilus) is normally present in large numbers in dried, stained preparations of vaginal mucus. This organism helps maintain a low pH.

Explaining the physiologic background of mucus production will reassure the patient, particularly if the advantage of the associated softening of the cervix as a prelude to delivery is stressed. Frequent bathing and thorough drying of the external parts, with application of bath powder, will reduce skin irritation due to moisture. Application of vinegar solution (white vinegar, 2-4 tbsp to one quart of water) may be soothing. A low-pressure vaginal douche (with a fountain syringe at an elevation of 18-24 inches) may be employed in troublesome cases.

Urinary Symptoms.

Urinary frequency, urgency, and stress incontinence are quite common, especially in advanced pregnancy. They are due to reduced bladder capacity and pressure of the presenting part upon the bladder.

Suspect urinary tract disease if dysuria or hematuria is reported.

88 Minor Discomforts of Normal Pregnancy

When urgency is particularly troublesome, limit caffeine, spices, and alcoholic beverages. Prescribe bladder sedative mixture:

> R̆ Tincture hyoscyamus   30
>   Potassium citrate   60
>   Water, q.s. ad   180

Give 4 ml in water orally every 4 hours as necessary. Urised® (a comparable preparation in tablet form), 1-2 tablets orally every 4 hours as necessary, may be preferred.

Heartburn.

Heartburn (pyrosis, "acid indigestion") results from gastroesophageal regurgitation. In late pregnancy this may be aggravated by displacement of the stomach and duodenum by the uterine fundus.

About 15% of all pregnant patients experience severe pyrosis (as well as nausea and vomiting) during the latter weeks of pregnancy because of diaphragmatic hiatus hernia. This develops with "tenting" of the diaphragm and flaring of the lower ribs after 7 or 8 months of pregnancy. This hernia is reduced spontaneously by parturition. Symptomatic relief, not surgery, is recommended.

Treatment is as follows:
A. Acidifying Agents: Glutamic acid hydrochloride, 0.3 gm 3 times daily before meals. (Hydrochloric acid solutions damage the teeth.)
B. Chewing gum, hot tea, and change of posture are helpful. In late pregnancy, antacids containing aluminum hydroxide gel preparations (e.g., Creamalin®, Gelusil®, Amphojel®) to reduce gastric irritation are beneficial. Avoid antacids during early pregnancy because gastric acidity is already low.

Constipation.

Bowel sluggishness is common in pregnancy. It is due to suppression of smooth muscle motility by increased steroid sex hormones, and pressure upon and displacement of the intestines by the enlarging uterus. Constipation frequently causes hemorrhoids and aggravates diverticulosis and diverticulitis.

A. General Measures: Stress good bowel habits; try for a bowel evacuation at the same time every day. The diet should consist of bulk foods, including roughage (unless contraindicated by gastrointestinal intolerance), laxative foods (citrus fruits, apples, prunes, dates, and figs), and a liberal fluid intake. Encourage exercise (walking, swimming, calisthenics).

B. Medical Treatment:
1. To soften the stool, give bulk laxatives and "smoothage" agents which are neither absorbed by nor irritating to the bowel. By accumulating fluid volume, they increase peristalsis. Dioctyl sodium sulfosuccinate (Colace®, Doxinate®) is a detergent. Psyllium hydrophilic mucilloid (Metamucil®) is hydrophilic.
2. Prescribe mild laxatives effective by stimulation of the bowel in more severe cases. These include cascara and phenolphthalein. Laxatives which increase the fluid content of the stool by osmotic means (milk of magnesia and Epsom salt) are also useful in small doses.
3. Avoid strong purgatives for fear of inducing labor. Do not prescribe mineral oil, which causes liver degeneration and prevents absorption of fat-soluble vitamins when administered in large amounts.

Hemorrhoids.

Straining at stool often causes hemorrhoids, especially in women prone to varicosities. For these reasons it is best to avoid and treat constipation early and to deliver by elective low forceps with episiotomy when feasible.

A. Medical Measures: Gently replace the hemorrhoid if this can be done easily. Warm (or cool) sitz baths or local witch hazel compresses are helpful. Soothing, astringent anal suppositories such as Anusol® or, if necessary, anesthetic ointments such as dibucaine (Nupercaine®) and cyclomethycaine (Surfacaine®) can be used for local relief of pain. If used sparingly, the following ointment is safe and most effective in relieving rectal pain:

℞ Cocaine hydrochloride	0.3 gm
Phenol	0.6 gm
Petrolatum	15 gm
Lanolin	15 gm

Apply an amount about the size of a pea to the anus 1-4 times daily as necessary.

B. Surgical Treatment:
1. Incise recently thrombosed, painful hemorrhoids under local anesthesia and evacuate the clot. Do not suture. Sitz baths, rectal ointments, suppositories, and mild laxatives are indicated postoperatively.
2. Injection treatments to obliterate hemorrhoids during pregnancy are contraindicated; they may cause infection and extensive thrombosis of the pelvic veins, and are rarely successful because of the great dilatation of many vessels.

Minor Discomforts of Normal Pregnancy

Breast Soreness.

Physiologic breast engorgement may cause discomfort, especially during early and late pregnancy. A well-fitted brassiere worn 24 hours a day affords relief. Ice packs or cold compresses are temporarily effective. Hormone therapy is contraindicated.

Headache.

Headache is most disturbing during the first and third trimesters. Emotional tension is the most common cause; consider anxiety, over-concern, uncertainty, etc, when headache is migrainous, band-type, occipital, or tends to be constant. Refractive errors and ocular imbalance are not caused by normal pregnancy. The pregnant woman is sedentary; she may read or sew more despite eyestrain. Hormonal stimulation causes vascular engorgement of the nasal turbinates, and the resultant congestion contributes to sinusitis and headache.

Severe, persistent headache in the last trimester must be regarded as symptomatic of toxemia of pregnancy unless toxemia can definitely be ruled out.

The belief that pituitary swelling during normal pregnancy causes headache is without foundation.

Treatment is as follows:
A. Discuss the patient's difficulties in an attempt to relieve her fears and resolve minor conflicts. "Work through" the major problem to a solution to relieve chronic psychogenic headache.
B. Ophthalmologic studies may reveal the need for corrective lenses for refractive error.
C. Nasopharyngeal examination may disclose abnormalities. Give phenylephrine (Neo-Synephrine®) nose drops, 0.25%, for acute nasal congestion.
D. Analgesics: Acetylsalicylic acid, 0.3-0.6 gm (5-10 gr) orally, for temporary relief.
E. Mild sedatives such as phenobarbital or meprobamate may provide temporary relief.
F. A low sodium diet (1 gm sodium/day) may be helpful.

Ankle Swelling.

Edema of the lower extremities not associated with toxemia develops in two-thirds of women in late pregnancy. Edema is due to sodium and water retention as a result of ovarian, placental, and adrenal steroid hormones; increased venous pressure in the legs, varicose veins with venous congestion, prolonged sitting or standing, and elastic garters.

Treatment is largely preventive and symptomatic, since nothing can be done about the effect of the pregnancy hormones. The patient should elevate her legs frequently and sleep in a slightly Trendelenburg position. Circular garters and clothing which interfere with venous return should not be worn.

Restrict salt intake and provide elastic support for varicose veins (see below).

Diuretics, particularly the thiazine compounds, may reduce edema considerably.

Varicose Veins.

Varicosities are usually a problem of the multipara, and may cause severe complications such as phlebothrombosis and embolism. Varices are due to congenital and acquired weakness of the vascular walls; increased venous stasis in the legs due to the hemodynamics of pregnancy; inactivity and poor muscle tone; and obesity, since the excessive tissue mass requires increased circulation and fatty infiltration of connective tissue impairs vascular support.

Although most varicose veins are asymptomatic, all are unsightly. Large or numerous varicosities cause muscle aching, edema, skin ulcers, and emboli. Venous stasis, trauma, and dermatitis contribute to phlebothrombosis and thrombophlebitis.

Phlebothrombosis is clinically silent, causing no local tenderness or swelling over the obstructed vein. Slight unexplained elevations in pulse rate and temperature are occasionally noted; fatal pulmonary emboli frequently result.

Thrombophlebitis, on the other hand, is a painful disorder, causing erythema, tenderness along the course of the involved vessels, pain in the leg, generalized enlargement of the part, tachycardia, fever, and leukocytosis. If the femoral vessels are involved, the leg may be pale, swollen, cool, and exceedingly painful, with diminution or absence of the ankle and popliteal pulses (phlegmasia alba dolens or "milk leg").

Serious phlebothrombosis and thrombophlebitis often complicate the puerperium, but they are uncommon during pregnancy. Pulmonary emboli are infrequent.

The vulvar, vaginal, and even the inguinal veins may be markedly enlarged during pregnancy. Damaged vulvovaginal vessels give rise to hemorrhage at delivery.

A. Prevention and Palliation:
   1. The patient should be instructed to exercise, rest in the recumbent position, elevate her legs above the level of her body, wear loose clothing, and control weight gain. Avoid vigorous massage and point-pressure over the legs.
   2. Fit elastic "stretch" stockings to patients with significant varices in the lower legs. Complete elastic leg hose are impractical. Cotton stockings are cooler and more absorptive than nylon hose.

      Have the patient lie flat with one leg raised for a few minutes to empty the veins, then roll the elastic

stocking on from the toe with the leg still elevated. Stockings should be worn at all times while the patient is up, but can be removed for 30 minutes several times each day during rest periods. In severe cases, elastic hose may even be worn during sleep.
  3. Large vulvar varices cause pudendal discomfort. A vulvar pad wrapped in plastic film, snugly held by a menstrual pad, belt, or T-binder, gives relief.

B. Definitive Therapy:
  1. Injection treatment of even small varicose veins during pregnancy is futile and hazardous.
  2. Ligation of veins is recommended only to prevent repeated emboli or thrombosis of a large venous system. Phlebothrombosis can rarely be treated surgically because it is almost impossible to diagnose until emboli occur. In severe pelvic thrombophlebitis, ligation of the vena cava and the ovarian vessels may be life-saving when septic emboli are dislodged.
  3. In severe thrombophlebitis, sympathetic nerve block by paravertebral or caudal injection of anesthetic improves the collateral circulation, relieves pain, and speeds healing. (Nerve block is contraindicated in patients taking anticoagulants since it may cause bleeding at the site of injection.)
  4. Require complete bed rest for thrombophlebitis. Elevate both legs even though only one extremity is apparently involved, since the other may also be affected. Apply a heat cradle; administer broad-spectrum antibiotics.
  5. Anticoagulants may be required in acute thrombophlebitis. Heparin is preferred to bishydroxycoumarin since it does not cause fetal damage, is more easily controlled, and is not excreted in the milk. However, neither drug, whether administered before or during labor, causes increased bleeding from the uterus; efficient mechanical compression of the myometrial vessels prevents excessive blood loss despite increased blood coagulation time. Cervical, vaginal, and perineal lacerations may bleed more briskly if the patient has received heparin or bishydroxycoumarin.
  6. Anticoagulant therapy is prophylactic for phlebothrombosis but is often therapeutic in thrombophlebitis.
  7. Heparin may be administered in doses of 0.5-0.75 mg /kg I.V. at intervals of 4 hours. A continuous drip is feasible, but cumulative effects occur easily. Depo-Heparin® is easier to administer: an initial dose of 200 mg subcut. or I.M. is repeated every 12 hours for at least 3 doses. The coagulation time should be held at about 15-20 minutes. Relief of pain indicates the end of the acute phase, whereupon 200 mg subcut.

or I.M. daily is generally adequate until recovery is complete.

Protamine sulfate I.V. is an almost immediate antagonist to heparin when abnormal bleeding occurs. Dilute 1% protamine sulfate with isotonic sodium chloride for slow administration. Give mg for mg heparin administered within the last 4 hours. Do not give more than 50 mg initially. Check coagulation time repeatedly.

8. The pregnant woman with probable phlebothrombosis or clinical thrombophlebitis may be given bishydroxycoumarin (Dicumarol®), 200-300 mg orally after delivery, assuming an initially normal prothrombin time. Bishydroxycoumarin need not be repeated until the second or third day. Prothrombin times should be determined daily and the level maintained at 20% of normal. As a rule, 200 mg will suffice for the second dose. Subsequent doses are gauged by laboratory control, but range from 25-75 mg. Re-evaluate the clinical circumstances after one week to determine whether the drug should be continued or not. The effect of bishydroxycoumarin is counteracted by the I.V. administration of phytonadione, 5 mg/kg.

Leg Cramps.

Cramping or "knotting" of the muscles of the calf, thigh, or buttocks occurs suddenly after sleep or recumbency in many women after the first trimester of pregnancy. For unknown reasons it is less common during the month before term. Sudden shortening of the leg muscles by "stretching" with the toes pointed precipitates the cramp. It is believed that one of the factors causing cramps is a reduced level of diffusible serum calcium or a relatively increased serum phosphorus. This follows excessive dietary intake of phosphorus in milk, cheese, meat, or dicalcium phosphate, or diminished intake or impaired absorption of calcium. Fatigue in the extremities is a contributing factor.

A. Immediate Treatment: Require the patient to stand barefooted on a cold surface (e.g., a tiled bathroom floor) and rub and "knead" the contracted, painful muscle. The husband should passively flex the foot to lengthen the calf muscles. Local heat is an effective palliative measure.

B. Preventive:
  1. Reduce dietary phosphorus intake temporarily by limiting meat to one serving daily and milk to one pint daily. Discontinue dicalcium phosphate and other medications containing large amounts of phosphorus.
  2. Eliminate excess phosphorus by absorption with aluminum hydroxide gel (Creamalin® or Amphojel®), 0.5-1 gm orally, in liquid or tablet form with each meal.

94 Minor Discomforts of Normal Pregnancy

    3. Increase calcium intake. Administer calcium lactate, 0.6 gm, or an equivalent, orally 3 times daily before meals. Even larger doses may be required because of limited absorption of calcium from the intestinal tract in some patients.
    4. Avoid walking with the toes pointed. ("Lead with the heel.")

Abdominal Pain.

Intra-abdominal alterations causing pain during the course of pregnancy include the following.
  A. Pressure: Pelvic heaviness, a sense of sagging or dragging, is caused by the weight of the uterus on the pelvic supports and the abdominal wall. Treatment consists of frequent rest periods in the supine or lateral recumbent position, and a maternity girdle.
  B. Round Ligament Tension: Tenderness along the course of the round ligament (usually the left) during late pregnancy is due to traction on this structure by the uterus with rotation of the uterus and change of the patient's position. Local heat and other measures as for pressure pain (see above) are effective.
  C. Flatulence, Distention, Bowel Cramping: Large meals, fats, gas-forming foods, and chilled beverages are poorly tolerated by pregnant women. Mechanical displacement and compression of the bowel by the enlarged uterus, hypotonia of the intestines, and constipation predispose to gastrointestinal distress. Dietary modifications give effective relief. Regular bowel function should be maintained, using mild laxatives when indicated. Exercise and frequent change of position are also of value.
  D. Uterine Contractions: So-called Braxton Hicks contractions of the uterus may be strong, sharp, and startling for some patients. The onset of premature labor must always be considered when forceful contractions develop. If they remain infrequent and brief in duration, the danger of early delivery is not significant. Phenobarbital, 30-60 mg orally 2-4 times daily; or sedatives such as meprobamate (Equanil®, Miltown®), 200 mg orally 1-3 times daily; or acetylsalicylic acid, 0.3-0.6 gm (5-10 gr) 2-3 times daily, may be of value. Codeine, 30-60 mg (1/2-1 gr), is rarely required.
  E. Intra-abdominal Disorders: Pain due to obstruction, inflammation, and other disorders of the gastrointestinal, urinary, neurologic, or vascular system must be diagnosed and treated specifically.
  F. Uterine or Adnexal Disease: Pain due to pathologic pregnancy and tubal or ovarian disease must be treated appropriately.

Fatigue.
The pregnant patient is more subject to fatigue during the last trimester of pregnancy because of altered posture and extra weight. Anemia and other systemic diseases must be ruled out. Frequent rest periods are recommended.

THE NEW OBSTETRIC PATIENT

Communication, understanding, and rapport between the patient and her physician are vital to good prenatal care. He must explain what is required of her during pregnancy and why her full cooperation is necessary.

Explanatory books or short reviews of obstetrics for the layman are available through most bookstores.

PROCEDURE AT THE INITIAL VISIT

After the history has been taken, the physical examination performed, and blood specimens obtained:

1. Request the patient to bring a first-voided urine specimen at each subsequent visit.
2. Supply her with written prenatal care instructions and a booklet or library reference. Ask the patient and her husband to read them carefully before the next visit.
3. Order a chest x-ray.
4. Prescribe a vitamin-mineral supplement and other necessary medications.
5. Instruct the patient regarding the date and time of her return visit.
6. Answer questions and explain the cost of obstetric care.
7. Order laboratory studies (see pp. 83, 84).

DIET & WEIGHT CONTROL

Diet is probably the most important single detail of antepartal care; nutritional deficiencies and excesses have significant implications for toxemia of pregnancy, postpartal hemorrhage, anemia, fetal abnormalities, and other complications.

Dietary Requirements During Pregnancy. (See Table 4-1.)
Certain minimal dietary requirements during gestation and lactation are well established; others must still be estimated.

Many women will overeat during pregnancy and require dietary restriction; some prefer or must accept a poorly balanced, partially deficient diet; others suffer from general dietary deprivation. It is not necessary for the pregnant woman to "eat for two."

Assuming that properly prepared fresh foods in adequate quantities are available and that dietary aversions and food faddism do not interfere, most healthy pregnant women will not need vitamin or mineral supplements. Poverty, social mores, cravings, unfavorable climate, and maternal disease affect so many women during pregnancy, however, that vitamin and mineral supplements are given to most obstetric patients to make certain that fetal and maternal deficiencies do not develop. If provided in half the daily requirement, a vitamin-mineral preparation may be most valuable and is never harmful. If the doctor stresses a high-protein, high-vitamin diet, caloric restriction (or increase) can be varied appropriately.

Although ample calcium and phosphorus are required by the mother for fetal anabolism, a relative excess of phosphorus may cause leg cramps. Large quantities of milk, meat, and dicalcium phosphate (taken as a supplement) provide too much phosphorus. Meat and milk are excellent sources of protein, however, and should not be drastically curtailed.

Milk is relatively inexpensive and contains 33 gm of protein per quart; therefore, prescribe one quart of milk per day. Skimmed or dried milk or buttermilk is best, especially when the cream content should be restricted for weight control. The milk need not always be in the form of a beverage but can be used in the preparation of food such as custard, junket, and soup. Low sodium milk (Lonalac®) may be prescribed when sodium restriction is necessary.

Most of the sodium in food is in table salt, although baking soda (bicarbonate of soda) also contains large quantities of sodium. The daily sodium chloride intake of an average woman in the USA is 3-7 gm. The type of food and individual preferences and habits determine the salt intake. In order to help avoid edema and eclamptogenic toxemia, sodium intake should be reduced during pregnancy to 0.8-1.5 gm (2-4 gm sodium chloride)/day.

Foods containing considerable salt (either naturally or to improve the taste or for preservation) include the following:
  All seafoods, meat, milk, processed cheese.
  Most frozen and canned vegetables—especially beets, carrots, celery, chard, kale, spinach.
  Yeast breads, crackers, potato chips.
  Butter, peanut butter, margarine.
  Pickles, catsup, other condiments.

Foods which are low in sodium content include the following:

Meat, fish, poultry (fresh or frozen, 3-4 oz/day): Lean beef, lamb, pork, veal, chicken, turkey, duck; fresh-water fish prepared without salt.

Eggs: One per day, poached or soft-boiled.

Vegetables (fresh only): Asparagus, beans, broccoli, cabbage, carrots, corn, cucumbers, leeks, lettuce, mushrooms, onions, peas, pumpkin, potatoes, turnips.

Cereal products: Barley, Cream of Wheat®, farina, macaroni, spaghetti, rice (plain or puffed), wheat (plain or puffed).

Bread: Specially prepared salt-free bread or rolls.

Dairy products: Sweet unsalted butter, cottage cheese (1 oz/day), cream (1 oz/day), Lonalac® (low-salt processed milk).

Table 4-1. Basic food requirements in pregnancy and lactation.

	Pregnancy	Lactation
Milk	1 pint	1 quart
Citrus fruit or tomato	1 serving	2 servings
Lean meat, fish, poultry, eggs, beans, cheese	1 serving	1 serving
Leafy green vegetables	1 serving	1 serving
Yellow vegetables	1 serving	1 serving

Skimmed milk or buttermilk is preferred in order to avoid unnecessary butterfat. Salty foods should be avoided. Entrees, vegetables, and fruits can be substituted freely (poultry for beef, etc). Butter and oils should be used sparingly; gravies and marinated foods should be avoided. Portions should be of average size, and between-meal snacks should not be permitted. (The patient may save food from one meal to be eaten between meals if desired.)

Block or processed commercial cheese should be limited to occasional small servings to prevent excess intake of sodium ion, phosphate radical, and butterfat. A calcium supplement (calcium lactate, carbonate, or gluconate), 1-2 tsp 3 times daily, is most desirable. (Dicalcium phosphate is poorly absorbed.)

Weight Control.

A. Significant Data Regarding Weight Gain During Pregnancy:
  1. A gain of 16-18 lb during normal gestation will permit a return to previous weight. With dietary supervision (control of caloric intake; additional protein, vitamins, and minerals), lactation can proceed successfully without maternal gain or loss of weight.

  If the patient is below her calculated ideal weight at the beginning of pregnancy, she should gain 16-18 lb plus the difference between initial weight and ideal weight. Women who are more than 20% under their calculated ideal weight for height and age are more likely to develop toxemia of pregnancy; urge such patients to make up much of their discrepancy during the first trimester and gradually limit their weight gain later in pregnancy.

If the patient is over her calculated ideal weight at the beginning of pregnancy, she should gain 16-18 lb minus the difference between initial weight and ideal weight. Patients who are overweight at the start of pregnancy are also more likely to develop toxemia. The incidence of toxemia among women who gain 25 lb more than their ideal calculated weight gain during pregnancy is about five times as high as in other women.

2. The rate of weight gain plays an important role in the development of toxemia. An increase of more than 4 lb/month in any 2 consecutive months will often be followed by toxemia.

Excess weight gain after midpregnancy is more likely to be followed by toxemia than weight gain which occurs early. Ideally, the average patient should gain approximately as follows:

1st trimester: about 3 lb (1 lb/month)
2nd trimester: about 9 lb (0.8 lb/week)
3rd trimester: about 5 lb (0.4 lb/week)

3. When weight gain is excessive, the likelihood of toxemia will be reduced by weight reduction through diet and the use of diuretics. Weight loss after excessive, abrupt gain usually represents edema. The weight loss should be pushed to a point well below the normal for that patient in the third trimester.

4. Excessive weight gain due to sodium and water retention is the most important single factor in predisposition to toxemia, but caloric weight also contributes to the incidence of toxemia. Since up to 10% of body weight in the form of retained fluids may be gained before peripheral edema can be demonstrated, the patient's weight and blood pressure must be checked carefully and repeatedly during pregnancy.

B. Methods of Weight Control:

1. Limitation of sodium intake - Table salt, bicarbonate of soda, and foods to which salt is added should be restricted during early pregnancy and curtailed severely after midpregnancy. A list of prohibited foods and beverages should be provided. If the choice of diet is otherwise free, sodium depletion is not likely to occur. Foods which are high in sodium are listed on p. 96.

2. Diuresis - For patients who gain weight abruptly or demonstrate generalized edema and those who report an excessive sodium intake, hydrochlorothiazide (Hydro-Diuril®) (or equivalent), 50 mg orally every other day upon arising, may be necessary. Allow a select diet, excluding only table salt and obviously salty foods. The chlorothiazides can be given in this manner for weeks, but not to diabetic women. The urine should be checked for glycosuria at regular intervals. With such a program, the low salt syndrome and potassium depletion almost never occur.
3. Adjustment of caloric intake - The normal weight gain during pregnancy is discussed above. Increase or decrease in weight can be achieved by varying the fats (9 Cal/gm) and carbohydrates (4 Cal/gm) in the diet. Many women have the misconception that they need only "cut out bread and potatoes" (starches). Others go on "crash" diets, subsisting on bananas and milk or other extremely deficient diets. Protein intake should remain above 85 gm/day, and a balanced diet is essential.
4. Dietary restriction by amphetamines[*] - The patient's motivation and determination must be mobilized in weight reduction regimens. Emotionally determined "hunger," peculiar food cravings, and the mistaken belief that a pregnant woman should "eat for two" require re-education and, occasionally, psychotherapy. Patients who become depressed while dieting need frequent encouragement. Although will power cannot be purchased in the pharmacy, amphetamines may help such patients by improving the mood while suppressing appetite. Dextro amphetamine sulfate (Dexedrine®), 2.5-5 mg orally one hour before meals, is helpful. If the patient becomes tense and is unable to sleep after taking this preparation, a mild sedative with dextro amphetamine sulfate, e.g., Dexamyl®, 5 mg 3 times daily orally well before the next meal, may be given.

    Methylcellulose, 200 mg taken with water 30-60 minutes before meals, develops a soft bulk in the stomach and so reduces appetite. Obocell®, a preparation of methylcellulose, methapyrilene, and dextro amphetamine sulfate, one tablet before meals, may be effective.
5. Hospitalization - In occasional cases a patient who is unable to control her weight at home must be admitted to the hospital for dietary assistance and treatment, particularly when toxemia or gastrointestinal diffi-

---

[*]See cautionary remarks on drug use in pregnancy on p. 86.

culties are imminent or clinically evident.
6. Fluids - At least 2-3 quarts of fluid per day should be taken during pregnancy to accommodate metabolic processes and to aid in elimination. This should normally include one quart of milk. Limitation of fluid will neither prevent nor correct fluid retention. Liquids containing no sodium will not contribute to edema in the absence of renal failure. Actually, increased intake of water aids slightly in the excretion of sodium.

Table 4-2. Recommended daily dietary allowances for nonpregnant, pregnant, and lactating women.*

	Nonpregnant	Pregnant	Lactating
Calories	2000	2200	3000
Protein	58 gm	78 gm	98 gm
Minerals†			
Calcium	0.8 gm	1.3 gm	1.3 gm
Iron	15 mg	20 mg	20 mg
Sodium	0.3 gm	0.2 gm	0.3 gm
Phosphorus	1-2 gm	2 gm	2.5 gm
Vitamins‡			
A	5000 I.U.	6000 I.U.	8000 I.U.
B_1 (thiamine)	0.8 mg	1 mg	1.2 mg
B_2 (riboflavin)	1.3 mg	1.6 mg	1.9 mg
B_6 (pyridoxine)	6 mg	8 mg	8 mg
C (ascorbic acid)	70 mg	100 mg	100 mg
D	—	400 I.U.	400 I.U.
Folic acid	1-2 mg	2 mg	2 mg
K (as menadione)	1-2 mg	2 mg	2 mg
Niacin (nicotinic acid)	14 mg	17 mg	21 mg

*Modified from Publication 589, National Academy of Sciences—National Research Council, 1963. Values for pregnancy are for the second and third trimesters; values for lactating women are based on the production of 850 ml of milk daily. **Note:** The caloric requirements listed are for an active woman 25 years old, 5 ft 4 in tall, weighing 128 lb. For many obstetric patients they will be too high and should be adjusted downward on an individual basis.

†The usual prescription vitamin-mineral mixture contains also iodine, manganese, magnesium, copper, molybdenum, zinc, and cobalt. Evidence for requirements of these minerals is equivocal.

‡The usual prescription vitamin-mineral mixture contains also vitamins B_{12} and E and pantothenic acid. Evidence for requirements of these vitamins is equivocal.

DENTAL CARE

The patient may neglect oral hygiene during early pregnancy, when nausea may be troublesome. Hormonal hypertrophy and turgescence of the gums (epulis of pregnancy) do permit irritation and infection of the gingivae, and alteration in food choices and variations in salivary pH during pregnancy may lead to dental caries. Nevertheless, even despite gross dietary calcium deficiency, decalcification of the mother's teeth does not occur as a result of pregnancy and there is no reason why dental care should be neglected. "For every child a tooth" is an old saying that has no basis in fact.

Dental anesthesia, repair, and extraction are rarely contraindicated during pregnancy. Abortion or premature labor and delivery are not caused even by extensive dental surgery. Septicemia as a sequel to dental abscesses may complicate maternal cardiovascular or renal disease; antibiotics should be administered prophylactically in such diseases.

TRAVEL

The pregnant woman should avoid long and arduous travel. If a long journey is essential, air travel is best. All commercial aircraft are now pressurized, so that even high-altitude flights are safe for the pregnant patient. Nevertheless, most airlines will not permit women to fly during the last month of pregnancy.

Travel will not cause abortion or premature labor, but the pregnant woman is jeopardized indirectly by travel in the following ways: (1) The patient may be far from competent medical care in the case of obstetric emergency. (2) Fatigue, overexertion, tension, and anxiety may be harmful. (3) Dietary control and regular personal habits are not easily maintained. (4) The patient is exposed to the risk of accident.

INTERCOURSE & VAGINAL HYGIENE

Coitus and douches very rarely contribute to spontaneous abortion and premature labor. However, intercourse and vaginal irrigation should be avoided during the first month by women who are habitual aborters. Forceful douches, especially with a hand bulb syringe, may produce air or fluid embolism. Tub baths, even late in pregnancy, probably are not a source of infection; fluid will not enter the vagina unless it is under increased pressure.

NURSING

Most women who breast feed their babies successfully do so naturally without preparation. The advantages of nursing should nevertheless be explained to the obstetric patient, and the final decision on whether or not to breast feed the baby should be reserved until the last trimester. Aversion and unwarranted objections may be dispelled, particularly if good doctor-patient rapport is established. If and when the patient decides to nurse, institute predelivery breast and nipple care (see pp. 90 and 205).

SMOKING

Smoking in moderation (less than one-half pack of cigarettes per day) does not appear to be harmful to the pregnancy. Insist upon further limitation or complete avoidance of smoking, however, when chronic respiratory irritation, asthma, or persistent indigestion are related to smoking. Multiparas who are moderate to heavy smokers bear an increased number of low birthweight infants. Although smaller, these neonates are not necessarily premature. Moreover, they seem to survive and flourish just as well as heavier controls. Lactation is not affected by smoking, nor is the nursing infant apparently harmed by limited smoking by the mother.

DRINKING

An occasional alcoholic beverage—e.g., one cocktail a day before dinner—may be permitted most pregnant patients. If weight reduction is a problem, however, it must be remembered that alcohol stimulates appetite and is itself a significant source of calories: there are 75-80 Calories in each cocktail or highball; 125-150 Calories per bottle of beer; and about 50 Calories per ounce of fortified or sweet dessert wines.

MEDICATIONS

In view of recent reports of teratogenesis referable to administration in early pregnancy of many drugs previously considered benign, it is probably wise to discourage the administration of drugs to pregnant women as much as possible. In general, give drugs only when urgently required; avoid new and experimental drugs and all drugs which have been suggested as possible teratogens; and give drugs, when needed, in the lowest dosage which is consistent with clinical efficacy.

Record **all** drugs taken by the patient during pregnancy, and caution her about taking any drug without first discussing it with her physician.

Most drugs taken regularly before pregnancy (thyroid, aspirin, laxatives) may be continued during pregnancy on approval of the obstetrician (but see above). It may be necessary, however, to vary the medication or dosage appropriately as pregnancy progresses.

A list of drugs with proved ill effects upon the fetus may be found on pp. 696-7.

EMPLOYMENT

Many expectant mothers can continue full or part-time employment during pregnancy. How long the pregnant woman may remain on the job safely depends upon her type of work, industrial hazards, the policy of the employer, and pregnancy complications. Sedentary workers may often work through the 28th week of pregnancy. Other more active employees may find it advisable to terminate their duties earlier. Rest periods during the day should be utilized to avoid undue fatigue.

THE FIGURE

Pregnancy need not "ruin" the figure. Excessive weight gain, change in body habitus, altered posture, and breast enlargement are temporary. Attention to personal appearance, avoidance of excessive weight gain, continued daily exercise, and a well-fitted brassiere worn much of the time will help to preserve the figure. Some loss of abdominal tone is inevitable, however, and the healthiest attitude is simply to minimize and accept it temporarily, with restoration planned postpartum (see pp. 195-201).

DANGER SIGNALS

Require the patient to report promptly any vaginal bleeding, abdominal or pelvic pain, fever, generalized swelling, blurred vision, markedly reduced urine output, escape of considerable fluid from the vagina, or other disturbing problems.

INSTRUCTIONS REGARDING ONSET OF LABOR

Nulliparas in particular are anxious about how to recognize the onset of labor so that they can get to the hospital in time. Explain the usual symptomatology.

5...
Course & Conduct of Normal Labor & Delivery

Labor is the process by which the products of conception are normally delivered. It requires a coordinated, effective sequence of involuntary uterine contractions, which are usually augmented by voluntary contractions of the abdominal muscles. Labor may begin at any time during pregnancy, but the likelihood increases as full term approaches. Endocrine alterations are partially responsible for its onset and probably for its maintenance. **True labor**, under normal conditions, implies dilatation of the cervix and proceeds in a definite sequence to recovery of the placenta. **False labor**, very common in late pregnancy, is characterized by irregular, brief contractions accompanied by a mild aching sensation confined to the lower abdomen. No change in the character of the cervix occurs, and the presenting part does not descend. False labor has no significance except as a frequent cause of premature admission to the hospital.

The beginning of true labor is marked by regular uterine contractions (pains) which become increasingly more frequent, more forceful, and more prolonged with the passage of time.

The patient is usually aware of the contractions during the first stage. The severity of pain depends upon the fetopelvic relationships, the quality and strength of uterine contractions, and the emotional and physical status of the patient. Very few women experience no discomfort during the first stage of labor. With the beginning of true normal labor, some women describe slight low back pain which radiates around to the lower abdomen. Each contraction starts with a gradual build-up of intensity, and rather prompt dissipation follows the climax. Normally, the contraction will be at its height well before discomfort is reported. Dilatation of the lower birth canal and distention of the perineum during the second stage of labor will almost always cause distress.

The tocograph, tocodynamometer, and pressure recordings using multiple intramyometrial microballoons will reveal contraction patterns typical of normal labor, but these are research procedures.

The fetal membranes, a protective barrier against infection, rupture before the onset of labor in about 10% of cases (premature rupture of the membranes). At full term, 9 pregnant women out of 10 will be in labor within 24 hours after rupture of the membranes. If labor does not begin within 24 hours after rupture, the case must be considered to be complicated by premature prolonged rupture of the membranes.

In rare instances, actual leakage of fluid ceases in premature rupture or premature prolonged rupture of the membranes, presumably as a result of sealing off of a small "high leak" in the membranes. More often, however, drainage ceases because the presenting part descends to obstruct the free egress of amniotic fluid.

Just before the beginning of labor, a small amount of red-tinged mucus may be passed ("bloody show"). This is a plug of cervical mucus mixed with blood, and is evidence of cervical dilatation and effacement and, frequently, descent of the presenting part.

THE COURSE OF NORMAL LABOR

There are 3 stages of labor: (1) The period from the onset of labor to full dilatation of the cervix; (2) the period from full dilatation of the cervix to the delivery of the fetus; and (3) the period from delivery to the recovery of the placenta. The hour immediately after the birth of the placenta, during which time the danger of postpartal hemorrhage is great, is often referred to as the 4th stage of labor; it will be considered here as part of the third stage.

The onset of the first stage begins with demonstrable, progressive dilatation and effacement of the cervix (see Figs 5-1 and 5-2). It is often difficult to determine the exact time of onset since the cervix may change so slowly (or so rapidly) that only an estimate of the time of onset is possible even when frequent vaginal examinations are done by an experienced physician.

The **first stage** of labor ends with complete (10 cm) dilatation of the cervix. This stage is by far the longest. The average duration of the first stage is about 15 hours for the primigravida and about 8 hours for the multipara. However, the first stage of labor may be less than one hour or more than 24 hours depending upon (1) parity of the patient, (2) the frequency, intensity, and duration of uterine contractions, (3) the ability of the cervix to dilate and efface, (4) fetopelvic diameters, and (5) the presentation and position of the fetus.

The **second stage** of labor begins when the cervix becomes fully dilated and ends with the complete birth of the baby. The second stage varies from a few minutes to several hours, depending upon (1) fetal presentation and position, (2) fetopelvic relationships, (3) resistance of maternal pelvic soft parts, (4) the frequency, intensity, duration, and regular-

106 Course of Normal Labor

Fig 5-2. Dilatation and effacement of the cervix in a primipara.

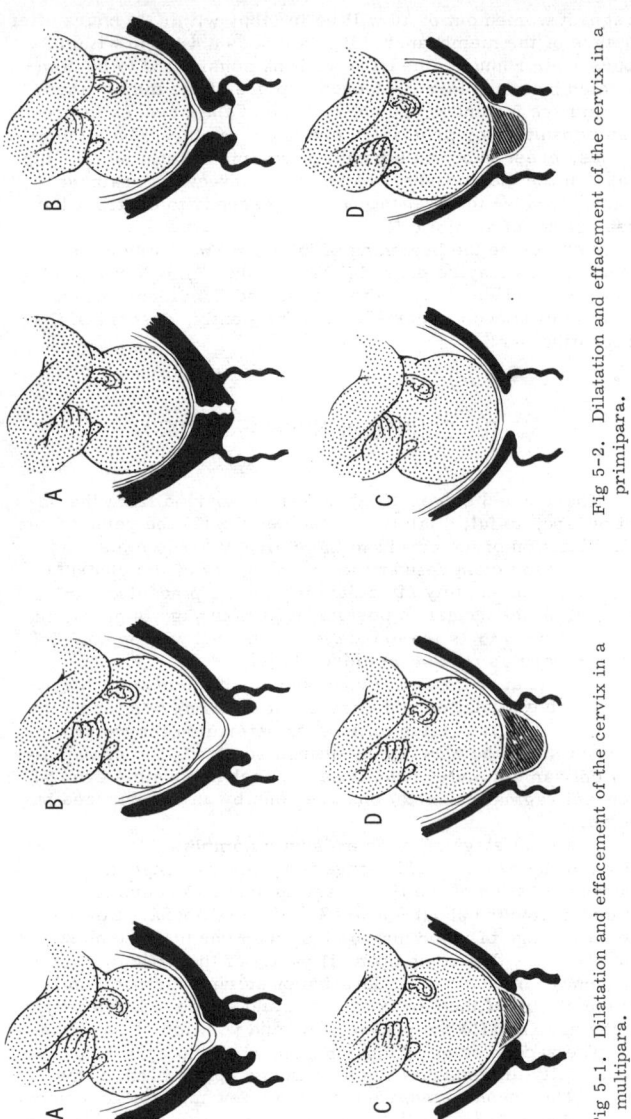

Fig 5-1. Dilatation and effacement of the cervix in a multipara.

Course of Normal Labor 107

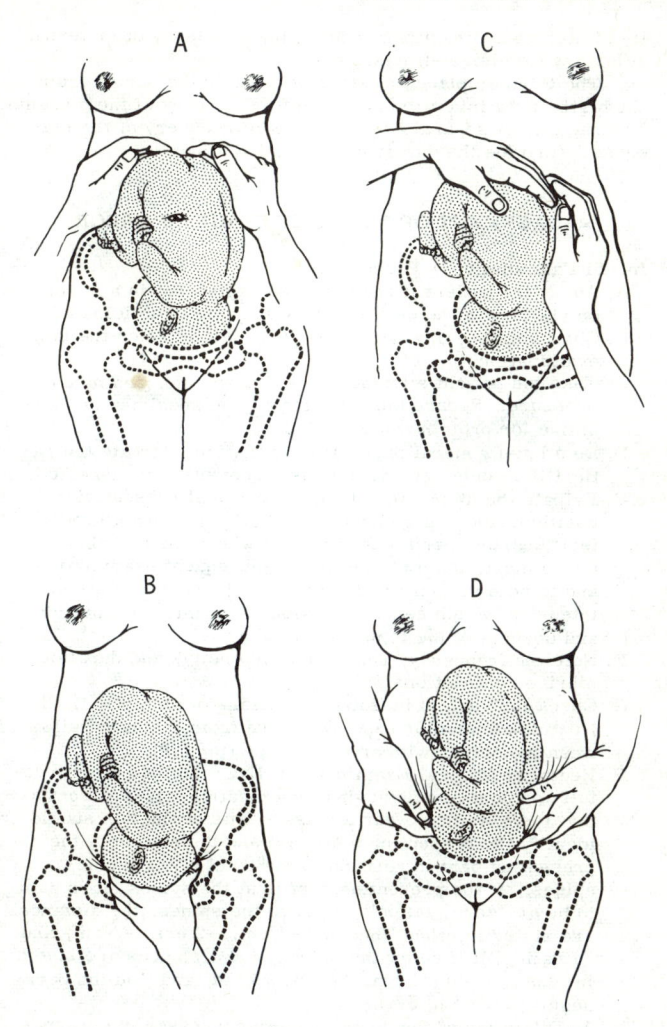

Fig 5-3. Determining fetal presentation (A, C), position (B), and engagement (D). (The 4 maneuvers of Leopold.)

108 First Stage of Labor

ity of uterine contractions, and (5) the efficiency of maternal voluntary expulsive efforts.

The **third or placental stage** of labor is the period from the birth of the infant to one hour after delivery of the placenta. The rapidity of separation and means of recovery of the placenta determine the duration of the third stage.

MANAGEMENT OF THE FIRST STAGE OF LABOR

Initial Examination & Procedures.
- A. Admit the patient if she has been registered in a hospital, or visit her at home if delivery at home is anticipated.
- B. Obtain history of relevant medical details since the last examination.
- C. Take the patient's temperature, pulse rate, and blood pressure. Secure a clean-catch urine specimen and examine for protein and glucose.
- D. Do a brief general physical examination. Isolate the patient if a contagious disease is discovered or suspected.
- E. Palpate the uterus to determine the fetal presentation, position, and engagement (see Fig 5-3). Auscultate the fetal heartbeat and mark the skin where the heartbeat is heard most clearly to facilitate subsequent examination and to note the shift and descent of the point of maximal intensity, which serves as evidence of internal rotation and descent of the fetus during labor.
- F. Note the frequency, regularity, intensity, and duration of uterine contractions.
- G. Check for vaginal bleeding or leakage of amniotic fluid. Nitrazine indicator paper will turn from green to yellow when moistened with amniotic fluid (pH 7.0).
- H. Rectal or Vaginal Examination: Examine the patient rectally or do a sterile vaginal examination. It is essential that the examiner wear a mask. This evaluation should identify the presenting fetal part and the station of the presenting part in relation to the level of the ischial spines. If the presenting part is at the spines, it is said to be at "zero station"; if above the spines, the distances are stated in minus figures (-1 cm, -2 cm, -3 cm, and "floating"); if below the spines, the distances are stated in plus figures (+1 cm, +2 cm, +3 cm, and "on the perineum") (see Fig 5-4).
    1. Dilatation of the cervical os is expressed in cm, indicating the diameter of the cervical opening. Ten cm constitutes full dilatation. A diameter of 6 cm or less can be measured directly; when the distance is more than 6 cm, however, it is often easier to subtract twice the width of the remaining "rim" from 10 cm. For example, if a 1 cm rim is felt anteriorly, posteriorly, and laterally, this indicates 8 cm dilatation.

First Stage of Labor 109

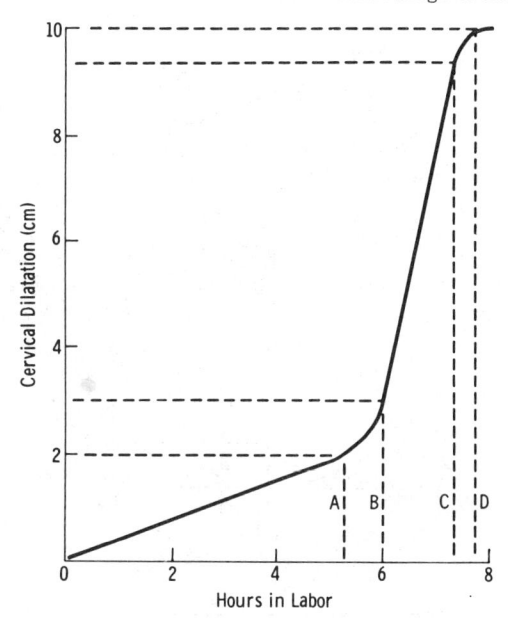

Mean Multiparous Labor Curve Based on the Study of Cervical Dilatation Time Relationships in a Group of 500 Multiparas. (A) Latent phase. (B) Acceleration phase. (C) Phase of maximum slope. (D) Deceleration phase. Curves (B) through (D) represent the active phase. (Redrawn and reproduced, with permission, from Friedman: Obstetrics and Gynecology **8**:691, 1956.)

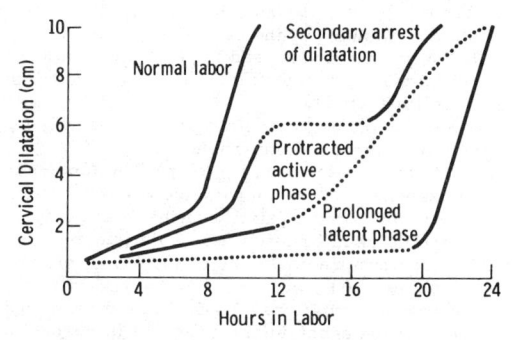

Three Major Aberrations May Be Detected by Comparing Progress of Dilatation With Normal Curve. (Courtesy of Wallace Laboratories.)

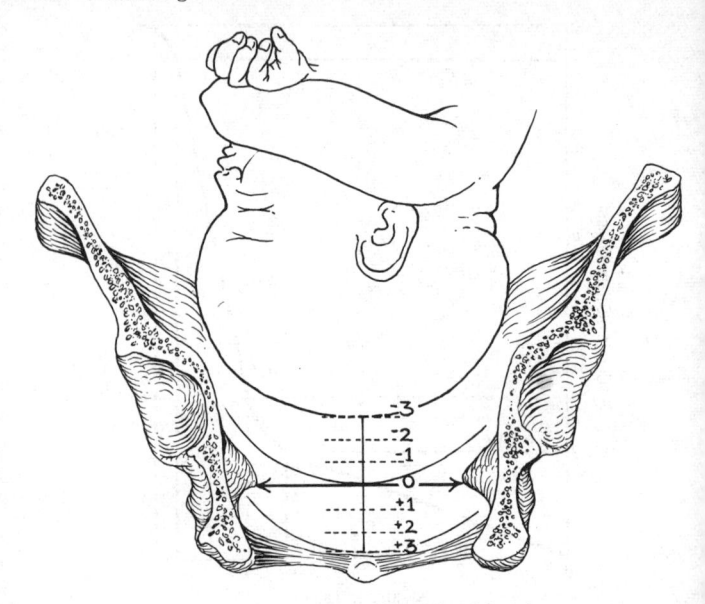

Fig 5-4. Stations of the fetal head.

2. Effacement of the cervix (Figs 5-1 and 5-2) is a process of thinning out which is accomplished before and, especially, during the first stage of labor. The cervix thins by retraction. In this manner, it "gets out of the way" of the presenting part, allowing more room for the birth process. Expression of mucus and compression aid in thinning of the cervix.

   Effacement is expressed in per cent. An uneffaced cervix is 0% and a cervix less than about 0.25 cm thick is 100% effaced.

3. The position of the presenting part can usually be confirmed by internal examination:
   a. Vertex presentations (Fig 5-5) - The fontanels and the sagittal suture are palpated. The position is determined by the relation of the fetal occiput to the mother's right or left side. This is expressed as OA (occiput precisely anterior), LOA (left occiput anterior), LOP, etc.
   b. Breech presentations (Fig 5-6) are determined by the position of the infant's sacrum in respect to the mother's right or left side. This is expressed as SA (sacrum directly anterior), LSA (left sacrum anterior), LSP, etc.

    c. Face presentations (Fig 5-7) - Extension of the fetal head on the neck causes the face to be the presenting part. The chin, a prominent and identifiable facial landmark, is used as a point of reference. As with vertex presentations, the position of the fetal chin is related to the mother's pelvis, left or right side, the anterior or posterior portion. This is expressed as RMP (right mentum posterior), etc.
    d. Brow, bregma, or sinciput presentation is a condition midway between flexion and extension. It usually is a temporary presentation which converts during labor to face or occiput presentation.
    e. Transverse presentations - The long axis of the body of the fetus is perpendicular to that of the mother. One shoulder (acromion) will occupy the superior strait, but it will be considerably to the right or left of the midline. Transverse presentations are designated by relating the child's inferior shoulder and back to the mother's back or abdominal wall. Thus, LADP (left acromio-dorso-posterior) indicates that the child's lower shoulder is to the mother's left and his back is toward her back.
    f. Compound presentations imply prolapse of a hand, an arm, or a foot or leg as a complication of one of the above presentations. These special or unusual presentations are generally recorded without abbreviations.

Preparation of the Patient in Labor.

The following should be done after the internal examination at admission or at the onset of labor to be conducted in the home:
  A. Preparation and Cleansing of the Pudendum: Shave the entire perineum and the labia and thoroughly wash with water and soap or surgical detergent.
  B. Enema: Administer a warm tap water or soapsuds enema to evacuate the lower bowel.
  C. Sedation: A barbiturate, e.g., pentobarbital sodium, 0.1-0.2 gm, or promazine (Sparine®), 50 mg, may be given to allay anxiety and to enhance relaxation. Sedatives should be administered before actual analgesia is required.
  D. Bed Rest: Keep the patient in bed after the membranes have ruptured or labor has definitely begun.
  E. Diet and Fluids: Allow only clear liquids by mouth during labor. Solid food is poorly assimilated, causes indigestion, and may be aspirated if vomiting occurs during general anesthesia or with eclamptic or epileptic convulsions. Offer tap water, tea, or fruit juices frequently to avoid dehydration.

Fig 5-5. Vertex presentations.

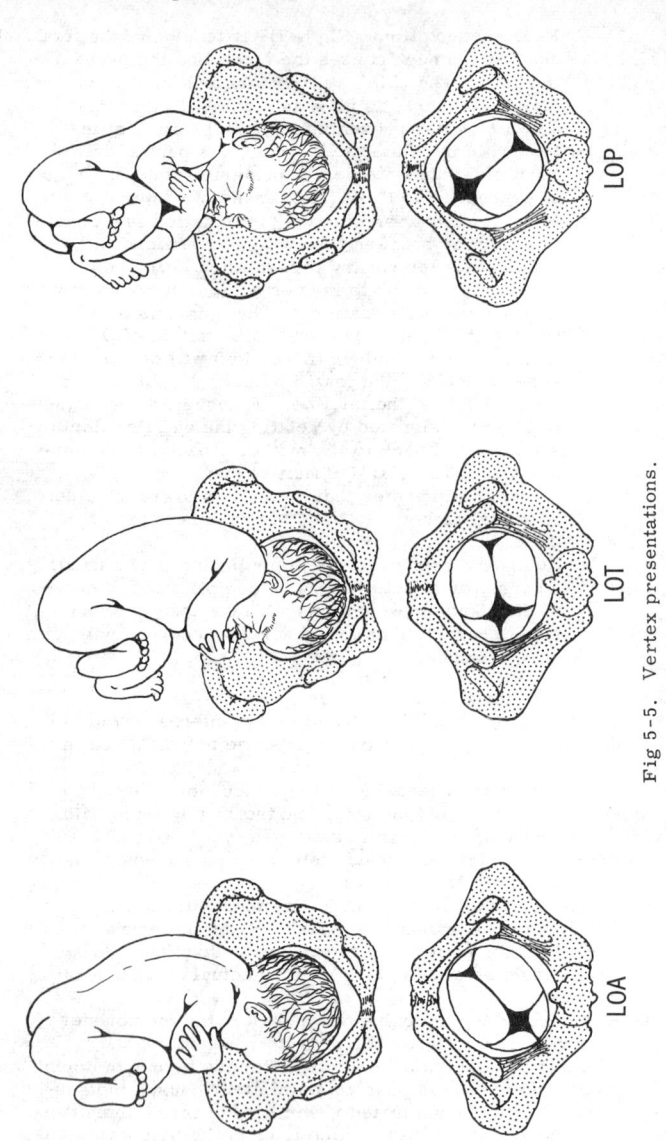

First Stage of Labor 113

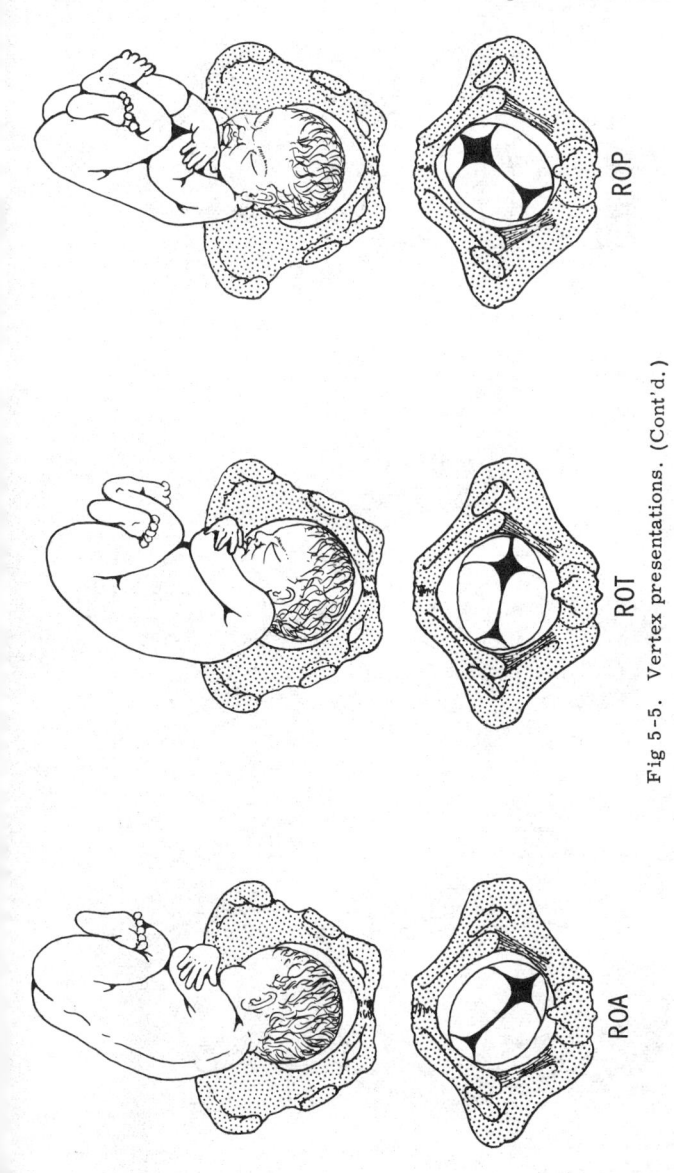

Fig 5-5. Vertex presentations. (Cont'd.)

114 First Stage of Labor

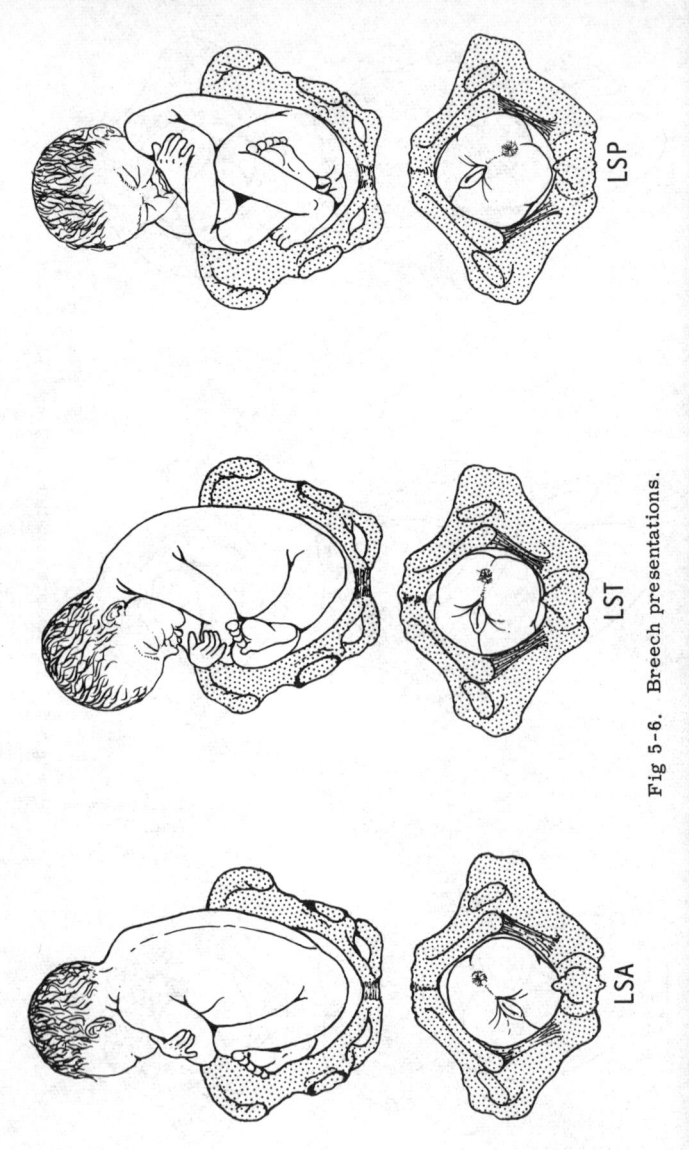

Fig 5-6. Breech presentations.

First Stage of Labor 115

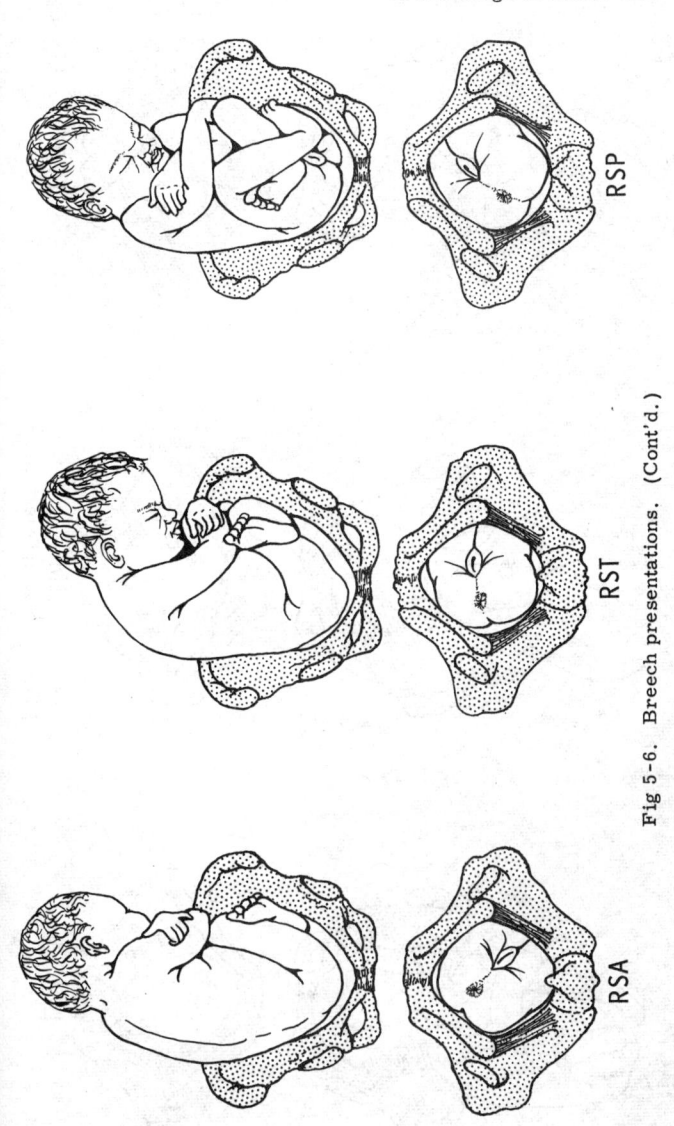

Fig 5-6. Breech presentations. (Cont'd.)

116 First Stage of Labor

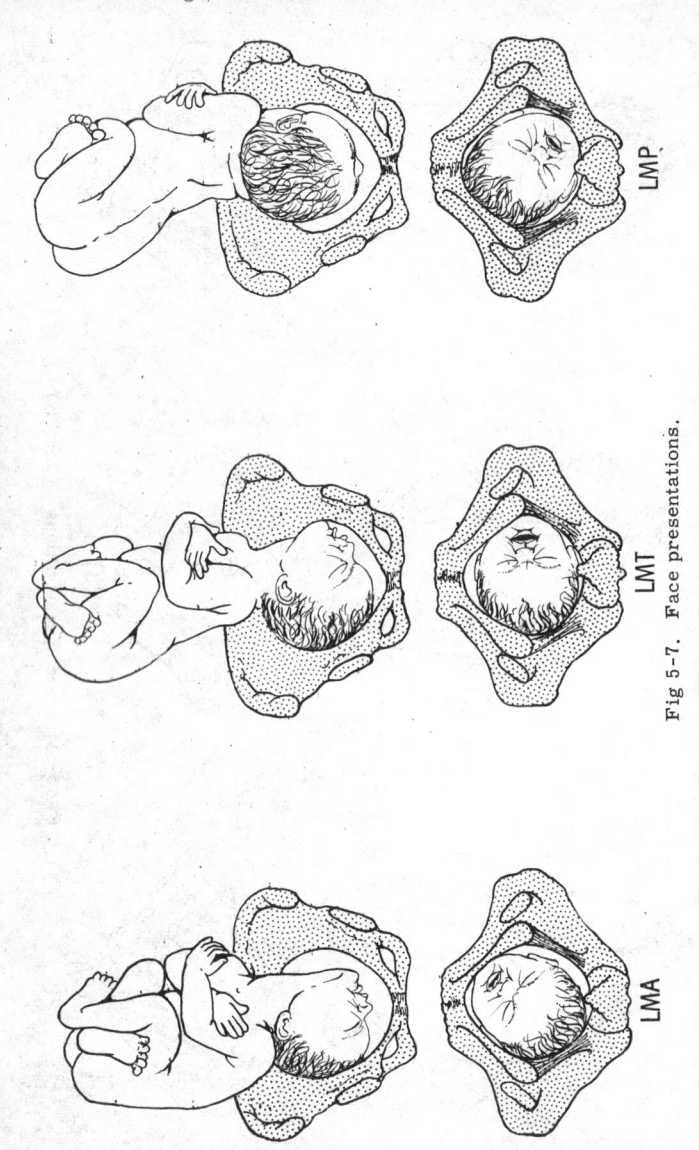

Fig 5-7. Face presentations.

LMP

LMT

LMA

First Stage of Labor 117

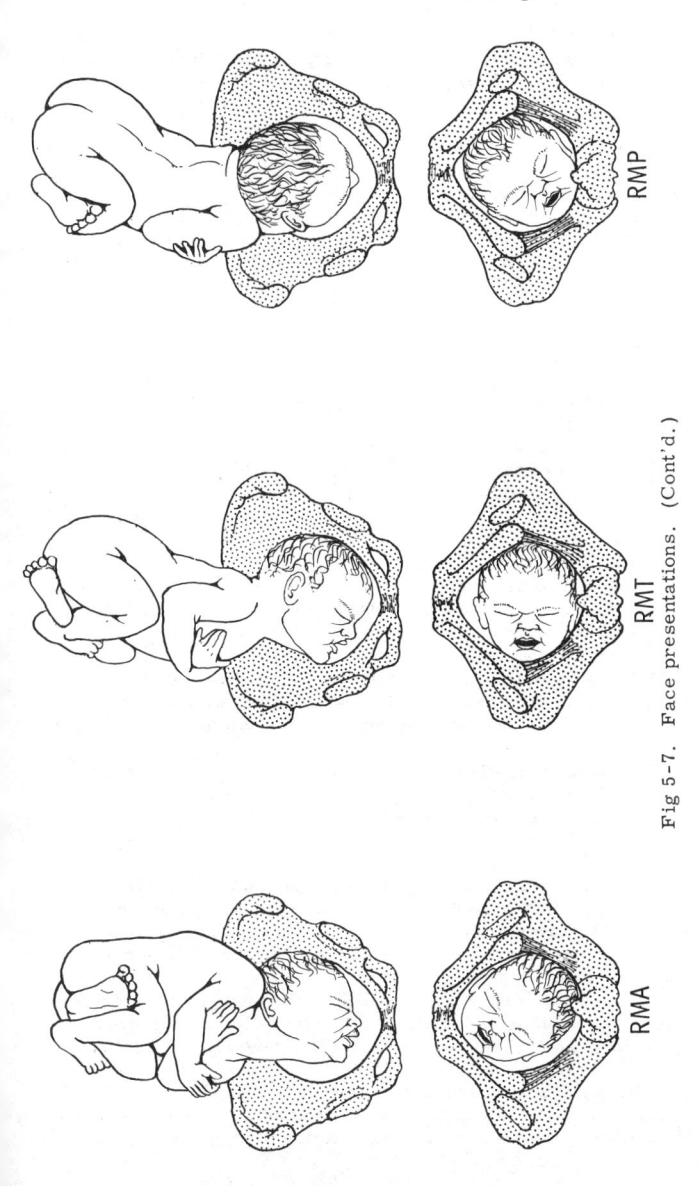

Fig 5-7. Face presentations. (Cont'd.)

118 First Stage of Labor

F. Analgesia: Analgesia should not be given until labor is definitely established. The cervix should be dilated to at least 3 cm. Analgesics must be ordered on an individual basis, considering each patient's anticipated obstetric problems, the quality of labor, her desire to be alert or subdued, etc.

Further Examinations & Procedures.

A. Record the fetal heart rate and rhythm every 15 minutes during the course of labor and also when the membranes rupture, if brisk bleeding occurs, or if meconium passes (in other than breech presentations).
B. Perform external and internal examinations as often as necessary to determine the progress of labor. In most instances several internal examinations are usually necessary during the course of labor. However, too frequent vaginal or rectal examinations cause the patient discomfort and increase the incidence of intra-uterine infection, particularly after rupture of the membranes. Descent of the fetus and internal rotation can often be determined by external palpation alone. The shift of the point of maximal impulse of the fetal heartbeat is a useful indication of fetal descent.
C. Record the frequency, intensity, and regularity of the uterine contractions, and note the tone of the myometrium between contractions. Observe the patient's reactions and her tolerance of labor. Restlessness and discomfort often develop as labor progresses.
D. Encourage the patient to void frequently. Palpate the abdomen occasionally for signs of bladder fullness. Catheterize if distention occurs or if voiding is obviously inadequate.
E. Cleanse the vulvar region before and after internal examination, defecation, and voiding, or when soiling by vaginal secretions occurs.

Preparation for Delivery.

The person conducting the delivery must designate the equipment, instruments, sutures, and other supplies to be used. (Most delivery rooms have a standard set-up, but variations in procedure are permissible when they are in conformity with good surgical principles.)

Place the patient in a modified lithotomy position for delivery. (Less preferable is the left lateral decubitus [Sims] position, but this may be used if a spontaneous uncomplicated birth is anticipated.)

Note: Strict asepsis is required:
A. Prepare the pudendum by washing again vigorously with water and soap or surgical detergent, e.g., hexachlorophene (pHisohex®).

B. Drape the patient with sterile towels and sheets, exposing only the introitus.
C. The physician and his assistants must carefully scrub their hands and wear masks and sterile gowns and gloves as for a major surgical procedure. Any delivery may become complicated. (See also p. 353.)

MANAGEMENT OF THE SECOND STAGE OF LABOR
(Vertex Delivery)

Spontaneous delivery of the fetus presenting by the vertex is divided into 3 phases: (1) Delivery of the head, (2) delivery of the shoulders, and (3) delivery of the body and legs.

Be alert to the imminence of delivery when the cervix becomes fully dilated. Final preparations for delivery should be completed by the time the presenting part reaches the pelvic floor (or sooner, if labor is progressing very rapidly):

(1) The physician should wear a mask, scrub his hands, and use sterile gown and gloves.

(2) Anesthesia is administered (pudendal block). Gown and gloves are changed if any contamination has occurred.

(3) Sterile instruments and necessary supplies should be arranged conveniently on a table or stand.

(4) An assistant should cleanse the pudendum with water and surgical detergent.

(5) Sterile drapes are applied.

During the late second stage, the head distends the perineum and vulva with each uterine contraction, aided by voluntary efforts. The presenting part recedes slightly during the intervals of relaxation but is said to "crown" when its widest portion (biparietal diameter) distends the vulva just prior to emergence.

Do not hasten delivery or serious damage to the mother and child may occur. As the head advances, control its progress by pressure applied laterally beneath the symphysis and maintain flexion of the head, when necessary, by pressure over the perineum. Steady and slow the speed of delivery as necessary to forestall pudendal laceration or unexpected extrusion of the fetal head. Sudden marked variations in intracranial pressure are capable of causing cerebral hemorrhage.

Gentle, gradual delivery is desirable. Draw the perineum downward to allow the head to clear the perineal body. Do not insert the fingers into the birth canal or anus to facilitate delivery at this time; trauma or infection may occur. Pressure applied from the coccygeal region upward (modified Ritgen's maneuver) will extend the head at the proper time and thereby protect the perineal musculature.

Episiotomy is done when the infant's head begins to distend the introitus.

Table 5-1. Mechanisms of labor.

VERTEX

Engagement	Flexion	Descent	Internal Rotation	Extension	External Rotation or Restitution
Generally occurs in late pregnancy or at onset of labor. Mode of entry into superior strait depends on pelvic configuration; posterior occiput is most common position.	Good flexion is noted in majority of cases. Flexion aids engagement and descent. (Extension occurs in brow and face presentations.)	Depends on pelvic architecture and cephalopelvic relationships. Descent is usually slowly progressive.	Takes place during descent. After engagement, vertex usually rotates to the transverse. It must next rotate to the anterior or posterior to pass the ischial spines, whereupon, when the vertex reaches the perineum, rotation from a posterior to an anterior or position generally follows.	Follows distention of the perineum by the vertex. Head concomitantly stems beneath the symphysis. Extension is complete with delivery of the head.	Following delivery, head normally rotates to the position it originally occupied at engagement. Next, the shoulders descend (in a path similar to that traced by the head). They rotate anteroposteriorly for delivery. Then the head swings back to its position at birth. The body of the baby is delivered next.

Table 5-1. Mechanisms of labor (cont'd).

FRANK BREECH

	Engagement	Flexion	Descent	Internal Rotation	Lateral Flexion	External Rotation or Restitution
Hips	Usually occurs in one of oblique diameters of pelvic inlet.		Anterior hip generally descends more rapidly than posterior, both at inlet and outlet.	Ordinarily takes place when breech reaches levator musculature. Fetal bitrochanteric rotates to AP diameter.	Occurs when anterior hip stems beneath symphysis; posterior hip is born first.	After birth of breech and legs infant's body turns toward mother's side to which its back was directed at engagement of breech. This accommodates engagement of the shoulders.
Shoulders	Bisacromial diameter engages in same diameter as breech.		Gradual descent is the rule.	Anterior shoulder rotates so as to bring shoulders into AP of outlet.	Anterior shoulder at symphysis and posterior shoulder is born first (when body is supported).	
Head	Engages in the same diameter as shoulders.	Flexes on entry into superior strait. Biparietal occupies oblique used by shoulders. At outlet, neck or chin arrests beneath symphysis and head is born by gradual flexion.	Follows the shoulders.	Occiput (if a posterior) or face (if an occiput anterior) rotates to hollow of sacrum. This brings presenting part to AP of outlet.		

Second Stage of Labor 121

122 Second Stage of Labor

Delivery of the Head. (See Figs 5-8 to 5-12.)

In vertex presentations, the forehead appears first (after the vertex) and then the face and chin. The neck then appears. The cord encircles the neck in about 20% of deliveries. Fortunately, the funis is rarely tight enough to cause fetal hypoxia. Gently slip the cord over the head. If this cannot be done easily, clamp the cord with forceps in 2 places, cut between the forceps, and proceed with the delivery. Wipe fluid from the nose and mouth, and then aspirate the nasal and oral passages with a soft rubber suction bulb or with a small catheter attached to a DeLee suction trap.

Before external rotation (restitution), which occurs next, the head is usually drawn back toward the perineum. This movement precedes engagement of the shoulders, which are now entering the pelvic inlet. From this time on, support the infant manually and facilitate the mechanism of labor.

Do not hurry. If the strength of the contractions seems to wane, be patient—labor will continue. Once the airway is clear, the infant can breathe and is not in immediate jeopardy.

Cautiously draw the head downward and backward until the anterior shoulder impinges against the symphysis. Then lift the head upward. This will aid in delivery of the posterior shoulder. One may slip several fingers into the vagina at this point to assist in delivering the posterior arm. The an-

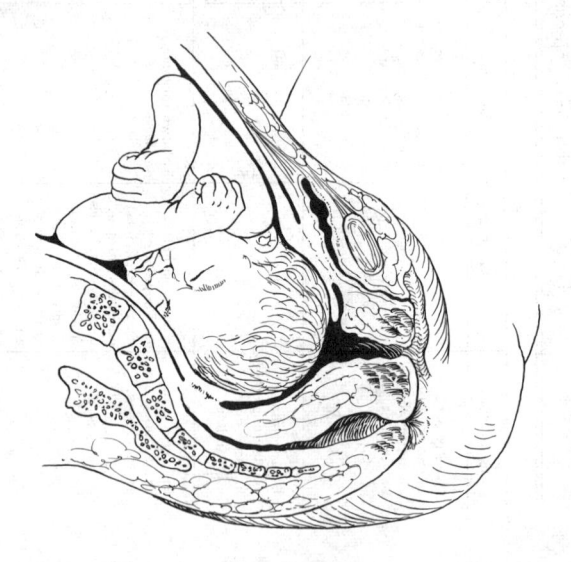

Fig 5-8. Engagement of LOA.

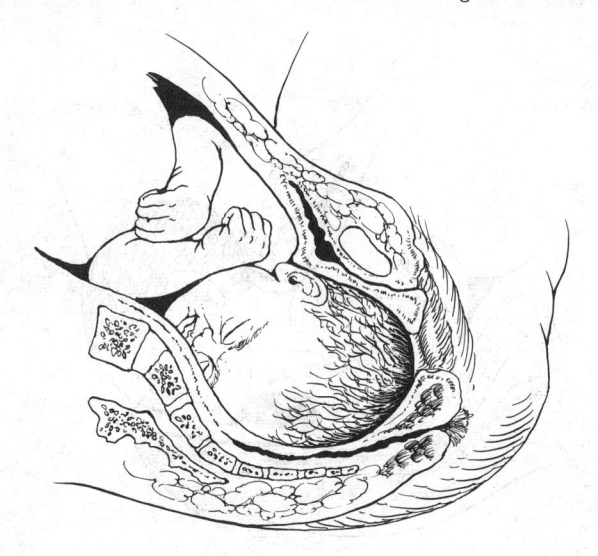

Fig 5-9. LOA position.

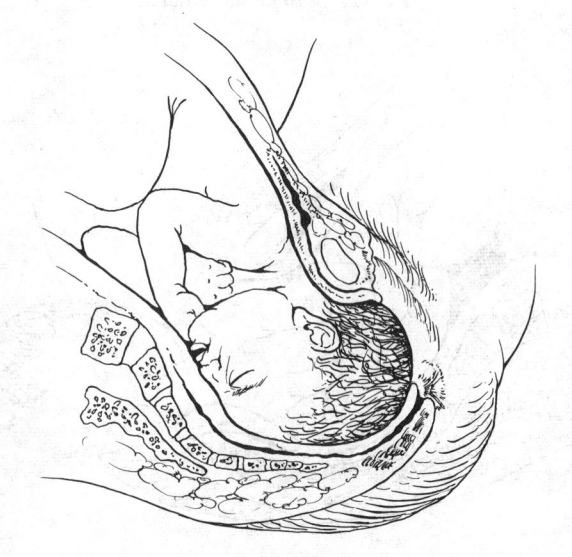

Fig 5-10. Anterior rotation of head.

124 Second Stage of Labor

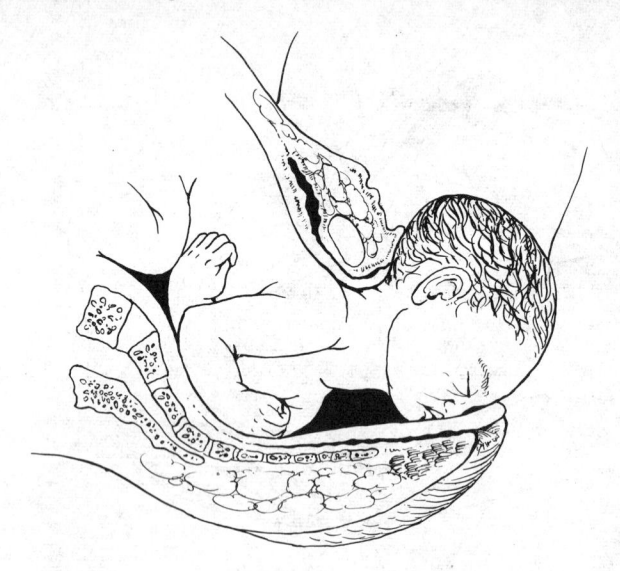

Fig 5-11. Extension of head.

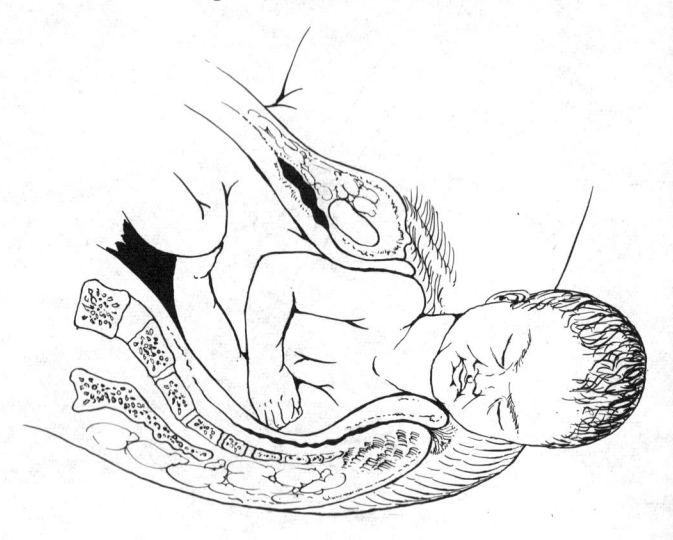

Fig 5-12. External rotation of head.

Fig 5-13. Delivery of anterior shoulder.

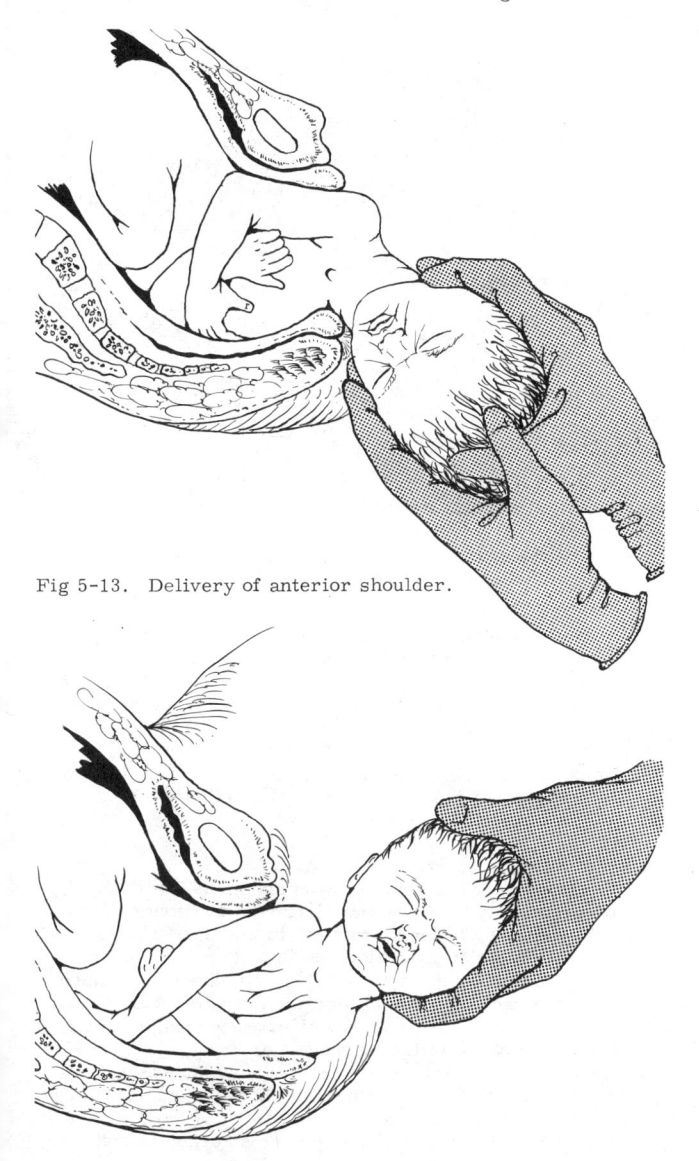

Fig 5-14. Delivery of posterior shoulder.

126 Second Stage of Labor

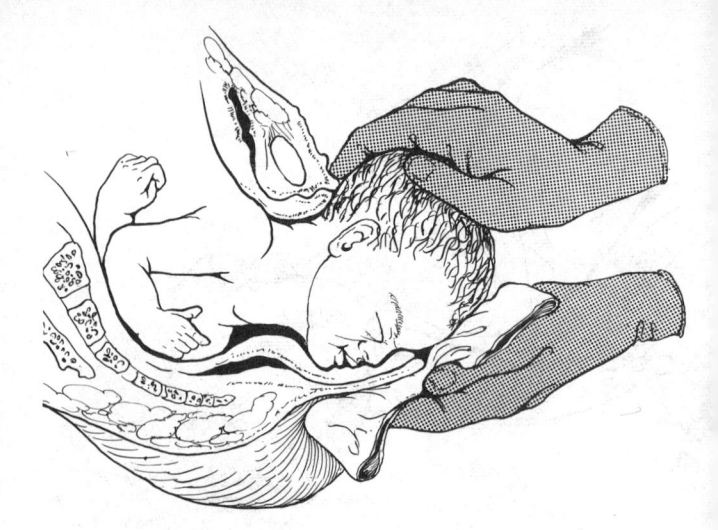

Fig 5-15. Modified Ritgen's maneuver.

terior shoulder is next delivered from behind the symphysis. (At times it may be easier to deliver the anterior shoulder first.)

Never exert strong anterior or posterior traction on the head. Do not hook a finger into the child's axilla to deliver a shoulder; a brachial plexus injury (Erb or Duchenne), a hematoma of the neck, or shoulder injury may result.

Deliver the body, hips, and legs by gradually lifting the child out of the birth canal.

Delivery of the Shoulders.

This portion of the birth process should be slow and deliberate to prevent fetal and maternal complications. The shoulders must rotate (or be rotated) to the anteroposterior diameter of the outlet for delivery. Once the head has emerged and a clear airway is established, there is no need for haste; the baby will usually breathe even before it is completely delivered. Deliver the shoulders after proper rotation, using one of the following maneuvers:
  A. Elevate the head toward the mother's symphysis for release of the posterior shoulder. This is often easily done and should be tried.
  B. Depress the head toward the mother's coccyx to bring out the anterior shoulder.

In vertex presentations, a hand may present after the head. This need not obstruct delivery of the shoulders. Merely sweep the baby's hand and arm over its face, draw the arm out, and deliver the other shoulder as outlined above.

Caution: Avoid undue pressure to and traction on the neck and shoulders, or injury to the brachial plexus and large vessels may occur.

Delivery of the Body & Extremities.

The body and legs of the baby should be delivered gradually by easy traction after the shoulders have been freed.

Immediate Care of the Infant.

As soon as the infant is delivered, it should be held with the head lowered (no more than 15 degrees) to remove fluid and mucus from the oropharynx. A rubber ear syringe or comparable suction device is useful in clearing the air passages. Place the baby on a wheeled stand or tray the height of the delivery table or slightly lower. If it is below the level of the placental insertion, blood will drain readily from the placenta and cord to the newborn. This will amount to 30-90 ml before the cord is clamped or the placenta separates.

Resuscitate if necessary (see p. 158).

Some physicians place the child on the mother's abdomen. This may contaminate the sterile field, however, and the baby is not secure there. The mother usually becomes concerned about its condition and safety. What is even more important, blood may actually drain from the baby into the cord and placenta.

Clamp and cut the cord as soon as the cord ceases to pulsate (or sooner if the infant is premature or distressed or if erythroblastosis is probable). Examine the umbilical cord for 2 arteries and one vein. Apply a sterile cord clamp, cord tie of umbilical tape, or a rubber band just distal to the skin edge at the cord insertion at the umbilicus. Cover the cord stump with a dry gauze dressing held by a belly band, preferably of elastic material.

Wipe the eyelids with moist cotton. Instill one drop of 1% aqueous silver nitrate solution into each eye. The medication must be freshly prepared or expressed from commercial wax "pearls" which maintain the safe concentration. Penicillin ophthalmic ointment is as effective as silver nitrate and is comparable in price, but penicillin is not as yet acceptable to numerous boards of health for prophylaxis of ophthalmia neonatorum.

Apply means of identification (necklace, bracelet, etc).

Thoroughly examine the infant and record its weight, total length, crown-rump length, shoulder circumference, the circumference of the head, and the cranial diameters. Transfer to the nursery for further observation and care.

After Delivery.

Carefully inspect the perineum, vagina, and cervix for lacerations, hematomas, or extension of episiotomy incisions.

The extent of laceration of the birth canal may be designated roughly in degrees: (1) In first degree lacerations only the mucosa or skin (or both) is damaged. Bleeding is usually minimal. (2) Second degree lacerations include tears of the mucosa or skin (or both) plus disruption of the superficial fascia and the transverse perineal muscle. (The sphincter ani muscle is spared.) Bleeding is often brisk. (3) Third degree lacerations involve the above structures plus the anal sphincter. Moderate blood loss is to be expected. (4) Fourth degree lacerations include the above structures plus entry into the rectal lumen. Bleeding may be profuse and fecal soiling is inevitable.

Sulcus lacerations, urethral and cervical damage, etc, are designated specifically.

The administration of oxygen to the mother after delivery of the child but before the cord is clamped is a useless gesture if one is attempting to increase the oxygenation of the infant's blood. Little or no oxygen can reach the baby from the mother after it has been delivered because of placental separation. However, oxygen given to the mother may aid in her recovery from the effects of analgesia and anesthesia.

MANAGEMENT OF THE THIRD STAGE OF LABOR

The third or placental stage of labor is the period from the birth of the infant to the delivery of the placenta, including recovery of the placenta and the hour thereafter (sometimes called the 4th stage of labor). The management of the placental stage of labor varies greatly in different localities. Many archaic and unsafe practices during the third stage, such as traction on the cord before placental separation and "kneading" the fundus to separate the placenta (Credé), contribute to maternal mortality as a result of hemorrhage, shock, and infection. More women die because of difficulties involving the third stage of labor than the other 2 stages combined.

Maternal morbidity and mortality increase in proportion to the degree of blood loss and the duration of the third stage of labor. The prognosis is excellent for the patient whose third stage is well managed, but guarded or grave for the woman with third stage complications. The uterus which contracts and remains contracted rarely bleeds excessively. Any condition or procedure which hinders or delays the prompt separation of the placenta, its delivery into the vagina, and its extraction from the lower birth canal may lead to postpartal hemorrhage. Any maneuver which expedites complete separation and delivery of the placenta serves to minimize bleeding. The immediate manual separation and extraction of the placenta from the fundus of the uterus is an effective direct technic, but strict asepsis and effective anesthesia are required. Less dangerous and generally satisfactory indirect methods are discussed below.

Delivery of the Placenta.

Normally, several uterine contractions following delivery of the infant cause the area of the placental site to become considerably smaller, and the placenta soon reaches its limit of elasticity. The placenta is attached to the uterine wall only by anchor villi and thin-walled blood vessels, all of which eventually tear. In some instances the placental margin separates first; in others, when the central portion of the placenta is freed initially, bleeding from the retroplacental sinuses may assist placental separation. In the average patient, the placenta is sheared off within 3-4 minutes after delivery of the fetus. Incomplete separation due to any cause or ineffectual uterine contractions keep the retroplacental blood sinuses open and often lead to blood loss, which may be severe.

Normal placental separation is manifested first by a firmly contracting, rising fundus. The uterus becomes smaller and changes in shape from discoid to globular. The umbilical cord becomes longer. There is a palpable and visible prominence above the symphysis (if the bladder is empty), and a slight gush of blood from the vagina. Cervical-vaginal fullness can be noted on rectal examination. Upon rectal or sterile vaginal examination the separated placenta can often be felt lying in the cervix or in the upper vagina.

These signs are not often confused with other conditions. However, it is well to remember that uterine anomaly or tumor, a second undelivered fetus, feces, a tumor, and lacerations of the birth canal can mimic many of the signs of normal placental separation.

Ideally, although the membranes still remain attached, the placenta should present at the internal cervical os after 4-5 firm postpartum contractions. It is then either expelled or expressed into the vagina for delivery; freeing of the membranes generally accompanies extrusion of the placenta.

In at least two-thirds of cases the presenting portion is the glistening fetal surface. This so-called Schultze mechanism was at one time erroneously believed to follow retroplacental bleeding and prompt separation. The Duncan mechanism, in which the placenta presented with the roughened maternal surface uppermost, was just as erroneously believed to imply delayed marginal separation, and was assumed to be associated with more severe bleeding. We now know that (1) retroplacental hematomas as such are rather rare and that (2) the placenta probably leaves the uterus the

130 Third Stage of Labor

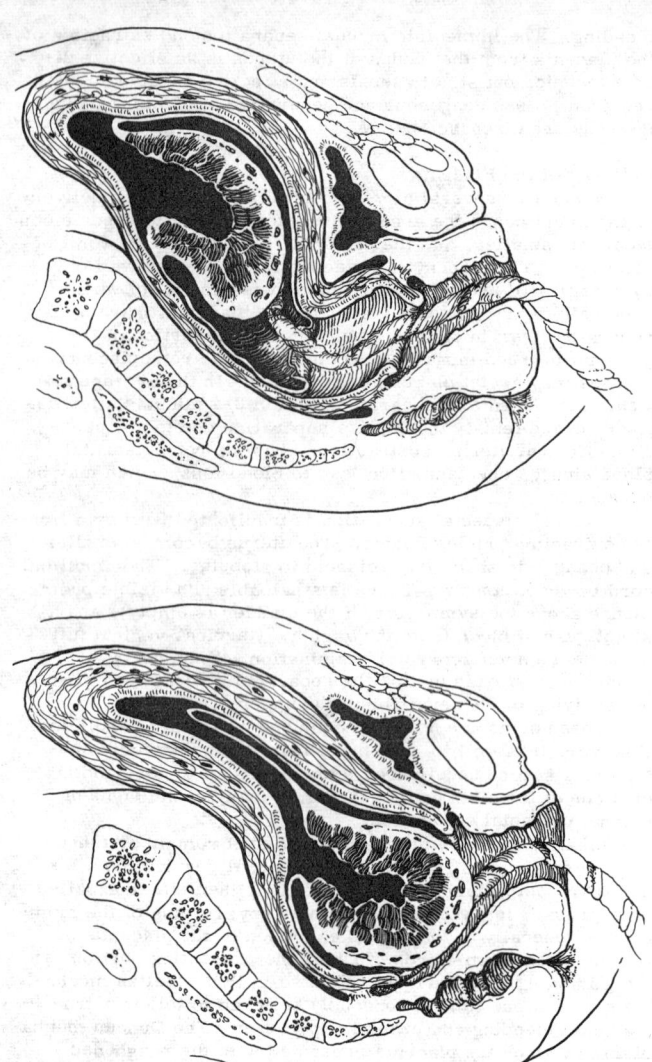

Fig 5-16. Delivery of the placenta (Schultz).

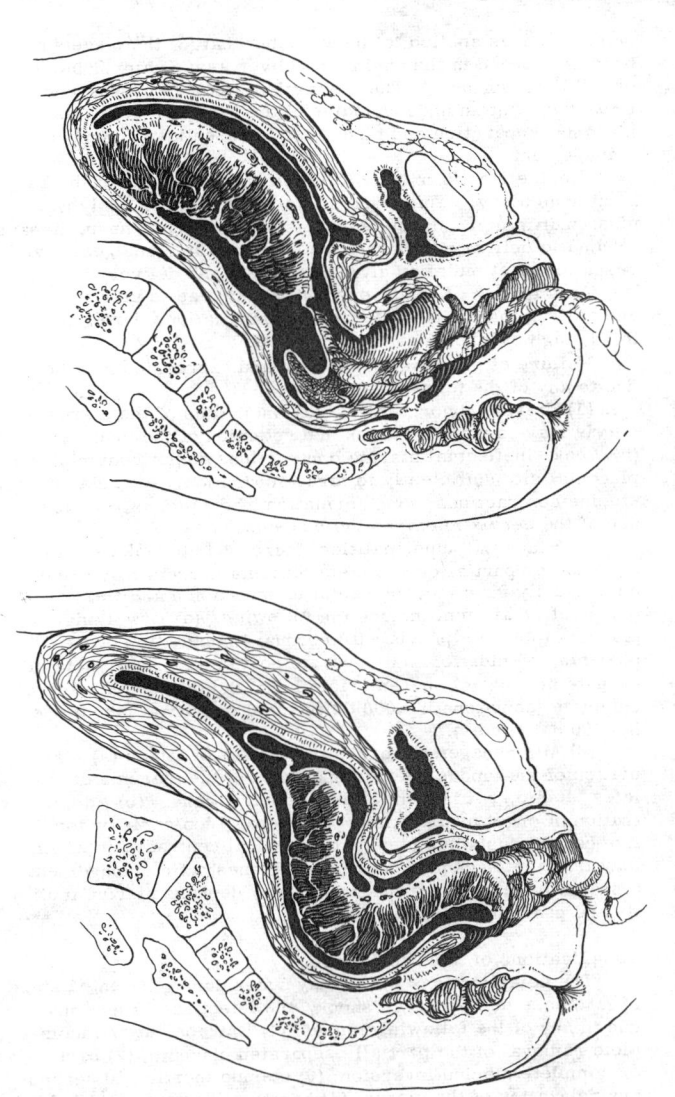

Fig 5-17. Delivery of the placenta (Duncan).

same way it is applied to the wall, but that (3) the placenta becomes turned in the vagina to deliver as a "shiny Schultze" or a "dirty Duncan." The mechanism itself is probably unimportant, but an understanding of the sequence of events of placental separation and blood loss is essential to correct management.

Uterine inertia may be followed after the birth of the baby by uterine atony. This occurs in prolonged labor, polyhydramnios, multiple pregnancy, myomas of the uterus, heart disease, traumatic delivery, hemorrhage and excessive analgesia, and cessation of stimulation after anesthesia and delivery.

Anticipation of conditions which may lead to uterine atony and aids to combat this will avoid complications during the third stage of labor.

Failure of placental separation and expression may be due to any of the following causes:

(1) Uterine abnormalities: (a) Anomalies of the uterus or cervix may cause restriction and retention of the placenta. (b) Weak, ineffectual uterine contractions do not constrict the placental site sufficiently to force separation. (c) Tetanic uterine contractions, ring-formation of the uterus, or closure of the cervix may trap the placenta.

(2) Placental abnormalities: Increased uteroplacental cohesion or partial or complete placenta accreta may create an unusually firm uteroplacental union. Abnormalities of placentation at term include the following: (a) Low-lying placenta (placenta previa); (b) cornual implantation of the placenta, or nidation in a separate portion of a subseptate or arcuate uterus; (c) succenturiate lobe; and (d) placenta accreta, complete (about one in 8000 deliveries) or partial (about one in 4000 deliveries).

(3) Mismanagement of the third stage of labor: (a) Manipulation of the fundus before separation of the placenta stimulates tetanic, not rhythmic fundal contractions. (b) Administration of ergot preparations parenterally too early or too late causes sustained uterine or cervical contractions which may trap the placenta. (c) Improper anesthetic management (especially deep ether anesthesia) may depress uterine motility and prevent contractions.

Complications of the Third Stage.

The complications which may occur during the third stage of labor are hemorrhage, shock, and infection. These may be due to any of the following causes: (1) Entrapment or incomplete removal of the partially separated placenta; (2) partial or complete uterine inversion; (3) uterine inertia and secondary relaxation of the uterus; (4) bacterial contamination of the cervix at the introitus when the fundus is used as a piston to expel the placenta; (5) failures of aseptic technic.

Emergency Treatment.

Sudden, massive hemorrhage, especially following instrumental vaginal delivery, requires immediate sterile exploration of the birth canal and uterus to control bleeding. Abruptio placentae, rupture of the uterus, and gross cervical or vaginal lacerations require immediate definitive treatment:

(1) Extract the separated placenta or manually separate and withdraw the afterbirth.

(2) Palpate the uterine cavity for tumors, defects, or anomalies.

(3) Administer oxytocin (Pitocin®), 0.5 ml I.M. stat. and 0.5 ml rapidly by I.V. drip.

(4) Examine the cervix and suture significant bleeding lacerations; inspect the vaginal canal and repair defects.

If rupture of the uterus is discovered, prepare for immediate laparotomy.

Obstetric Procedures Which Minimize Complications During the Third Stage.

In vertex presentations administration of ergonovine (Ergotrate®), 0.2 mg I.V., at the time of delivery of the baby's anterior shoulder has been shown to augment uterine contractions, which greatly facilitates prompt separation of the placenta and prevents considerable loss of blood. Timing and route of the injection are extremely important; if the injection is given too late or if it is not all given I.V., the cervix may contract and trap the separated placenta. When this happens, manual extraction and often additional anesthesia will be required, and some undesirable delay will be inevitable. Amyl nitrite (2-3 inhalations of an ampule held in a sponge) may relax the cervix sufficiently to permit recovery of the placenta.

The following program will usually prevent entrapment of the placenta and conserve blood:

(1) Give oxytocin (Pitocin®), 0.5 ml I.M., immediately after delivery of the infant.

(2) Recover the placenta by Pastore's or Brandt's technic.

(3) After delivery of the placenta, give ergonovine (Ergotrate®), 0.2 mg I.M.

(4) Elevate and compress the uterus manually to express all clots. (Clots may form when brisk bleeding occurs, especially from vaginal and cervical lacerations. Slight bleeding from the uterus ordinarily clots and liquifies to pass finally as fluid blood.)

(5) If bleeding continues and intravenous fluids have not been started, insert a No. 16 or No. 18 needle into a large vein and administer 5 units (0.5 ml) oxytocin in one liter of 5% glucose in water. Have crossmatched blood available.

(a) Examine the lower genital tract for lacerations.

(b) Explore the uterus **without anesthesia,** if possible,

for retained products of conception and rupture of the uterus.
- (6) Give a second dose of ergonovine intravenously.
- (7) Repair lacerations quickly.

Technics of Recovery of the Placenta.

A. Pastore Technic:
1. Stand to the patient's left and elevate the fundus with the fingers of the right hand.
2. If the placenta separates, massage the fundus gently; otherwise, leave it alone until contractions occur.
3. Place the left hand flat over the abdomen with the fingers superior to the symphysis.
4. When contractions occur and the placenta separates, squeeze the fundus gently and push it downward slightly with the right hand.
5. Prevent the fundus from entering the pelvis by holding the left hand above and behind the symphysis. The placenta can be felt to slide beneath the hand through the lower uterine segment into the cervix or vagina.
6. Lift the fundus upward to leave the placenta free in the vagina.
7. Extract the placenta from the vagina by gentle cord traction.

B. Brandt Technic (Modified):
1. Immediately after delivery of the infant, clamp the umbilical cord close to the vulva. Palpate the uterus gently without massage to determine whether firm contractions are occurring.
2. After several uterine contractions and a change in size and shape indicate separation of the placenta, hold the clamp at the vulva firmly with one hand, place the fingertips of the other hand on the abdomen, and press between the fundus and symphysis to elevate the fundus. If the placenta has separated, the cord will extrude into the vagina.
3. Further elevate the fundus, apply gentle traction on the cord, and deliver the placenta from the vagina.

C. Manual Separation and Removal of the Placenta:
1. Prepare the perineum and vulva again with detergent and antiseptic solution. Change gloves and re-drape the operational field.
2. Making the hand as narrow as possible, insert it gently into the vagina and palpate for defects in the vagina and cervix. Slowly probe through the cervix with the fingers, taking care not to lacerate or forcefully dilate the canal. (Moderately deep anesthesia may be required.)
3. Locate the placenta and separate it if this can be done easily. (Do not attempt to force separation against unusual resistance.)

4. Palpate the fundus for defects or tumors.
5. Remove the hand, grasping the completely separated placenta, or leave the placenta in the uterus if it is firmly adherent. Hysterectomy will probably be required in the latter case.

Treatment of Complications.

When hemorrhage is due to hypofibrinogenemia, replace blood loss and administer Fibrinogen, U.S.P. (Parenogen®), 4-10 gm I.V., to restore the clotting mechanism. **Caution:** Never operate until the coagulation mechanism is restored to normal. If the patient continues to bleed excessively, prepare for hysterectomy. In most instances, packing the uterus is only a temporary expedient. One cannot insert enough packing and the pack may hold the sinuses open rather than closed.

Blood replacement is almost invariably inadequate. Estimates are often only half or less than half of the actual loss. Using skin color, pulse, respiration, blood pressure, patient response, etc, as guides, replace blood loss and treat shock.

In certain cases of postpartal hemorrhage, conservative measures will not prevent death, whereas timely hysterectomy may be life-saving. Fortunately, these cases are rare. If, after correction of the blood coagulation defect, the patient continues to bleed excessively, hysterectomy is indicated—even in a primipara—preferably under cyclopropane or other light anesthesia. Do not give spinal, ether, or—unless in combination with another agent—thiopental anesthesia since these types of anesthesia tend to be associated with hypotension and prolonged depression of vital functions.

Consider uterine (and often vaginal) packing in the following cases: (1) Gross cervical laceration when insufficient assistance for repair is not immediately available. (2) Rupture of the uterus while waiting for an operating room in which to do a laparotomy. (3) Cases of placenta previa after placental extraction when bleeding continues from blood vessels in the lower uterine segment which are not collapsed even when the fundus is well contracted. (4) When it is necessary to retain a uterus replaced after inversion. (5) When it is necessary to temporarily control paravaginal and vulvar hematomas. (6) After evacuation of a large hydatidiform mole.

In general, packing can be avoided by the proper use of intravenous oxytocics, elevation and gentle massage of the uterus, and proper management of the third stage of labor.

AIDS TO NORMAL DELIVERY

EPISIOTOMY (PERINEOTOMY); REPAIR OF EPISIOTOMY & LACERATIONS

An episiotomy is a pudendal incision designed to widen the vulvar orifice to permit the easier passage of the fetus. It is used in the majority of primigravidas and in many multiparas.

The advantages of episiotomy are that it prevents perineal lacerations, relieves compression of the fetal head, and shortens the second stage of labor by removing the resistance of the pudendal musculature. Furthermore, a surgical incision can be repaired more successfully than a jagged tear.

Episiotomy is indicated (1) when a tear is imminent, (2) in most forceps and breech deliveries, and (3) to facilitate delivery of a premature infant.

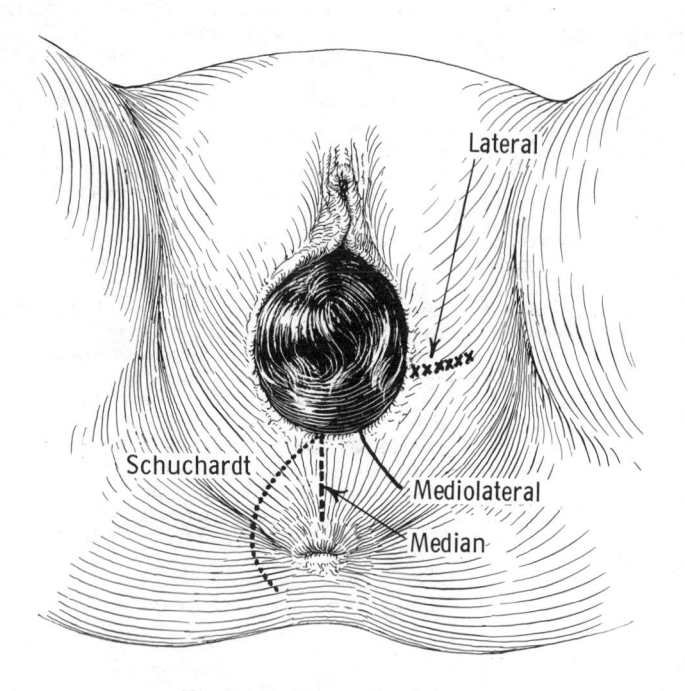

Fig 5-18. Types of episiotomy.

Types of Episiotomy.

The tissues incised by an episiotomy are (1) skin and subcutaneous tissues, (2) vaginal mucosa, (3) the urogenital septum (mostly fascia, but also the transverse perineal muscles), (4) intercolumnar fascia or superior fascia of the pelvic diaphragm, and (5) the lowermost fibers of the puborectalis portions of the levator ani muscles (if the episiotomy is mediolateral and deep).

- A. Median: This is the easiest episiotomy to accomplish and to repair and is certainly the most bloodless. It consists of incising the median raphe of the perineum almost to the anal sphincter. The disadvantage of this procedure is the occasional accidental extension of the incision through the sphincter (third degree laceration) or through the sphincter and into the lumen of the rectum (4th degree laceration).
- B. Mediolateral: The mediolateral incision is the most widely used, especially in operative obstetrics, because of its safety. Incise downward and outward in the direction of the lateral margin of the anal sphincter. The choice of a right or a left incision depends upon the position of the presenting part and the surgical facility of the operator in repairing an oblique defect. A right mediolateral episiotomy widens the introitus slightly more (on the right) than a left mediolateral episiotomy does if the infant presents in an LOA, LOP, LSA, LMA, or any position in which the small parts are to the right. This is particularly important in forceps delivery and when the infant is large because it relieves stretch where the tension is greatest, thereby preventing lacerations. It also avoids the extension of an episiotomy when placed on the opposite side.

  Bilateral mediolateral episiotomies are not recommended since they cause excessive blood loss, marked discomfort during healing, and an ultimately unsatisfactory anatomic result.
- C. Schuchardt Incision: This is a maximally-extended mediolateral episiotomy which is carried deep into one vaginal sulcus and is curved downward and laterally part way around the rectum. Although rarely required, it is of great help in the difficult delivery of a large head, a restricted decomposition of a breech, and in the correction of shoulder dystocia. It is also employed in vaginal surgery requiring wide exposure.
- D. Lateral: Lateral episiotomy affords very little relaxation of the introitus, is associated with profuse bleeding, and is difficult to repair. This incision has no merit and should be abandoned.

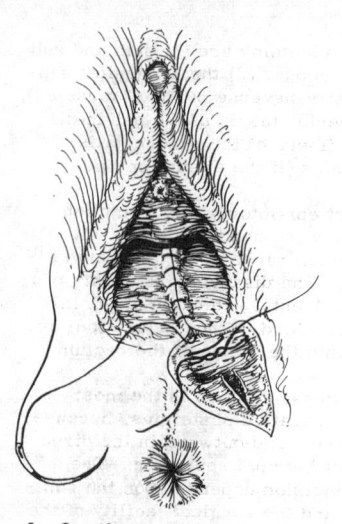

138 Episiotomy

1. Continuous suture of mucosa with inverted suture of perineal body
2. Mucosal suture continued in skin and tied with inverted suture 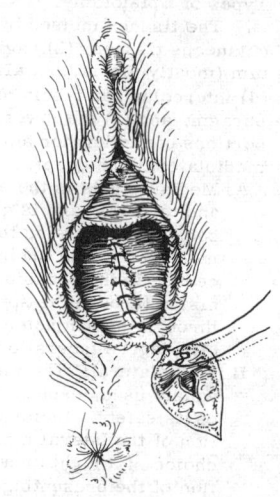
3. Closure of levator ani and perineal tissue 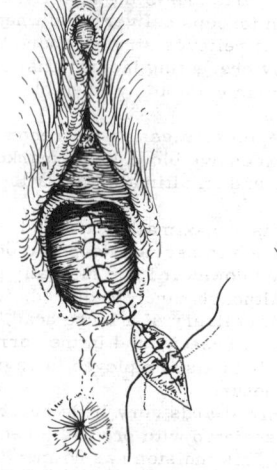
4. Skin closed subcutaneously 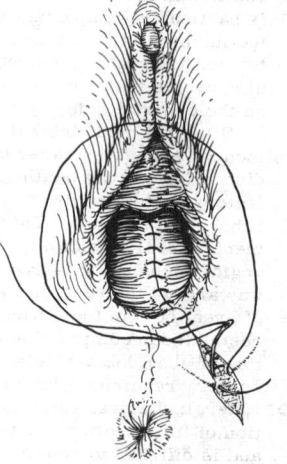

Fig 5-19. Episiotomy repair.

Episiotomy 139

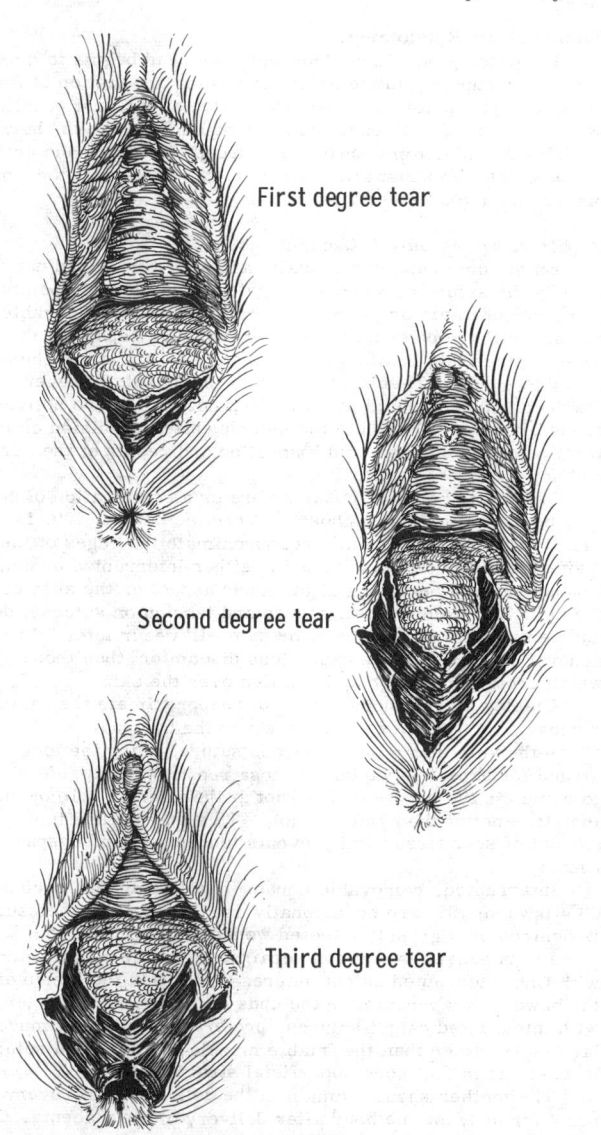

Fig 5-20. Perineal tears.

140 Episiotomy

Timing of the Episiotomy.

Episiotomy should be done when the head begins to distend the perineum, immediately preceding application of forceps, and just prior to breech extraction or internal podalic version. The slight reduction in blood loss which is achieved by delaying episiotomy until after forceps insertion and articulation is less important than a satisfactory application of the blades and a good episiotomy repair.

Repair of Episiotomy & Lacerations.

Episiotomy repair is actually a fascial repair and not merely the suture of muscle. Ligate freely bleeding points, using 000 chromic or plain catgut sutures. It is preferable to wait until the placenta is recovered before repairing the defect, since this limits blood loss and encourages the best possible surgical result. If speed is important, however, the deep sutures should be placed but not tied before delivery of the placenta. Complete the suturing after expulsion or extraction of the placenta and inspection and repair of the cervix and upper vaginal canal.

Interrupted or continuous suture or a combination of both may be used if catgut is chosen. Chromic catgut, 000, is usually selected. Carefully reapproximate the edges of the divided muscles and fascia, using either interrupted or continuous sutures beginning at the inner aspect or the apex of the defect. Avoid mass ligatures and tension on sutures; do not tie the sutures too tightly or pain will occur later. In general, buried sutures cause less discomfort than those which protrude through and are tied over the skin.

Employ a continuous suture to reapproximate the vaginal mucosa from the apex of the defect to the hymenal ring. Close the skin with a subcutaneous suture, using the long strand left from the vaginal mucosa repair. It is preferable to complete the repair with a knot at the inferior pole of the incision—not at the hymenal ring. This may reduce the amount of scar tissue and prevents tenderness and dyspareunia.

Interrupted, removable nonabsorbable sutures, such as 00 silkworm gut, are occasionally used when a rapid closure is desired or a grossly infected wound is to be repaired.

In 4th degree laceration repairs, close the rectal wall with fine interrupted catgut sutures tied within the lumen of the bowel. Reapproximate the ends of the rectal sphincter with interrupted catgut sutures, preferably in the perimuscular fascia rather than the friable muscle itself. Then suture lacerations in the more superficial structures.

The mother should remain in the delivery or recovery room for at least one hour after delivery of the placenta. Observe her vital signs and note her reactions. Record the blood pressure and the pulse rate and regularity every 15 minutes, or oftener if necessary.

Be alert to reports of severe perineal pain suggestive of hematoma formation. Consider a rapid pulse and increasing hypotension as evidence of impending shock, usually due to continued or excessive blood loss. Severe headache and hyperreflexia may precede eclampsia.

Support the uterine fundus, and massage it gently and frequently to maintain its firm contraction. Express clots occasionally and estimate blood loss.

Do not release any patient to ward or room care until her condition is sufficiently improved and stable to permit convalescent status.

USE OF OXYTOCICS

Oxytocics are employed after delivery to reduce blood loss and to prevent subinvolution of the uterus and the spread of endometritis. Two principal products are used: the ergot preparation and oxytocin (natural or synthetic).

Pitocin® or Syntocinon®, nearly pure oxytocin, is used in amounts of 0.5 ml (5 units of extract) with or immediately after delivery of the infant and repeated in the same dose following the recovery of the placenta (see p. 133). **Caution**: Never use pituitrin because it contains vasopressin, which is capable of causing sudden hypertension, coronary occlusion, and asthmatic crises.

Ergonovine maleate (Ergotrate®) or methylergonovine maleate (Methergine®), 0.2 mg I. M., may be given immediately after the placenta is delivered. **Caution**: Do not administer these drugs to patients with toxemia because of their pressor effect. Avoid intravenous administration (unless diluted in 50 ml or more of fluid) for fear of hypertensive reactions and cardiovascular accidents.

OUTLET FORCEPS
(Elective Outlet Forceps)

Outlet forceps are employed to extend the head and to guide the fetus beneath the symphysis and over the perineum. An outlet forceps is employed only when the vertex is on the perineum and extension is beginning.

Outlet forceps are used in the following circumstances: (1) When spontaneous expulsion is inhibited by analgesic or anesthetic drugs. Caudal or spinal anesthesia diminishes the patient's voluntary expulsive efforts. Outlet forceps are used in the majority of these cases. (2) When uterine inertia delays or prevents delivery of an infant whose vertex is distending the perineum. (3) When fetal distress is discovered during the late second stage. (4) When laceration of the introitus is likely. In such cases prophylactic episiotomy is also utilized.

142 Analgesia, Amnesia, Anesthesia

Caution: Outlet forceps, like other surgical devices, can be used safely only by the skilled operator. An experienced obstetrician can reduce fetal and maternal mortality and morbidity by outlet forceps delivery. In the hands of an inexperienced physician, the reverse will be true. The availability of outlet forceps delivery does not justify shortening the second stage by means of low- or midforceps extraction.

OBSTETRIC ANALGESIA, AMNESIA, & ANESTHESIA

Pain in childbirth is due to traction upon the adnexal, uterine, and cervical supports; pressure upon the ureters, bladder, urethra, and bowel; dilatation of the cervix and the lower birth canal; hypoxia and the accumulation of catabolites in the myometrium; and fear, severe tension, and anxiety. The type of pain reported may be an ache in the back or loins (referred pain, perhaps from the cervix), a cramp in the uterus (due to fundal contraction), or a "bursting" or "splitting" sensation in the distal genital canal or pudendum (due to dilatation of the cervix, vagina, and introitus).

Many patients are tense and apprehensive at the onset of labor, although there may be little or no discomfort.

Dystocia, usually quite painful, may be due to cephalopelvic disproportion; tetanic, prolonged, or dysrhythmic uterine contractions; intrapartal infection, and many other causes.

Hundreds of procedures and agents have been used to assuage pain in childbirth. Every method and drug used probably has some advantage, but a "perfect" method has not yet been discovered and probably will not be. The following types of pain relief are in use today: (1) positive conditioning of the patient; (2) hypnosis; (3) analgesics, which reduce the patient's pain threshold; (4) amnesics, which obscure the memory of pain and associated disagreeable experiences; (5) regional anesthesia, which interrupts afferent pain pathways; and (6) general anesthesia, which prevents central perception of discomfort. Some of these are useful in home as well as in hospital delivery. Others can be used only in maternity hospitals where equipment and specially trained professional personnel are available.

Types of Analgesics, Amnesics, & Anesthetics.*
A. Narcotic Analgesics: The commonly employed analgesics are narcotic drugs. Many are synthetic opium derivatives.

---

*Although many effective drugs and combination of drugs are available to obstetricians, the preferences at the author's institution are secobarbital as a sedative and meperidine (Demerol®) and trichloroethylene (Trilene®) as analgesics. Of the

Injectable narcotics are pharmacologically similar to morphine. In the usual doses they elevate the pain threshold by 50% or more; establish a state of relaxation, indifference, and euphoria or apathy; and induce lethargy and sleep. Most drugs in this group have a peak action in about 90 minutes and a duration of effect of at least 2-3 hours. Nausea, vomiting, cough suppression, intestinal stasis, and diminution in the frequency, intensity, and duration of uterine contractions in the early first stage of labor are common undesirable effects. Minimal or no amnesia is achieved.

B. Inhalant Analgesics: Most narcotics affect the fetus adversely by depressing all of its central nervous system functions, especially the activity of the respiratory center. Gestational age, weight, trauma, and long labor enhance the susceptibility of the fetus to narcosis.

Inhalant analgesics include trichloroethylene (Trilene®) and nitrous oxide. Both of these gases are nontoxic if given with adequate air or oxygen. Inhalators for the self-administration of these gas mixtures for brief periods during labor contractions are most useful and popular.

Do not prescribe morphine or comparable opiates to interrupt premature labor or for analgesia within 2 hours of delivery. The infant may die of asphyxia.

C. Sedatives (Hypnotics): The sedatives slow mentation, reduce perception of sensory stimuli, and increase receptivity to suggestion. They are poor analgesics and do not raise the pain threshold appreciably in conscious subjects. Amnesia does not occur. Labor may be slowed by large doses of sedatives, especially when they are given too early in the first stage.

Barbiturates are frequently given with, or before, a narcotic or other analgesic. Secobarbital, 0.1 gm, may be administered orally in early labor followed by meperidine or morphine when progress is more advanced. However, because serious fetal depression occurs, the barbiturates and narcotics should rarely be administered together.

The use of barbiturates alone for obstetric analgesia is not warranted because the required dosage is dangerous to the fetus, which is extremely sensitive to central nervous system depression by these drugs. Periodic

---

phenothiazine potentiators, one of the piperidine compounds (e.g., mepazine [Pacatal®] or thioridazine [Mellaril®]) is preferred. The amnesics are rarely used in our institution today. Regional anesthesia is often used, paracervical and pudendal or spinal anesthesia being the most favored types. Levallorphan (Lorfan®) is our choice of the narcotic antagonists.

apnea and even abolition of all movements outlast the effects of the barbiturates on the mother.

Paraldehyde is a reasonably safe and effective obstetric sedative-amnesic. Its disagreeable odor and taste may be disguised in the following "cocktail":

℞	Paraldehyde	20
	Port wine or syrup elixir	20
	Ice water, q.s. ad	60

This drink may be repeated every 2 hours as necessary, or the drug may be given rectally with an equal part of vegetable oil.

D. Amnesics: (**Note:** Although amnesia during labor and delivery may have technical advantages, there is also evidence that a woman who is "spared" recollection of her delivery experience may be harmed psychologically to the extent that she may reject her offspring.) The prototype of this group of drugs is scopolamine, which blots out memory astonishingly well. Unfortunately, this drug has no analgesic action and sometimes actually seems to lower the pain threshold. Furthermore, its effects are unpredictable: some patients become somnolent or stuporous; others restless, hallucinating, and delirious. For these reasons, combinations of drugs are used to enhance the desirable and minimize the undesirable effects. For example, synergistic analgesia and amnesia is achieved with meperidine and scopolamine, as follows: meperidine, 100 mg, and scopolamine hydrobromide, 0.6 mg, slowly I.V. when the cervix becomes 4 cm dilated. Repeat meperidine, 100 mg I.M., every 3 hours as necessary for pain, but give scopolamine, 0.6 mg, again in one hour and then 0.3 mg every 2 hours (by the clock) until the cervix is completely dilated. Variations in the metabolism of these drugs require such a program to maintain analgesia and amnesia.

It is usually the meperidine (or other additive), not the scopolamine, which delays the course of labor and depresses the fetus. The patient is completely uncooperative under adequate doses of scopolamine, however, and instrumental delivery is required.

E. Potentiating Drugs: Phenothiazine drugs potentiate certain of the desirable (as well as a few of the undesirable) effects of the analgesics, amnesics, and general anesthetics.

F. Inhalation Anesthetics: This group includes a number of potent agents which can often be used for major operative procedures.

The inhalants discussed with analgesic drugs are not used as general anesthetics because they are too dangerous to be used alone to induce deep surgical anesthesia.

Analgesia, Amnesia, Anesthesia 145

G. Thiobarbiturates: Intravenous anesthetics such as thiopental (Pentothal®) and thiamylal (Surital®) are widely employed in general surgery. However, in about 7 minutes after injection into the mother's vein the concentrations of the drug in the fetal and maternal blood will be equal. Even when a very rapid delivery is accomplished under thiopental anesthesia, for example, the baby may be so severely narcotized that it cannot be resuscitated. Intravenous anesthesia should therefore not be employed in obstetric delivery.

H. Regional Blocks: A needle guide called the "Iowa trumpet" Fig 5-21) is useful in pudendal and paracervical anesthetic blocks. A thumb ring with a trumpet-shaped opening facilitates the entry and direction of the needle. The standard Iowa trumpet is 5 1/2 inches long; a 6 1/2 inch 22-gauge spinal needle will protrude slightly beyond the guide.

1. Paracervical anesthesia - Paracervical anesthesia is administered when the cervix is 4 cm or more dilated. It relieves pain until the presenting part reaches the introitus, whereupon a pudendal and perineal block or other anesthetic procedure will be required. It is simple and effective and rarely disturbs the mother. The infant is not affected. Labor may be retarded briefly. Exceptional instances of sensitivity to the medication (tachycardia, syncope, convulsions) require supportive measures. A five- or six-inch needle with a guide or a lead shot affixed to it is used so that the point can be inserted 2 cm into the tissues. Inject 5 ml of a 2% aqueous solution of lidocaine (Xylocaine®) or other long-acting local anesthetic about 1-2 cm lateral to the cervix on both sides. If the presenting part is too far down to reach the lateral fornix easily, 5 ml injected as high as possible into the lateral vaginal wall will give considerable relief of discomfort during the second stage of labor.

2. Pudendal and perineal block - This permits spontaneous, breech, low, or even midforceps delivery with little or no pain. It is extremely safe, simple, and uncomplicated, and the patient maintains her ability to cooperate. The infant is not depressed, and blood loss is minimal. The disadvantages include regional discomfort during the injection and the five-minute wait necessary for the anesthetic to take effect. Knowledge of the nervous innervation of the lower birth canal is required for successful pudendal and perineal local anesthesia.

The 2 important nerves to be blocked on each side of the vagina are the pudendal and the posterior femoral cutaneous nerves. The pudendal nerve lies near the inner aspect of the ischial spine and should be blocked

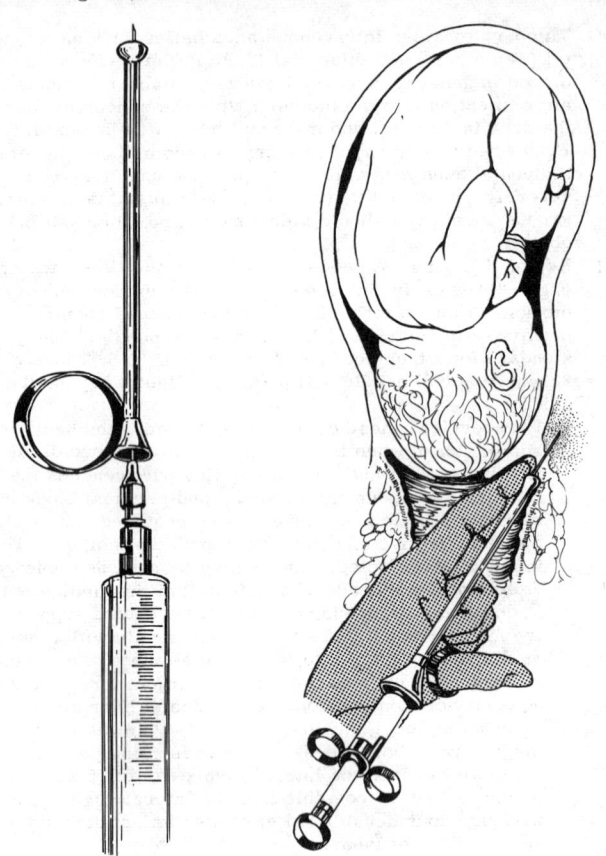

Fig 5-21. "Iowa trumpet" assembled.

Fig 5-22. Paracervical block.

there. The posterior femoral cutaneous nerve may be injected beneath the inferior medial border of the tuberosity of the ischium. The descending branches of the ilioinguinal nerve supply the clitoral region. The pudendum and the perirectal zone are innervated by the hemorrhoidal nerve. The procedure is as follows:
a. Develop a wheal of 0.5-1% procaine (or equivalent) at the base of each labium majus. Perform all injections through this site.

Analgesia, Amnesia, Anesthesia 147

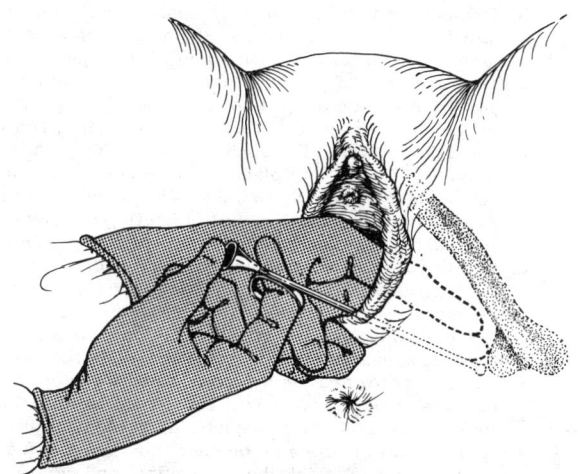

Needle guide in place on ischial spine

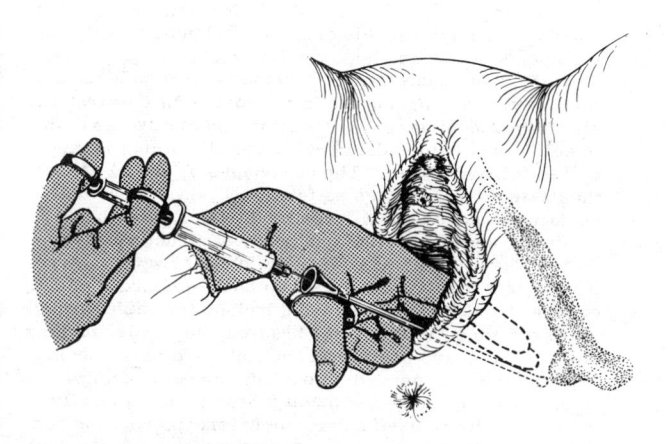

Needle inserted through needle guide

Fig 5-23. Use of needle guide ("Iowa trumpet") in pudendal anesthetic block.

b. Palpate the ischial spines vaginally (or rectally). Slowly guide a four- or five-inch, 20- or 21-gauge spinal needle toward each spine while injecting a small amount of procaine ahead of the advancing point. Aspirate and, if not in a vessel, deposit 5 ml below each spine. This blocks the right and left pudendal nerves. Refill the syringe when necessary, leaving the needle in place, and proceed in a similar manner to anesthetize the other areas specified. Keep the needle moving while injecting and avoid the vaginal mucosa and periosteum (which are sensitive).
c. Withdraw the needle about 3 cm and redirect it toward an ischial tuberosity. Inject 3 ml near the center of each tuberosity to anesthetize the inferior hemorrhoidal and lateral femoral cutaneous nerves.
d. Withdraw the needle almost entirely and then slowly advance it toward the symphysis pubis almost to the clitoris, keeping it about 2 cm lateral to the labial fold and about 1-2 cm beneath the skin. The injection of 5 ml of procaine on each side beneath the symphysis will block the ilioinguinal and genitocrural nerves.

If the above procedure is unhurried and skillfully done, there will be slight discomfort during injections only. Prompt flaccid relaxation and good anesthesia for one-half to one hour can be expected.

I. Caudal Anesthesia: Caudal anesthesia may be given continuously, i.e., during the latter portion of the first and all of the second stage of labor; or terminally, as a single injection just before delivery. Special training is required for both types. The advantages of caudal anesthesia are that it causes no fetal asphyxia, the mother remains conscious to witness the birth, blood loss is minimal, and the vaginal and perineal structures are quite relaxed. The technic is difficult, however, and inadvertent massive (high) spinal anesthesia occasionally occurs. Undesirable reactions include the rapid absorption syndrome (hypotension, bradycardia, hallucinations, convulsions), and postpartal backacke and paresthesia. The incidence of persistent occiput posterior positions is increased because the infant's head is not normally rotated on the relaxed pelvic floor; forceps rotation and delivery is therefore more often necessary. A considerable quantity of anesthetic agent must be injected: 35 ml of 1.5% piperocaine (Metycaine®) or equivalent.

The procedure is as follows: Inject 8 ml of a 1.5% aqueous solution of piperocaine (Metycaine®), or a similar agent, into the caudal canal as a test dose. If spinal anesthesia does not result after 10 minutes, assume that the solution was injected extradurally. Inject 30-35 ml of the anesthetic solution slowly to accomplish an adequate degree and suitable level of caudal anesthesia. This constitutes a single injection for terminal caudal anesthesia. A special caudal catheter or malleable caudal needle should be inserted and left in the caudal canal for continuous caudal anesthesia. Injections of 15-35 ml are required every 2-3 hours, depending upon the need.

J. Spinal Anesthesia: Spinal anesthesia is widely employed not only to alleviate the pain of delivery but also to relieve pain during the late first and entire second stages of labor. Short-acting agents are employed in the first instance; more potent and long-acting drugs are necessary in the second. Brief or minimal spinal anesthesia is far safer than prolonged spinal anesthesia, which is not recommended for obstetric use. The advantages of spinal anesthesia are that no fetal hypoxia occurs, blood loss is minimal, the mother remains conscious to witness delivery, no inhalation anesthetics or analgesic drugs are required, the technic is not difficult, and good relaxation of the pelvic floor and lower birth canal is achieved. Prompt anesthesia is achieved within 5-10 minutes, and there are fewer failures than with caudal anesthesia. The dosage of spinal anesthetic is small. Complications are fewer and easier to treat. Hypotension is rare with these doses. Spinal headache occurs in 5-10% of patients, however, and operative delivery is more often required because voluntary expulsive efforts are eliminated. Drug reactions (e.g., hypotension) may occur. Respiratory failure may occur if the anesthetic ascends within the spinal cord as a result of rapid injection or straining by the patient.

The procedure is as follows:

1. Inject 40 mg of procaine (0.8 ml of a 5% solution) or 20 mg of piperocaine (Metycaine®) (4 ml of a 0.5% solution), or comparable drug, slowly into the third or 4th lumbar interspace between contractions. Have the patient lying on her side or sitting up. Elevate her head on a pillow immediately after the injection. Tilt the table up or down to achieve a level of anesthesia at or near the umbilicus. Anesthesia will be maximal in 10-15 minutes and will last for one hour or longer.

2. Obtain and record the blood pressure and the respirations every 10-15 minutes.

3. Give oxygen for respiratory depression and mild hypotension. In addition, administer vasopressors such as ephedrine, 25 mg I.V., if a marked fall in blood pressure occurs.

General Comments & Precautions.

A. If the patient is prepared psychologically for her experience she will require far less medication. Anticipate and dispel her fears during the antenatal period and in early labor. Never promise a painless labor.
B. Nurse anesthetists, trained by and working under the close supervision of physician anesthesiologists, generally function very well in obstetrics. They must be thoroughly indoctrinated regarding obstetric problems and must be capable of functioning efficiently whenever emergency resuscitation is required. Although nurse anesthetists are commonly restricted from instituting regional anesthetics because of legal liabilities, they are usually permitted to administer inhalation or parenteral analgesia and anesthesia.
C. Individualize the treatment of every patient, because each one reacts differently. Unfavorable reactions occur to all drugs.
D. Always think in terms of normal maternal-fetal physiology rather than the requests of the patient and her family. The overly-demanding patient and the yielding physician are a perfect combination for tragedy.
E. Know the drug you intend to administer. Be familiar with its limitations, dangers, and contraindications as well as its advantages.
F. Do not render the patient unconscious in the first stage of labor. Some pain relief may be desirable, and relaxation may speed labor; but total amnesia and analgesia may be detrimental to the mother and her infant. Mild degrees of fetal asphyxia are not easily discernible but are often harmful.
G. Avoid injections in an area of skin infection.
H. Spinal, caudal, and other anesthetic blocks are surgical procedures requiring scrupulous preparation and aseptic technic.

Treatment of Complications.

A. If labor terminates earlier than planned, a narcotic antagonist may reverse the depressive effect of an opiate but, unfortunately, will intensify the barbiturate effect.
B. Resuscitation of the Mother: Most anesthetic deaths are the result of 2 successive misfortunes: (1) a potentially lethal dose is given, and (2) successful resuscitation is not accomplished.
  1. Establish a patent airway (hyperextend the head; if necessary, insert a tracheal tube).
  2. Aspirate mucus, blood, vomitus, etc, with tracheal suction. Utilize a laryngoscope for direct visualization of air passages.

3. Administer oxygen by artificial respiration if respirations are absent or weak. If high spinal anesthesia has occurred, continue to "breathe" for the patient until paralysis of the diaphragm has dissipated.
4. Give antihistamines intravenously (e.g., diphenhydramine, 15-25 mg) and oxygen by mask for drug sensitivity.
5. Give vasopressors intravenously (e.g., methoxamine, 10 mg, or ephedrine, 25 mg). Place the patient in Trendelenburg's position and give plasma, plasma expanders, and blood transfusion for traumatic or hemorrhagic shock.
6. Specifically treat cardiac arrhythmias, arrest, failure, etc, if a heart disorder is the basic problem.

C. Resuscitation of the newborn is discussed on p. 158.

Prognosis.

Excellent for mother and infant when physician anesthesiologists and obstetricians work as a team, and a 24-hour anesthesiology service is available.

INDUCTION OF LABOR

Induction of labor by medical or surgical means should be performed only upon specific indications. Elective induction or induction for minor or controversial reasons ("meddlesome obstetrics") often increases maternal and fetal mortality and morbidity. Fundamentally, the decision to induce labor implies that the problem is so serious that the patient should be delivered within 24 hours and termination of pregnancy should be pursued by all available means until the fetus is delivered successfully. This means that if labor cannot be induced easily by relatively safe procedures, a more dangerous procedure will be required. Unless the reason for inducing labor in the first place was a logical and acceptable one, the physician risks the accusation of malpractice or, at best, bad professional judgment for having started on a course which led him and his patient into avoidable difficulties. X-ray studies (pelvimetry, fetometry, fetal ossification centers) are useful before elective induction.

Indications.

Indicated induction of labor, especially in the treatment of abnormal pregnancy (toxemia, pyelonephritis), usually reduces maternal and fetal mortality and morbidity. The following indications for induction of labor are valid in 5-8% of pregnancies.
A. Maternal infections (pyelonephritis, diverticulitis), which often fail to resolve and are likely to become more severe unless pregnancy is interrupted.

152 Induction of Labor

B. Uterine bleeding with partial placental separation or partial placenta previa.
C. Toxemia of pregnancy which is unresponsive or only temporarily responsive to therapy.
D. Diabetes mellitus.
E. Renal insufficiency.
F. Premature rupture of the membranes after the 37th week.
G. Previous precipitate delivery in a woman who cannot be transported quickly to a hospital.
H. Marked polyhydramnios.
I. Placental insufficiency.
J. Isoimmunization (erythroblastosis).

Contraindications.
A. Cephalopelvic disproportion.
B. A floating or deflected vertex, or an unfavorable presentation (including breech and multiple pregnancy).
C. A firm, closed, uneffaced posterior cervix. (A vaginal examination must be performed before induction so that "ripeness" of the cervix can be confirmed.)
D. Previous cesarean section or extensive myomectomy.
E. Maternal cardiac disease (functional class III or IV).

Dangers of Induction of Labor.
A. For the Mother: In many cases induction of labor exposes the mother to more distress and discomfort than judicious delay and subsequent vaginal or cesarean delivery. The following hazards must be borne in mind:
 1. Emotional crisis (fear and anxiety).
 2. Failure of induction and subsequent attempts to institute labor or to deliver the fetus.
 3. Uterine inertia and prolonged labor.
 4. Tumultuous labor and titanic contractions of the uterus, causing premature separation of the placenta, rupture of the uterus, and laceration of the cervix.
 5. Intrauterine infection.
 6. Postpartal hemorrhage.
 7. Hypofibrinogenemia.
B. For the Fetus: An induced delivery exposes the infant to the risks of prematurity if the EDC has been inaccurately calculated. Violent labor or trauma in delivery may result in damage due to hypoxia or physical injury. Prolapse of the cord and infection may follow amniotomy.

Methods of Induction.
A. Medical:
 1. Oxytocin - Parenteral administration of a very dilute solution of oxytocin is the most effective medical means of inducing labor. (**Note**: Ergot preparations cause sustained contractions and must not be used before de-

livery for any reason. Posterior pituitary extract [Pituitrin®] should never be used because of the vasoconstricting and antidiuretic effect of the vasopressin which it contains.) Oxytocin exaggerates the inherent rhythmic pattern of uterine motility, which often becomes clinically evident during the last trimester and increases as term is approached.

The dosage of oxytocin must be individualized. The administration of oxytocin is really a biologic assay: the smallest possible effective dose must be determined and then utilized for each patient to initiate labor.

Note: Constant observation by the physician himself is required if this method is used.

The intravenous route is preferred. (Intramuscular administration of oxytocics is too dangerous.) Oxytocin (Pitocin®, Syntocinon®), 0.5 ml, is mixed with 250 ml of 5% dextrose in water and administered slowly by I. V. drip (20-40 drops/minute) until regular, forceful, sustained contractions begin, whereupon the drip is discontinued. If labor does not begin after 250 ml of this solution have been administered, further attempts to induce labor should be abandoned for 24 hours. If contractions cease or become weak and ineffectual after a satisfactory start, the infusion may be resumed.

2. Reflex hyperactivity of the uterus occurs after intestinal and ureteral hyperactivity. (Patients with colitis or pyelonephritis complicating pregnancy often develop uterine contractions which lead to premature labor.) This is the basis for the use of enemas and purges for the induction of labor, but this method is often unsuccessful and is not recommended.

B. Surgical:
1. Amniotomy is the easiest and surest way to induce labor. Release of amniotic fluid shortens the muscle bundles of the myometrium; the strength and duration of the contractions are thereby increased and a more rapid contraction sequence follows. Amniotomy causes few complications and is not painful.

The membranes should be ruptured at the internal os with a hook or other sharp instrument. Make no effort to strip the membranes, and do not displace the head upward to drain off amniotic fluid. Keep the patient in bed in Fowler's position after amniotomy so that drainage of fluid can occur. Anticipate labor within 6 hours if the patient is at term.

2. Drainage of the hindwaters with a Drew-Smythe S-shaped metal catheter is an effective induction technic. Several pints or more of amniotic fluid may be drawn off without releasing the forewaters and without seri-

ously dislodging the presenting part. A breech presentation can often be accommodated in this way. Cautious insertion of the catheter is required to avoid the placenta and to prevent perforation of the uterine wall.
3. Stripping of the membranes (alone) is not recommended since it is unpredictable, increases maternal morbidity, may lead to bleeding from a low-lying placenta, may cause rupture of the membranes and prolapse of the cord with a high presenting part, and is painful.
4. A bougie or Voorhees bag inserted through the cervix into the uterus is a foreign body which causes the uterus to contract to expel it along with the uterine contents. This method is not recommended since it displaces the presenting part, is traumatic to the cervix, and increases the risks of infection.
5. Transuterine injection of hypertonic (irritating) solutions into the amniotic cavity is unnecessarily dangerous for the fetus and is not sanctioned for induction of labor except after death in utero.

• • •

"NATURAL CHILDBIRTH"

In modern obstetrics numerous procedures and drugs are used for the purpose of reducing discomfort and shortening labor. These technics range from elective induction of labor to continuous conduction analgesia-anesthesia and prophylactic forceps delivery. Admittedly, over-enthusiastic or ill-advised use of such methods may complicate parturition and, perhaps, "cheat" the mother of the satisfaction to be gained from a significant natural experience. For these reasons, Grantly Dick Read postulated that fear results in tension which, in turn, causes pain, and that this can retard and intensify the discomforts of labor and delivery. Adequate knowledge about the mechanics of childbirth, emotional and physical preparation, and the confidence thus gained will often reduce pain and tension. Read urged the abandonment of "meddlesome midwifery" and a return to supportive therapy based upon good doctor-patient rapport and positive psychologic and physical conditioning of the patient. Good antenatal care is implied, and suitable pain relief is given when necessary even though the patient is encouraged to rely largely upon her own resources. Read's precepts are sound and should continue to receive the respectful attention of the profession. However, so many individual variations and interpretations of these concepts have evolved that exactly what is meant by the term "natural childbirth" must always be carefully defined by the patient or physician using it.

6...
The Full-Term Infant

NURSERY CARE OF THE NEWBORN

Immediate Care.
- A. Place the infant supine on a flat surface or with the head slightly lowered in a heated crib. Avoid contamination. Irrigate the eyes with sterile normal saline solution. Administer vitamin K, 1 mg I. M., if the mother has not received vitamin K during labor or as a dietary supplement.
- B. Observation: Aspirate mucus with a suction tube. Maintain the infant in a slightly head-down position for evacuation of fluid from the nose and throat. Examine the cord tie (or clamp) occasionally and retie or reclamp if oozing occurs.

  Record the infant's temperature every hour until the temperature has stabilized. Maintain the crib temperature at 75-78° F (24-25.5° C) or higher if the infant's temperature does not remain within the normal range.

  Record the time, relative amount, and character of urine and feces passed.

Fluid & Food.
- A. Do not feed the infant or offer water for 12 hours. Then give 5% carbohydrate solution according to the hospital schedule (every 3-4 hours). If the mother is a rooming-in patient, feedings may be on demand.
- B. After 24 hours, begin periodic breast or formula feeding.

Skin Care & Bathing.
- A. Wipe away excess vernix. Cleanse the skin daily (and when soiling occurs) with moist gauze dipped in liberal amounts of a hexachlorophene preparation such as pHisohex®. Allow some of the cream to remain on the skin as a bacteriostatic unction. Do not bathe the baby for at least 4-5 days.
- B. Routine application of antiseptic preparations should be avoided because of the danger of irritation or sensitization. Powders and oils are usually not necessary.

Medications.

Consider prophylactic antibiotic therapy in the following circumstances:
- A. If the membranes had been ruptured for over 24 hours before delivery (especially when frozen section of the cord reveals vasculitis or when clinical antepartal amnionitis is likely).
- B. If laryngoscopy, intratracheal intubation, or prolonged resuscitation was required, or if the infant has severe respiratory distress.
- C. When the stomach aspirate contains considerable numbers of bacteria at birth.

ASPHYXIA NEONATORUM & RESUSCITATION

Most babies breathe in less than one minute after birth. Those who do not react within 1-2 minutes, for whatever cause, will develop asphyxia. Asphyxia may cause neurologic deficits, e.g., cerebral palsy, mental retardation, or epilepsy, or death will occur in uncorrected cases.

Etiology.

Asphyxia of the newborn may be due to maternal, fetal (or neonatal), placental, or cord disorders:
- A. Maternal Disorders: Marked anemia, severe toxemia of pregnancy, uterine tetany, severe hypotension and shock, hemorrhage.
- B. Fetal or Neonatal Disorders: Central nervous system disorders (cysts and tumors), pulmonary hypoplasia, congenital cardiovascular anomalies; depression of respiratory center during labor and delivery due to maternal analgesics, general anesthetics, intrauterine hemorrhage, shock from traumatic delivery; obstructed airway (mucus, blood); erythroblastosis fetalis, syphilis.
- C. Placental and Umbilical Disorders: Hydatidiform mole, intervillous fibrin deposition, infarction; hemorrhage due to premature separation, placenta previa, laceration of placenta; cord occlusion due to entwinement or true knot with compression, angulation of cord, prolapse and obstruction of the cord.

Appraisal of the Newborn.

The following factors are evaluated one minute after complete delivery of the infant and again at 2 and 5 minutes unless the infant is severely depressed at birth, in which case he should be observed constantly. The degree of response in each category is recorded as 0, 1, or 2.

Heart rate: None to 100+/minute.
Respiratory effort: None to loud crying.

Table 6-1. Apgar score of newborn infant.

	Score 0	Score 1	Score 2
A Appearance (color)	Blue, pale	Body pink; extremities blue	Completely pink
P Pulse (heart rate)	Absent	Below 100	Over 100
G Grimace (reflex irritability in response to stimulation of sole of foot)	No response	Grimace	Cry
A Activity (muscle tone)	Limp	Some flexion of extremities	Active motion
R Respiration (respiratory effort)	Absent	Slow, irregular	Strong cry

Muscle tone: Flaccidity to vigorous movements.
Reflex irritability: None to cough or sneeze (with stimulation of catheter passed into the nasal pharynx).
Skin color: Pale, cyanotic, or pink.

A rating of 10 indicates an infant in the best possible condition, but this is rarely achieved because slight peripheral cyanosis is present in most newborns.

Clinical Classification of Depressed Infants (Apgar).

Severely depressed = Apgar 0-3
Moderately depressed = Apgar 4-6 (good heartbeat but slightly pallid or cyanotic; gasping or shallow breathing)
Normal or slightly depressed = Apgar 7-9
"Perfect" infant score = Apgar 10, an uncommon rating even in the mature infant spontaneously delivered.

Eight or 9 out of 10 normal infants will score 7 or above at birth.
Babies with Apgar scores of 6 or above usually do not require immediate treatment.
The Apgar rating at birth should be made a part of the permanent health record.

Prevention of Asphyxia.

Prolonged hypoxia during or after delivery is almost always associated with central nervous system damage. Expert obstetric management and skillful handling of the asphyxiated newborn infant will minimize the incidence of permanent neurologic sequelae due to hypoxia.

Avoid giving large, frequent doses of analgesics to the woman in labor, especially within one hour of delivery. Curtail sharply all medications for relief of pain in premature labor or when operative obstetrics is likely. Use conduction anesthesia, especially pudendal and paracervical block, whenever possible.

High pressure insufflation of air or oxygen and inept instrumentation should be avoided since they may cause emphysema, pneumothorax, or pneumomediastinum.

Rectal stimulation, "jack-knifing" the infant in an attempt at artificial respiration, and hot and cold tub baths should never be used to resuscitate the newborn.

Resuscitation of the Newborn.

A pediatrician, anesthesiologist, or other person skilled in resuscitation should be present if operative delivery, premature birth, or a serious obstetric problem is anticipated. Efficient gentle management of the infant in the delivery room is essential.

The following equipment should be on hand in every delivery room for emergency use:

 Oxygen source with pressure-reducing valve system and hydration attachment.
 Assorted infant masks with connective tubing.
 Sterilized Rausch two-hole catheter with DeLee suction trap attached.
 Infant laryngoscope with blades for premature and term infants.
 Dry-sterilized Cole endotracheal tubes (sizes 10, 12, 14).
 Plastic pharyngeal airways in assorted sizes (00, 0, 1).
 Safar double mouthpiece for insufflation.
 Soft rubber bulb syringe for aspiration.
 Stethoscope (chained to the bassinet or incubator to prevent misplacement).

A. Emergency Treatment:
 1. Severely depressed infant (Apgar 0-3) - Support the infant in the head-down position to drain amniotic fluid, blood, and mucus from the nasopharynx. Gently aspirate the infant's nose and throat with a small, soft rubber catheter attached to a DeLee mucus trap. Avoid rough handling; keep the infant warm. If meconium has been passed in utero or if thick viscid mucus is difficult to aspirate, perform direct laryngoscopy.

    If the heartbeat cannot be heard, begin external cardiac massage by applying moderate finger pressure over the midsternum (depress the sternum about 2 cm) 30-40 times a minute. Follow with laryngoscopy (see below) and oxygen therapy.

 2. Moderately depressed infant (Apgar 4-6) - Support the infant, aspirate the nose and throat, handle gently, and

Asphyxia Neonatorum & Resuscitation 159

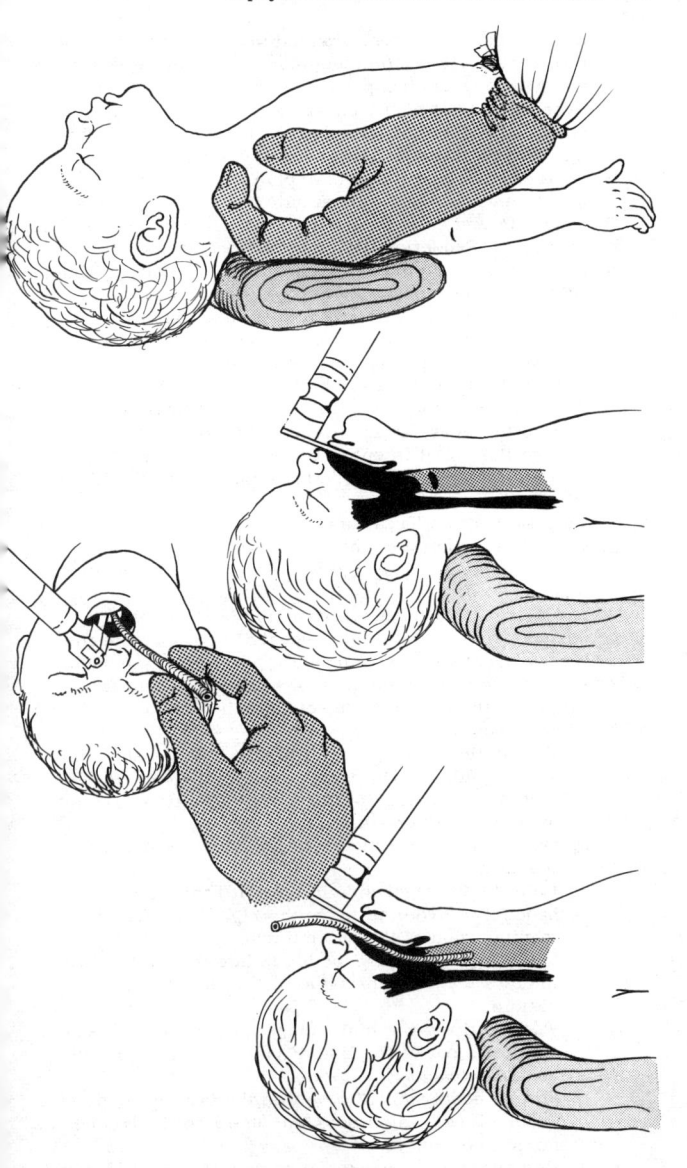

Fig 6-1. Resuscitation of the newborn.

keep warm, as above. Extend the neck and insert a pharyngeal airway (see below). Apply an oxygen mask and give oxygen at a pressure of 15-20 cm of water. Note movement of the chest wall, heart rate, and skin color. Continue oxygen therapy until breathing is normal and the heart rate is over 110/minute.

B. General Measures: Delay clamping the cord in most instances until it ceases to pulsate. Allow fetal blood in the placenta and cord to flow into the newborn circulation by gravity. (**Exception**: Clamp the cord at once if the infant is premature or immature; if he is behaving abnormally though apparently not asphyxiated ["distressed infant"]; or if erythroblastosis fetalis is a possibility.) Transfer the infant to a warmed incubator, bassinet, or crib. Have an assistant determine the Apgar rating at one, 2, and 5 minutes after birth.

Tie and dress the cord, instill silver nitrate or penicillin into the eyes, apply an identification bracelet, etc, only when the infant is out of danger. Observe every infant closely for at least one hour for signs of cardiorespiratory distress.

C. Special Methods of Treatment:
  1. Laryngeal intubation and aspiration - Utilize in instances of meconium passage in utero or if thick viscid mucus is difficult to aspirate; if depression (asphyxia) is severe; if pulmonary expansion is incomplete or unequal; or if persistent, repeated retraction of the thorax occurs in the immediate postdelivery period.
  2. Prepare for transfusion or blood replacement for infants with serious erythroblastosis fetalis.
  3. Laryngoscopy -
     a. Extend the neck by elevating the infant's shoulders with a folded towel or by allowing the head to extend over the edge of the table. (**Caution**: Do not overextend the neck.)
     b. Open the infant's mouth by applying pressure on the chin.
     c. Hold the laryngoscope in the left hand (if right-handed) in order to leave the right hand free for manipulation of the suction tube.
     d. Insert the laryngoscope blade into the angle of the infant's mouth; center the blade when the glottis is visible.
     e. Tilt the tip of the instrument upward to raise the epiglottis out of the line of vision. This will expose the trachea.
     f. Slip an endotracheal tube into the laryngoscope slot; under direct vision pass the tube into the trachea as far as the flange.
     g. Remove the laryngoscope carefully so as to leave the endotracheal tube in place.

    h. Gently aspirate any free fluid or mucus.
    i. Direct short puffs of hydrated oxygen into the tube (at a pressure of 15-20 cm of water for one second, 10-15 times/minute). If the chest wall rises, the lungs are inflating. Check heart action by auscultation. If the thorax does not move, the tube may be plugged or in the esophagus. Continue regular, brief insufflations until spontaneous breathing occurs and a heart rate of greater than 110/minute is achieved.
4. Mouth-to-mouth breathing - Aspirate fluid and insert a pharyngeal airway or Safar mouthpiece. By cheek action, gently blow a small quantity of **mouth** air (never air exhaled from the lungs) into the child's air passages (mouth and nose) 10-15 times/minute. Allow time for release of air between puffs.
5. Consultation and x-rays - When depression persists despite the above measures, secure further consultation and obtain an x-ray of the chest to note the expansion of the lungs, congenital anomalies, or pneumothorax.
6. Aspirate the stomach (**after** resuscitation) if the infant was delivered by cesarean section, if placental insufficiency is a possibility (see p. 65), or if the abdomen is markedly distended or the infant chokes repeatedly. (**Caution:** Do not aspirate the stomach of a small premature infant under any circumstances; little fluid will be present and the danger of trauma is great.) Apply suction through a No. 10 or No. 12 Rausch or other soft rubber catheter with a DeLee mucus trap attached. Use slight epigastric pressure.

    Suspect intestinal atresia or tracheo-esophageal fistula when obstruction to the catheter is met or when the aspirate is 30 ml or more.
7. Transfusion - For pallid infants who have probably lost blood as a result of laceration or cord injury, promptly give a transfusion of whole blood (type O, Rh-negative) into the umbilical vein. Do not wait for a crossmatch.
8. Drugs -
    a. Narcotic antagonists - Administer opiate antagonists such as levallorphan (Lorfan®), 0.05 mg, or nalorphine (Nalline®), 0.1-0.2 mg, I.V. or I.M., to combat the effect of narcotics. (**Caution:** Do not give these drugs if barbiturates have been given or the infant will become more depressed.)
    b. Inject epinephrine, 1:1000 aqueous solution, 0.15 ml, into the umbilical vein in moderately asphyxiated infants, or directly into the heart through the 4th interspace to the left of the sternum if the baby is severely asphyxiated.

162 Full-Term Infant

    c. Inject 10 ml of 10% glucose solution in water into the umbilical vein in instances of severe anoxia.
    d. Respiratory stimulants are of no value in initiating breathing. Caffeine and sodium benzoate, 6-10 mg/kg into the umbilical vein or I. M., may stimulate the baby once breathing begins.
    e. Administer antibiotics to the newborn when severe intrapartal infection occurs or when prolonged, difficult resuscitation is required. Procaine penicillin G, 20,000 units/lb, and streptomycin, 5 mg/lb, given daily in 2 doses for 3-4 days, are usually effective.

Prognosis.

Prognosis depends upon the mother's health, complications of labor and delivery, the maturity and condition of the newborn, and the success of resuscitation.

Infants scoring 7 or above on the Apgar scale will probably not suffer from the effects of hypoxia. Those with scores of 0-6 may develop temporary or permanent central nervous system damage depending upon the severity and duration of oxygen lack.

EXAMINATION OF THE FULL-TERM INFANT

The Infant at Birth.
A. Position After Delivery: Attitude is determined largely by the infant's presentation in utero. Babies which presented by the vertex tend to assume the flexed "fetal position"; those delivered after face presentation maintain the extended head; breech babies extend the legs.
B. Skin:
    1. Vernix caseosa—a white, creamy material composed of sebaceous secretions, exfoliated cells, and lanugo—covers the skin of most infants.
    2. Slight initial cyanosis is common. With adequate oxygenation and normal cardiopulmonary function, the skin becomes ruddy within moments after birth, although the extremities may remain dusky or mottled for several hours.
    3. The skin is usually dry, with superficial cracks, especially in the folds of the body and over the hands and feet.
    4. Milia—distended sebaceous glands—appear over the forehead, nose, and sides of the face as minute unpigmented papules.
    5. Lanugo or downy hair is often scattered over parts of the face, back, and extremities.
    6. Petechiae, erythematous patches, and even frank port wine spots (birthmarks) may be present, with a pre-

Full-Term Infant 163

    dilection for the face, the nape of the neck, and the scalp.
- 7. Abrasions, contusions, and forceps impressions represent delivery trauma.

C. Head:
1. The head is obviously large in proportion to the body. "Molding" and even slight overlapping of the cranium may be noted in babies presenting by the vertex, especially after a difficult operative delivery. Nevertheless, the largest diameters of the infant are those of the skull. Two frontal, parietal, and temporal bones, one occipital bone, and the wings of the sphenoid bones compose the cranium. Only the bones of the base of the skull are firmly joined at term.
2. Caput succedaneum is a soft swelling of the scalp, sometimes ecchymotic, which represents the actual site of presentation at the cervix. A comparable edematous zone may develop over the sacrum or one buttock in complete breech presentation.
3. Craniotabes, or thinning of the bones of the vault of the skull, is common and usually not significant.
4. Cephalhematoma - Blood between periosteum and skull which does not cross suture line. Needs no treatment.
5. In striking contrast with that of the adult, the infant's face is much smaller than its cranium.
6. Wide, unossified, slightly depressed areas over the cranium are termed fontanels. These are mainly at the juncture of the principal bones of the vault. The frontal or large fontanel is between the parietal and frontal bones; the occipital, small, or posterior fontanel is at the point of convergence of the 2 parietal and the single occipital bones. There are also 2 mastoid and 2 sphenoid fontanels, but these are smaller and are unimportant obstetrically. The fontanels are small and slightly depressed at birth. If they are wide and full, suspect increased intracranial pressure.
7. The fibrous unions between the bones of the head are called cranial sutures. The principal sutures are easily palpable: The coronal suture lies between the frontal and parietal bones in the anterior portion of the skull; the sagittal suture lies between the parietal bones extending from the frontal bone to the occiput. These sutures cause the anterior fontanel to be diamond-shaped and the posterior fontanel triangular.
8. The major diameters of the cranium: (See Fig 6-2.)
   a. The occipitofrontal (OF) diameter is the distance from the prominence of the occipital bone to the frontal bone at the base of the nose. Average normal: 11.75 cm.
   b. The biparietal (BP) diameter is the distance between the parietal bones at the widest point. It represents

164 Full-Term Infant

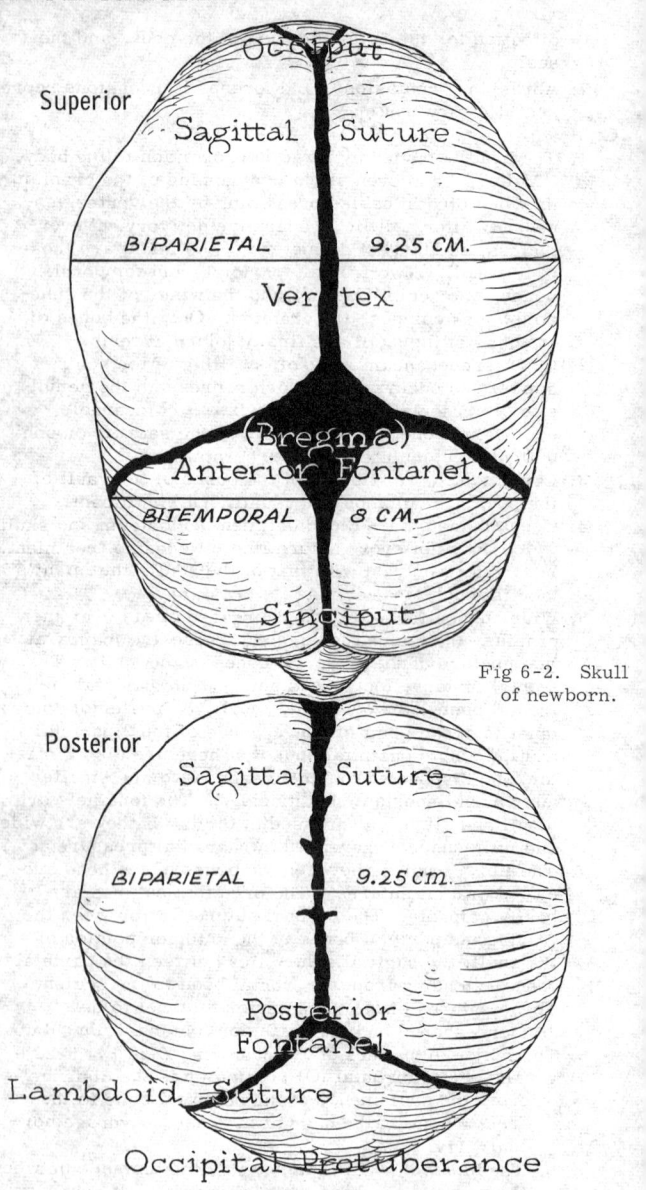

Fig 6-2. Skull of newborn.

Full-Term Infant 165

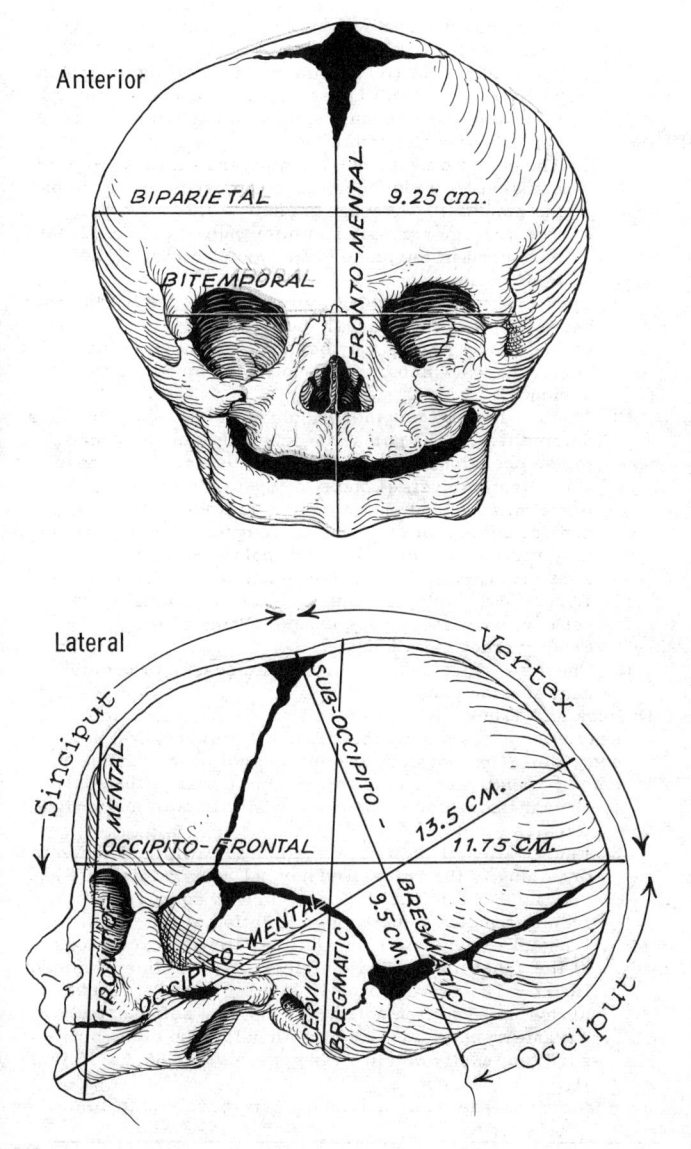

Fig 6-2. Skull of newborn (cont'd.).

the greatest transverse diameter of the head. Average normal: 9.25 cm.
   c. The bitemporal (BT) diameter is the greatest distance between the frontal bones and is measured from the midpoint of the coronal suture on each side of the head. Average normal: 8 cm.
   d. The occipitomental (OM) diameter is a linear dimension from the occipital prominence to the tip of the mandible. Average normal: 13.5 cm.
   e. The average normal circumference of the head, measured in the plane of the occipitofrontal diameter, is 34.5 cm.
 9. Eyes - The iris is blue-gray in white babies but blue-brown in pigmented races. Subconjunctival and even retinal hemorrhages may be noted. Minute retinal hemorrhages which do not involve the macula are not serious.
 10. Mouth - Harelip or other nasolabial defects are obvious deformities. The gums are generally smooth except for an occasional small papule at the margin. These are retention cysts (Bohn's or Epstein's pearls). A few similar elevations may also be present over the central portion of the palate. Tonguetie (short frenulum) may restrict the tongue. Cleft palate is often associated with harelip or other head and neck anomalies.
 11. Ears - Maldevelopment of the ears or unusually low-set ears may accompany abnormalities of the genitourinary tract in both sexes.
 12. Cheeks - The cheeks are rounded because of prominent sucking pads.
D. Neck and Trunk: At birth the neck is very short; the head almost rests upon the infant's shoulders, which are not wide. The thorax is narrow and not deep, but the trunk is relatively long in proportion to that of the adult.
 1. Breast tissue can be palpated easily in both males and females.
 2. Lungs - Respirations are shallow at first, and abdominal breathing is the rule. The normal respiratory rate at rest is 38-44/minute. Coarse breath sounds and harsh fremitus indicate incomplete inflation of the lungs. Unequal expansion or persistently limited excursions of the chest may indicate atelectasis or maldevelopment.
 3. Heart - The average rate is 120-140/minute. Sinus arrhythmia is often noted. Transient, soft murmurs without transmission are functional. The blood pressure (not easily obtained) is generally 80-85/50-55 mm Hg.
E. Abdomen*: The liver and kidneys are barely palpable.

---

*For Umbilicus, see p. 127.

Occasionally the experienced examiner will feel the tip of the spleen in a normal infant.
F. Genitalia: In the male the prepuce is long and completely covers the glans, to which it is adherent. The testes are usually within the scrotum at term. In the female the labia minora are prominent. A whitish mucoid discharge may be noted at the introitus.
G. Anus: The anus should be patent and the rectal sphincter competent at birth.
H. Extremities:
 1. The arms are relatively longer than the legs in comparison with adults. Subcutaneous fat over the extremities obscures the musculature.
 2. The fingers and toes are short. The feet are stubby. Talipes or clubfoot must be distinguished from mere relaxed flexion.
I. Reflexes: The following reflexes are normally present in the newborn: grasping, sucking, rooting, Moro, Chvostek, Babinski, tonic neck, deep tendon, abdominal, and cremasteric.
J. Temperature: The mature newborn's temperature ranges between 98-99°F (36.7-37.1 C); the premature's temperature is usually 1°, and often 3-4°, lower.
K. Weight: Male infants outweigh females. Caucasian newborns weigh more than those of the darker races; second and subsequent infants are often heavier at birth than the firstborn.
L. X-Ray Determination of Ossification Centers:
 1. At birth the average full-term infant has 5 ossification centers demonstrable by x-ray: distal end of femur, proximal end of tibia, calcaneus, talus, and cuboid.
 2. The clavicle is the first bone to calcify in utero, calcification beginning during the 5th fetal week.
 3. Epiphysial development of girls is consistently ahead of that of boys during all of childhood.
M. Laboratory Data:
 1. Blood findings at birth -
     Red blood count: 4.1-7.5 million/cu mm (avg, 5.9 million).
     Hgb: 14-24 gm (avg, 19 gm), of which one-half to three-fourths are fetal hemoglobin.
     White blood count: 8000-38,000/cu mm (avg, 17,000)
       PMN's: 60%
       Lymphocytes: 20%
       Monocytes: 10%
       Immature white cells: 10%
     Platelets: 350,000 cu mm
     Nucleated red cells: < 500/cu mm
     Reticulocytes: 3%
     Sedimentation rate: Markedly accelerated

168 Full-Term Infant

Hematocrit: 54±10 mm
MCV: 85-125 cu μ
MCHC: 36%
MCH: 35-40 $\gamma\gamma$
Prothrombin, plasma thromboplastin component (factor IX), proconvertin (factor VII), and Stuart factor (factor X) are low. Proaccelerin (factor V) is either normal or slightly elevated.

2. Urine - About 30-60 ml of urine with low specific gravity are normally passed the first day. Protein and acetone are often present. Occasional casts, red cells, and white cells may be present. Uric acid crystals are often the cause of pink urine.
3. Stools - Meconium may be passed at birth or soon after.

Changes Which Occur During the First Week After Birth.

A. Position: A more relaxed posture is assumed, although the fetal position is still favored by most infants.
B. Weight: All newborn infants lose weight during the first week. Almost 10% of the birth weight is lost by the 4th-5th day. Early inability to retain and digest milk retards stabilization of metabolism and delays weight gain. Premature, damaged, and maldeveloped babies lose as much as one-fourth of their original weight despite supportive measures. If the milk supply is abundant and there are no complications, most newborns regain their birth weight by the beginning of the second week.
C. Skin: The color changes from ruddy to flesh-pink. Most petechiae and erythematous patches fade or vanish.

Lanugo begins to disappear, particularly from the face.

Peeling of the superficial layers of the skin, which is particularly noticeable over the hands and feet, begins on about the 5th day. Large patches of surface cells are exfoliated. Occasional fissures form, particularly at the wrists. The new surface is of fine texture.

About 2-4 days after delivery, slight jaundice is recognizable in about 40% of newborn infants. Jaundice, especially when it appears earlier than normal, may indicate erythroblastosis. Jaundice usually disappears by the 7th day.
D. Head and Face: Deformity due to molding and caput succedaneum disappears by the end of the first week.
E. Chest: Slight breast engorgement and prominence of the nipples are noted 2-3 days after birth in most mature newborns of both sexes. Minimal whitish, viscid fluid ("witch's milk") may even leak from the nipple ducts. This secretion is the result of breast stimulation by maternal hormones in utero and endocrine alterations after delivery.
F. Abdomen: Drying and contraction reduce the cord stump

to a shriveled, brown crust which usually drops off on about the 7th day.

Gastrointestinal problems may develop. Vomiting may be due to swallowed blood, air, or other irritants and overfeeding; colic may be due to intolerance to the formula or ileus due to firm plugs of meconium obstructing the bowel.

G. Genitalia: Vulvar engorgement and leukorrhea may be recognized in female infants after 3-4 days. One in 50-60 of these babies will have slight uterine bleeding (pseudomenstruation). Discharge is caused by maternal estrogen stimulation of the fetal genital canal during pregnancy; bleeding is the result of sudden reduction of the blood titer beginning at birth.

H. Stools: Feces are dark, greenish, pasty, or tarry meconium until 3-4 days after birth, when softer, green-yellow stools begin. The movements may become curdy and yellow on about the 6th day. Brownish movements are the rule after 7-8 days. Large babies, formula-fed babies, and those delivered with considerable difficulty have larger and more numerous stools than other infants. Initially, the stools are only slightly fetid. When yellow, they have a faint odor of sour milk. Normal stools never contain blood or mucus, and very little liquid should separate from the movement on standing. Foul-smelling, whitish, very dark, slimy, thin, or frothy stools are suggestive of disease.

I. Laboratory Data: Hematologic studies reveal a reduction in hemoglobin, marked rise in serum bilirubin (up to 13 mg/100 ml), and elevation of the icteric index. Peak liver function, even in the mature newborn, is not reached for some time after delivery (and is further delayed in the premature).

There is a gradual increase in urinary output until it reaches 200-300 ml/day by the end of the first week.

During the first week after delivery, the spinal fluid is normally xanthochromic and contains a few white cells together with an elevated protein content (mean: less than 100/ml).

THE PREMATURE INFANT

An infant is considered premature when it is born before the 37th-38th weeks of gestation. Other criteria of prematurity are as follows:
Weight: 2500 gm (5 lb 8 oz) or less.
Crown-heel length: < 47 cm (18.2 inches)
Occipitofrontal diameters: < 11.5 cm (4.6 inches)
Circumference of head: < 33 cm (13.2 inches)
Circumference of thorax: < 30 cm (12 inches).

The premature infant has prominent eyes and a large head in proportion to its body. The skin is red, wrinkled, and thin, with little covering vernix. Minimal subcutaneous fat is present, and slight generalized edema is often noted. The thorax is soft; chest expansion limited; and the breasts are neither developed nor engorged. The abdomen is protuberant, often with an umbilical hernia. The genitalia are small, and the testes are frequently undescended. The nails are delicate and do not extend to the fingertips. Body temperature is usually subnormal.

ERYTHROBLASTOSIS FETALIS
(Hemolytic Disease of the Newborn,
Rh or ABO Incompatability)

Erythroblastosis fetalis is a disorder of the fetus and newborn which is manifested by hemolytic anemia and compensatory erythropoiesis due to maternal isohemagglutinins. Incompatibility between the mother and fetus develops as the result of passive transfer of hemolytic antibodies from the patient to the fetus during the latter portion of pregnancy. Isoimmunization with the Rh antigen (attached to the red cells), ABO, or other blood protein sensitization may cause this disease. Slightly over 85% of the white population of the USA are Rh-positive. The Rh trait is rare (< 10%) in other races.

The incidence of clinical erythroblastosis fetalis is about one in 200 pregnancies in the USA.

Pathology.
A. Rh Factor: The injection of Rhesus monkey blood into rabbits has been found to produce antibodies capable of agglutinating the red cells of all Rhesus monkeys and the majority of white people. The first 2 letters of the word Rhesus designate the antigen (Rh factor); agglutinins are known as anti-Rh antibodies.

The Rh antigen is actually a group of specific proteins. Three principle subtypes are recognized: Rh' (now usually called C), Rh_0 (D), and Rh'' (E). These are commonly found in combination with other antigenic substances. If the 3 major antigens are not present, it is likely that Hr (now usually called c), Hr_0 (d), or Hr'' (e) will have been substituted.

B. Inheritance of Blood Factors: Allelic genes permit the inheritance of Rh and Hr factors. Each gene determines the presence of one antigen. One gene of each pair is transmitted to the child by the father and one by the mother Hence, every individual will have 3 pairs of genes related to the Rh, Hr pattern. The letters C, D, E, etc are now more commonly employed to designate the above combination than Rh_0, Rh'', etc. Transmission of the genes is determined by the homozygous (dominant) (CC), (EE), etc, or the heterozygous (recessive) (cc), (dd), etc character of the genes.

Pathologic Physiology.

Those persons who carry the Rh factor are described as Rh-positive; those who do not are Rh-negative. When the Rh antigen is introduced into the tissues or blood stream of an Rh-negative individual, such a person will become sensitized to the antigen and produce blocking or agglutinating antibodies depending on the quantity of antigen injected and the frequency of its administration. Agglutinating antibodies will agglutinate or hemolyze red cells carrying the Rh antibody in vitro or in vivo.

The mating of 2 Rh-negative or Rh-positive individuals is not dangerous.

Rh incompatibility is the most serious cause of erythroblastosis; ABO incompatibility is more common and is generally the least serious. Erythroblastosis due to incompatibility to the Kell, Duffy, and similar uncommon blood factors has been reported also. The Rh_0 (D) factor is by far the most frequently found in Caucasians and is more potently antigenic than Rh' (C) or Rh'' (E).

Slightly over 10% of marriages are between an Rh-negative woman and an Rh-positive man. This is termed an Rh incompatibility mating. Two-thirds to three-fourths of the children of these couples will be Rh-positive. Other combinations (both Rh-positive, both Rh-negative, or woman Rh-positive and man Rh-negative) are not clinically significant.

ABO sensitization develops in a manner similar to Rh incompatibility except that antigens to group A or B substances rather than Rh substance are involved. Incompatibility to B factor is more serious than anti-A, which is often subclinical. Even first-born infants may develop ABO erythroblastosis.

The production of Rh antibodies by an Rh-negative person predisposes to severe, often fatal reactions to transfusions of Rh-positive blood and erythroblastosis fetalis in the infants of sensitized women. Erythroblastosis typically occurs in the following way: (1) An Rh-negative woman becomes sensitized by Rh-positive cells (by transfusion, placental leakage of red cells in a previous pregnancy, etc). (2) Marked production of anti-Rh agglutinins follows. (3) Transfer of the anti-Rh agglutinins from the mother to the fetus across (or through) the placental barrier occurs. (4) Agglutination or hemolysis of fetal erythrocytes occurs. (5) Compensatory fetal hematopoiesis occurs. (6) Kernicterus follows the deposition of the bile pigments in the nuclear zones of the midbrain and brain stem.

ABO incompatibility may cause hemorrhagic disease of the newborn in a similar fashion.

Clinical Findings.

A. Diagnosis of Rh Negativity in the Woman:
 1. First pregnancy, no previous transfusions or intramuscular blood - Type the patient and her husband to determine their Rh status. If the husband is Rh-positive, check the patient's agglutinating and blocking antibody titers each month after the 7th month.
 2. Second and subsequent pregnancies (husband Rh-positive, or previous transfusions of possibly incompatible blood) - Test the woman's blood each month for antibody titer. Note the date of first appearance of antibodies; clinical hemolytic disease of the newborn does not usually develop for at least 10 weeks thereafter. (This may be important in the timing of termination of pregnancy.)

B. Diagnosis of Erythroblastosis Fetalis in the Newborn:
 1. Mild erythroblastosis - There might be only slight to moderate hemolytic anemia and early jaundice.
 2. Moderately severe erythroblastosis - The placenta is large (weighs considerably more than one-sixth of the birth-weight of the infant). Abnormal central nervous system signs consist of spasticity, inactivity, and stupor. Jaundice appears within the first 12-18 hours after delivery. Slight generalized edema is present. Moderate hepatomegaly and splenomegaly are noted.
 3. Severe erythroblastosis - The fetus may be stillborn, or the above signs will be much more marked. Gross edema is present. Marked jaundice constitutes icterus gravis neonatorum.

C. Laboratory Findings:
 1. The mother is Rh-negative and the infant Rh-positive. (Rh-positive infants are occasionally typed as Rh-negative initially because of blocking antibodies.)
 2. Increased anti-Rh titer in mother's blood.
 3. Infant's blood - The bleeding time is prolonged. Progressive anemia is noted from birth or in the first few days of life. The Coombs test (anti-human globulin) and the Witebsky test (coating of fetal red cells by maternal Rh antibodies) are positive. Increased numbers of nucleated red cells are present in peripheral blood. The indirect serum bilirubin is increased. Anti-Rh agglutinins are present in the serum.

Hemantigen® Testing.

About 40 blood antigens which may cause isoimmunization are now recognized. With regard to the prediction of erythroblastosis, many antibodies other than anti-RhO can be responsible for this disorder: anti-D is much more common; next is anti-C, then anti-A and Kell antigens. Actually, 20% of antibodies identifiable in the blood of pregnant women are other than D and A, which are the most frequent.

A cell pool which contains all of the common antigens, called Hemantigen®, is now produced commercially. If, upon mixing the patient's serum and Hemantigen®, any agglutination occurs, it is apparent that the subject has one or more antibodies which may or may not be serious for the fetus. The antibodies usually can then be identified by specific cell panel testing. The most frequent are D, C, E, K, and Fy[a].

If one uses this newer approach, routine ABO and Rh typing of the mother and father is no longer necessary. Instead, all antigens are sought and the patient's serum is tested against Hemantigen® at about the 5th month, when considerable antibody production is to be expected. If agglutination occurs, the antibody or antibodies are then identified. Maternal serum specimens are frozen and stored for titer comparison with subsequent specimens. When delivery is anticipated, and erythroblastosis seems likely, compatible blood is obtained and held for possible exchange transfusion of the fetus.

If a negative Hemantigen® test is reported at the 5th month in pregnancy, the patient should be retested at 8-9 months.

Prevention.
  Avoid giving unnecessary blood transfusions. Give Rh-positive blood to an Rh-negative woman only in extreme emergencies.

Treatment.
A. Management of the Rh-Negative Obstetric Patient: Obtain consultation, if necessary, concerning management of pregnancy and time and method of termination of pregnancy. Two or more transuterine amniocenteses and spectrophotometry evaluations (at intervals of 2-4 weeks) should be performed in all women with anti-D, anti-c, and anti-Kell antibodies to a titer of > 1:8 by direct Coombs test whose husbands have similar antigens. If severe isoimmunization is likely on the basis of the history or is suspected, the first amniocentesis may be done as early as the 22nd week of pregnancy. Prior to viability, consider intrauterine fetal transfusion by a specialist experienced in the procedure when the prognosis for live birth seems hopeless, i.e., when spectrophotometric examination of specimens free of blood at 450 mμ shows extreme deviations from normal or when severe scalp edema or fetal ascites is observed on x-ray.

  A plot of the degree of abnormal spectral absorption after the 28th-32nd week usually will indicate whether it is safe to continue the pregnancy or whether prompt delivery is required because of critical erythroblastosis.

  It is best to wait until the 36th-38th week to induce labor, but if the last baby died at the 36th week, for example, it may be necessary to deliver before that time to avoid severe damage or fetal death in utero. Be prepared to exchange transfuse all babies of pregnant women whose Rh antigen titers are persistently elevated.

B. Management of the Infant With Probable Erythroblastosis Fetalis:
1. Administer oxygen to the mother during the second stage of labor and whenever fetal distress occurs. Withold depressant drugs to the woman in labor.
2. Transfusions (generally into the umbilical artery) - Use only Rh-negative, specific type or type O blood. Give 11-22 ml of blood/kg (5-10 ml/lb). Replacement transfusions are required in severe cases; no transfusions may be needed or small transfusions may be sufficient in mild or moderate cases.

Consider **exchange transfusion** of the infant when any of the following are noted (in order of seriousness): (1) Evidence of erythroblastosis at birth, particularly when the duration of pregnancy is under 37 weeks. (2) Serum bilirubin of 3.5 mg/100 ml or more on cord blood, or over 20 mg/100 ml in the first 24 hours or in the 24 hours after a transfusion. (3) Positive Coombs test on cord blood. (4) Jaundice in the first 12 hours of life. (5) Hemoglobin < 15 gm/100 ml and reticulocyte count > 5%. (6) History of previous erythroblastosis in infants born of the same parents, especially when the father is Rh-positive. (7) Consistently elevated maternal anti-Rh titer of 1:16 or more.

Prognosis.

First trimester abortion is almost never due to Rh incompatibility because severe antibody damage to a fetus requires more time. However, fetal death in utero or premature termination of pregnancy does occur later. Fetal death in utero near term or death in the neonatal period is the usual prognosis for infants with hydrops fetalis. Choreo-athetosis often results if kernicterus develops in a newborn with icterus gravis.

If the infant with serious erythroblastosis fetalis survives, there are no sequelae.

7...
Complications of the Third Stage of Labor

POSTPARTAL HEMORRHAGE

Postpartal hemorrhage is the major cause of maternal deaths in the USA. Five to 8% of all patients delivered at term develop some degree of postpartal hemorrhage, which is defined arbitrarily as the loss of at least 500 ml of blood following delivery of the fetus. Unfortunately, this distinction is not helpful in treatment or prognosis because it does not allow for the small woman, who cannot lose that amount safely, nor for the large woman, who may lose more than 500 ml without disastrous consequences. A far more useful definition of postpartal hemorrhage would be loss of blood in an amount equivalent to 1% or more of body weight, which relates readily with blood volume.

It is essential to measure (1 ml blood = 1 gm) or weigh blood loss accurately. Estimates are grossly inaccurate.

Postpartal hemorrhage may be sudden, massive, and exsanguinating or slow, continuous, and only slight to moderate in amount at any one time. The total amount of blood lost, however, will eventually be excessive if allowed to continue. Postpartal hemorrhage may be early, from delivery until 24 hours afterward; or late (secondary), from 24 hours to 4 weeks after delivery. Secondary postpartal hemorrhage occurs in patients who lose more than 1% of their body weight in blood. Of these, 2% require hospitalization and often surgery or blood replacement (or both).

Uterine bleeding is normally controlled after delivery of the fetus by the ligature effect of the intertwining contracted myometrial muscle bundles.

Etiology.

Many causes have been determined for postpartal hemorrhage: (1) Mismanagement of the third stage of labor. (2) Incomplete separation of the placenta. (3) Uterine atony due to excessive analgesia or anesthesia, prolonged labor, retained adherent placental fragments (partial placenta accreta, adherent succenturiate lobe), or excessive uterine distention (as in multiple births, polyhydramnios). (4) Laceration of the birth canal, e.g., perineal-vaginal lacerations, cervical lacerations. (5) Complications of pregnancy such as abruptio placentae, placenta previa, inversion or rupture of the uterus.

176 Postpartal Hemorrhage

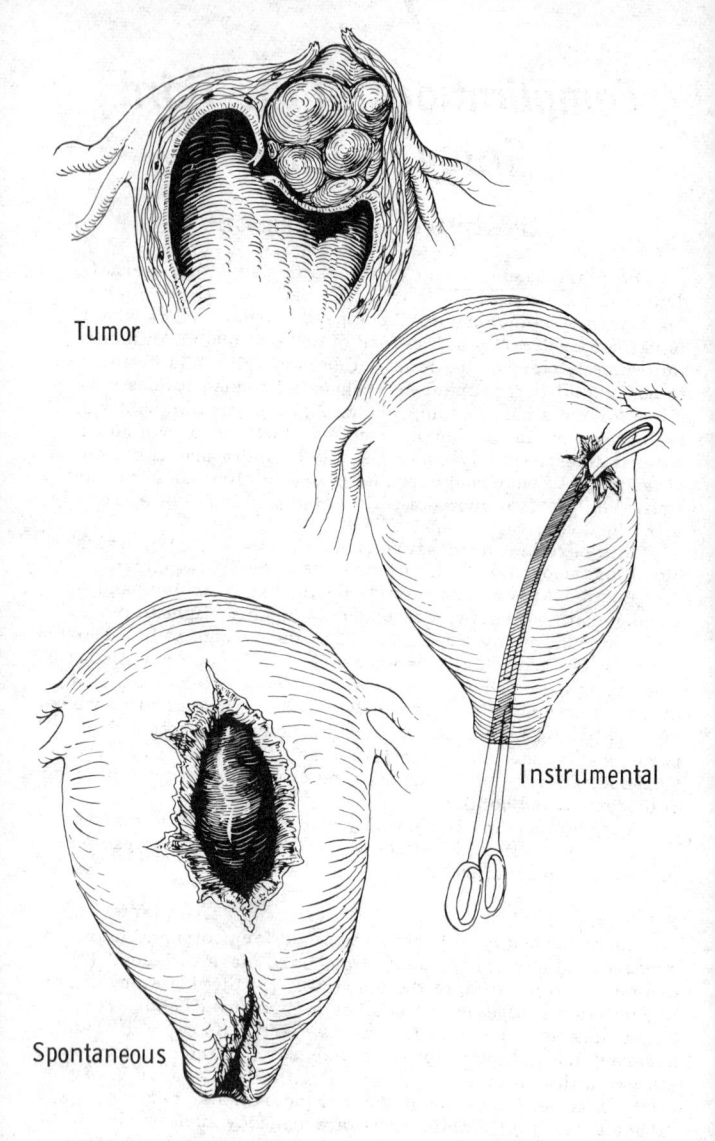

Fig 7-1. Sites of uterine rupture.

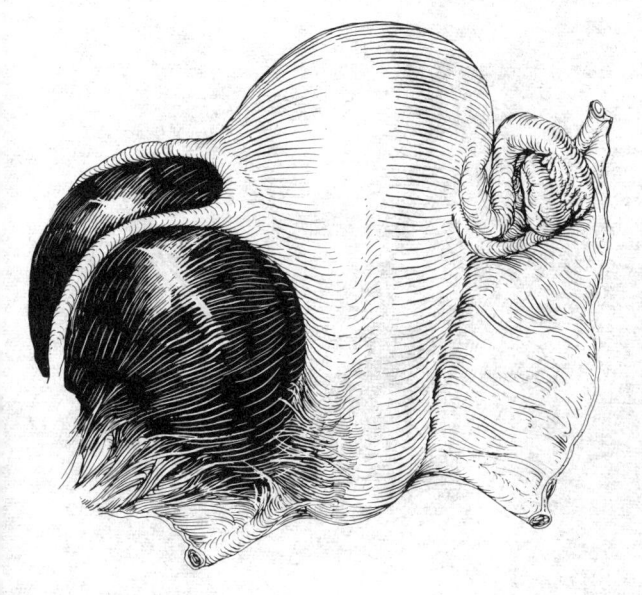

Fig 7-2. Rupture of lower uterine segment into broad ligament.

(6) Tumors of the cervix and uterus, e.g., myomas, adenomyosis, chorio-epithelioma, endometrial carcinoma, carcinoma of the cervix, hemangioma or aneurysm of a uterine vessel. (7) Hematologic disorders, e.g., hypofibrinogenemia, leukemia, thrombocytopenic purpura. (8) Medical complications during pregnancy, e.g., hypothyroidism, vitamin B complex deficiency, vitamin K deficiency, perhaps vitamin P deficiency. (9) Placenta accreta. (10) Infections of the genital tract, e.g., endometritis, parametritis.

Almost all cases of early postpartal hemorrhage are due to uterine atony, lacerations, or bleeding or coagulation defects.

Late postpartal hemorrhage is often due to noninvolution of the placental site. A large, adherent blood clot, when dislodged from the placental area for any reason, causes bleeding from thrombosed thin-walled blood vessels protruding from the shrunken endometrium. Other causes are retained placental fragments and infection.

Clinical Findings.

Three phases of the third stage of labor are related to excessive bleeding:

178 Postpartal Hemorrhage

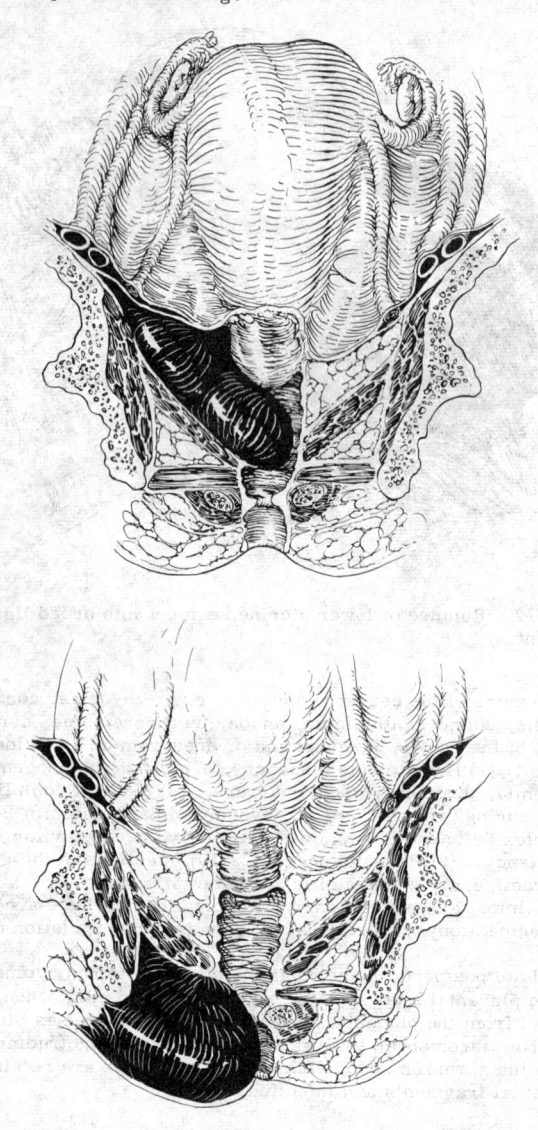

Fig 7-3. Hematoma in supralevator space (above) and infralevator space (below). (After Melody.)

A. From Delivery to Separation of the Placenta:
   1. Episiotomy, perineal or vaginal lacerations, or rupture of varices are usually accompanied by a steady ooze of dark red blood.
   2. Cervical lacerations cause a free flow of bright red (arterial) blood.
   3. Incomplete separation of the placenta or partial placenta accreta causes loss of dark blood in spurts with uterine manipulation or fundal contraction.
B. From Separation to Expression of the Placenta: Delay in expression of the separated placenta may occur when the free placenta in the uterus covers the cervix, so that the fundus cannot contract well, bleeding continues, and blood is trapped. Large clots accompany the placenta when the afterbirth is finally expelled or extracted.
C. Following Recovery of the Placenta:
   1. Atony of the uterus causes steady, persistent bleeding, with additional gushes during uterine contractions.
   2. Prolapse of the uterus into the pelvis causes a profuse continuous flow of blood not related to uterine contractions.
   3. Lacerations of the birth canal—particularly those of the uterus—cause continuous hemorrhage, principally of arterial blood.

Complications.

Postpartal hemorrhage predisposes to puerperal infection, embolism, and anemia.

Prevention.

Faulty technic in expression of the placenta contributes to blood loss. The Pastore or Brandt method of placental expression is preferred. The Credé maneuver is always contraindicated, and the fundus should never be used as a piston to push the placenta out.

It is essential to anticipate postpartal hemorrhage if possible so that preventive steps can be taken as outlined below. A history of postpartal hemorrhage in prior deliveries is an obvious indication for careful preventive management. Others include multiple pregnancy, cesarean section, and infection of the uterus. Conditions which are often associated with postpartal hemorrhage but which may be difficult or impossible to anticipate before the event are polyhydramnios, primary or secondary uterine inertia, desultory or prolonged labor, placenta previa, and abruptio placentae.

In these cases postpartal hemorrhage can be prevented by the following measures:

(1) Near the end of the first stage of labor, begin a slow I.V. infusion of 5% glucose in water (500 ml) through a No. 18 needle.

180 Postpartal Hemorrhage

(2) Immediately after delivery, add 0.5 ml (5 units) of oxytocin to the bottle. (**Caution**: Do not inject oxytocin into the tubing or massive administration will result.)

(3) On completion of the third stage, inject 0.2 mg of ergonovine (Ergotrate®) directly into the tubing near the needle so that the patient will receive the drug promptly.

(4) Elevate the fundus out of the pelvis; massage the uterus until it becomes firm and remains so.

(5) Keep the patient in the delivery room (or recovery room) for at least one hour after delivery and until vital signs are stable.

Treatment.
   A. Emergency and Specific Measures: (See also Management of the Third Stage of Labor, p. 128.)
      1. Repair episiotomy incisions, perineal, vaginal, or cervical lacerations, and ruptured varices promptly.

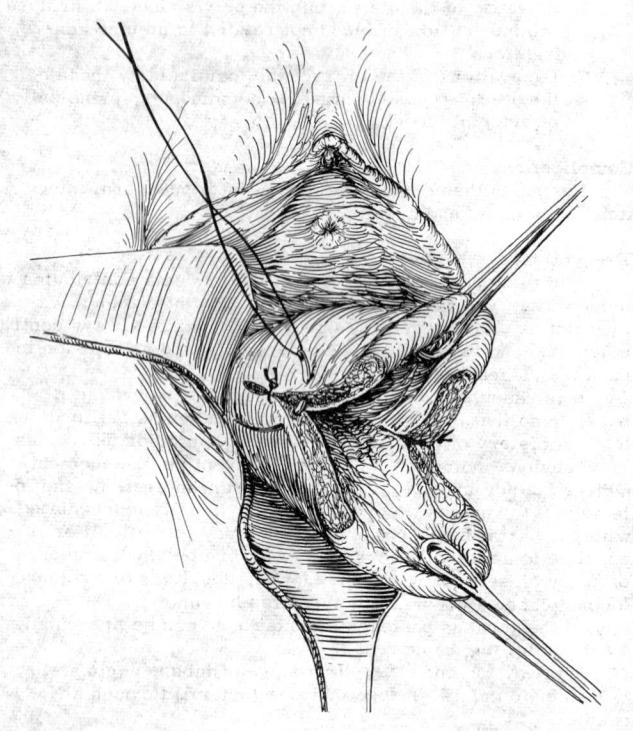

Fig 7-4. Repair of cervical lacerations. (After Edgar.)

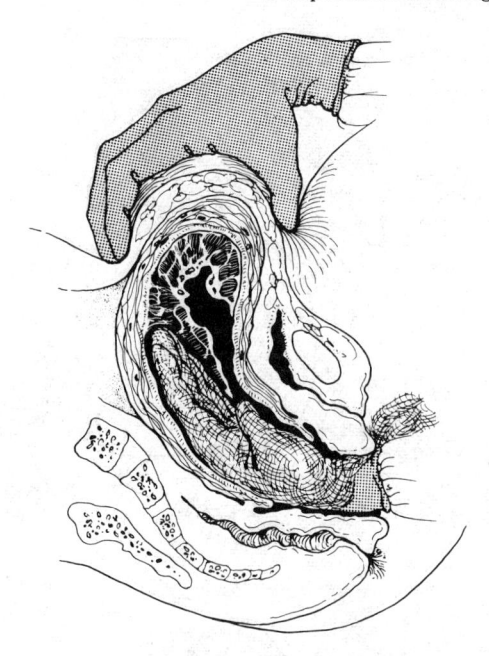

Fig 7-5. Finger and gauze curettement of uterus.

2. Incomplete separation of the placenta or partial placenta accreta accompanied by uterine bleeding - If slight, wait until the placenta separates. If profuse, remove the placenta manually (without additional anesthesia, if possible), using the ulnar edge of the gauze-covered hand from above downward to avoid perforation of the uterus (Fig 7-5).
3. Delay in expression of separated placenta - Express the placenta when the signs indicate it has separated. Do not delay recovery of the placenta until perineal repair is complete. Use the Pastore or Brandt technic for placental expression.
4. Atony of the uterus -
    a. Hold the uterus out of the pelvis and massage the fundus gently. If bleeding is profuse, give oxytocin, 0.5 ml (5 units) in an I.V. infusion.
    b. Prolapse of the uterus into the pelvis - Lift the uterus and support the fundus. Elevate the cervix and uterus with gauze on a sponge-stick, if necessary.

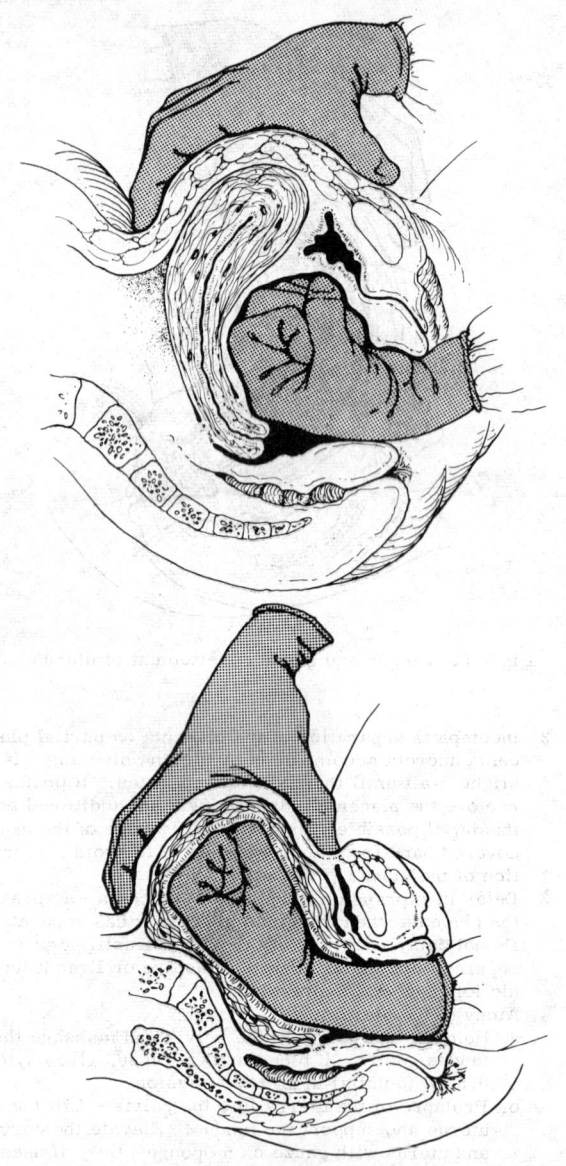

Fig 7-6. Bimanual compression of uterus.

c. Packing the uterus - The purpose of packing the uterus is to check bleeding by compression of points of hemorrhage and to cause the uterus to contract around the foreign body (the packing). However, packing has the following disadvantages: (1) The uterus relaxes slowly and bleeding often recurs, even when the uterus is very tightly packed. (2) If the uterus is packed too tightly it may be so full that further contraction is not possible. (3) Initial packing of the uterus often fails to check the bleeding, and further blood loss may make a necessary hysterectomy even more hazardous. (4) In order to close all potential bleeding points and aid in contraction, it is logical to pack the vagina also; this is rarely done. (5) The risk of infection is greater with than without packing.

Experience is required to pack a uterus properly, but this emergency procedure may be life-saving.

Be prepared to pack the uterus if uterine blood loss reaches 400-500 ml. Have available several

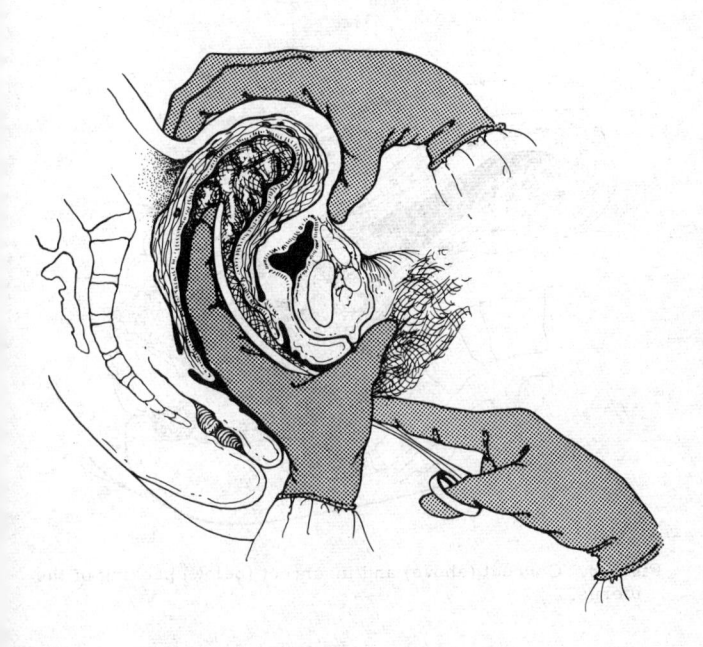

Fig 7-7. Packing the uterus with forceps.

184 Postpartal Hemorrhage

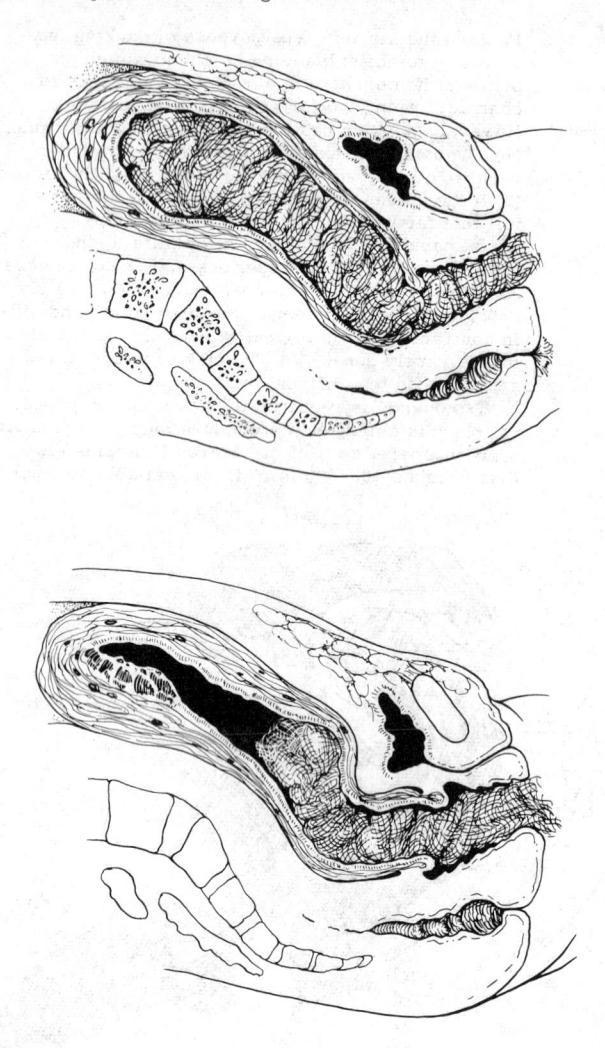

Fig 7-8. Correct (above) and incorrect (below) packing of the uterus.

jars of dry gauze, one yard wide and 5 yards long, previously folded into a four-inch strip and sterilized in a wide-mouthed glass container. A Holmes tubular packing instrument may be helpful but it is not essential.

Procedure for Packing the Uterus:

(1) Insert the left hand (if right handed) into the vagina and on up into the lower uterine segment.

(2) Require the assistant or nurse to feed the gauze from the opened jar held over the patient's lower abdomen.

(3) Deliver the gauze into the left palm with a uterine dressing forceps in the right hand (Fig 7-7).

(4) Carry the folds of packing to the fundus by extending the fingers of the hand within the uterus.

(5) During packing, set the dressing forceps aside from time to time and place the right hand over the uterine fundus to control the direction and pressure of packing.

(6) Pack the fundus, starting in the cornual area, working across to the other cornu, then back and forth, until even the lower segment is firmly packed also.

(7) Continue the packing to include the vagina if the fundus cannot be held out of the pelvis easily; if there are lower birth canal lacerations; or if a perivaginal hematoma complicates the problem.

(8) Remove the packing cautiously in 8-12 hours or less if indicated. When removed after correct packing, the gauze from the fundus will be blood-stained but not saturated; the lower gauze may be moist.

Caution: Do not mistake an hour-glass contraction ring for the fundus and pack only to this point, or hemorrhage will continue from above and the patient will finally "bleed through the pack."

B. General Measures: See Management of the Third Stage of Labor, p. 128.

C. Treatment of Complications: Further hemorrhage, shock, air hunger, and death due to vasomotor or cardiovascular collapse require replacement of blood immediately, correction of the bleeding problem, and other antishock therapy.

Prognosis.

The prognosis depends upon the cause of bleeding, the amount of blood lost, and the rapidity with which it is lost (in proportion to the patient's weight); the patient's general health; and the choice, speed, and completeness of therapy.

Maternal mortality and morbidity rise in direct proportion to the amount of blood lost. A febrile puerperium is 4

INVERSION OF THE UTERUS*

Inversion of the uterus—the extrusion of a portion or all of the body of the uterus into the vagina—is a rare but very dangerous condition. **Puerperal** inversion is a critical emergency; it usually occurs just after delivery but may occur within 6 weeks after delivery. The incidence is about one in 15,000 of all deliveries, and is lowest where obstetric care is of the highest quality. **Nonpuerperal** inversion is a less serious disorder which occurs in one in 25,000 adult gynecologic or nonpuerperal patients.

Partial inversion (Fig 7-9) is herniation of the fundus into the uterine cavity. **Complete** inversion is extrusion of the corpus through the cervix into or beyond the vagina. Either type may be acute or chronic and spontaneous or induced.

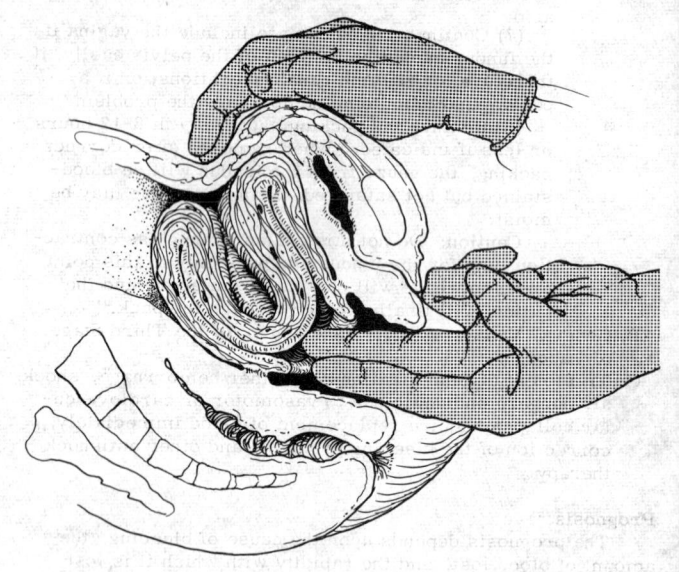

Fig 7-9. Partial inversion of the uterus.

---

*For convenience both puerperal and nonpuerperal inversion will be discussed in this chapter.

Spontaneous acute puerperal inversion is due to straining by the patient after delivery or pulling by the infant on the cord and placenta (e.g., when delivery is spontaneous and precipitous with the patient in a standing position and unattended).

Induced acute puerperal inversion is the result of (1) traction on the cord before placental separation, (2) severe "kneading" of the fundus (unrestrained Credé maneuver) by the physician to induce placental separation and expulsion, (3) excessive pressure on the uterine fundus by the physician (Kristellar maneuver), (4) delivery of an infant with a short cord or one which has been shortened by coiling, or (5) separation and extraction of an adherent placenta—done manually and in haste.

Induced chronic puerperal inversion is due to the same causes as acute induced puerperal inversion but may not be recognized until more than one month after delivery.

Acute nonpuerperal inversion of the uterus may occur as a result of extrusion of a uterine tumor (most often a large pedunculated myoma) or as a complication of the extraction of a sizable, tesselated fibroid tumor. **Chronic nonpuerperal** inversion is due to the same causes but is not promptly recognized.

Clinical Findings.

Acute complete inversion of the uterus causes sudden, agonizing pain with an explosive sensation of "fullness" extending downward to the vagina. Brisk bleeding and profound shock occur in over half of patients; exsanguination may occur. If inversion is partial, pain and bleeding are less severe.

Bimanual examination is necessary. Abdominally, the depressed fundus or absent corpus is revealed by "dimpling" or a crater-like depression. Vaginally, complete inversion is apparent by the presence of a large bleeding mass outside the introitus which may have the placenta attached; in partial inversion a cup-shaped mass can be palpated just above or bulging through the cervix.

Chronic partial uterine inversion is characterized by persistent unexplained bleeding and discharge accompanied by discomfort.

Differential Diagnosis.

A large submucous myoma at the external cervical os may cause the same symptoms as inversion, but the fundus is larger than normal and there will be no umbilication of the mass above the symphysis.

Complications.

Anemia, infection, and embolism may follow inversion of the uterus.

Inversion of Uterus

Prevention.

Do not pull on the cord unless the placenta has separated; do not push on the fundus or use the Credé maneuver; do not leave the patient until the uterus is contracted and rounded; and do not place a pad or roll beneath the abdominal binder postpartum.

Treatment.

In acute puerperal inversion the maternal mortality is high. Obtain consultation and assistance immediately.
- A. Before attempting definitive treatment, control shock with I.V. fluids, plasma, whole blood, and oxytocin (Pitocin®). Avoid giving ergot preparations, which cause continued tetanic contracture of the cervix and uterus, until the uterus is replaced (see below).
- B. Replace the uterus by abdominovaginal manipulation, developing countertraction on the cervix while directing the inverted portion upward. Deep general (ether) anesthesia is required. Leave the placenta attached, compress the fundus in the anteroposterior diameter, and apply a ring forceps to the cervix. Cervical constriction may be relaxed with whiffs of amyl nitrite vapor or 0.3-0.6 ml of epinephrine, 1:1000, I.M.
- C. Retain the fist within the uterus until contraction is effected with oxytocics (ergot) to prevent recurrence of inversion. Packs are not effective; they usually maintain uterine distention.
- D. If correction is not accomplished easily and quickly by manipulation, immediate surgery is mandatory.
    1. Houltain technic (transabdominal) - Incise the posterior wall of the inverted uterus, replace the fundus with towel clamps placed hand-over-hand, and suture.
    2. Spinelli technic (transvaginal) - Transect the cervix anteriorly to replace the fundus from below, and suture.
    3. Kustner technic (transvaginal) - Incise through the cervix posteriorly, replace the fundus, and suture.
- E. Chronic inversion of the uterus is corrected by vaginal hysterectomy.
- F. Postoperatively, administer broad-spectrum antibiotics; replace blood, fluid, and electrolytes; and decompress the stomach with a nasogastric tube.

Prognosis.

Manual replacement of the uterus, when correctly employed, is successful in about 75% of patients with inversion. If precautions are ignored, mortality will be about 30%.

It is not likely that inversion of the uterus will recur, though it is possible.

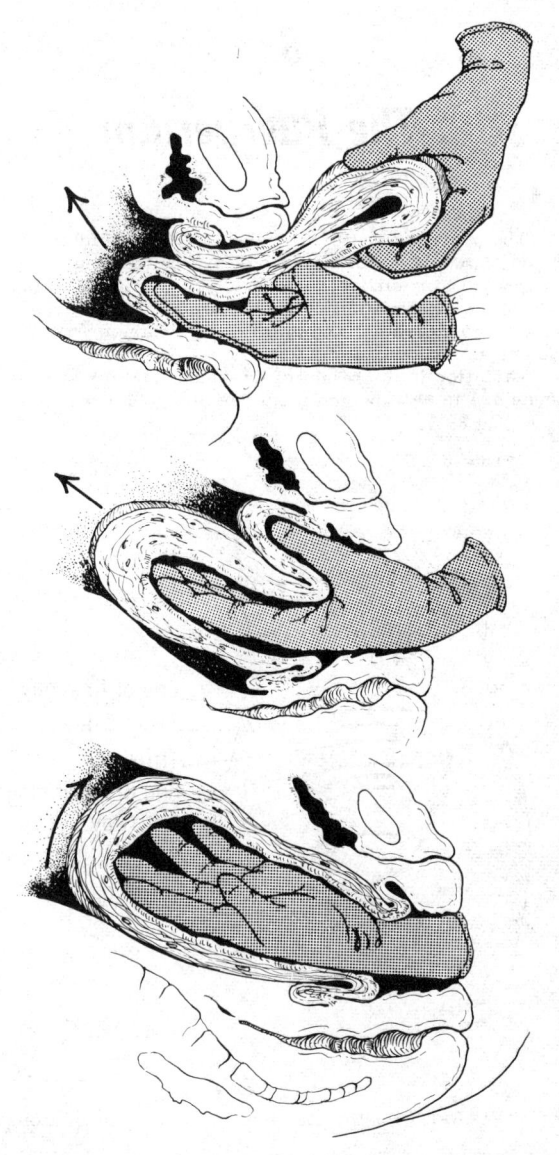

Fig 7-10. Replacement of inverted uterus.

8...
The Puerperium

The puerperium (the 6 weeks following childbirth) is the period of recovery during which time the maternal organism is expected to return to its normal prepregnancy status. However, menstruation is not restored for 6-8 weeks in women who do not nurse and for 6-12 months or more in those who do.

Variation in the height of the fundus and the size of the uterus are to be expected from delivery to 1-6 weeks thereafter (Fig 8-1).

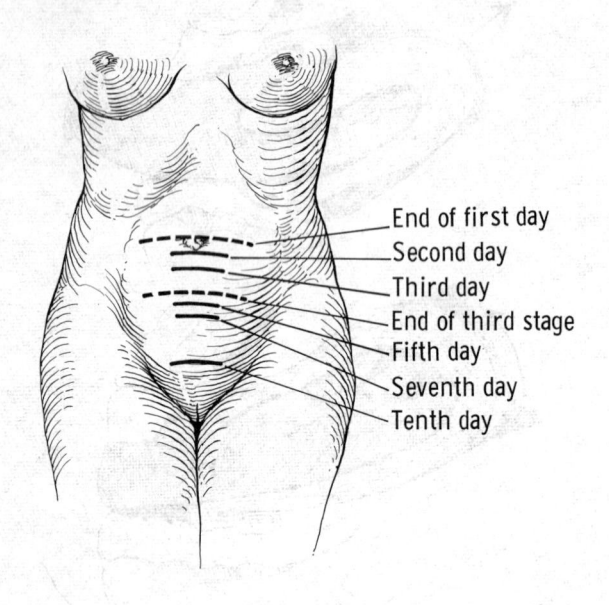

Fig 8-1. Postpartal levels of uterine involution.

CARE IMMEDIATELY AFTER DELIVERY

Transfer the patient to a recovery room or keep her in the delivery room for constant observation and treatment for at least one hour after delivery.

Uterine Massage & Management of Bleeding.

After the third stage of labor the uterus must be palpated frequently for several hours to make certain that the fundus remains firm and that vaginal bleeding is not abnormal in amount. Estimations of blood loss are inaccurate, especially when clots are passed; but the loss of about 300 ml or more of blood constitutes excessive loss, and if more than 500 ml are lost frank hemorrhage has occurred.

When excessive bleeding occurs:

(1) Elevate the fundus slightly and massage the uterus gently to stimulate its continued firm contraction. Maintain uterine support and massage for 15-30 minutes, or longer if necessary.

(2) Administer ergonovine (Ergotrate®) or equivalent, 0.2 mg orally immediately, or give I.V. slowly and well diluted in normal saline solution. Repeat every 4 hours for 4 doses.

(3) Obtain venous blood for typing and crossmatching if this was not done before delivery. Check bleeding and clotting time and note clot retraction time. Have 2-3 units of blood ready for transfusion.

(4) Start an I.V. drip of oxytocin, 1 ml (10 units) in 1 liter of 5% glucose in water, administered through a No. 18 needle.

(5) If bleeding is not controlled promptly, return the patient to the delivery room for inspection of the birth canal. Be prepared to suture lacerations or remove placental fragments.

Pulse & Blood Pressure.

A. Pulse: Record the pulse rate and rhythm whenever the uterus is palpated—at least every 15 minutes for the first hour after delivery. The first warning of excessive blood loss may be a rise in the pulse rate of 10-15/minute. If this change is maintained, begin antishock therapy and treat for postpartal hemorrhage.

B. Blood Pressure: A fall in blood pressure may also presage shock. Elimination of placental circulation and contraction of the uterus after separation and delivery of the placenta restores at least 300 ml of blood to the maternal system. This normally causes an elevation of blood pressure of 10-20 mm Hg and is helpful in supporting the diastolic pressure for several hours after delivery. The temporary rise then slowly dissipates.

Record the patient's blood pressure immediately upon her return to the ward and then every 12 hours for the first 24 hours and daily thereafter for several days. Toxemia, infection, or other complications may require more frequent determinations.

HOSPITAL (OR HOME) CARE DURING THE FIRST WEEK OF THE PUERPERIUM

Length of Hospitalization.

All patients would derive benefit from at least one week of hospitalization after delivery, but the expense involved and the shortage of accommodations preclude a convalescence of this duration for many women. Most patients can return home safely 3-5 days after delivery. Earlier discharge is generally considered to be unwise, especially for primiparas who may not have learned to care for the baby, how to avoid the complications of lactation, etc.

Exercise & Early Ambulation.

The incidence of prolapse of the uterus, bleeding, embolism, and puerperal infection is not increased by early resumption of activity. Encourage the mother to turn in bed and move her extremities as soon as she is able. She should be allowed to lie on her abdomen or assume any comfortable position, but pressure beneath the knees for long periods should be avoided to prevent vascular stasis and thrombosis.

Caution: Early ambulation does not mean return to normal activity or work.

Early ambulation gives a psychologic lift and a sense of well being, hastens involution of the uterus, improves uterine drainage, and may reduce the incidence of phlebothrombosis and thrombophlebitis by increasing circulation to the pelvis and lower extremities.

A recommended schedule of activity after delivery is as follows:

(1) First 24 hours after delivery: Complete freedom of movement in bed.

(2) Postpartal Day I: Out of bed and to the lavatory with help.

(3) Postpartal Day II: Out of bed as desired with help.

(4) Postpartal Day III on: Out of bed as desired.

Precautions: Rest is essential, and no patient should be forced to get out of bed against her will; encourage but do not force her to be active. She should avoid lifting, straining, and pushing and should not be allowed to become fatigued.

Diet.

Provide a regular diet as soon as the patient desires food and is free from the effects of analgesics, amnesics, and anesthetics. The menu should emphasize high-protein foods, fruits, vegetables, and milk products. Avoid overfeeding. Even nursing women probably require no more than 2600-2800 Calories/day despite reports to the contrary. If required, continue the daily vitamin-mineral supplement for about 2 weeks for women who do not nurse and throughout the nursing period for those who do.

Restrict sodium intake for toxemia patients for at least 3 days or longer, as indicated.

Vital Signs.

Record the temperature, pulse, and respiration every 4 hours for 2-3 days at home or in the hospital.

Bladder Care.

It is essential to avoid overdistention of the bladder, which is normally atonic during pregnancy and immediately after delivery. If the bladder fills to 1000 ml or more, at least 3 days of decompression by catheter may be required to establish voiding without significant residual urine. Normally, the marked polyuria notable for several days after delivery causes the bladder to fill in a relatively short time. It is therefore usually necessary to resort to catheterization more frequently than is required for most other surgical patients with urinary retention. Catheterize the patient every 6 hours after delivery if she is unable to void or empty her bladder completely. If a woman requires catheterization 3 or more times per day during the first several days after delivery, insert a retention catheter for 2-3 days. Sulfisoxazole (Gantrisin®) or a similar chemotherapeutic agent, 1 gm orally 3 times daily, will usually prevent a clinically evident urinary infection while the catheter is in the bladder.

Bowel Function.

If an enema was effectual before delivery, do not expect the patient to have a bowel movement for 1-2 days after childbirth.

The mild ileus which usually follows delivery can generally be reversed by administering a mild laxative such as milk of magnesia, 15-20 ml orally on the evening of the second postpartal day (day III). If a bowel movement does not occur by the next morning, order a rectal suppository such as bisacodyl (Dulcolax®) or administer a small tap water or soapsuds enema. Occasional laxatives may be required subsequently, while the patient is sedentary. Avoid mineral oil because it absorbs fat-soluble vitamins. Phenolphthalein, senna, and jalap laxatives should not be used if the patient is nursing because of the slight contamination of milk which occurs.

First Week of Puerperium

Oxytocics.

Oxytocics are valuable in the treatment of postpartal hemorrhage and endometritis, but their value as extended therapy after delivery is questionable. Oxytocics should be prescribed only when indicated for specific problems in individual patients.

Heretofore, ergot preparations such as ergonovine (Ergotrate®) or methylergonovine (Methergine®) were often given routinely every 4-6 hours for at least 4-6 doses, supposedly to limit bleeding and to speed the uterine involution. However, continued administration of oxytocics will conserve only 100-200 ml of blood, and involution is not materially hastened by brief ergot therapy. Ergot poisoning may occur if prolonged therapy is permitted.

Analgesics.

Discomfort is easily controlled by simple analgesics, e.g., acetylsalicylic acid, 0.6 gm (10 gr), with codeine, 30-60 mg (1/2-1 gr), orally every 4 hours as necessary. Meperidine (Demerol®) and morphine should be avoided.

Sedation.

Hospital procedures, noise, and strange surroundings are not conducive to sleep at night. Sedatives such as phenobarbital, 30 mg (1/2 gr) orally at bedtime as necessary, will generally ensure a good night's rest.

Care of Episiotomy Incisions & Lacerations.

Perineal wounds heal best if not overtreated. Gently cleanse the area with medicated soap or detergent and water at least once or twice each day and after voiding or defecation. It is impossible to keep the pudendum sterile, but if it is kept clean and dry healing will occur rapidly. Dry heat applied to the perineum with an infrared lamp for 20-30 minutes 3 times daily will relieve discomfort and promote healing.

Avoid the use of sanitary napkins for 1-2 days after delivery. Clean absorbent pads should be placed beneath the patient's hips while she is a bed patient.

Inspect the perineotomy or repaired lacerations daily. Perform vaginal or rectal examination if hematoma or infection seems likely. Open and drain the sutured area if suppuration develops.

Avoid applying greasy ointments or salves to the perineum because skin maceration may develop and infection is fostered by the protective oily film. Painting or spraying the area with antiseptic solutions is probably of no value.

Baths.

Daily bed baths are prescribed for the first several days. As soon as the patient is able, she may take a shower. Sitz or tub baths after the second postpartal day are probably safe if the tub is kept scrupulously clean. Although perineal pain is alleviated by wet as well as dry heat, showers are preferred to tub baths because of the profuse flow of lochia during the early puerperium.

POSTPARTAL EXERCISES

Restorative exercises will have no permanent effect on uterine position but will "tone" the skeletal muscles and improve the physique. Repeat each exercise 4 times twice daily and add another exercise each day. Continue daily for one month or longer (see Fig 8-2).

The so-called "monkey-walk" and knee chest position have no therapeutic value and may be harmful. They have been eliminated from modern obstetrics.

POSTPARTAL CARE DURING THE FIRST THREE WEEKS AT HOME
(8th-28th Postpartal Days)

Hygiene is essentially the same as practiced in the hospital.

Inform the patient at the time of her dismissal from the hospital that she will note decreasing amounts of sanguineous vaginal discharge for about 3 weeks and possibly a "small period" during the 4th-5th week after delivery (bleeding from the placental site). She should wear a brassiere constantly, especially if she is nursing, to preserve her figure, but will require a girdle only if necessary or if this is her custom. Vaginal douches should be used only upon specific indications, perhaps after the third week following delivery. Coitus should not be resumed for 4-6 weeks, depending upon the results of the postpartal examination.

A gradual increase in activity and responsibility is planned for the recovery period at home. During 3-4 weeks after discharge from the hospital, a typical regimen is as follows:

First Week.
Caring for the new baby should be the mother's sole responsibility. If possible, domestic help should be provided to care for the other children, help about the house, do the laundry, and cook and shop for 1-2 weeks or longer if necessary.*

---

*The author realizes that this represents a financial burden for many young couples and is completely out of the question in some instances. Nevertheless, the ideal thus outlined has many advantages for all concerned and should be pursued.

196 First Three Weeks at Home

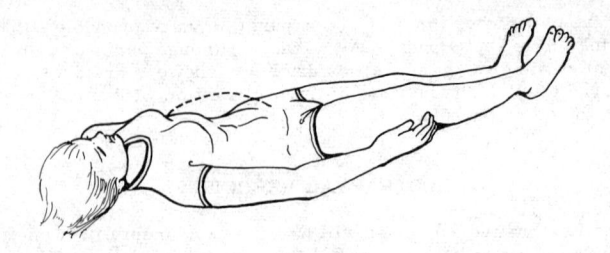

First Day: Breathe in deeply; expand the abdomen. Exhale slowly, hissing; draw in abdominal muscles forcibly.

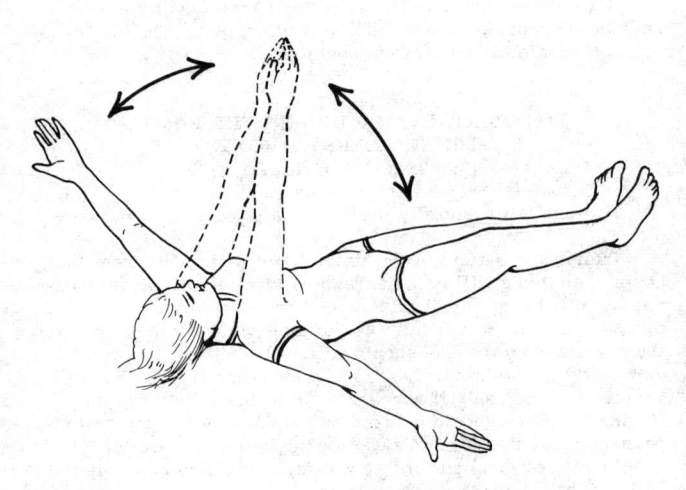

Second Day: Lie flat on the back with the legs slightly apart. Hold arms at right angles to the body; slowly raise the arms, keeping the elbows stiff. Touch hands together and gradually return arms to their original position.

Fig 8-2. Postpartal exercises.

Note: Repeat each exercise 4 times twice daily and add a new exercise each day.

First Three Weeks at Home 197

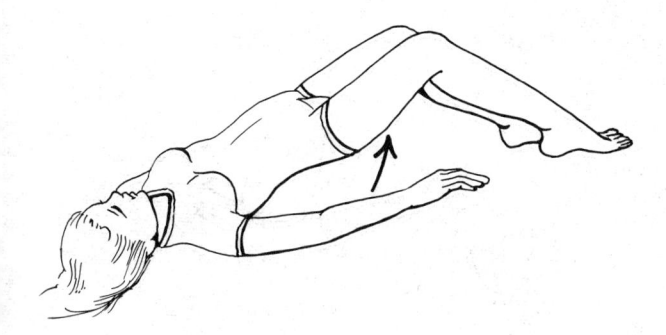

Third Day: Lie flat on the back with the arms at the sides. Draw the knees up slightly. Arch the back.

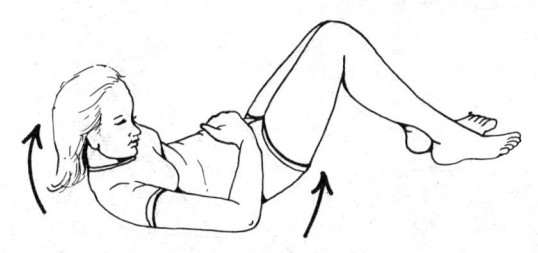

Fourth Day: Lie flat on the back with the knees and hips flexed. Tilt the pelvis inward and contract the buttocks tightly. Lift the head while contracting the abdominal muscles.

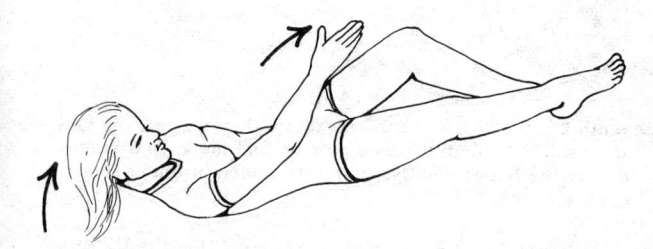

Fifth Day: Lie flat on the back with the legs straight. Raise the head and one knee slightly. Then reach for, but do not touch, the knee with the opposite hand. Alternate with the right and left hand.

Fig 8-2. Postpartal exercises. (Cont'd.)

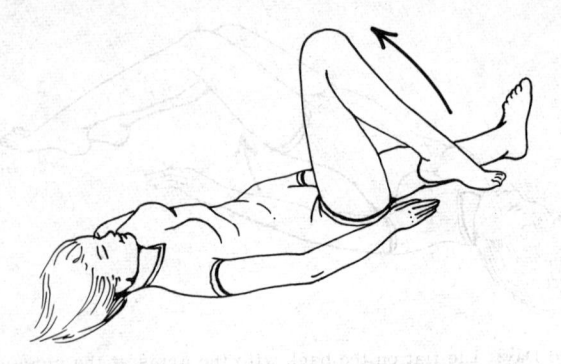

Sixth Day: Slowly flex the knee and then the thigh on the abdomen. Lower the foot to the buttock. Straighten and lower the leg to the floor.

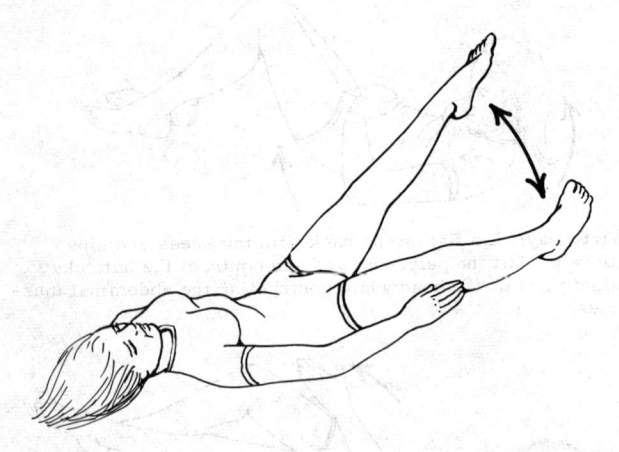

Seventh Day: Raise first the right and then the left leg as high as possible. Keep the toes pointed and the knee straight. Lower the leg gradually, using the abdominal muscles but not the hands.

Fig 8-2. Postpartal exercises. (Cont'd.)

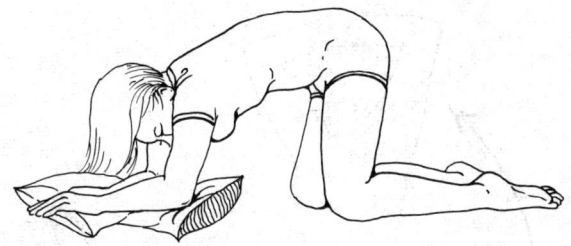

First Three Weeks at Home 199

Eighth Day: Rest on the elbows and knees, keeping the upper arms and legs perpendicular with the body. Hump the back upward. Contract the buttocks and draw the abdomen in vigorously. Relax, breathe deeply.

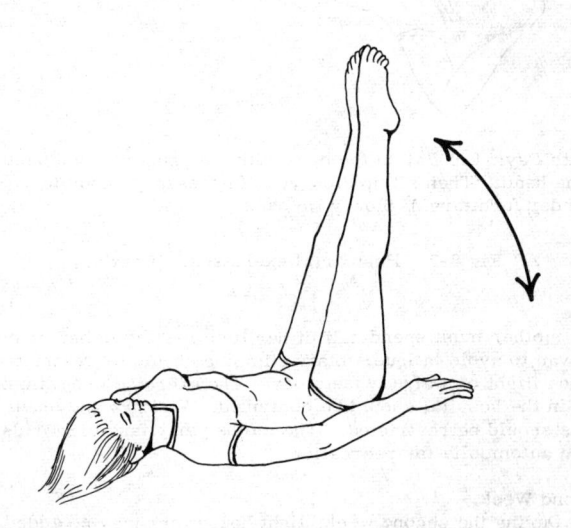

Ninth Day: Same as seventh day, but raise both legs at the same time, etc.

Fig 8-2. Postpartal exercises. (Cont'd.)

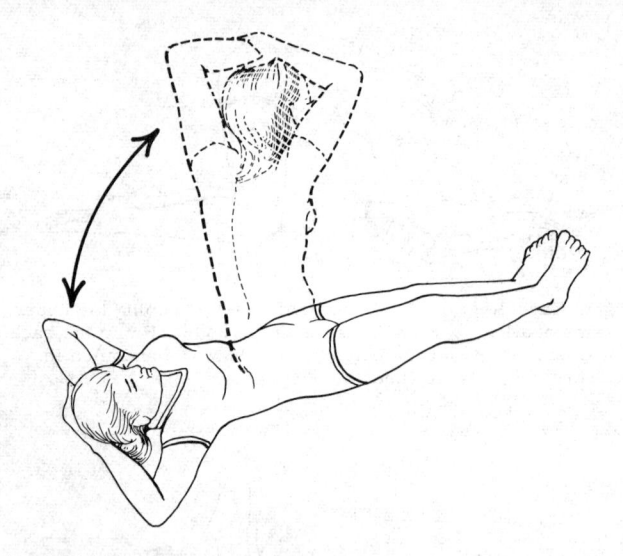

Tenth Day: Lie flat on the back with the arms clasped behind the head. Then sit up slowly. (If necessary, hook feet under furniture.) Slowly lie back.

Fig 8-2. Postpartal exercises. (Cont'd.)

The mother must spend half of her time resting in bed or on a divan to avoid fatigue. Stair climbing should be restricted to one flight of stairs twice a day. The exercise program begun in the hospital should be continued. Visitors and phone calls should be restricted. The mother may take brief rides in an automobile for recreation.

Second Week.
During the second week, light housework may be added to the program, and the mother may drive her car occasionally and prepare a simple lunch and dinner for the family. She must rest 2 hours twice daily and be in bed by 9:00 p.m.

Third Week.
Activities should be generally curtailed. The mother may prepare meals of moderate complexity, wash baby clothes, and shop with someone who can carry heavy packages, but she should rest one hour twice daily and be in bed by 10:00 p.m.

Fourth Week.

During the fourth week the mother should restrict activities slightly, avoiding unnecessary duties, and rest one hour in the afternoon. Daily low-pressure acetic acid douches may be helpful for vaginal hygiene.

During the 4th or 4th week a postpartal examination should be scheduled with the obstetrician.

POSTPARTAL EXAMINATIONS

Examine the patient during the 4th week or so after delivery if possible. This is somewhat earlier than examinations have been scheduled in the past, but it is advisable to begin therapy (e.g., for cervicitis) as soon as possible and still have an opportunity for a second examination before the 6th week, when most patients can return to full activity or employment. The first postpartal examination should include the following:

Weight.

The patient should have returned to her approximate prepregnancy weight by this time. A suitable diet may have to be prescribed if she has not done so. Assuming that she has performed her exercises faithfully, the muscles will be firm and fatty tissue distribution will have returned to its prepregnancy configuration.

Breasts.

Note the adequacy of support, abnormalities of the nipples, the presence of tenderness or mass formation, and lactation.

Uterine Bleeding.

Persistence of uterine bleeding may demand definitive investigation and treatment. A course of ergonovine (Ergotrate®) may be required. In extreme cases, dilatation and curettage are necessary.

Vaginal Discharge.

Profuse leukorrhea ceases in about two-thirds of patients by the 4th-5th week unless vaginitis, cervicitis, or chronic uterine subinvolution is present. Vaginitis will generally yield to specific treatment. For minimal cervicitis, daily acetic acid douches may be all that is required. Antibiotic therapy or coagulation is necessary when cervicitis is more extensive. Subinvolution may be the result of infection, retroposition, or retained products of conception; treatment must be directed toward correction of the specific problem, but douches and antibiotics are often helpful. Dilatation and curettage are occasionally required when endometritis seems to be the result of retained afterbirth. A vaginal pessary may support a retroposed uterus, improve the circulation of the internal genitalia, and enhance involution generally.

Pelvis.

Do a complete rectovaginal evaluation. Perineovaginal support should be adequate. Examine the episiotomy incisions and repaired lacerations.

If uterine malposition is present, review the record to see if the patient had a uterine retroposition or descensus before or during early pregnancy. If so, and if there are no symptoms referable to the "tipped uterus," it is likely that this position is physiologic for her. About 20% of all women have a congenital, symptomless retroposition, and replacement of the organ is not necessary in these cases. If pain, abnormal bleeding, or other findings are present, insert a vaginal pessary as a trial procedure to encourage anteversion of the fundus. If uterine prolapse (descensus) is present, its degree should be noted and, if possible, related to individual symptoms. Pessary support offers only temporary relief in such instances. If prolapse is marked, consider surgical correction.

Observe and, when necessary, treat cervical lesions until they are completely healed. Examine all multiparas at least once a year to detect and correct significant cervical disorders.

Repeat specific laboratory studies which were definitely abnormal during pregnancy.

Contraception.

Advise the patient regarding family planning. Prescribe the contraceptive method most suitable and acceptable to the couple if asked to do so.

Further Examinations.

Release the patient to full activity or employment if her course to this point has been uneventful, or schedule another visit after appropriate therapy.

A gynecologic examination and cytologic vaginal examination is desirable 6 months after delivery. At that time, all of the above items must be evaluated again.

LACTATION

Lactation begins about 48-72 hours after delivery with sudden engorgement of the breasts when the milk "comes in." However, the baby can begin nursing almost immediately after birth and will receive colostrum.

Physiology of Lactation.

Estrogen and progesterone, present in large amounts during pregnancy, stimulate the ductal and alveolar systems of the breast, respectively. This causes proliferation and differentiation of the mammary glands and the production of clear, thin, serum-like colostrum as early as the second month of pregnancy. Colostrum continues to be secreted to term, but the steroid sex hormones inhibit formation of lactogenic hormone (LH, prolactin), which causes actual milk production. After the birth of the baby and delivery of the placenta, estrogen and progesterone titers fall sharply and LH released by the anterior lobe of the pituitary gland acts upon the mammary alveoli to produce milk. Optimal thyroid and adrenal hormone levels play a secondary but necessary role in lactation. All of this is accomplished without the nursing effort.

Nursing stimulates the posterior lobe of the pituitary gland by neural mediation to release oxytocin into the circulation. In addition to its oxytocic effect, oxytocin is a galactokinetic hormone. It contracts the periacinar muscle fibers of the breast. This is the milk ejection or milk let-down reflex whereby milk is actually forced down into the major collecting sinuses which converge on the nipple where it can be expressed by the mother or withdrawn by the baby.

Advantages of Breast Feeding.
A. For the Mother: Breast feeding is convenient, costs nothing, is emotionally satisfying for most women, and speeds uterine involution.
B. For the Child: The food is digestible, readily available, at the right temperature, and free from bacterial contamination. Errors in formula preparation do not occur. The child receives passive antibodies and emotional satisfaction.

Disadvantages of Breast Feeding.
A. For the Mother: Regular nursing is restrictive, and mastitis may develop.
B. For the Child: None, if the mother is healthy, willing, and strong and the supply of milk is adequate.

Principles of Breast Feeding.

The normal, average mother's yield of breast milk is directly proportionate to the baby's demand, assuming that free secretion has been established and feedings are given every 3-4 hours.

The baby does not nurse so much by developing intermittent negative pressure as by a rhythmic biting action; he "works" the milk into his mouth. Very little force is required in nursing because the breast reservoirs can be emtied and refilled independently of suction.

Nursing mothers develop a sensation of "drawing" and tightening—a "draught" or concentration—within the breast at the beginning of suckling after the initial breast engorgement disappears. They are thus conscious of the milk ejection reflex, which may even cause milk to spurt or run out. It can be augmented by physical and emotional preparation during pregnancy as well as by good postpartal management.

The milk let-down phenomenon is inhibited by such factors as pain, breast engorgement, embarrassment, or adverse psychic conditioning.

For several days after the initial breast filling, the milk ejection reflex may be deficient. The breasts become so full and distended that the nipples appear retracted, the areolas are unyielding to the infant's efforts, and the baby obtains little or no milk. Manual expression of milk or the administration of oxytocin (or both) will usually start the flow and relieve the engorgement, whereupon nursing may be more successful.

The mother should nurse her infant at both breasts at each feeding because overfilling of the breasts is the main danger to the maintenance of milk secretion. Nursing at only one breast at a feeding inhibits the reflex, which is provoked simultaneously in both breasts. Thus, nursing at alternate breasts at each feeding may increase engorgement distress and reduce milk output.

Milk Production.

With nursing, the average milk production on the second postpartal day is about 120 ml; on the third postpartal day, it will have risen to at least 180 ml; by the 4th day, the mother will usually provide a total of 240 ml of milk, etc, up to about 300 ml/day.

A good rule of thumb for calculation of milk production for a given day during the first week after delivery is to multiply the number of the day by 60. This will equal the approximate number of milliliters of milk secreted in that 24-hour period.

Assuming that everything goes well, sustained milk production will be achieved by most patients after the first 10-14 days. A yield of 120-180 ml of milk per feeding is common by the end of the second week. Once free secretion is established, marked increases are possible; a wet nurse often can suckle even 3 babies successfully for weeks.

Early diminution in milk production may be due to failure to empty the breasts (weak efforts by the baby or ineffectual nursing procedures), psychic problems such as aversion to nursing, or medical complications (e.g., mastitis or debilitation). Late diminution in milk production results from too generous complimentary feedings, emotional or other illness, and pregnancy.

Stimulation of Lactation.
A. Reinforce the patient's maternal instinct and inherent desire to nurse her baby. During pregnancy (if the patient is receptive), make frequent references to the advantages of breast feeding for mother and infant.
B. Prepare and "toughen" the nipples during the third trimester.
  1. Have the patient wash the nipples daily with unscented mild soap and water, using a washcloth. After drying, she should apply liquid petrolatum. Scented soaps and skin or hand creams should not be used because they may contain irritants or allergens such as perfume. Alcohol should not be used because it dries and hardens the skin.
  2. Inverted or short nipples should be drawn gently outward every day to temporarily increase their length.
  3. Protect the nipples with plastic film, oiled silk, or nipple shields. Have the patient wear a well-fitted brassiere even at night to support the breasts, improve circulation, and avoid trauma.
  4. Teach the patient how to express colostrum gently from the breasts. This should be done several times a day during the last 4-6 weeks of pregnancy to open ducts blocked by inspissated secretions and to stimulate the flow of fluid. This manipulation will not cause premature labor.
C. Beginning on the first postpartal day, if the mother's condition permits, allow the mature, normal newborn to nurse at each breast on demand or approximately every 3-4 hours for 3 minutes' total nursing time. Increase the time by one minute each day, but never exceed 7 minutes. Sixty to 90% of the milk is obtained by the average baby in 4 minutes of nursing. Suckling for longer than 7 minutes may cause maceration and cracking of the nipples and mastitis.
D. Give the mother a glassful of cool water 5 minutes before nursing or utilize other suggestions to strengthen the reflex of milk ejection.
E. Avoid engorgement and trapping of milk by gentle expression of excess milk before nursing with or without oxytocin, 0.5 units in 1 ml of normal saline I.M., or 10 units in 0.25 ml of normal saline as a nasal spray just before infant feeding.

Suppression of Lactation.
If the patient does not suckle her infant and wishes to "dry up" her breasts, this can be done in one of the following ways:
A. Oral estrogen, e.g., ethinyl estradiol, 1.3 mg (26 tablets, containing 0.05 mg each) may be administered as follows:

(Diethylstilbestrol may also be used in comparable doses.)
1. Four tablets (0.2 mg) twice daily on the first day after delivery.
2. Three tablets (0.15 mg) twice daily on the second day.
3. Two tablets (0.1 mg) twice daily on the third day.
4. One tablet (0.05 mg) twice daily on the 4th-7th days.

B. Depot estrogen, e.g., estradiol valerate (Delestrogen®), 10 mg/ml, or an androgen-estrogen such as Deladumone® (testosterone enanthate, 90 mg, and estradiol valerate, 4 mg/ml), 3 ml of either injected immediately after delivery, will prevent lactation in the great majority of patients. An occasional patient will have increased uterine bleeding in the late puerperium, possibly as a result of estrogen stimulation of the endometrium. An androgen-estrogen combination for suppression of breast engorgement and lactation such as Deladumone® seems less likely to cause this type of abnormal flow than estrogen alone.

C. Oral androgens are also effective in suppressing lactation. Give methyltestosterone, 10 mg buccal tablets dissolved in the cheek pouch 5 times daily on the second and third days.

D. Mechanical suppression of lactation is successful whether or not the patient attempts to nurse. This is the only method feasible if mastitis develops or if weaning of the baby obviates lactation; hormonal suppression is not effective after the early puerperium. The patient should cease nursing, expression, and pumping, and apply a tight compression binder (with elevation of the breasts) to be worn constantly for 72 hours and a snug brassiere thereafter. Analgesics such as acetylsalicylic acid, 0.3 gm (5 gr), with codeine, 30-60 mg ($1/2$-1 gr) orally every 4 hours as necessary, may be given for pain.

Apply ice-packs to the breasts as necessary.

Fluid restriction and purging do not contribute to the "drying up" process.

The breasts will become distended, firm, and tender. After 48-72 hours, lactation and discomfort will cease as pressure within the breast ductal and alveolar systems stops the secretion of milk. Involution of the breasts will be complete in about one month.

9...
Multiple Pregnancy

Twin pregnancy is the result either of retarded segmentation of a single fertile ovum (identical, monovular, or monozygotic twins) or fertilization of two ova by 2 spermatozoa (fraternal or dizygotic twins). Multiple births account for about one in every 90 confinements in the USA.

Twenty-five per cent of twins are derived from one ovum and 75% develop from 2 ova.

An approximate estimate of the frequency of occurrence of multiple pregnancies can be stated as follows:

    Twins   1:90
    Triplets   1:90^2 = 1:8100
    Quadruplets 1:90^3 = 1:729,000, etc

Though the relative number of females increases with the number of fetuses in multiple births, males predominate over females, but to a lesser degree than with single births.

The parents' race and the mother's age and parity are important in the incidence of double ovum and triple ovum pregnancies. These factors do not pertain to single ovum twinning, in which the rate is almost the same for all races. It is not known why older women who have had numerous babies should produce more fraternal twins than young women of lesser parity.

Negro couples have a 20-25% greater likelihood of conceiving twins, a 70-75% greater likelihood of conceiving triplets, and a 4 times greater likelihood of conceiving quadruplets than Caucasian couples. Multiple pregnancy is most common in Negroes and least common in the Oriental race.

Both males and females carry the plural pregnancy trait. Marriages between twins of different families and even individuals whose families have produced numerous multiple pregnancies have a greater than normal likelihood of producing twin and triplet offspring.

Identical twins result from fertilization of a single ovum by a single sperm: they are always of the same sex. Fraternal twins result from the fertilization of 2 or more ova by 2 or more single sperms. Two ova may be released from separate follicles (or, very rarely, from the same follicle) at approximately the same time. Fraternal twins may be of the same or of different sexes.

Double ovum twinning is in large part genetically determined; we can only speculate about other causative factors.

Single ovum twinning results from temporary delay of development of the ovum prior to implantation. Postulated causes include reduced oxygen tension of the tube and alteration in nutrition during transmigration.

Triplets may result from repeated twinning of one ovum (also called double twinning or supertwinning) and later death of one embryo. Twinning by 2 ova and elimination of one embryo or development of these fetuses from 3 simultaneously expelled and fertilized ova is also possible. Quadruplets arise from one, 2, 3, or 4 ova.

If division occurs early in the second week, conjoined (Siamese) twins develop; if cleavage is further postponed, incomplete twinning (two heads, one body) occurs.

Double ovum twins have 2 placentas (often fused to resemble one), 2 chorions, and 2 amniotic sacs. In contrast with single ovum twin placentas, there is no anastomosis between the venous or arterial placental channels in fraternal twin placentas.

At delivery, the membranous septum between the twins should be inspected and sectioned to note the probable type of twinning. Single ovum twins have a transparent (thin) septum made up of 2 amniotic membranes only (no chorion and no decidua). Double ovum twins have an opaque (thick) septum made up of 2 chorions, 2 amnions, and intervening decidua (see Fig 9-2).

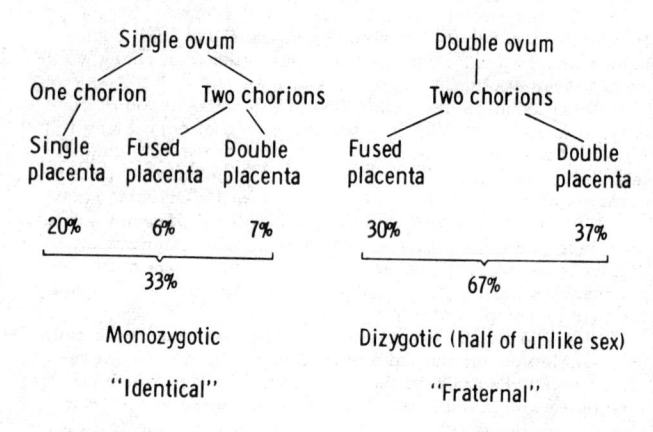

```
              Single ovum                      Double ovum
             /          \                           |
      One chorion    Two chorions              Two chorions
         |            /        \                /          \
      Single      Fused      Double         Fused         Double
     placenta   placenta    placenta       placenta      placenta

       20%         6%          7%            30%            37%
       _____/        _____/
                   33%                              67%

              Monozygotic                  Dizygotic (half of unlike sex)

              "Identical"                         "Fraternal"
```

Fig 9-1. Placental variations in twinning. (After Potter.)

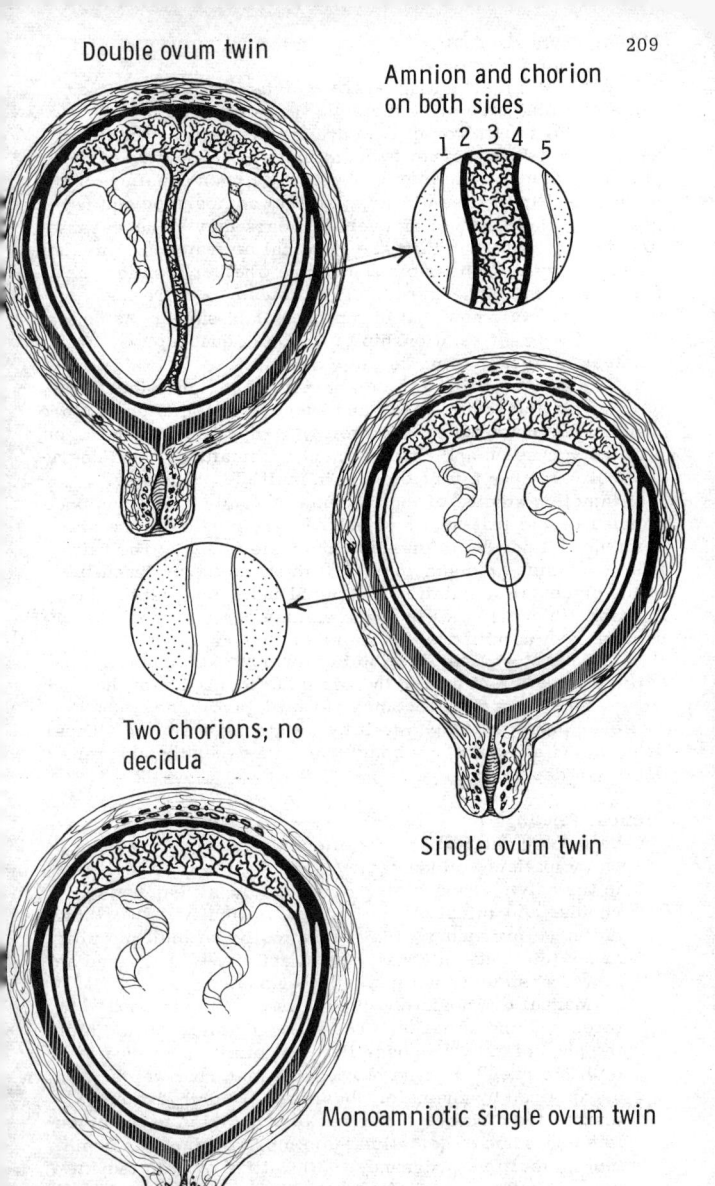

Fig 9-2. Amniotic membranes of twins.

210 Multiple Pregnancy

Each twin placenta generally weighs less than the placenta of a singleton after the 30th week of pregnancy.

Almost two-thirds of twin pregnancies can be identified as single or double ovum twins at birth by inspection of the placenta, study of the membranes, and finger-, palm-, and footprints. In the remainder, physical comparison and repeated psychologic testing over the years may be necessary to determine whether they are identical or fraternal. In some cases it may be impossible to be sure whether identical or fraternal twinning occurred. The problem is more than merely academic now that organ transplant surgery is possible. The exact relationship of triplets, quadruplets, or quintuplets to each other is often doubtful.

Single ovum twins are smaller, have a higher incidence of congenital abnormalities, and succumb more often in utero than double ovum twins. Crowding, competition for nutrition, cord compression and entanglement, prematurity, and operative delivery take a terrible toll in multiple pregnancy.

Injection studies of the placenta in single ovum twin pregnancies reveal that the arteries from the portion of the placenta underlying each fetus communicate freely. The veins from each side also anastomose with each other. Inequities of the placental circulation (marginal insertion, partial infarction, thinning, etc) in one area may destroy one fetus or deprive it of nutrition while the other thrives.

The heart will not develop in a twin whose circulation is extremely deficient during the period of formation of the viscera. This fetus then becomes parasitic and is nourished by whatever blood is pumped to it by its stronger sibling. Other deformities are also commonly present, depending upon the degree of deprivation.

Clinical Findings.

A. Symptoms and Signs: The effects of multiple pregnancy on the patient include earlier and more severe pressure in the pelvis, nausea, backache, varicosities, hemorrhoids, abdominal distention, and difficulty in breathing. A ''large pregnancy'' may be indicative of multiple pregnancy (distended uterus). Fetal activity is increased and more persistent than in single pregnancy.

Manual diagnosis of twinning is possible in about three-fourths of cases. The following signs should alert the physician to the possibility or definite presence of multiple pregnancy: (1) Excessive maternal weight gain unexplained by edema or obesity. (2) Polyhydramnios, manifested by uterine size out of proportion to the calculated duration of gestation, is almost 10 times as common in multiple pregnancy. (3) Outline or balottement of more than one fetus. (4) Multiplicity of small parts. (5) Uterus containing 3 or more large parts. (6) Simultane-

Multiple Pregnancy 211

ous recording of different fetal heart rates, each asynchronous with the mother's pulse and with each other and varying by at least 8 beats per minute. (Irritate the fetus mechanically, by pressure or displacement, to accelerate its heart rate.) (7) Palpation of one or more fetuses in the fundus after delivery of one infant.

B. Laboratory Findings: The hematocrit, hemoglobin, and red cell count are usually considerably reduced. Maternal anemia is common in multiple pregnancy, beginning during the second trimester as the fetal demand for iron increases beyond the mother's ability to assimilate it.

C. X-Ray Findings: Films of the uterus usually reveal the number of fetuses and their presentation in plural pregnancy after the 20th week. Both twins will present by the vertex in almost one-half of cases (Fig 9-3). One will be a vertex and the other a breech in slightly over one-third of cases (Fig 9-4). Both fetuses will be breech presentation in one-tenth of the total, and almost that many will be single (or double) transverse presentations. In multiple pregnancy, vertex presentation occurs only two-thirds as often as breech presentation; transverse presentation occurs 10 times as often in plural pregnancy as in single fetus pregnancy.

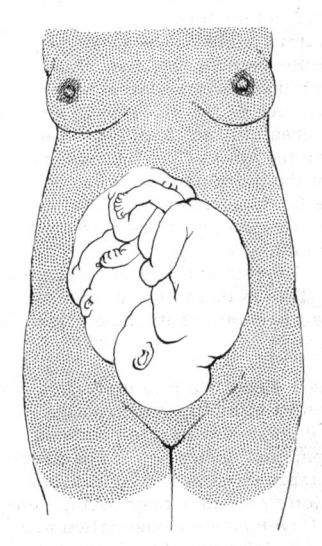

Fig 9-3. Both twins presenting by the vertex.

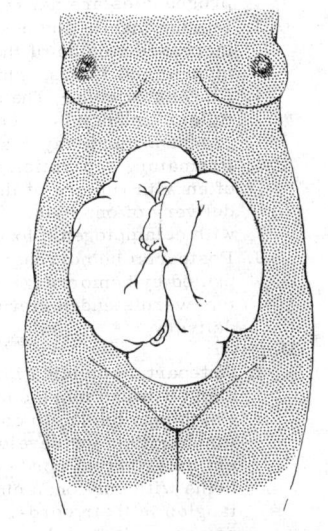

Fig 9-4. One vertex and one breech presentation.

D. Electrocardiographic Findings: Electrocardiography, utilizing electrodes placed on the mother's abdomen in midline positions, may be used to diagnose multiple pregnancy after the 20th week. Individual fetal electrocardiography will be superimposed upon the mother's. During the last 2 months of pregnancy, breech and vertex presentation can also be determined with great accuracy: if the baby's cardiac axis is similar to the mother's, then their R waves will be in the same direction and the fetus must be a breech. The R waves are in the opposite direction if the presentation is vertex.

E. Weights of Twins: The median weight of twins at birth is just over 5 lb (2270 gm). Male infants weigh slightly more than female. Nevertheless, single fetuses weigh more than individual multiple fetuses after the 30th week.

Complications.

A. Maternal:
1. Toxemia occurs 3 times as often in multiple pregnancy as in single fetus pregnancies.
2. Premature labor and delivery - The overdistended uterus finally reaches its limit of tolerance, and uterine contractions or premature rupture of the membrane (or both) occurs. Three-fourths of all multiple pregnancies are delivered before term.
3. Uterine inertia and desultory labor - The greatly increased volume of the uterus overstretches the myometrial fibers, which then cannot contract.
4. Placenta previa - The surface of the placenta in multiple pregnancy is often greater than in single fetus pregnancy and may reach the zone of the internal os.
5. Premature separation of the placenta occurs more often with rupture of the first bag of waters or after delivery of one twin. (It also occurs more frequently with eclamptogenic toxemia.)
6. Postpartal hemorrhage - Uterine atony is often accompanied by hemorrhage. This is due to the inability of the overdistended uterus to remain contracted after delivery.

B. Fetal:
1. Antepartal complications - Fetal death in utero is about 3 times more common in multiple pregnancy. Death may be due to cord compression, competition for nutrition, or developmental anomalies. The greatest hazard from cord compression is in single ovum twins with only one amniotic sac; they may become entangled in their cords. Developmental anomalies are common with single ovum twins and polyhydramnios. Almost twice as many single ovum twins than double ovum twins die in the perinatal period, and many of

Multiple Pregnancy 213

these die before delivery. Attrition is even greater for triplets, quadruplets, etc.
2. Intrapartal complications - These are the most common causes of fetal loss in multiple pregnancy. Delivery one month before term is often due to premature labor, premature rupture of the membranes, cervicitis, or vaginitis, which occur in about 25% of twin, 50% of triplet, and 75% of quadruplet pregnancies. Abnormal and breech presentation, circulatory interference by one fetus with the other, and operative delivery all increase fetal loss. Prolapse of the cord occurs 5 times as often as during a single pregnancy. Premature separation of the placenta before delivery of the second twin may cause death of the second twin by asphyxia. One twin may obstruct the delivery of both fetuses: in locked twins (Fig 9-5), the first is always a breech and the second a vertex presentation. The heads become impacted in the pelvis and one or both fetuses may die despite operative intervention. Conjoined twins, united at the chest (thoracopagus), the sacrum (pygopagus), or the head (craniopagus), may be undiagnosed prior to labor. Dystocia occurs and the twins may die during attempts at delivery.
3. Postpartal complications - Survival depends upon obstetric and pediatric difficulties and their solution. Immaturity and prematurity claim twice as many twins as single-born infants. Intracranial injury is more common in premature infants—even those delivered spontaneously—and often leads to death in the neonatal period.

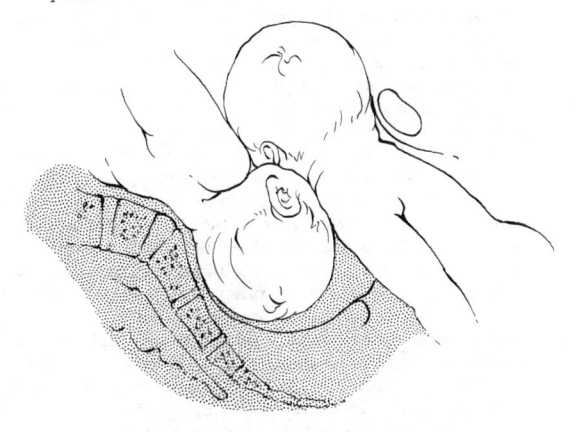

Fig 9-5. Locked twins.

214 Multiple Pregnancy

Differential Diagnosis.

Multiple pregnancy must be distinguished from the following:

A. Single Pregnancy: Only one fetus can be palpated and only one fetal heart heard. Inaccurate dates may give a false impression of the duration of pregnancy and the fetus may therefore be larger than expected.

B. Polyhydramnios: Either single or multiple pregnancy may be associated with excessive fluid accumulation. Careful examination may distinguish one or more fetuses. Obtain x-ray films if the number and normality of the fetuses is still in doubt during the last trimester.

C. Abdominal Tumors Complicating Pregnancy: Numerous fibroid tumors of the uterus are usually felt when present, but ovarian tumors are generally single and discrete.

D. Complicated Twin Pregnancy: If one double ovum twin dies and the other lives on, the dead fetus may become flattened and mummified (fetus compressus or fetus papyraceus). Its portion of the fused placenta will be pale and atrophic, but remnants of 2 sacs and 2 cords will usually be found.

E. Hydatidiform degeneration of the placenta of one fetus of a double ovum pregnancy may occur. The surviving fetus may be thought to be a primary single fetus until delivery.

Treatment.

A. Delivery: An assistant—scrubbed, gowned, and gloved—should always be present for delivery of a patient with multiple pregnancy. Intravenous glucose, 5% in water (1 liter) through a No. 18 needle, should be started during the latter part of the first stage of labor and continued until the third stage is completed. Blood or specific medication can then be administered when indicated without delay. The patient should be typed and crossmatched, and several units of blood should be available in the delivery room for emergency transfusion.

Note: Do a cesarian section only for accepted obstetric reasons. Multiple pregnancy itself is not an indication, but disproportion (e.g., conjoined twins) is.

1. Admit the patient to the hospital at the first sign of labor or leakage of amniotic fluid.
2. Anesthesia - Limit analgesia drastically during labor. Infants are usually premature, and operative intervention is often necessary. Employ pudendal block anesthesia if possible; spinal, intravenous, and deep intravenous, and deep inhalation anesthesia may be dangerous. Give oxygen to the mother by face mask during the second stage of labor.
3. If the first fetus presents by vertex or breech, deliver it in the usual manner. Avoid a difficult forceps or

rapid breech delivery. If the fetus is in transverse presentation, do an internal version and a slow, gentle extraction when the cervix is fully dilated. Make a deep episiotomy incision to minimize constriction of the head.
4. Clamp the cord promptly to prevent the second twin of a single ovum pregnancy from partially exsanguinating through the first cord. Leave 4-6 cm attached to each twin for transfusion purposes later if required. Label the twins and the cords attached to the placenta A and B.
5. Examine the patient vaginally immediately after delivery of the first infant to note presentation of the second. Rupture the second bag of waters. If there is no second amniotic sac (monoamniotic single ovum twins), deliver the second twin at once to prevent asphyxia (premature separation of the placenta or cord entanglement). About half of such second twins die promptly unless the delivery is expedited.
6. Do not give ergot or posterior pituitary injections after the birth of the first twin. Reduction of the uteroplacental circulation will jeopardize the second twin.
7. Avoid haste, but try to deliver the second twin within 10-15 minutes of the first to prevent death due to hypoxia. Cautiously administer dilute oxytocin intravenously to stimulate uterine contractions when uterine inertia becomes a problem. The second twin may present as a transverse. Attempt to guide it into the birth canal as a vertex or breech by fundal pressure. If this is not possible, do an internal version and breech extraction.
8. Manage the third stage of labor cautiously. Administer oxytocin (Pitocin®), 1 ml I.M. immediately after delivery of the second twin, or start an intravenous oxytocin drip. Elevate but do not massage the fundus until after the uterus contracts and expels the separated placenta. Then give an ergot preparation such as ergonovine (Ergotrate®), 0.1 mg I.M., and gently massage and elevate the fundus for 15-30 minutes.

If bleeding is excessive before separation of the placenta, separate and extract the placenta manually. Minimal inhalation anesthesia (trichloroethylene or nitrous oxide) will suffice for placental removal.
9. Locked twins - With the patient under deep anesthesia, have an assistant support the twin already partially delivered as a breech. Push both heads upward out of the pelvis, and then try to deliver its head. If this is not feasible, apply forceps to the other twin and try to deliver both twins together. If this cannot be done, elevate the partially delivered twin, establish an air-

way, and protect the cord. When the undescended twin dies, decapitate it, deliver twin A, and then deliver the body and head of the dead twin. In most instances, both fetuses will die if one takes time to set up for a cesarian section.
- B. General Measures: Maintain optimal weight during pregnancy: ideal weight for height and build plus 16-18 lb. Prevent anemia, toxemia, and vaginal infections, and treat them early when they do occur.
- C. Treatment of Complications: Toxemia, premature labor and delivery, etc are managed as outlined elsewhere in this book. If dystocia occurs, obtain x-ray films to rule out malpresentation or conjoined twins and to determine if malpresentation has occurred. Explore the cervical canal and lower uterine segment vaginally for soft tissue dystocia.

Prognosis.
- A. Mother: Maternal morbidity (fever, infection) is 4-8 times higher with multiple pregnancy than with average term vaginal delivery, but mortality is only slightly increased. Toxemia, hemorrhage, and the complications of operative obstetrics increase the hazard to the mother.
- B. Fetuses: The neonatal mortality for twins is 4-5 times that of single infants born at term. More single ovum than double ovum twins die in the neonatal period. The fetal mortality rate for triplets is twice that of twins. Rarely do triplets, quadruplets, etc all live.

If the fetus is delivered alive, its weight is the best criterion of survival. A twin or triplet weighing over 2500 gm has a better prognosis than a singleton of the same weight.

The best outlook is for both twins to present by the vertex. Twins or other multiple fetuses delivered by spontaneous means do better than those extracted by forceps or after version.

The second twin is in greater danger than the first because it is usually smaller and because circulatory problems and the trauma of delivery may be more damaging.

10...
Obstetric Complications of Labor & Delivery

ECTOPIC PREGNANCY

A fertilized ovum implanted outside the uterine cavity is an ectopic pregnancy. This occurs once in 150-200 conceptions. Ninety per cent occur in the fallopian tube, and 60% of these are on the right side. Eighty per cent are diagnosed within the first 2 months after conception. Ectopic pregnancy may occur at any time from menarche to menopause, but 90% occur in women between the ages of 20 and 40. The incidence of extrauterine pregnancy is inversely proportionate to parity, i.e., it is higher in infertile (especially "one child sterility") patients. There is no racial predisposition, but the frequency is greater in lower socioeconomic groups.

Ectopic pregnancy may be classified according to frequency of site of implantation as follows:

(1) Tubal: Ampullary, infundibular, isthmic, interstitial (angular, cornual), and bilateral.
(2) Abdominal
(3) Ovarian
(4) Cervical
(5) Combined extrauterine and intrauterine

Delay in passage of the ovum from the ovary to the uterine cavity predisposes to ectopic pregnancy. At least 50% of cases are caused by tubal inflammatory lesions.

(1) **Tubal factors:** (In order of frequency.)
  Agglutinated luminal folds (postinflammation)
  Congenital diverticula, accessory ostia, or atresia
  Peritubal adhesions
  Pelvic tumors
  Excessive length or tortuosity
(2) **Ovarian factors:**
  Abnormal ovum
  Transmigration of ovum
  Abnormally early implantation
  Tubal abortion and reimplantation elsewhere

Gestation becomes pathologic when a fertilized ovum implants outside the uterus because organs other than the uterus are not adaptable to pregnancy. In a sense, the conceptus behaves like a malignant neoplasm. No barrier to the tropho-

218 Ectopic Pregnancy

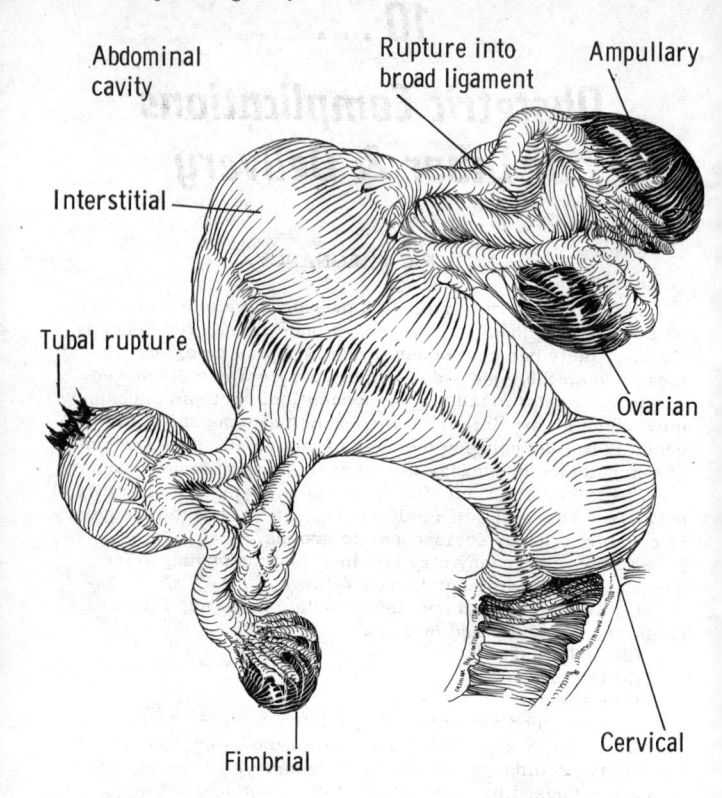

Fig 10-1. Sites of ectopic pregnancies.

blast develops. Sparse decidua formation is likely, and there is only slight muscular hypertrophy for accommodation. Rapid invasion of the muscle ensues, with invasion of the large vessels; internal hemorrhage then occurs.

In tubal pregnancy, distention and weakness of the tube predispose to rupture due to slight trauma. Extracapsular rupture occurs when a portion of the villous ovum extrudes through the tubal wall. In intracapsular rupture, the embryo, fluid, and blood are expelled from the tube after the amniotic and chorionic membranes tear.

Bleeding may cease temporarily after either extracapsular or intracapsular rupture, but the embryo rarely survives. In occasional cases pregnancy may continue if an adequate portion of the placental attachment is retained or if secondary implantation occurs elsewhere.

Abdominal pregnancy may be primary, with the fertilized ovum implanting initially in the abdominal cavity, but it is more often secondary to rupture of a tubal pregnancy with the trophoblast maintaining its tubal attachment or the entire ovum implanting de novo elsewhere after the rupture. The incidence of abdominal pregnancy is 1:15,000 pregnancies; the fetal mortality rate is at least 75%.

The corpus luteum of pregnancy continues to develop as long as the trophoblast is viable. The uterus becomes slightly enlarged and is soft; it contains decidua but no trophoblast. Decidual separation and bleeding occur when the conceptus dies. Only in interstitial pregnancy does blood from the tube drain via the uterus.

Ectopic pregnancy can terminate as follows:

(1) Tubal: Tubal abortion, missed tubal abortion, rupture into the broad ligament, rupture into the peritoneal cavity.

(2) Abdominal: Rupture into the peritoneal cavity, rupture into the retroperitoneum, lithopedion, a viable infant.

(3) Ovarian: Rupture into the peritoneal cavity.

(4) Cervical: Rupture into the vagina.

(5) Combined (usually tubal and intrauterine): Same as (1) above and uterine abortion, or same as (1) above and a viable infant.

Isthmic rupture usually occurs at 6 weeks. Ampullary rupture may ensue at 8-12 weeks. Interstitial rupture may occur at about 4 months, depending upon such factors as the size of the uterus and whether trauma occurs.

If intra-abdominal pregnancy occurs and death comes to an advanced fetus, it cannot be absorbed. It may become infected; it may become mummified; or it may be converted into a grayish, greasy mass called an adipocere.

Clinical Findings.

No specific signs or symptoms are diagnostic. Ectopic pregnancy should be suspected when bleeding or pain occurs within the first 7-8 weeks after the missed period. The pregnancy may be acute (ruptured), chronic (threatened or atypical), or unruptured.

A. Symptoms and Signs: The following symptoms and signs (in the order noted) are present in 75% of cases. (1) Amenorrhea due to increasing chorionic gonadotropin. (2) Uterine bleeding following failure of pregnancy, irrespective of its situation. (3) Abdominal pain due to rupture of the amnionic-chorionic sac, with local bleeding or an enlarging pregnancy, pulsion, and traction. (4) Pelvic mass caused by growth of the conceptus, hematoma from placental separation or host organ, adherence of bowel and omentum, or infection.

1. Tubal pregnancy -
    a. Acute - (Almost 40% of tubal pregnancies.) The complications threaten life. Sharp pain in the ab-

domen and backache are the most common complaints. Scant but persistent uterine bleeding occurs in 80% of patients; 70% have a pelvic mass. A history of abnormal menstruation and infertility is present in about 60% of cases. Collapse and shock, often precipitated by vaginal examination, occur in 10%. Shock may follow sudden massive hemorrhage or severe pain, and is characterized by weakness, thirst, profuse perspiration, "air hunger," vomiting, and oliguria.
- b. Chronic - (About 60% of tubal pregnancies.) The complications may be incapacitating. Blood escapes from the tube, pelvic discomfort increases, and a mass develops. Blood pigmentation of the umbilicus may be present, indicating hematoperitoneum (Cullen's sign). Separation or extrusion of the pregnancy and hypotension reduce the bleeding area of the placental attachment. Clots compress the placental site and the bowel and omentum become adherent to the hematoma, but blood often liquefies and is absorbed before infection develops.
- c. Unruptured - (About 2% of tubal pregnancies.) Brief amenorrhea, tenderness, or adnexal fullness is present before the acute or chronic stage.
- d. Advanced unilateral and bilateral tubal pregnancy is rare. Delivery of a viable fetus is exceptional.

2. Abdominal pregnancy - Because abdominal pregnancy is usually secondary to rupture of a tubal pregnancy, a history of the rupture can usually be elicited. As the pregnancy progresses following secondary abdominal implantation, there is often pressure and peritoneal irritation, causing nausea, vomiting, diarrhea, and abdominal pain, the latter especially notable with fetal movement. In late pregnancy the fetal small parts are more readily palpable and the fetal heartbeat is louder than when the pregnancy is intrauterine. The position is usually abnormal in that transverse lies are common. Braxton Hicks contractions are not present, and the small, empty uterus may occasionally be palpable by abdominal examination.

The usual criteria for abdominal pregnancy are as follows: (1) Normal appearing tubes, ovaries, and broad ligaments. (2) No evidence of penetration of the space between the broad ligament and the fimbriated extremity of the tube. (3) No intraligamentary rupture of the tube. (4) No evidence of escape of the ovum from the uterine cavity.

3. Combined extrauterine and intrauterine pregnancy, a variety of double ovum twins, has been reported in over 100 patients. One or the other is usually diagnosed, but rarely both. The extrauterine fetuses

usually die, and only 60% of the intrauterine fetuses survive to viability.
   4. Ovarian pregnancy is so rare that only about 50 cases have been authenticated. They usually terminate at 6-8 weeks, but a few have gone to full term. Ovarian pregnancy is generally mistaken for early tubal pregnancy or ovarian cyst, and the exact diagnosis is not ascertained until after laparotomy. Secondary ovarian pregnancy usually follows rupture of a tubal pregnancy, but in rare cases it may be primary, i.e., fertilization of the ovum within its follicle.
   5. Cervical pregnancy is very rare. Progression beyond 2-3 months is uncommon. It is always acute and is often misdiagnosed as advanced carcinoma of the cervix. Bleeding is excessive.
B. Laboratory Findings: Pregnancy tests are not useful because they are positive in only 35-40% of cases, and in any event do not identify the site of pregnancy; furthermore, negative tests do not exclude an aborted ectopic pregnancy with hematoma.
   1. Blood - Anemia is often sudden and severe as a result of intraperitoneal bleeding. The icterus index is elevated. The white blood count is elevated if infection is present. Serum amylase may be as high as 1600 Somogyi units/100 ml (normal = 80-180 units) if narcotics have not been given. Reticulocytosis (due to bleeding) is present; reticulocytes may increase to 2.2% (normal = < 1%). Hematin is detected by spectroscopy in peripheral blood 2 days after 100 ml or more of blood accumulate intraperitoneally.
   2. Urine - Urine urobilinogen is elevated, indicating decomposition of blood. Slight porphyrinuria is present with hematocele and hematoperitoneum, but may also indicate a twisted ovarian cyst.
C. X-Ray Findings: Hysterosalpingography may permit a diagnosis of tubal pregnancy, but it is **dangerous** since the injected fluid may rupture the tube or aggravate bleeding. It will not identify an abdominal pregnancy. A flat film (AP) with pneumoperitoneum or pneumocolon may disclose a mass, fluid level (after rupture), and fetal bones. Arteriography defines ectopic pregnancy but is too dangerous to employ routinely.
D. Special Examinations: Blood recovered by culdocentesis is evidence of hematoperitoneum if red cell rouleau is absent; if red cells are crenated; if blood is dark and viscid and contains small clots; or if blood is noncoagulable (having already clotted and liquefied). Culdoscopy permits aspiration, inspection, and tubal surgery. Culdoscopy or peritoneoscopy may identify an unruptured or early aborting tubal pregnancy, but large collections of

Table 10-1. Differential diagnosis of ectopic pregnancy.

	Ectopic Pregnancy	Appendicitis	Salpingitis	Ruptured Corpus Luteum Cyst	Uterine Abortion
Pain	Unilateral cramps and tenderness before rupture.	Epigastric, periumbilical, then right lower quadrant pain; tenderness localizing at McBurney's point. Rebound tenderness.	Usually in both lower quadrants, with or without rebound.	Unilateral, becoming general with progressive bleeding.	Midline cramps.
Nausea and vomiting	Occasionally before, frequently after rupture.	Usual. Precedes shift of pain to right lower quadrant.	Infrequent.	Rare.	Almost never.
Menstruation	Some aberration: missed period, spotting.	Unrelated to menses.	Hypermenorrhea or metrorrhagia, or both.	Period delayed, then bleeding, often with pain.	Amenorrhea, then spotting, then brisk bleeding.
Temperature and pulse	99-100 °F. Pulse variable: normal before, rapid after rupture.	99-100° F. Pulse rapid: 90-100.	99-104° F. Pulse elevated in proportion to fever.	Not over 99° F. Pulse normal unless blood loss marked, then rapid.	To 99° F if spontaneous; to 104° F if induced (infected).
Pelvic examination	Unilateral tenderness, especially on movement of cervix. Crepitant mass on one side or in cul-de-sac.	No masses.	Bilateral tenderness on movement of cervix. Masses only when pyosalpinx or hydrosalpinx is present.	Tenderness over affected ovary. No masses.	Cervix slightly patulous. Uterus slightly enlarged, irregularly softened. Tender with infection.
Laboratory findings	White cell count to 15,000. Red cell count strikingly low if blood loss large. Sedimentation rate slightly elevated.	White cell count 10,000-18,000 (rarely normal). Red cell count normal. Sedimentation rate slightly elevated.	White cell count 15,000-30,000. Red cell count normal. Sedimentation rate markedly elevated.	White cell count normal to 10,000. Red cell count normal. Sedimentation rate normal.	White cell count 15,000 if spontaneous; to 30,000 if induced (infection). Red cell count normal. Sedimentation rate slightly to moderately elevated.

blood render these procedures useless and dangerous.
Dilatation and curettage and endometrial biopsy may disclose decidual endometrium (without chorionic villi). If trophoblast is recovered, uterine pregnancy is established. Inadequate, degenerated tissue will be obtained after 4-5 days of continued bleeding. A steroid sex hormone shift, as reflected by vaginal smears, may indicate abortion but does not identify the site of pregnancy. Exploratory laparotomy establishes the presence or absence of internal (but not cervical) ectopic pregnancy. Laparotomy is indicated (1) when the diagnosis of ectopic pregnancy has been made but culdotomy does not permit adequate exposure for removal of the conceptus; or (2) when an acute abdominal emergency necessitates investigation.

A special test for abdominal pregnancy requires the I.M. injection of 0.1 unit of oxytocin. Within 2 minutes, the uterus will contract but no change will be felt in the structures overlying an extrauterine fetus.

Differential Diagnosis.

About 50 pathologic conditions are clinically similar to extrauterine pregnancy. The most common of these are appendicitis, salpingitis, ruptured corpus luteum cyst or ovarian follicle, and uterine abortion (see Table 10-1). Twisted ovarian cyst and urinary tract disease are infrequently confused with ectopic pregnancy.

Complications.

Without surgery a ruptured ectopic pregnancy may cause exsanguination and death. Chronic salpingitis often follows neglected ruptured ectopic pregnancy. Infertility develops in 50% of patients who have undergone surgery for extrauterine pregnancy; 30% of these become sterile. Chronic urinary tract infection and ureteral stricture may occur after infection. Intestinal obstruction and fistulas may develop after hematoperitoneum and peritonitis. Lithopedion (a mummified, calcified fetus) is the result of an unrecognized abortion of an advanced ectopic pregnancy.

Prevention.

Avoid adhesions at surgery; treat salpingitis early and vigorously; perform dilatation and curettage promptly for incomplete abortion.

Treatment.

Operate immediately after the diagnosis is made. Delay is justified only to correct shock.

A. Emergency Treatment: Hospitalize the patient if ectopic pregnancy is suspected. Insert a large needle into a large vein and transfuse 4-6 pints of blood, under pres-

sure if bleeding is massive and facilities are available. Administer antishock measures as indicated: Keep the patient comfortably warm, give morphine and oxygen, and apply moderately snug tourniquets around the upper legs.
- B. Surgical Treatment: **Control hemorrhage.** Remove the products of conception and evacuate gross blood and clots. **Caution:** If the pregnancy is advanced, do not disturb an adherent placenta but leave it in situ. Do not insert drains. If necessary, give autotransfusions, using the patient's own fresh, citrated blood. Use stimulant anesthetics (ether or cyclopropane); avoid depressants (spinal, thiopental).
  1. If the tube is grossly distorted, dilated, or damaged (as in pregnancy of over 3 months' duration), perform salpingectomy by cornual excision (not resection) to prevent repeat ectopic pregnancy and endosalpingosis of the stump.
  2. If the pregnancy is early (small) or if tubal missed abortion has occurred, perform salpingostomy to enucleate the pregnancy. Ligate bleeding points; suturing is not necessary.
  3. Hysterectomy is usually required in ruptured interstitial or cervical pregnancy.
  4. Oophorectomy is necessary in ovarian pregnancy.
- C. Supportive Treatment: If symptoms and signs of infection are present, give broad-spectrum antibiotics; prescribe oral or I.M. iron therapy (or both); order a high-protein diet with vitamin and mineral supplements as soon as the patient is able to take foods by mouth.

Prognosis.

Maternal mortality due to ectopic pregnancy in the USA is 1-2%; fetal mortality is almost 100%. Ectopic pregnancy does not prevent subsequent normal pregnancy: normal pregnancies are later achieved by more than half of patients who have had one ectopic pregnancy.

Ectopic pregnancy recurs in about 8% of cases.

CAUSES OF THIRD TRIMESTER BLEEDING

Obstetric bleeding is the major cause of maternal mortality and morbidity and is also a significant factor in fetal mortality and morbidity. Five to 10% of women complain of vaginal bleeding in late pregnancy. Multiparas are more commonly affected.

Antepartal bleeding may be classified as placental or nonplacental. Placental bleeding is most often due to placenta previa and premature separation of a normally implanted placenta, including marginal sinus rupture. Nonplacental bleeding is usually due to blood dyscrasia or lower genital tract disorders, including cervical or vaginal infections, neoplasia, and varices. It is essential to distinguish between these 2 large groups.

Placental causes of bleeding often threaten the life of both mother and child, whereas most of the nonplacental bleeding problems—with the exception of cancer—are annoying but not serious. **Nonplacental** bleeding is generally slight; even carcinoma of the cervix or a ruptured vaginal or vulvar varix usually does not cause frank hemorrhage. The same may be true of premature separation of the placenta and placenta previa, however, and vaginal or rectal examination is therefore necessary to make the differentiation. Rupture of the uterus, which occurs in about 1% of patients previously delivered by cesarean section, may cause excessive bleeding; most of the blood lost will be concealed.

Diagnosis of the Cause of Bleeding.

Two attitudes are distinguished in the diagnosis of antepartal bleeding: (1) The radical approach is to require immediate vaginal examination in virtually every patient with third trimester bleeding. (2) The conservative approach is to insist on a regimen of study, purposeful delay, and adequate preparation of the patient, with pelvic examination under the best circumstances. In the author's experience, the latter is infinitely better. If the patient is seen at home, rectal or vaginal examination should be withheld and the vagina or cervix should not be packed. The patient should be hospitalized at once, preferably by ambulance.

Because of the extreme hazard of uncontrollable antepartal uterine hemorrhage, it is vital to avoid a vaginal or even a "gentle rectal examination" since either may cause critical bleeding. Only fragmentary and unreliable information is obtained in most cases by these procedures, and they usually must be repeated.

Procedure on admission to the hospital: (1) Place the patient at complete bed rest, flat in bed. (2) Perform a complete, gentle abdominal examination. (3) Do not perform rectal or vaginal examination. (4) Obtain a crossmatch and have 2-4 units of blood ready for immediate transfusion if necessary. (5) Give a liquid diet of clear fluids only. (6) Reassure the patient and give mild sedation. (7) Observe closely for increasing or decreasing signs of bleeding or fetal distress.

Note: Over 90% of patients with third trimester bleeding will cease to bleed in 24 hours on bed rest alone, no matter what the cause.

The abdominal examination should indicate the size and position of the fetus, the approximate duration of the preg-

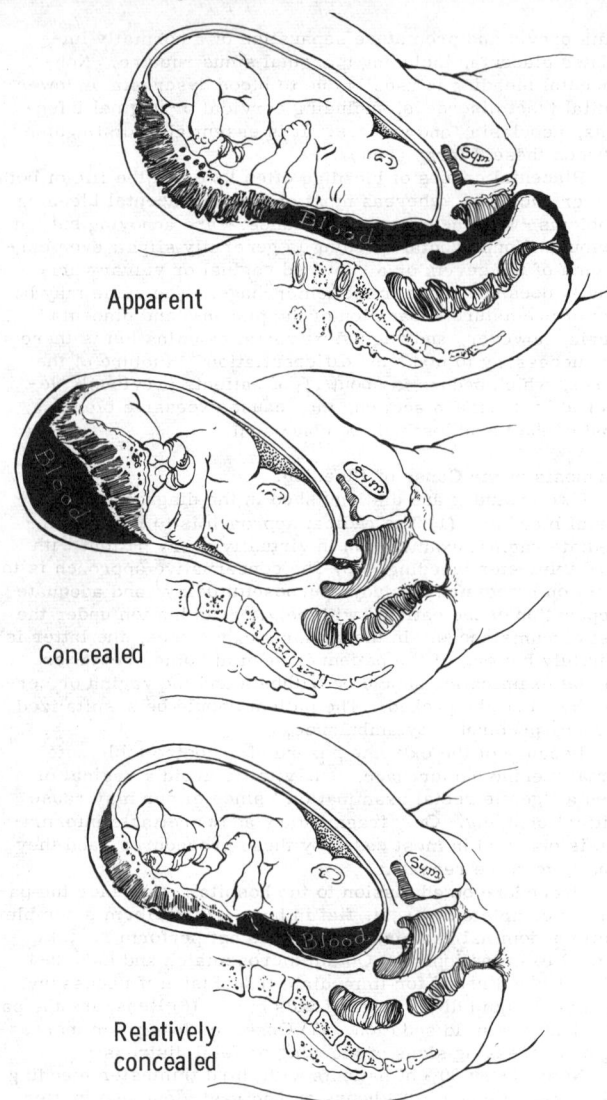

Fig 10-2. Types of premature separation of the placenta. (Redrawn and reproduced, with permission, from Beck and Rosenthal: Obstetrical Practice, 7th ed. Williams and Wilkins, 1957).

nancy, the presentation and position of the infant, the presence or absence of tenderness, uterine resting tone and contractions, and the rate and regularity of the fetal heartbeat.

It is wise to have the nurse save all perineal pads so that a reasonably accurate estimate of blood loss can be made.

Observe the patient for 24 hours if bleeding is not excessive or if hemorrhage ceases, assuming she is at or near term. If hemorrhage is profuse and persistent, however, prompt vaginal examination under the traditional "double set-up" with the operating room readied for possible cesarean section is accomplished after preparation and blood replacement therapy.

If the patient is less than 36 weeks pregnant and the fetus is too small to have a reasonable likelihood of survival, obtain placentograms and avoid more than initial speculum examination. Penetration of the cervical canal may initiate hemorrhage from a placenta previa, and often requires delivery of the premature infant too early for its survival.

There are times when extended hospitalization or bed rest at home will be required for delivery of a viable infant. Recurrent, spontaneous, exsanguinating hemorrhage from placenta previa or premature separation is exceedingly rare. The calculated risk of later bleeding and the uncertainties of an incomplete or presumptive diagnosis are far outweighed by the decreased fetal and maternal mortality and morbidity with a conservative, nonaggressive program of management of antepartal bleeding.

PREMATURE SEPARATION OF THE PLACENTA
(Abruptio Placentae, Ablatio Placentae, Accidental Hemorrhage)

Premature separation of the placenta accounts for 30% of all cases of antepartal bleeding before the delivery of the fetus. Two types are recognized: (1) concealed, painful hemorrhage (retroplacental bleeding without avenue of escape); and (2) external, painless hemorrhage (bleeding from the separated edge or lateral portion of the placenta with drainage of blood through the cervix).

Premature separation of the placenta occurs most often after the 28th week of pregnancy. If it develops before this time, the problem is usually classified as abortion. The placenta detaches in about 50% of patients before the onset of labor and in 10-15% during the second stage of labor.

Vascular injury and vasodilatation are the major causes of premature separation of the placenta. This disorder is not influenced by race. About 80% of patients are multiparas. Over two-thirds of women with premature separation of the placenta also have toxemia of pregnancy. Premature separa-

228 Premature Separation of Placenta

tion of the placenta occurs approximately once in 175-200 pregnancies.

Predisposing factors include overdistention of the uterus, toxemia, renal disease, hypertension, shortness of the umbilical cord, vascular stasis, malnutrition, advanced age, and multiparity. Precipitating factors include the following: (1) Sudden disturbance of the vascular equilibrium, as in vasodilatation secondary to shock. (2) Abrupt increase in blood pressure, as in paralytic vasodilatation or block or compression of the aorta. (3) Passive engorgement of the uterus and placenta, as in the "supine hypotensive syndrome," in which the vena cava is compressed by the enlarged uterus when the patient lies on her back, or due to torsion of the uterus by adnexal or uterine tumors. (4) Abdominal trauma, either due to a direct blow to the uterus or as a result of secondary transmission of force to the uterus. (5) Placental circulatory insufficiency, as in preeclampsia, chronic renal disease, or diabetes mellitus. (6) Rapid decrease in uterine volume, such as follows hasty delivery of the first twin or sudden drainage of hydramnios.

External hemorrhage is due to marginal or partial premature separation of the placenta. Further separation of the placenta, with labor and rupture of the membranes, may occur. Concealed hemorrhage may be associated with retroplacental bleeding when the margins are adherent; complete separation of the placenta but continued attachment of the amnion to the decidua parietalis; complete separation of the placenta and laceration of the membranes following bleeding into the amniotic cavity; or engagement of the presenting part and complete or incomplete separation of the placenta, permitting blood to collect between the membranes.

The most serious type, concealed hemorrhage associated with adherent placental margins, occurs in about 20% of cases. The bleeding is within the decidua basalis, not the placenta itself. Infiltration of the uterine wall behind the placenta by extravasated blood follows. Intramyometrial bleeding eventually results in uteroplacental apoplexy, the so-called Couvelaire uterus, a purplish, copper-colored, ecchymotic, indurated organ which all but loses its contractile power because of disruption of the muscle bundles.

With retroplacental hemorrhage, hematoma develops and general uterine spasm follows. The blood pressure is thus increased in the intervillous spaces and blood is forced into the uteroplacental vessels, bursting these channels. Before delivery, the distended uterus cannot contract to control the bleeding. As uterine contractions subside, blood from the retroperitoneal hematoma ruptures the decidual basal plate, completing the placental separation in that area.

Premature separation of the placenta causes colicky uterine pain, tenderness, and increased tone. Contractions are dysrhythmic and very painful; the patient may develop shock out of proportion to the amount of blood lost.

Hypofibrinogenemia may develop in extreme cases of premature separation. Petechiae appear over the peritoneum, skin, and mucous surfaces; hemorrhage into internal organs occurs, and bleeding may occur in the gastrointestinal, respiratory, and genitourinary tracts.

A completely separated placenta may present before an unengaged (dead) fetus. This is called **prolapse of the placenta**.

Degrees of Premature Separation of the Placenta.
Grade 0: (About 30%.) No diagnostic signs or symptoms are present. Premature separation is not recognized until the placenta is examined after delivery.

Grade 1: (About 45%.) External bleeding is present; uterine tetany and uterine tenderness may or may not be present. Shock does not occur, and there is no fetal distress. (Grade 1 rarely progresses to grade 2.)

Grade 2: (About 15%.) External bleeding may or may not be present. Uterine tetany and tenderness develop. Maternal shock does not occur, but fetal distress is always present and fetal death in utero may occur. (Grade 2 frequently increases in severity, becoming grade 3.)

Grade 3: (About 10%.) External bleeding may or may not be present. Uterine tetany is marked. Maternal shock and fetal death in utero are the rule. A coagulation defect is usually present.

Clinical Findings.
A. Maternal Symptoms and Signs: Patients with marginal premature separation of the normally implanted placenta who report external bleeding generally describe no unusual pain, only blood loss. Those with concealed hemorrhage have great pain when a retroplacental hematoma develops. If blood extravasates from the placental site, with blockage of the blood above the engaged presenting part, uterine discomfort may or may not be described.

The severity of the symptoms depends upon the degree of placental bleeding, the speed of separation, and the retention or pocketing of blood. If blood is retained, regional or generalized uterine pain or tenderness usually is sudden and severe. In extreme cases, agonizing generalized uterine pain and shock are reported. In mild cases there may be localization of the discomfort, particularly if the placenta is implanted anteriorly; persistent, deep pelvic discomfort is described if the placenta is implanted posteriorly. Other manifestations of premature separation with blood retention are a tender, firm (often board-like) uterus which fails to relax, and constant lumbosacral backache of increasing severity.

Uterine bleeding is rarely evident until advanced. The uterus may enlarge slightly if considerable blood is retained.
B. Fetal Signs: Auscultation of the fetal heartbeat discloses evidence of fetal distress due to hypoxia. Tachycardia is first noted; then slowing and irregularity of the heartbeat; and finally disappearance of the heartbeat if fetal death occurs. Unexpected, sudden fetal activity ceases with fetal death due to hypoxia.
C. Laboratory Findings: Anemia may be noted (despite hemoconcentration); in concealed hemorrhage, anemia is often more severe than would be expected in view of the apparent blood loss. The capillary fragility test is positive when the coagulation time is increased. Plasma fibrinogen levels should be determined.

Coagulation time is frequently increased in patients with severe concealed hemorrhage.

Differential Diagnosis.

A. Nonplacental Causes of Bleeding: Nonplacental bleeding is usually not painful. It may be due to cancer of the cervix, urethra, or vagina; vulvar varices, vaginitis or cervicitis, cervical polyps, blood dyscrasias, and vaginal or other trauma. "Bloody show" due to cervical dilatation and effacement just before or during early labor may also be responsible for vaginal bleeding. Rupture of the uterus may cause vaginal bleeding, but is associated with pain, shock, and death of the fetus. Vaginal and cervical speculum examination will reveal most of these entities. Laboratory studies may confirm the diagnosis of infection or neoplasia.
B. Placental Causes of Bleeding: Placenta previa is associated with painless hemorrhage and is diagnosed by palpation.
C. Undetermined Causes of Bleeding: In at least 20% of cases the precise cause of antepartum bleeding during the last trimester of pregnancy is never determined. If one can rule out serious problems, however, undiagnosed bleeding should cause little concern.

Complications.

A. Maternal: Complications include shock out of proportion to the degree of hypotension, dissemination of fibrin emboli, defibrination of blood, renal cortical ischemia followed by renal cortical necrosis, lower nephron nephrosis, and activation of a fibrinolytic system in the maternal plasma.
B. Fetal: Premature separation of the placenta causes fetal hypoxia which, if prolonged, results in cerebral damage which is often irreversible. Hypoxia may lead to cerebral

Premature Separation of Placenta 231

palsy and mental deficiency if the infant survives. More severe degrees of hypoxia cause fetal asphyxia and death.

Prevention.

Improved obstetric care will reduce the incidence and severity of toxemia of pregnancy, but otherwise it does little to prevent premature separation of the placenta. Prompt diagnosis and treatment of retroplacental (concealed) hemorrhage will usually reduce the seriousness of uteroplacental apoplexy. Rupture of the membranes often prevents the more serious complications of premature separation of the placenta. Although the danger of shock decreases after the uterus is emptied, postpartal hemorrhage may be a critical problem if hypofibrinogenemia is not corrected.

Treatment.
  A. Emergency Measures: The clotting mechanism must be restored before any attempt is made to deliver the patient. Eight to 10 gm of fibrinogen should be available in all hospitals for such emergencies. Institute antishock therapy (give transfusions, intravenous plasma expanders, and mild sedation, and prevent heat loss).

  Rupture the membranes, if possible, irrespective of the probable mode of delivery.
  B. Specific Measures:
    1. Premature separation of the placenta with external bleeding can usually be managed by rupture of the membranes to speed labor and delivery from below. If excessive, uncontrollable hemorrhage persists or if fetal distress is apparent, rapid cesarean section is often justified.
    2. An estimate of the magnitude or grade of premature separation is of great value in prognosis and therapy.
      a. Grade 0 - No specific measures are required. Premature separation is not recognized until after delivery.
      b. Grade 1 - When the patient is not in labor, watchful expectancy is indicated; bleeding ceases spontaneously in many cases. When labor begins, prepare for delivery from below in the absence of further complications.
      c. Grade 2 - Anticipate vaginal delivery if labor is expected within 6 hours, especially if the fetus is dead. Cesarean section is justified if fetal distress occurs but the child is likely to survive.
      d. Grade 3 - The patient is always in shock, the fetus has died, the uterus is tetanic, and a coagulation defect may be present. After correction of the coagulation defect, deliver the patient vaginally if this can be done within about 6 hours. (Vaginal

delivery is probably possible for the multiparous patient.) Otherwise, do a cesarean section.
C. General Measures: Prophylactic transfusion of patients who are slightly anemic and are actively bleeding often prevents shock; the availability of 3 or more units of bank blood for immediate transfusion is essential. Avoid excessive analgesia despite patient discomfort since hasty delivery may be required. Give oxygen, 6 liters/minute, by nasal tube or face mask for fetal distress. A fetal heart chart should be kept. Record the rate and rhythm every 5 minutes in patients who are actively bleeding and every 15 minutes if bleeding has ceased and fetal distress is not evident.
D. Surgical Measures: Cervical incision and forceps delivery are rarely indicated in premature separation of the placenta because of fetal and maternal damage, even though the patient is a multipara and the fetal heart tones deteriorate suddenly. Cesarean section is indicated (1) when labor is expected to be of long duration (over 6 hours), but after restoration of the coagulation defect; (2) when hemorrhage does not respond to amniotomy and cautious administration of dilute oxytocin; (3) in cases of early (not prolonged) fetal distress when the fetus is mature and is likely to survive.

Hysterectomy for the removal of a Couvelaire uterus, the source of hemorrhage, is rarely indicated. Such a uterus will contract and bleeding will almost always cease when the coagulation defect is corrected.
E. Treatment of Complications:
  1. Defibrination syndrome - Bank blood, because its fibrinogen has been denatured, will replace the volume of blood lost but not the fibrinogen removed by intravascular clotting. Even if direct transfusions were a practical source of fibrinogen in premature separation of the placenta with a bleeding diathesis, very large amounts of fresh blood (8-10 units) would have to be given. Concentrated fibrinogen is therefore required. In grade 2 and grade 3 premature separation with a deficient clotting mechanism, transfuse with fresh blood to replace blood lost, using a large needle (No. 16 or No. 18); and administer 5 gm of Fibrinogen, USP (Fibrinogen [Human]®, Parenogen®), I.V., in 250 ml of diluent. This will correct most cases of deficient coagulation. Ten gm will fully restore clotting in the vast majority of patients with severe hypofibrinogenemia.
  2. Fibrinolysins - Epsilon-aminocaproic acid (EACA, Amicar®) is a specific antagonist of plasminogen activator. If toxicity can be controlled, excessive fibrinolysis may be prevented by this drug. Nevertheless,

interference with prompt lysis of thrombi in vital areas by dissolution of fibrin could inhibit the defensive function of fibrinolysin. Further study of EACA is indicated.

3. Viral hepatitis may occur in patients who receive blood transfusions and intravenous fibrinogen. This is a calculated risk. Gamma globulin, 5-10 ml I. M. may be of value in prevention. If viral hepatitis develops, isolate the patient and place her on a low protein, high carbohydrate diet.

   Because lyophilized fibrinogen is very expensive, it is not always available in quantity in smaller hospitals. It is available, however, through the Red Cross and other blood bank depots. It may be possible to obtain concentrated plasma, a substitute for purified fibrinogen, in double or even quadruple strengths. One unit of fresh blood contains about 1.1 gm of fibrinogen. One pint of quadruple strength plasma, therefore, would provide about 4.4 gm of fibrinogen. If blood volume becomes excessive, as much as 1 liter of concentrated plasma will correct most cases of coagulation deficiency.

4. Renal cortical necrosis is secondary to marked prolonged hypotension. Give hydralazine (Apresoline®), 25-40 mg by slow I. V. drip, to reduce renal cortical ischemia.

5. Acute cor pulmonale secondary to fibrin embolization to the lung reduces pulmonary ventilation. Oxygen therapy by face mask or tent is required. Avoid excessive amounts of intravenous fluid or blood.

6. Lower nephron nephrosis and anuria - Many patients with toxemia of pregnancy develop premature separation of the placenta. The toxemia may result in lower nephron nephrosis and anuria. It is necessary to measure daily fluid intake and output and to avoid giving excessive amounts of sodium and potassium. Plasma dialysis may be required in extreme cases when serum potassium rises above 7 mEq/liter. Peritoneal dialysis for the removal of excessive blood metabolites is now an established procedure in many hospitals.

Prognosis.

External or concealed bleeding, excessive blood loss, shock, nulliparity, a closed cervix, absence of labor, and delayed diagnosis and treatment are unfavorable prognostic factors.

Maternal mortality rates between 0.5-5% are currently being reported from various parts of the world. Most women die of hemorrhage (immediate or delayed) or cardiac or renal failure. A high degree of suspicion, early diagnosis, and definitive therapy will reduce maternal mortality to 0.5-1%.

Fetal mortality ranges between 50-80%. About 30% are delivered at term. In about 20% of patients no fetal heartbeat is heard on admission to the hospital, and in another 20% fetal distress is noted early. In cases where transfusion of the mother is urgently required, the fetal mortality rate will probably be at least 50%.

Forty to 50% are premature births. Infants die of hypoxia, prematurity, and delivery trauma.

PLACENTA PREVIA

In placenta previa the placenta develops within the zone of dilatation and effacement of the lower uterine segment so that the placenta precedes the fetus at delivery. The cause is not known, but decreased vascularity of the endometrium in the fundus is assumed to be one factor. Placenta previa is most common among older women and those who have borne many children, and occurs once in every 200-225 pregnancies which continue beyond the 28th week. The placenta completely covers the cervical os in only 10-15% of cases.

The relative size of the placenta and its site of insertion are important factors in the development of placenta previa. The lower the insertion, the less suited is the uterine mucosa for nidation. The surface area of the placenta in placenta previa is generally 30-40% greater than that of a normal placenta. The placenta is inserted on the anterior wall of the uterus in 60% of cases (twice the normal incidence).

Bleeding in placenta previa may be due to any of the following causes:

(1) Mechanical separation of the placenta from the uterus near the cervical os, following retraction of the uterine wall during the formation of the thinner lower uterine segment, effacement and dilatation of the cervix, or intravaginal manipulation.

(2) Placentitis.

(3) Variability of vascular pressures is a possible cause of bleeding for which the following mechanism has been adduced: (a) Erosion of the trophoblast produces secondary venous lakes in the decidual basalis. (b) Maternal blood floods these lakes instead of leaving the placenta from the decidual area into which it originally entered. (c) The blood then enters the many uterine veins at the periphery of the placenta, and from here returns to the general circulation. (d) Decreased venous pressure occurs in an area of the placenta deficient in underlying maternal arterioles. (e) Maternal blood tends to fill such a low-pressure zone; it may even break through a poorly supported area to escape from the maternal surface of the placenta.

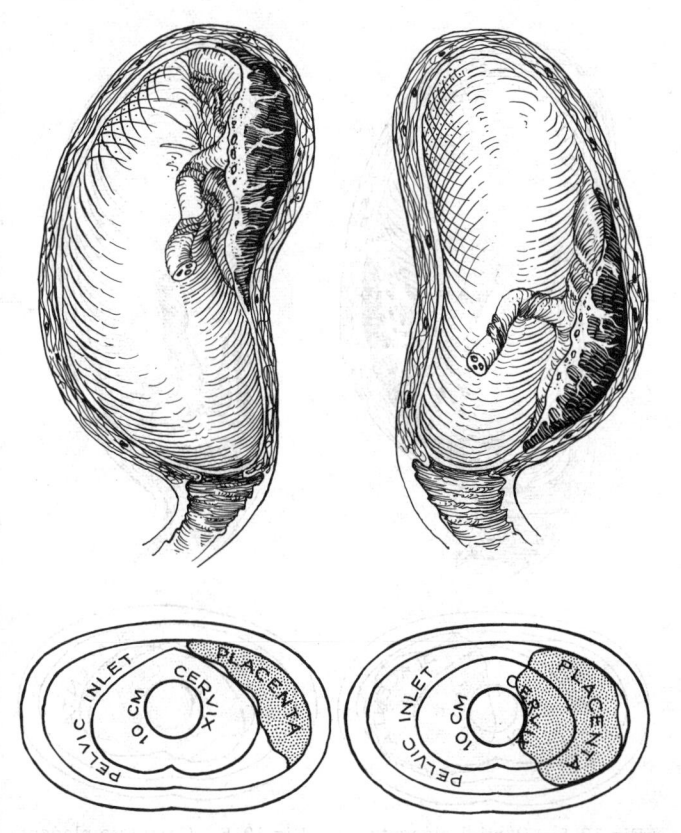

Fig 10-3. Normal placenta.   Fig 10-4. Low implantation.

Placenta previa is now classified on the basis of the approximate area of the internal cervical os which would be covered by the placenta if the cervical os were permitted to become completely dilated (10 cm).* The cervix, but not the placenta, will retract as the internal cervical os dilates and the lower uterine segment develops. This causes a shearing of the placental-cervical attachment.

---

*Placenta previa was formerly classified as (1) central or complete, in which the placenta covers the entire internal osteal area; (2) partial, in which the placenta incompletely cov-

236 Placenta Previa

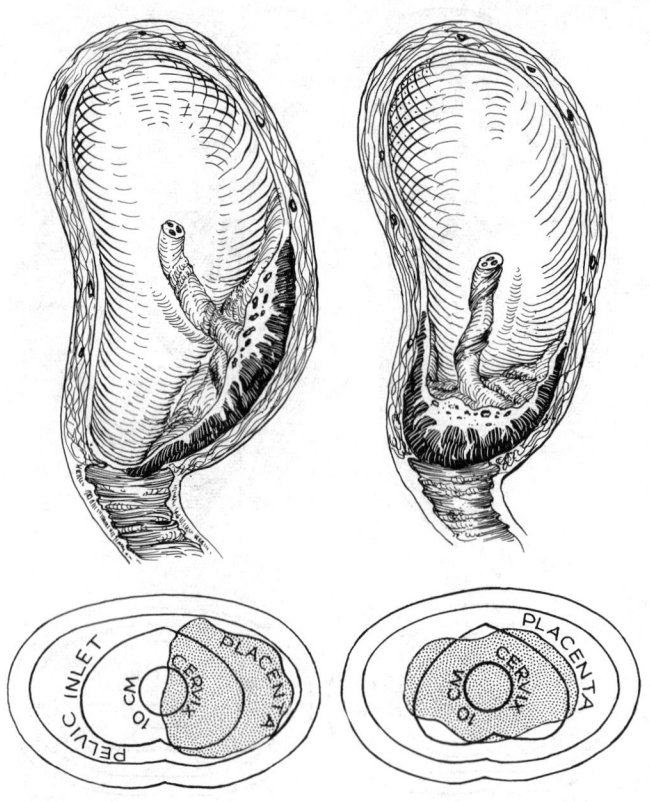

Fig 10-5. Partial placenta previa.

Fig 10-6. Complete placenta previa.

In Fig 10-7, the internal os at term is represented at varying degrees of dilatation. If the edge of the placenta can be palpated at the center of the internal os, then about half of

ers the os; and (3) marginal, in which only the edge of the placenta can be felt at the margin of the os. The disadvantage of this classification is that the relationships depend upon the extent of dilatation of the internal cervical os at examination. Since complete placenta previa may become partial after dilatation of the internal os, and marginal placenta previa may also become partial, the classification does not permit valid comparisons and should be abandoned in favor of that given above.

Placenta Previa 237

EDGES OF PLACENTA PALPATED THROUGH CERVIX

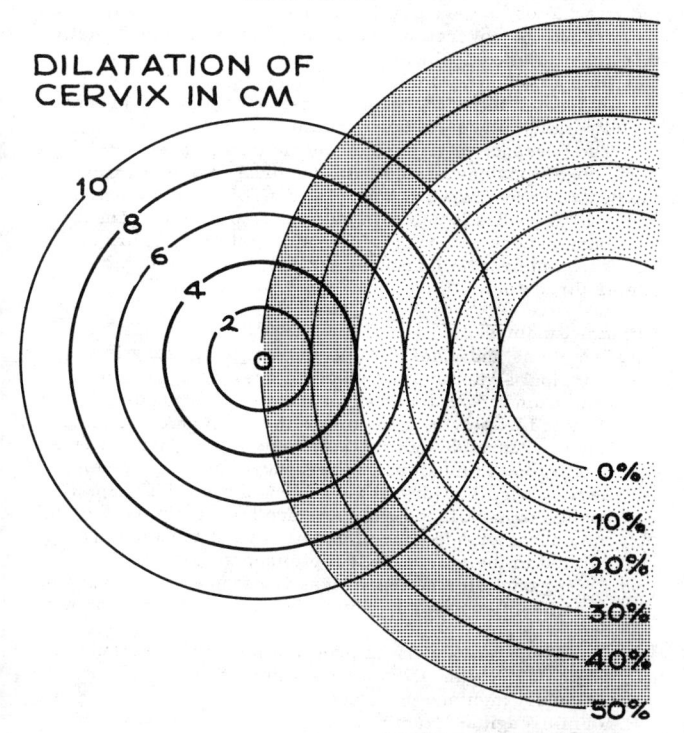

DILATATION OF CERVIX IN CM

10
8
6
4
2
0

0%
10%
20%
30%
40%
50%

PERCENTAGE PLACENTA PREVIA

MANAGEMENT:
LESS THAN 30% VAGINAL DELIVERY
MORE THAN 30% ABDOMINAL DELIVERY

Fig 10-7. Relation of placenta previa to the cervix. (After Tatum.)

the area represented by the internal os should be covered by
placenta (assuming that the internal os were allowed to dilate
completely); this constitutes 50% placenta previa. If the placental edge can be palpated 3 cm laterally from the center of
the internal os, an area of the internal os having a radius of
2 cm should be covered by the placenta at complete dilatation;
this constitutes 20% placenta previa.

Note: Do not try to determine any degree of placenta
previa greater than 60% before delivery. This may produce
uncontrollable placental hemorrhage.

The presence of tumors, atrophic changes, scars, and
other conditions associated with impaired vascularization of
the decidua encourages the development of placenta previa.
Almost 10% of cases occur in patients who have had cesarean
sections, especially lower segment operations. A low cervical cesarean section increases the chances of later placenta
previa three-fold.

Clinical Findings.

A. Symptoms and Signs: Painless uterine bleeding is the
   principal symptom, but placenta previa rarely causes
   exsanguinating antepartal bleeding unless bleeding is
   initiated by pelvic or rectal examination before onset of
   labor. Although spotting may occur throughout the first
   and second trimesters of pregnancy, marked bleeding
   usually begins after the 28th week of gestation. Small
   gushes of dark blood and clots are frequently passed, but
   the character and time of occurrence of bleeding are not
   related to the type or extent of placenta previa.

   Regional uterine tenderness is not present. Occasional contractions may be noted, but normal relaxation will
   occur.

   Breech and abnormal presentations are common with
   placenta previa. Even a presenting vertex will remain
   unusually high and unengaged.

B. Sterile Vaginal Examination: A positive diagnosis of
   placenta previa can be made only by sterile vaginal examination in the so-called "double set-up" procedure.
   The patient should be in the hospital and prepared for
   vaginal or cesarean delivery, with typed and crossmatched
   blood available.
   1. Inspect the lower genital tract for varicosities, ulcerative areas, neoplasms, or other sources of bleeding.
      Visualize the cervix and observe its apparent degree
      of dilatation, its thickness, and any bleeding from beyond the internal os.
   2. Gently feel around the cervix and attempt to elicit
      ballottement of the presenting part. Note any soft
      mass between the presenting part and the cervix or in
      the lower uterine segment.

3. Palpate the cervix to determine its consistency, degree of dilatation, and effacement.
4. Carefully insinuate the finger into the cervical os. Gently feel for spongy tissue partially or completely covering the internal os.
5. Ascertain whether the membranes are intact or ruptured.

C. X-Ray Findings: Direct or indirect placentography may supplement vaginal examination in the diagnosis of placenta previa, but clear relationships cannot usually be observed except with vertex presentation, in which the baby's head normally rests symmetrically on the pelvic brim when the mother is erect and the juncture of the upper and lower uterine segments are in the vicinity of the pelvic brim. When the placenta is implanted low or over the os, the fetal head is displaced from its normal position at the brim. Placenta previa may be missed on soft tissue radiography with breech, transverse, or oblique presentation; polyhydramnios, abruptio placentae, bipartite placenta, placenta totalis, twins with 2 placentas, pelvic tumor, and lateral oblique malposition of the uterus.

A crescent-shaped mass in the body of the uterus whose normal outlines are adjacent is probably the placenta, and almost completely rules out the possibility of placenta previa.

X-rays facilitate the vaginal examination by reducing the risk of severe hemorrhage, since the probable site of attachment of the placenta can often be ascertained before digital exploration.

1. Direct placentography - Soft tissue radiography is useful in outlining the placenta after the 32nd week of pregnancy. It is employed mainly to rule out placenta previa rather than to diagnose the placental site as such. Two lateral views of the uterus, one with the patient recumbent and the other with the patient erect, will allow identification of the placenta when it is in the fundus in 95% of term pregnancies.

   Translumbar and retrograde-femoral aortography have both been used with great success to identify the vascular pattern of the placenta after the 24th week, but this method is hazardous and should not be used except by a specialist.

2. Indirect placentography employing cystography allows a diagnosis of placenta previa by demonstrating excessive displacement of the presenting vertex. In the management of placenta previa it is often more important to know the relationship of the presenting part to the pelvic brim than that of the placenta to the internal os. To obtain a cystogram for the diagnosis of

placenta previa, inject 120-140 ml of a 10% aqueous sodium iodide solution into the bladder; inject 200 ml of air into the rectum; and secure AP and lateral x-rays with the patient erect. The distance from the presenting part to the bladder; the distance between the presenting part and the anterior rectal wall; and the distance between the presenting part and the sacral promontory are then measured. Placenta previa may be present if these measurements are each over 2 cm during the 10th lunar month or 3 cm during the 9th lunar month. This method is accurate in about 80% of cases of vertex presentation after the 36th week. It cannot be used with breech, oblique, or transverse presentations.
D. Radioisotope Localization: Radioactive isotope localization of the placenta is an accurate and safe procedure if done by a radiologist. Preferably, minute amounts of pure gamma emitters such as I^{125} bound to serum albumin (RISA) or red cells tagged with Cr^{51} are injected into the mother's circulation and calculations of radioactivity are made over various abdominal segments.

Differential Diagnosis.

Extrauterine causes of bleeding may be revealed by vaginal and cervical inspection. If the bleeding is intrauterine, it may be of placental or nonplacental origin. Blood which is observed to flow through the cervical canal is probably from within the uterus (although a cervical cancer or infection high in the canal must be considered). Placental causes of bleeding other than placenta previa include premature separation of the normally implanted placenta and rupture of the "marginal sinus" of the placenta.

The only certain method of distinguishing between placenta previa and premature separation of the placenta is palpation of the placenta through the cervical os. One cannot distinguish premature separation of the margin of the placenta and rupture of the "marginal sinus" before delivery and inspection of the placenta.

Before examination is attempted, one must determine whether the fetus is sufficiently large to survive if delivered at that time. Palpation through the cervix may cause such profuse bleeding as to require immediate vaginal delivery or cesarean section. One may decide to withhold digital examination at that time and to admit the patient to a hospital until the fetus is viable, assuming that excessive bleeding does not develop.

Complications.
A. Maternal: Maternal hemorrhage, shock, and death may follow severe antepartal bleeding from placenta previa.

Death may also occur as a result of intrapartal and postpartal bleeding, operative trauma, infection, or embolism.

Premature separation of a portion of a placenta previa occurs in virtually every case, and causes excessive external bleeding without pain. However, complete or wide separation of the placenta before full dilatation of the cervix is not common.

Rupture of the lower uterine segment may follow version or the insertion of an intra-ovular Voorhees bag (now rarely used in the treatment of hemorrhage from placenta previa).

Intrapartal and postpartal endometritis, parametritis, and peritonitis commonly occur following placentitis.

Placenta previa accreta is a rare but serious abnormality in which the sparse endometrium and the myometrium of the lower uterine segment are penetrated by the trophoblast in a manner similar to placenta accreta higher in the uterus.

B. Fetal: Prematurity due to placenta previa is the major cause of fetal mortality, accounting for 60% of perinatal deaths. The fetus may die as a result of intrauterine asphyxia or birth injury. Fetal hemorrhage due to tearing the placenta occurs with vaginal manipulation and especially upon entry into the uterine cavity at cesarean section done for placenta previa. About half of these cesarean babies lose some blood. The fetal blood loss is directly proportionate to the time which is allowed to elapse between laceration of a cotyledon and clamping the cord.

Treatment.

The type of treatment given depends upon the amount of uterine bleeding, the duration of pregnancy and viability of the fetus, the degree of placenta previa, the presentation, position, and station of the fetus, the gravidity and parity of the patient, the status of the cervix, and whether or not labor has begun.

Once the diagnosis of placenta previa is made, the patient should stay in the hospital until delivered. Two or more units of bank blood should be typed, crossmatched, and ready for transfusion. Be prepared to replace twice as much blood as the estimated loss.

Great gains in fetal survival can be achieved by postponing delivery for one week to 5 months. If at all possible, the baby should not be delivered before the 36th week. If severe hemorrhage occurs between 37-40 weeks, consider emptying the uterus. Earlier in pregnancy, a more conservative program is recommended. Maturity is a prime requisite for fetal survival.

Seventy-five per cent of cases of placenta previa are now terminated artificially between the 36th and 40th week of pregnancy.

A. Mode of Delivery: **Caution:** Because uterine contractions are a major cause of hemorrhage, do not stimulate labor except by rupturing the membranes if this can be done easily. Because distention of the lower segment may rupture the uterus, avoid manipulative vaginal delivery.

The modern treatment of placenta previa is essentially institutional. There are 3 choices in therapy: (1) expectant treatment in the hospital, terminating in vaginal delivery; (2) artificial rupture of the membranes; and (3) cesarean section. Most patients with 20-30% placenta previa (marginal or minimally partial) should be delivered vaginally unless hemorrhage is excessive. If placenta previa is more than 30% (complete or extensively partial), cesarean section will probably be required. Regardless of the degree of placenta previa, prompt abdominal delivery is indicated if the patient's status or that of the viable infant deteriorates rapidly. For breech, transverse, or oblique presentations, abdominal delivery will probably also be necessary.

1. Vaginal delivery - If vaginal delivery is decided upon, amniotomy should be done immediately. Although prolapse of the cord is a calculated risk, this probably will not occur if the patient is placed in the semi-Fowler position during drainage. Tamponade of the presenting part against the placental edge usually reduces bleeding as labor progresses.

   The vacuum extractor (see p. 370) is most useful for expediting delivery in placenta previa.

   Willett scalp traction forceps may be employed, especially in multiparous patients with minor degrees of placenta previa, for control of bleeding and acceleration of labor. Superficial injury to the fetal scalp occurs in one-third of cases, but serious damage is not common. The forceps (Fig 10-8) is passed into the uterus and a generous fold of the fetus's scalp is grasped. One to 2 lb of traction force are then applied.

   Unless an extreme degree of placenta previa is present, multiparous patients will usually go into labor promptly; most of these can be delivered safely from below.

   If labor does not follow rupture of the membranes within 6-8 hours, cautious stimulation with intravenous oxytocin (Pitocin®, Syntocinon®), 5 units (0.5 ml) in 1 liter of 5% glucose, may be given at a rate of 1-2 ml/minute.

   Deliver the patient in the easiest and most expeditious manner as soon as the cervix is fully dilated and

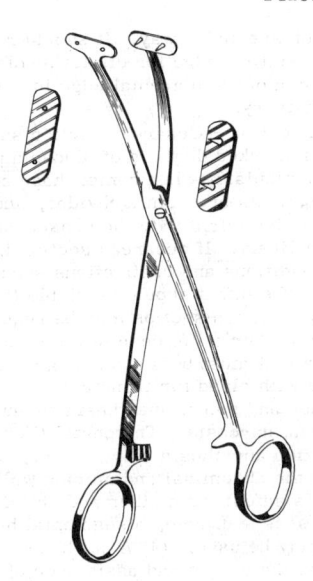

Fig 10-8. Willett placenta previa forceps. The Willett forceps is passed into the uterus and a generous fold of the fetal scalp is grasped. Traction (1-2 lb) is then applied. This forceps may cause scalp laceration and infection, but it is used to correct malposition of the vertex, to check bleeding and expedite delivery in partial placenta previa, to facilitate extraction of the vertex at cesarean section, and to hasten delivery, especially of a dead fetus.

the presenting part is on the perineum. Check the fetal heartbeat regularly every 15 minutes during the course of labor. If fetal distress develops, conclude vaginal delivery if possible; otherwise, perform immediate cesarean section. If bleeding continues, auscultate the fetal heartbeat every 3-5 minutes during the second stage.

Bipolar (Braxton Hicks) version should not be attempted even if the infant is dead. Rupture of the lower uterine segment, cervical lacerations, and severe hemorrhage may occur.

Internal podalic version is contraindicated in the treatment of placenta previa. Laceration of the placenta and the maternal soft parts frequently results even in the multiparous patient.

An intra-ovular Voorhees bag may be used to control bleeding temporarily while preparations for cesarean section are under way. It should rarely be used as a hydrostatic wedge for dilatation of the cervix and compression of the placental edge in anticipation of vaginal delivery.

2. Cesarean section - Cesarean section should be reserved for marked degrees of placenta previa (30% or more), particularly when hemorrhage continues. Many of these patients are primigravidas, and prompt delivery of a live infant with the conservation of maternal blood is unlikely. If cesarean section is decided upon, certain conditions and restrictions should be kept in mind: (1) The infant should be viable (although in rare instances cesarean section may be required to preserve the mother's life despite fetal death in utero). (2) The patient must be a good surgical risk (not in shock and with blood for transfusion available). (3) Avoid ether and spinal anesthesia because of the hazards of fetal narcosis. Thiopental (Pentothal®) or light nitrous oxide anesthesia may be used, but local infiltration of the abdominal and uterine wall with 0.5-1% procaine is safest for mother and child. If an anesthesiologist is available, a segmental block or cyclopropane may be used. (4) A skillful surgical team is necessary; the advice and assistance of an obstetrician may ensure a favorable outcome for mother and child.

The classical operation is preferred in the treatment of placenta previa because (1) it is more advantageous in an emergency; (2) entry is rapid and exposure is good; (3) the placenta is rarely torn; and (4) the lower segment is easily exposed for suture of the large sinuses from within the uterus.

To avoid fetal hemorrhage during lower uterine segment cesarean section for placenta previa, separate the placenta gently, if at all; rupture the membranes; rotate the infant's face into the incision, aspirate its mouth and throat, and establish an airway; clamp the cord; deliver the infant and cut the cord.

If a delay of one minute after visible damage to the placental blood vessels occurs, the infant may lose enough blood to require transfusion. A fall of hemoglobin in venous blood below 14 gm/100 ml within 24 hours suggests such blood loss. If the hemoglobin reaches 10 gm/100 ml within 24 hours, the infant should probably be transfused. If the hemoglobin drops to 12 gm or lower 3 hours following delivery, transfusion is urgently required.

B. Treatment of Complications: Treat hemorrhage and shock promptly and adequately. Ample blood for transfusion is vital. Rupture of the uterus requires laparotomy for suture of the rent or hysterectomy. The latter is generally

Abortion 245

necessary. Puerperal infection is treated with massive doses of broad-spectrum antibiotics and correction of anemia. Placenta previa accreta is an indication for total hysterectomy via the abdominal approach.

Prognosis.

Placenta previa is more common in repeat cesarean sections, and occurs in at least 5% of these cases.
  A. Maternal Mortality: Maternal mortality in placenta previa has dropped from 1% to 0.5-0.8% during the past 10 years with modern therapy in the larger hospitals in the USA. Unfortunately, fetal mortality and morbidity have not paralleled this improvement.
  B. Fetal Mortality: Fetal mortality is approximately 20% in most medical centers. The likelihood of an infant dying when placenta previa complicates the pregnancy is at least 10 times that in normal pregnancy. The minimal fetal mortality can probably be reduced ultimately to 10-15% (corrected for living viable infants without serious anomalies).

SPONTANEOUS & HABITUAL ABORTION

Abortion is the termination of pregnancy before the fetus becomes viable. Viability is usually reached at 28 weeks, when the infant weighs slightly more than 1000 gm; with proper care in the neonatal period, the infant may survive. Abortion may occur early, before the 16th week; or late, from the 16th to 28th weeks. About 75% of abortions occur before the 16th week; of these, 75% occur before the 8th week.

The relative incidence of abortion is highest in early adulthood and just prior to the menopause. About 12% of all pregnancies terminate in spontaneous abortion.

Etiology.

About 50-60% of spontaneous abortions result from ovular defects; 15% are caused by maternal factors; the cause of the remainder is not known.

Random cases occur without predisposition (10%); recurrent cases are the result of chronic germ plasm defects in ovum or sperm (0.5%). Habitual abortion (loss of 3 or more consecutive previable pregnancies) is usually secondary to recurrent causes.
  A. Ovular Factors: Organization of an early conceptus (even in a favorable site) may be faulty; a normal infant cannot develop and abortion ensues. This is especially true if implantation occurs outside the uterus.
    1. First trimester - 40% of abortuses show characteristics of hydatidiform mole, but many pregnancies are

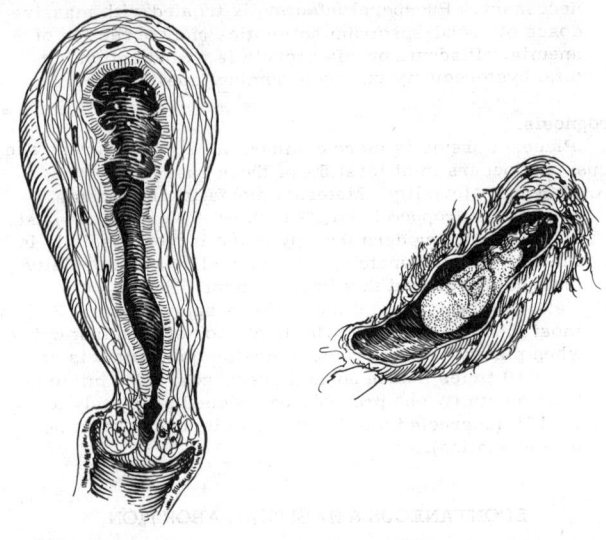

Fig 10-9. Complete abortion. At right: Product of complete abortion.

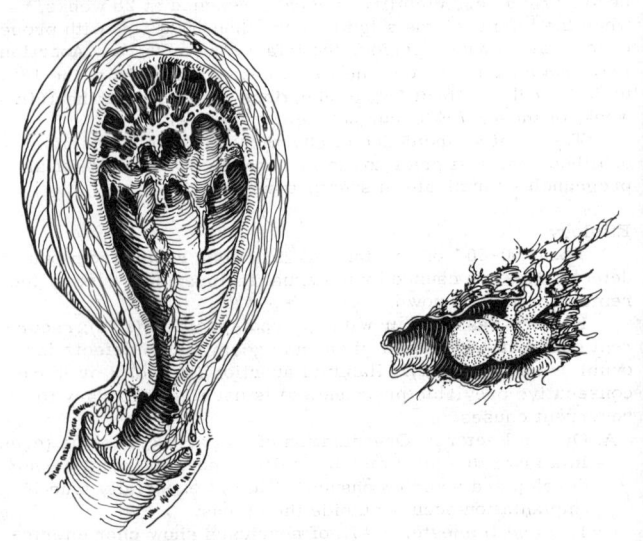

Fig 10-10. Incomplete abortion. At right: Product of incomplete abortion.

expelled so early that deficiencies cannot be accurately determined. Congenital absence of the embryo is common. Cleavage defects of the ovum, absence of the chorionic cavity, and a hypoplastic trophoblast are found occasionally.
  2. Second trimester - Shallow circumvallate implantation of the placenta is the major fetal cause of abortion. Erythroblastosis and other fetal anomalies are less frequently responsible.
B. Maternal Factors:
  1. Indirect trauma - Abortion may be induced by medical or surgical shock, total body irradiation greater than 3000 r, or electric shock (lightning or power-line contact).
  2. Direct trauma - Concussion of the lower abdomen after the 4th month may injure the uterus, causing placental separation. Abdominal surgery or coitus may excite uterine irritability and induce abortion.
  3. Infections - Rubella, syphilis, brucellosis, or toxoplasmosis increases the likelihood of abortion.
  4. Diet - Avitaminosis C and B or severely deficient protein or caloric intake.
  5. Endocrine - Hypothyroidism, diabetes mellitus.
  6. Toxic - Folic acid antagonists (aminopterin), lead poisoning, maternal hypoxia.
  7. Psychic - There is no good evidence to support the concept that abortion may be induced by psychic stimuli such as severe fright, grief, anger, or anxiety.
  8. Uterocervical - Incompetence of the cervix as a result of previous pregnancies and lacerations causes second trimester abortion. Uterine anomalies may result in first or second trimester abortion.

Clinical Findings.
A. Symptoms and Signs: Abortion is classified clinically as (1) complete, (2) incomplete or inevitable, and (3) missed. In threatened abortion the previable gestation is in jeopardy but the pregnancy continues.
  1. Complete - In complete abortion all of the conceptus is expelled. When complete abortion is impending, the symptoms of pregnancy often disappear and sudden bleeding begins, followed by cramping. The fetus and the rest of the conceptus may be expelled separately. When the entire conceptus has been expelled, pain ceases but slight spotting persists.
  2. Incomplete or inevitable - In incomplete abortion, portions of the conceptus have already been passed; in inevitable abortion, evacuation of part or all of the conceptus is momentarily impending. Bleeding and cramps do not subside. Abortion is inevitable when

248 Abortion

> 2 or more of the following are noted (Brown): (1) Moderate effacement of the cervix, (2) cervical dilatation > 2 cm, (3) rupture of the membranes, (4) bleeding for > 7 days, (5) persistence of cramps despite narcotics, (6) signs of termination of pregnancy.

Fever and generalized pelvic discomfort indicate infection. Retained tissue is evidenced by a patulous cervix and an enlarged, boggy uterus.

3. Missed - In missed abortion the pregnancy has been terminated for at least one month but the conceptus has not been expelled. Symptoms of pregnancy disappear; basal body temperature is not elevated. There is a brownish vaginal discharge but no free bleeding. Pain is not present. The cervix is semi-firm and only slightly patulous; the uterus becomes smaller and irregularly softened; the adnexa are normal.

B. Laboratory Findings:
1. Urine - The Friedman and Aschheim-Zondek tests are negative or equivocally positive. On a stained smear of centrifuged sediment the epithelial cells are similar in staining properties to those seen on smears of vaginal discharge.
2. Blood - If significant bleeding has occurred, blood studies will show anemia. If infection is present, the white count will be elevated (12-20 thousand). The sedimentation rate, already elevated by pregnancy, increases rapidly with infection and anemia. The serum Friedman test is usually negative.
3. Hormones - With the exception of hypothyroidism, it is unlikely that abnormalities in hormone secretion cause abortion. Elevated blood and urine hormone levels in pregnancy are almost always physiologic. (1) Chorionic gonadotropin is produced by the cytotrophoblast (Langhans' cells). It is present in the urine in diminished amounts in failing pregnancy; absent after pregnancy ceases. (2) Estrogen: The greatest source of estrogen is the trophoblast; a small amount is secreted by the ovary. A falling blood or urine estrogen titer may signify impending abortion. (3) Progesterone: During the first trimester the principal source of progesterone is the corpus luteum. Thereafter, the principal source is the chorioplacental system. Pregnanediol (the major catabolite of progesterone) drops precipitously in abortion.

C. X-Ray Findings: X-rays are of no value in the diagnosis of early abortion. In advanced missed abortion, x-rays may reveal a distorted fetal skeleton and intrauterine gas.

Differential Diagnosis.

A. Ectopic pregnancy is the probable cause of menstrual abnormality, unilateral pelvic pain, uterine bleeding, and a tender adnexal mass.
B. Unopposed estrogen stimulation or hyperestrinism causes abnormal uterine bleeding in the nonpregnant patient.
C. Membranous dysmenorrhea is characterized by cramps, bleeding, and passage of endometrial casts. Decidua and villi are absent; amenorrhea does not occur.
D. Hydatidiform mole usually ends in abortion before the 5th month. Theca lutein cysts, when present, cause bilateral ovarian enlargement; the uterus may be unusually large. Bloody discharge may contain hydropic villi.

Complications.

Hemorrhage is a major cause of maternal death. Infection is most common after criminally induced abortion; death results from salpingitis, peritonitis, and septicemia or septic emboli. Perforation of the uterus, accompanied by injury to the bowel and bladder, hemorrhage, infection, and fistula formation, may occur during dilatation and curettage because of the soft and vaguely outlined uterine wall. About three-fourths of cases of chorio-epithelioma follow abortion, 30% within 4-6 months. Infertility may result from tubal occlusion or chronic cervicitis following uterine abortion.

Prevention.

Many abortions can be prevented by study and treatment of maternal disorders before pregnancy; early obstetric care, with adequate treatment of maternal diabetes, hypertension, etc; and by protection of pregnant women from hazards to health in industry, from exposure to rubella, etc. Cerclage (Shirodkar) during the second trimester for closure of an incompetent cervix will prevent many abortions.

Treatment.

Successful management of abortion depends upon early diagnosis. Every patient should receive a general physical (including pelvic) examination, and a complete history should be taken. Laboratory studies should include cultures of cervical mucus to determine pathogens in case of infection, antibiotic sensitivity tests, blood typing and crossmatching, and a complete blood count. Thyroid deficiency should be determined by appropriate tests.

A. Emergency Measures: If abortion has occurred after the first trimester, the patient should be hospitalized. In all cases, give oxytocics, e.g., oxytocin (Pitocin®, Syntocinon®), 1 ml/500 ml of 5% dextrose in water I.V., or 0.5 ml I.M. every 30 minutes for 2-4 doses, to contract the uterus and limit blood loss and aid in the expulsion of

250 Hydatidiform Mole

      clots and tissues. Ergonovine (Ergotrate®) should be
given only if the diagnosis of complete abortion is certain.
Give antishock therapy, including blood replacement, to
prevent collapse after hemorrhage.
- B. Specific Measures: Endocrine therapy has theoretical
value in about 15% of abortions (those due to maternal
hormonal deficiencies), but has not proved clinically use‐
ful. Do not give steroid sex hormones.
- C. General Measures: Place the patient at bed rest and give
sedatives to allay uterine irritability and limit bleeding.
Coitus and douches are contraindicated.
- D. Surgical Measures:
  1. Dilatation and curettage for possible retained tissue.
  (Start an oxytocin [Pitocin®] intravenous drip prior to
  surgery to prevent uterine perforation.)
  2. Uterine packing to control bleeding and promote sepa‐
  ration and evacuation of fragments. Remove packing in
  6-8 hours to allow drainage.
- E. Treatment of Complications:
  1. Uterine perforation - Observe for signs of intraperi‐
  toneal bleeding, rupture of the bowel or bladder, or
  peritonitis. Exploratory laparotomy may be necessary.
  2. Pelvic thrombophlebitis and septic emboli are critical
  sequelae. Consider antibiotics, anticoagulants, and
  ligation of the internal iliac veins and vena cava.

Prognosis.

    Correction of maternal disorders may make future suc‐
cessful pregnancies possible.

HYDATIDIFORM MOLE
(Vesicular Mole, Hydropic Mole, Cystic Degeneration of the Chorion)

Hydatidiform mole is a degenerative disorder of the chori‐
on which occurs as a complication of about one in 1500 preg‐
nancies in the USA, almost always during the first 18 weeks.
It is characterized by prominent, white grape-like vesicular
enlargements of the villi and vascular incompetence of the vil‐
lous tree. Although it is assumed to be of placental origin,
the etiology is not known. Hydatidiform mole is more common
among women under 20 and over 40, and is more than 5 times
as prevalent in the Orient as in the west. In the Philippines,
at least 15% of hydatidiform moles are regarded as malignant
either initially or subsequent to definitive therapy. In the
USA, malignancy (chorio-epithelioma) is reported in about 4%
of cases.

    It is not known whether hydatidiform mole is a primary
ovular defect, an intrauterine abnormality, or both. Maternal

Hydatidiform Mole 251

constitution and age seem to play a part in the pathogenesis; nutritional deficiency may be a contributory cause. Viral infections are capable of producing villar hydrops in experimental animals and perhaps in humans.

Most or all of the villi show minute to extreme swelling. The smaller blebs are pale, shiny, translucent, and yellowish-brown, resembling cooked tapioca; the larger hydatids resemble seedless white grapes. Some villi reach a diameter of more than 1 cm. Here and there, enlarged vesicles are supported by strands or stalks of connective tissue. They contain small amounts of clear, pale amber fluid. A containing amniotic membrane is usually not present. In the majority of cases no conceptus is found. If hydatidiform mole occurs in a double ovum twin pregnancy, one placenta is usually spared. In a single ovum twin pregnancy the entire chorion is diseased and both embryos are destroyed.

Polycystic ovaries are observed in molar pregnancies associated with abnormally high levels of chorionic gonadotropin.

On microscopic examination the villi are greatly altered and enlarged. Although most are superficial, others are deep within the endometrium or even in the inner myometrium. The syncytial investment is complete. The cytotrophoblast is generally prominent and persists well after the 4th month if evacuation of the mole does not occur. An edematous, avascular stroma is typical of hydatidiform mole. Bleeding and infection may be observed also.

Ovarian cystic changes include various degrees of luteinization of thecal elements, mainly luteinization of normal-sized follicles with or without luteinization of the stroma. In addition, there may be large, scattered cystic follicles, and true follicle cysts which cause gross enlargement of the gonads.

Failure of development of the fetal blood vessels may be primary or may be secondary to the hydropic changes in the villi.

The cytotrophoblast is the source of chorionic gonadotropin (CG). When the mole is proliferating, the urinary CG is usually elevated—often far higher than in normal pregnancy. Pregnancy tests based upon the effects of this hormone are therefore strongly positive (even in high dilution) in patients with hydatidiform mole except in the case of a grossly degenerated, largely evacuated mole or a decomposed, missed abortion of a molar pregnancy.

Clinical Findings.
A. Symptoms and Signs: Excessive nausea and vomiting occur in over one-third of patients with hydatidiform mole. Uterine bleeding, beginning at 6-8 weeks, is observed in virtually all instances and is indicative of threatened or

252 Hydatidiform Mole

incomplete abortion. Most hydatidiform moles cause bleeding by the 18th week. In about one-fifth of cases the uterus is larger than would be expected in a normal pregnancy of the same duration; this is due to the great volume of the vesicular villi. Uterine discomfort due to overstretching of the myometrium is reported in one-third of patients. Fullness, softness, and thinning of the entire lower uterine segment often occurs in early pregnancy. Bilateral cystic ovarian enlargement develops in one-fifth of cases as a result of gonadotropin stimulation of the ovaries. Eclamptogenic toxemia, frequently of the fulminating type, may develop during the second trimester. Hypertension, generalized edema, and proteinuria will be observed. Intact or collapsed vesicles may be passed through the vagina during episodes of spotting, since there is no amniotic membrane to prevent evacuation. A sound introduced through the cervix will not meet the resistance of membranes. (**Caution:** One may interrupt a nonmolar pregnancy in this way.) Vesicular changes may be noted in curettings from incomplete abortions not suspected of being molar pregnancies.

B. Laboratory Findings:
  1. Routine urinalysis may reveal protein in the absence of significant formed elements, which suggests toxemia.
  2. Reduced Hct, Hgb, and red cell count are the result of bleeding and infection. Elevation of the sedimentation rate and the white count and the presence of numerous immature cells in the differential count are due to infection.
  3. Hydatidiform mole, malignant mole, or chorio-epithelioma is probably present when the FSH exceeds 500,000 rat units/liter and the LH titer is above 200,000 rat units/liter. (A positive pregnancy test is generally obtained when 3000+ rat units/liter of CG are present.)
  4. The urinary 17-ketosteroid level is often twice the normal pregnancy level, but pregnanediol excretion is within the normal pregnancy range.
  5. In some cases thyroid hormone analogues (as estimated by the serum PBI) may reach thyrotoxic levels although there is no clinical evidence of toxic goiter. The reasons for this are obscure.
  6. The vaginal smear reveals distinct, heavy cell groupings, predominance of superficial cells, and acidophilia and pyknosis in approximately 50% of the exfoliated cells.
  7. Identification of placental hydatids will establish the diagnosis. Any tissue passed spontaneously should be preserved for pathologic examination.

C. X-Ray Findings: Hysterography after the third month, either by the transcervical or transcutaneous route, util-

Hydatidiform Mole 253

izing intravenous urographic media, may demonstrate a honeycomb appearance of the uterine contents. There is no indication of a distinct amniotic cavity, and usually no outline of a conceptus. Chest x-ray may reveal metastases.

Differential Diagnosis.

Hyperemesis gravidarum may occur as a complication of any pregnancy. (Abortion due to other causes than hydatidiform mole is discussed on p. 245.) The fundus will also be larger than expected in multiple pregnancy, polyhydramnios, and uterine tumor complicating intrauterine pregnancy. Resilience and distention of the lower uterine segment (usually with cervical dilatation or effacement) are generally related to imminent abortion due to any cause. Consider bilateral dermoid or other cystic enlargement of the ovaries during gestation as well as theca lutein cysts of hydatid mole. The sudden appearance of adnexal enlargement during an abnormal pregnancy suggests a mole.

Flecks of mucus and yellowish fragments of blood clot may simulate placental vesicles. Identification by microscopic examination of extruded tissues is required to prove hydatidiform mole.

Complications.

A. Nonmalignant Complications: Hemorrhage, especially in advanced molar pregnancy, is common before, during, and even after evacuation of the uterus by spontaneous or operative means. A mole frequently distends the uterus excessively, so that the uterine musculature may respond poorly to oxytocics. Infection is a major problem, since there is no barrier to cervical or vaginal contamination of the uterine cavity. Perforation of the thin-walled uterus during surgical evacuation may lead to widespread infections. Spontaneous rupture of the uterus may occur with benign or malignant mole, especially when the fundus is greatly distended.

Hydatidiform moles are benign and do not invade nor metastasize; however, they may undergo malignant degeneration (see below).

B. Malignant Complications: Invasive or **malignant mole** (also called mole destruens) may actually grow through the uterine wall to cause perforation and rupture of the uterus. It may also metastasize occasionally, usually to the lung, where it may cause chest pain, cough, or hemoptysis. **Chorio-epithelioma** may be manifested by uterine bleeding, continued or recurrent, after evacuation of a mole; or by the presence of an ulcerative vaginal tumor, pelvic mass, or evidence of distant metastatic tumor.

A distinction between invasive mole and chorio-epithelioma is often difficult, and grading of the malignancy may be impossible. Half of all cases of chorio-epithelioma occur as a complication of hydatidiform mole; about one-fourth follow abortion, and one-fourth complicate term pregnancies.

Invasive moles may resemble those of the vesicular type grossly and microscopically. Others may reveal proliferation of both cyto- and syncytiotrophoblastic cells which invade the myometrium. Villi are often seen deep in the uterine wall. Inflammation is frequently observed. Hemorrhage and necrosis are not conspicuous.

Grossly, a chorio-epithelioma is a reddish, moderately well demarcated, irregular, soft tumor, often necrotic and hemorrhagic. It may resemble a partially organized hematoma. Chorio-epithelioma often involves the cervix or vagina, but in other instances only the uterine wall or other pelvic structures will be involved. This malignancy metastasizes early via the blood stream to involve the lungs, liver, and brain. Ovarian lutein cysts are usually present.

Microscopically, sheets and strands of trophoblastic cells of variable size and maturity which reveal numerous mitoses and hyperchromatism are noted. It is often difficult to distinguish cytotrophoblastic from syncytiotrophoblastic cells. Little stroma is present. Villi are never seen. Inflammation is minimal. Invasion of the myometrium, hemorrhage, and widespread coagulation necrosis are obvious.

The microscopic appearance of evacuated molar tissue will not reveal its malignant potential. Sections from the uterine wall or from a metastasis may disclose the malignant characteristics and lead to a correct diagnosis.

Following spontaneous evacuation of an early pregnancy, the uterus may remain boggy and bleeding often persists. This may indicate retained products of conception, the development of a syncytioma, or even a chorio-epithelioma. Subinvolution of an otherwise normal, empty uterus may present similar symptomatology.

A syncytioma is a benign process in which persistent survival of nonproliferative, noninvasive trophoblast in the placental site results in delayed involution and continued bleeding.

A chorio-epithelioma causes bleeding and occasionally softness of the uterus because of malignant, invasive trophoblast in and perhaps beyond the placental site.

Treatment.

Do not strive too long to "preserve" a questionable pregnancy; it may be a mole.

A. Emergency Measures: Hemorrhage indicative of abortion requires immediate hospitalization. Type and crossmatch

the patient's blood, and have at least 2 units of blood available for transfusion. Bleeding will cease as soon as the uterine contents are evacuated and firm uterine contraction is established. Encourage spontaneous expulsion of most of the molar tissue by stimulation with intravenous oxytocin (see p. 181). Curettage will probably be required for removal of adherent tissue.
B. Specific (Surgical) Measures:
   1. Empty the uterus as soon as practicable after the diagnosis of hydatidiform mole is established. Spontaneous evacuation followed by careful dilatation and curettage is the preferred method of treatment in 75% of cases. Pack the uterus for 6-12 hours after curettage to reduce further bleeding and aid in the removal of tissue missed by the curet. Give ergonovine (Ergotrate®), 0.2 mg orally, every 4 hours after curettement until 4 doses have been given.
   2. Hysterotomy - If the uterus is larger than a five-month pregnancy and the cervix is resistant to wide dilatation, hysterotomy is indicated (vaginal if infection is clinically evident; anterior abdominal if infection is probably not present). Do not resect ovarian cysts and do not remove the ovaries; spontaneous regression will occur with elimination of the mole.
   3. Hysterectomy may be the treatment of choice in older patients.
C. General Measures: Evaluate all products of conception for evidence of benign or malignant mole. Order a chest x-ray and examine for pulmonary or other metastases. Insist that the patient avoid pregnancy for at least 6 months. Determine CG titers once each month for 6 months after evacuation of the mole. A rising titer indicates chorio-epithelioma or a new pregnancy. It is best to use serum (not urine) assays and to employ immature rats (Aschheim-Zondek test) rather than rabbits (Friedman test), or to use immunologic tests (see p. 44).
D. Supportive Measures:
   1. Replace blood and administer iron if the patient is anemic. Ensure a proper diet with vitamin supplementation.
   2. Prescribe a broad-spectrum antibiotic for 24 hours before and for 3-4 days after surgery if infection is suspected.

Treatment of Complications.

A. Nonmalignant Complications: Hemorrhage is usually due to retained products of conception and is an indication for dilatation and curettage. If salpingitis or other infection develops, treat intensively with antibiotics. Rupture of the uterus is an indication for laparotomy and consideration of hysterectomy. Perforation of the uterus without infection or intraperitoneal bleeding probably will not necessitate laparotomy. Treat cautiously.

Syncytioma and subinvolution of the uterus are self-limited. Prescribe ergonovine (Ergotrate®), 0.01 gm orally every 4 hours for 6 doses, and warm acetic acid vaginal douches daily for one week.

B. Malignant Complications: Malignant change is rarely diagnosed from curettings alone. Continued or repeated brisk bleeding after dilatation and curettage; prolonged subinvolution of the uterus; visible, palpable, radiographic, or neurologic evidence of metastases; and a persistently elevated CG titer 3 months after uterine evacuation of mole are presumptive evidence of malignant mole or chorio-epithelioma. (About 20% of patients will have a positive pregnancy test 2 months after surgery.)

Repeat dilatation and curettage after 3 months if malignancy is suspected (assuming another pregnancy has not occurred).

1. Malignant mole - Total hysterectomy (preserving the tubes and ovaries if they are not affected) is indicated. Metastases of malignant moles disappear by spontaneous regression, perhaps after removal of the primary lesion, or following irradiation or chemotherapy as outlined below for treatment of chorio-epithelioma.

2. Chorio-epithelioma of the uterus - Consider total abdominal hysterectomy and bilateral salpingo-oophorectomy. If metastases are large or widespread, spare the patient futile surgery and treat with chemotherapy, x-ray therapy, or both.

    a. Irradiation therapy consists of a tumor dose directed to the site of residual or metastatic cancer (e.g., pelvis, lung).

    b. Chemotherapy - Methotrexate (amethopterin) is the most promising agent. Administer a total of 2.5 mg/kg over a five-day period by slow intravenous drip or give orally in divided doses. Side effects (usually reversible) include stomatitis, bone marrow depression, rash, anorexia, nausea and vomiting, and diarrhea. Death occasionally occurs from toxic hepatitis or agranulocytosis. Repeat the course of therapy several times if improvement occurs, allowing stomatitis and other side reactions to resolve during each interval. If the tumor reappears, give repeat courses of methotrexate. In resistant cases, administer dactinomycin (actinomycin D, Cosmegen®), 10 μg/kg intravenously (well diluted) over a period of five days.

        Diethylstilbestrol (or equivalent), 200-300 mg orally daily, may suppress certain malignant moles, but estrogen therapy should be used only when methotrexate is not well tolerated or is ineffective.

Prognosis.

Repeated (even sequential) molar pregnancy is occasionally reported, but the risk of chronic abortion is not great in women who have had hydatidiform mole.

The presence or absence of ovarian cystic enlargement has no prognostic value relative to malignant trends.

A positive pregnancy test, even 3 months after evacuation of a mole, may not indicate a malignant trend unless it is persistent and in high dilution.

Occasionally, a hydatidiform mole may prove fatal because of its malignant course (and the complications of treatment) even though it may be histologically benign. Nevertheless, most patients with malignant mole treated promptly and adequately will recover.

Until recently almost 90% of patients with chorio-epithelioma died in less than one year even with the best care. With the advent of methotrexate therapy, the prognosis is expected to improve.

VOMITING OF PREGNANCY & HYPEREMESIS GRAVIDARUM

Vomiting of pregnancy—including its most pernicious form, hyperemesis gravidarum—affects almost 75% of pregnant white women in the USA. About two-thirds of these are primiparas. Most cases are very mild, but in the USA one in about 200 patients requires hospitalization. Intractable vomiting may be fatal, but therapeutic abortion is justified only in extremely rare instances.

Significant vomiting of pregnancy is uncommonly reported by indigent, Negro, and Oriental patients, and is not a serious problem among unmarried pregnant women.

There are no proved causes of vomiting of pregnancy. Psychically unstable women whose established reaction patterns to stress involve gastrointestinal disturbances are often affected. Many of these patients have unresolved sex problems, including relative frigidity. They frequently display immature personality traits to which pregnancy adds forebodings regarding labor and the dangers of childbirth; concern about loss of personal attractiveness and independence; and resentment of the husband's indifference toward the pregnancy. Fears of inadequacy, insecurity, and emotional conflicts lead to subconscious resentment and the figurative rejection of pregnancy symbolized by vomiting.

Innumerable—often tenuous—hypotheses of somatic causes include the following: (1) Allergic or toxic factors (degradation products of corpus luteum hormone, decidua, or trophoblast). (2) Hormonal imbalance (CG elevation, depression of adrenocortical function). (3) Nutritional deficiency (pregnancy needs may lead to methionine and tryptophan deficiency). (4) Metabolic alteration (diminished liver glycogen and lessened carbohydrate reserves, low BUN).

Most persons have different thresholds for vomiting and respond differently to the varied methods of treating emotional problems. Personal variations and degrees of disability are therefore to be expected.

Dehydration leads to fluid and electrolyte complications, particularly acidosis. Starvation causes hypoproteinemia and hypervitaminosis. Degenerative myocarditis, hepatitis, nephritis, and polyneuritis produce characteristic signs and symptoms. Jaundice and hemorrhagic diatheses secondary to vitamin C and B complex deficiency as well as hypoprothrombinemia lead to bleeding from mucosal surfaces. The embryo or fetus may die in utero, and the patient sometimes succumbs to irreversible metabolic alterations or to visceral involvement.

Three stages in the development of severe vomiting of pregnancy are recognized: (1) Psychogenic: The act of vomiting is a symptom of displeasure. (2) Metabolic: The results of excessive vomiting are dehydration, hypochloremia, acetonemia, hypokalemia, hypoglycemia, and hypoproteinemia. Liver and occasionally kidney damage occur, and are followed by hyperketosis, hyperbilirubinemia, nitrogen retention, vitamin deficiency, and jaundice. (3) Toxic: This may be critical. Death occurs from cardiac, hepatic, or adrenocortical failure, singly or in combination.

Clinical Findings.

A. Symptoms and Signs: Many patients are "high-strung" or neurotic. The gastrointestinal symptoms vary in severity from occasional to protracted vomiting. Nausea and vomiting usually begin about 5-6 weeks after conception (when the patient realizes that she is pregnant). In most cases, vomiting persists only until the 14th-16th week, though it may continue throughout pregnancy.

Nausea and vomiting usually occur in the morning upon arising, but evening nausea and vomiting are almost as common and develop with fatigue, food odors as the patient prepares the evening meal, household confusion, or the husband's return home. In most cases, despite the severity of subjective complaints, there are few or no signs of nutritional deficiency.

The mild form of this illness is characterized by occasional vomiting; the moderately severe form, by constant nausea and frequent vomiting; the severe form (hyperemesis gravidarum), by intractable vomiting which may be fatal. If a less severe form gets out of hand it

progresses to a more serious stage.
B. Laboratory Findings: In severely ill patients, hemoconcentration is reflected in a relative elevation of the hemoglobin, red cell count, and hematocrit. There is a slight increase in the white count and shift to the left of the differential count, with increased numbers of eosinophils and band forms.

Ketone bodies (acetone) will be found in the urine, which is usually concentrated. Slight proteinuria (trace to 1+) is a frequent finding.

In very ill patients, depletion of the serum proteins and alkali reserve is common. If the patient is oliguric, the BUN, serum sodium, and serum potassium may be elevated.

With advanced liver disease, serum proteins, prothrombin, and fibrinogen will be decreased.
C. X-Ray Findings: Hypermotility of the upper gastrointestinal tract may be revealed by x-ray films following a barium meal. If nausea and vomiting are severe, this study should be done to disclose possible hiatal hernia, peptic ulcer, or gastric carcinoma.
D. Special Examinations: Periodic ophthalmoscopic evaluations are required if the patient is seriously ill. Retinal hemorrhage and detachment of the retina are most unfavorable prognostic signs.

Complications.

Neuritis and bleeding due to hemorrhagic diatheses associated with vitamin deficiency may occur. Stress ulcers of the stomach may develop. Jaundice due to so-called toxic hepatitis is particularly ominous.

Treatment.
A. Ambulatory Treatment: (For the patient with slight to moderate nausea and vomiting of pregnancy.)
  1. General measures - Provide reassurance and relieve the patient's fears of pregnancy. Schedule frequent office visits during the period when the patient is nauseated.
  2. Medical measures - Ensure rest and reduce the work load. Prescribe sedation, e.g., phenobarbital, 30-60 mg ($1/2$-1 gr) orally or rectally 2-3 times daily. The phenothiazines should be used only if necessary because of their potential teratogenic effects. Perphenazine (Trilafon®), 8 mg as an oral Repetab® or rectal suppository on arising and again at bedtime, is an effective phenothiazine antinauseant. Promazine (Sparine®), 50 mg orally or rectally 2-3 times daily, is also of value.

  A sedative-antispasmodic mixture such as the following is beneficial:

R̆ Tincture of belladonna   30
   Elixir of phenobarbital, q.s. ad 240

   Sig: One tsp every 4 hours or one hour
        before meals.

Amphetamines, e.g., dextro amphetamine sulfate, 5 mg orally twice daily, are of indirect value for their psychic stimulant effects.

Vitamins are of value only if specific deficiencies exist. The antihistamines are beneficial in nausea and vomiting of pregnancy in proportion to their sedative effects. Narcotics have no place in the treatment of digestive problems during pregnancy.

B. Hospital Treatment: (For severe nausea and vomiting [hyperemesis gravidarum].)
  1. General measures - Place the patient in a quiet, cheerful, well ventilated private room. Insist upon complete bed rest without bathroom privileges until improvement occurs and record fluid intake and output accurately. Give antiemetics by rectum or parenterally. Allow no visitors, not even the husband, until vomiting ceases and the patient is eating. Inform the family of the rationale of therapy and enlist their cooperation. Report to the husband daily regarding his wife's progress. Encourage the patient, emphasizing an early, complete recovery. Give protracted moderate sedation parenterally or rectally.
  2. Medical dietary measures - Permit nothing by mouth for the first 48 hours. Order adequate parenteral fluids, electrolytes, carbohydrates, and protein: (1) Intravenous glucose, 10% in water (2000 ml) and 5% in normal saline (1000 ml) daily, with potassium added, plus vitamins. (2) If the serum proteins are depleted, intravenous amino acid preparations, e.g., Amigen®, 500 ml twice daily. (Blood transfusion should be used only if the patient is markedly anemic.) Vitamins—especially B complex, C, and K—should be added to the infusion. Many injectable B complex preparations are available to which ascorbic acid and vitamin K can be added.

Nasogastric tube feeding of a well balanced liquid baby formula by slow drip should be instituted if the patient cannot retain food by mouth after 48 hours. If she responds to the above regimen after 48 hours, prescribe a dry diet in 6 small feedings daily with clear liquids one hour after meals.

If severe vomiting recurs before dismissal from the hospital, repeat parenteral therapy from the beginning. Re-admission to the hospital may be required.

C. **Therapeutic Abortion:** Obtain medical and psychiatric consultation if the patient's condition deteriorates despite the above or comparable therapy. Delirium, blindness, tachycardia at rest, jaundice, anuria, and hemorrhage are ominous manifestations of severe organ toxicity; therapeutic abortion may be required in order to save the patient's life.

Prognosis.

Vomiting of pregnancy is self-limited, and the prognosis is good. Intractable hyperemesis gravidarum is a real threat to the life of the mother and the fetus.

PROLAPSE OF THE UMBILICAL CORD

The umbilical cord may protrude through the cervix or become compressed by the presenting or other prominent fetal part. Prolapse of the cord occurs about once in 200 advanced pregnancies and may be due to any of the following factors: (1) Abnormal presentation (breech, shoulder, face, brow, transverse, compound). (2) Multiple pregnancy. (3) Immaturity and premature rupture of the membranes prior to engagement of the vertex or breech. (4) Contracted pelvis (fetopelvic disproportion). (5) Polyhydramnios. (6) Low implantation of the placenta. (7) Abnormally long cord (75 cm or more).

There are 3 types of prolapsed cord: (1) The forelying cord, which precedes the presenting part, is held within intact membranes but can be felt through the cervix. (2) Occult prolapse, in which the cord lies over the face or head of the fetus but cannot be felt on internal examination. The membranes may be intact or ruptured. (3) Complete prolapse of the cord, in which the membranes are ruptured so that the cord extrudes through the cervix into the vagina or beyond the introitus.

Partial compression of the cord by virtue of its forelying position or prolapse causes fetal hypoxia. Complete cord obstruction results in rapid death of the fetus.

Clinical Findings.

A. **Symptoms and Signs:** In complete prolapse the patient may feel the cord slide through the vagina and over the vulva after rupture of the membranes. Compression of the cord often causes violent fetal activity, obvious to the patient and even to the observer. Marked rapidity and then slowing of the fetal heartbeat may be noted. The cord may be seen or felt by the patient or by an attendant or physician during external or internal examination, or it may be palpated during rectal or vaginal examination. Auscultatory signs of fetal distress (e.g., slowing or ac-

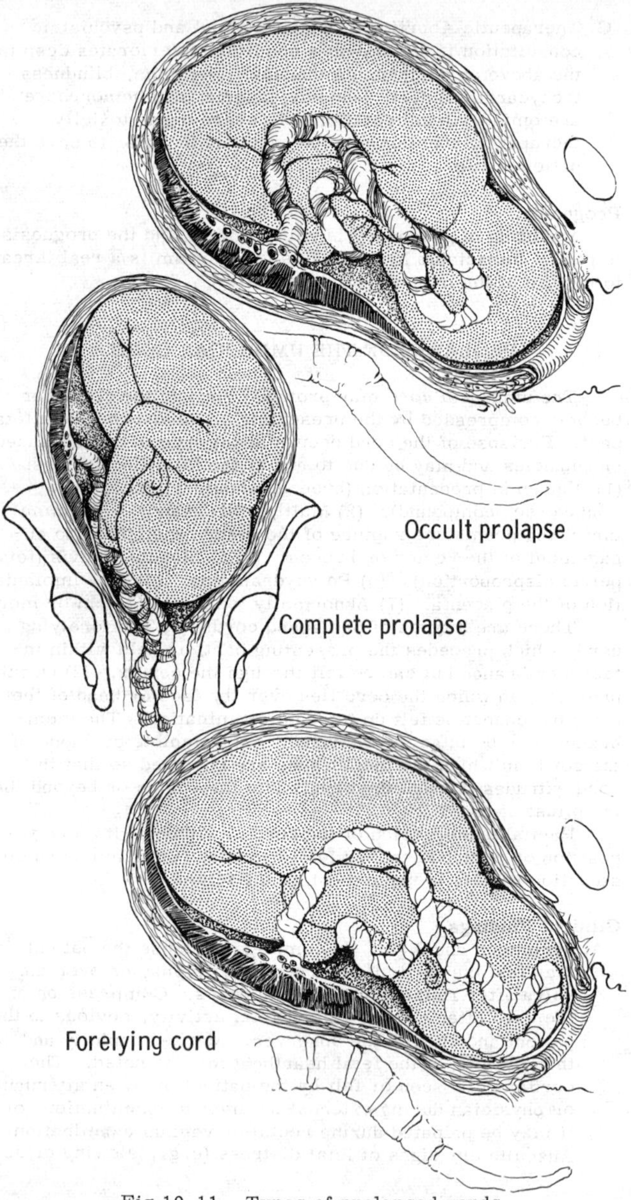

262 Prolapse of Umbilical Cord

Occult prolapse

Complete prolapse

Forelying cord

Fig 10-11. Types of prolapsed cords.

Table 10-2. Suggested mode of delivery in prolapse of the umbilical cord.

	Vertex	Presentation Breech	Transverse
Primipara			
Cervix < 5 cm dilated	Cesarean section	Cesarean section	Cesarean section
Cervix > 5 cm dilated	Cesarean section	Bring down a foot and leg (Pinard)	(1) Cesarean section (2) Bring down foot and leg
Multipara			
Cervix < 5 cm dilated	Cesarean section or vacuum extractor	Cesarean section or hydrostatic bag, bring down a leg	Cesarean section or hydrostatic bag, internal version, breech extraction
Cervix > 5 cm dilated	Duhrssens incision, then forceps delivery	Bring down a leg or slow breech extraction	Internal version, breech extraction

celeration of the fetal heartbeat during a contraction) are often present.

B. Special Examinations: Sterile vaginal examination may confirm the presence of occult or complete prolapse of the umbilical cord.

Complications.

Cord obstruction causes fetal hypoxia or anoxia. Hypoxia, if mild and not prolonged, may cause no fetal damage. Marked or prolonged hypoxia causes fetal neurologic deficit or death.

Prevention.

If the membranes rupture spontaneously and prematurely while the patient is in bed, have her stand up at once despite gross leakage of fluid. The presenting part may gravitate over the inlet and block the cord. If she remains in bed, the cord may work its way down and out through the cervix.

Examine the patient rectally or vaginally promptly after rupture of the membranes, especially when a breech or transverse presentation is known to exist, to determine if prolapse is a possibility.

Treatment.

A. Emergency Measures: Cord compression results from pressure by the presenting part against the cervix with the cord between. For any type of prolapsed cord, place the patient in the knee-chest or deep Trendelenburg position and have her remain so. Using aseptic technic, attempt to slip the cord back into the uterus. (Cord repositors almost never replace and retain the cord within the uterus.) On rare occasions, it is possible to push the cord back and to loop the cord above the ear of the fetus. This may retain it inside the uterus. If this maneuver is successful, rest the patient on her side in the Sims position with her hips elevated and her head and body at a lower level. If the presenting part then engages, the danger of recurrent prolapse of the cord may be over.

B. Mode of Delivery: (See Table 10-2.) The mode of delivery in emergencies such as prolapse of the umbilical cord is a matter of judgment and experience. The following measures are to be condemned: Manual dilatation of the cervix (accouchement forcé); incision of a rigid, thick cervix less than 5 cm dilated; version and extraction without a well dilated, effaced cervix; and deep anesthesia. Management depends upon the following factors:
1. Duration of pregnancy - If the pregnancy is of less than 30 weeks' duration, it is probably inadvisable to increase the maternal risk in an effort to salvage a very immature fetus. It may be necessary to abandon the fetus and allow labor and delivery to proceed.
2. Parity of the patient - Multiparous women have shorter labors and softer, more dilatable cervices than primigravidas, and fewer maternal complications usually result from operative delivery.
3. Quality of labor - The patient may not be in labor, or the labor may be desultory in contrast with strong labor close to the time of delivery. The mode of delivery may depend upon the proximity of delivery.
4. Fetal presentation - A footling breech may be a more favorable presentation than a transverse presentation.
5. Dilatation and effacement of the cervix - The proximity to delivery and the "negotiability" of the cervix will determine the course of action when there is a fetal indication for delivery.

C. Treatment of Complications: Lacerations of the birth canal must be repaired promptly. Blood transfusion may be required. Give oxytocics if uterine atony develops.
Resuscitation of the newborn is often a problem because of hypoxia, the trauma of delivery, and prematurity.

Prognosis.

A. Fetal: Brief (< 5 minutes), partial cord compression probably is not harmful. Complete occlusion for the same period or partial occlusion for a longer time will cause death or severe central nervous system damage.
B. Maternal: Infection or trauma associated with attempts at replacement of the cord or operative vaginal delivery of the fetus may complicate the puerperium.

PUERPERAL SEPSIS

Any infection in the genital tract which occurs as a complication of abortion, labor, or delivery is termed puerperal sepsis. Streptococci, staphylococci, clostridia, coliforms, and neisseriae are the pathogens most often identified. Debility (anemia, undernutrition), serious systemic disorders, premature or prolonged rupture of the membranes, protracted labor, and traumatic examinations or delivery predispose to puerperal infection.

The incidence of puerperal sepsis in hospitals in the USA has been variously estimated to be 1-8%. Puerperal sepsis is exceeded only by hemorrhage and toxemia of pregnancy as a cause of maternal death in this country.

The infection is acquired from hospital personnel or from an endogenous source in circumstances where scrupulous aseptic technic is not observed. Cellulitis resulting from vaginal or cervical contusions or lacerations favors the spread of the infection—as does endometritis also, particularly when it occurs in the zone of placental attachment (the equivalent of a large surface wound). Salpingitis, peritonitis, lymphangitis, and pelvic lymphadenitis may then occur, and vasculitis in pelvic arteries and veins, thrombophlebitis, and embolization often result. Septicemia may develop, and local or distant abscesses may form.

Clinical Findings.

Many genital tract infections are so mild as to cause few or slight symptoms. Others are violent, fulminating, and fatal within a short time.

- A. Symptoms and Signs: Malaise, headache, anorexia, and remittent slight elevations in temperature and pulse generally begin 3-4 days after delivery. Vague discomfort in the perineum or lower abdomen, nausea, and vomiting may follow. High fever ("childbed fever"), rapid pulse, ileus, and localization of pain and tenderness in the pelvis may be observed during the next 1-2 days. The lochia is foul or profuse. Bacteremic shock may occur. If improvement does not occur in 48-72 hours with antibiotic therapy, the alarming progress of the infection will be obvious.
- B. Laboratory Findings: Polymorphonuclear leukocytosis and increased sedimentation rate are indications of infection. Reduced hematocrit and hemoglobin values indicate anemia. Identification of pathogens by culture and sensitivity tests from cervical and uterine lochia will require 36-48 hours.
- C. X-ray Findings: X-ray studies are not helpful except to exclude nonpuerperal problems such as pneumonia or infarction.

Complications and Sequelae.

Genital tract infections commonly progress to peritonitis, pelvic cellulitis and abscess formation, septicemia, pulmonary embolism, and death. Other extremely serious problems secondary to such infections include dynamic or adynamic ileus, anemia, hepatitis, pneumonia, empyema, and meningitis. Any of these disorders may prove fatal.

If the patient recovers, chronic salpingitis may cause recurrent disability. Tubal occlusion may be the cause of "one child sterility." Femoral thrombophlebitis ("milk leg") is often followed by chronic pain and swelling of the leg.

Differential Diagnosis.

Febrile complications of the puerperium unrelated to genital tract infection include mastitis, urinary and respiratory infection, and enteritis, in that order of frequency.

Prevention.

The prevention of puerperal sepsis consists of good obstetric care from the time the patient is first seen until she is discharged from the hospital, with particular emphasis on strict aseptic technic during manual examination and delivery.

Treatment.

A. Emergency Measures: Treat shock. Early recognition of incipient shock is important. Institute preliminary broad-spectrum antibiotic therapy pending the results of bacteriologic studies. Give hydrocortisone or its equivalent in doses of 250-500 mg I.V. every 8-12 hours for 3 days and supportive measures such as oxygen, parenteral fluids, and vasopressor drugs together with specific anti-infective therapy.

B. General Measures:
  1. Isolate the patient. Utilize gown and glove technic, and sterilize bedpans and dishes. Obtain specimens of cervical, uterine, and other discharges for culture and sensitivity studies.
  2. Place the patient in the semi-Fowler position. Give a clear liquid diet for several days at least. Give I.V. fluids to maintain electrolyte and fluid balance.
  3. Give an ergot preparation to improve drainage and speed uterine involution.
  4. Give analgesics, hypnotics, and laxatives as required.

C. Specific Measures: Initially, give antibiotics in large doses, e.g., penicillin G, 1 million units or more I.M., plus streptomycin, 1 gm I.M. Stat. followed by penicillin, 600,000 units, with streptomycin, 0.5 gm 4 times daily; or chloramphenicol (Chloromycetin®), 1 gm orally Stat., followed by 500 mg 4 times daily on the first day and 250 mg 4 times daily on the following day. When bacteriologic reports are received, continue therapy with the antibiotic of choice in large and repeated doses. Give tetanus toxoid and antitoxin if Clostridium tetani infection is suspected.

D. **Surgical Measures:** Hysterectomy is indicated for a ruptured infected uterus, postabortal uterine abscess associated with abortion, hydatidiform mole, or myoma. Ligation of the vena cava and ovarian veins may be life-saving in case of repeated (often septic) pulmonary embolization.

Prognosis

The susceptibility of the pathogenic microorganism, the extent of involvement, the patient's resistance, and the promptness and adequacy of treatment determine the outcome. In 1962 the maternal mortality rate due to puerperal sepsis in the USA was 0.4%, but in some areas of the world the death rate is much higher.

11...
Toxemia of Pregnancy

Toxemia of pregnancy is a syndrome characterized by hypertension, edema, and proteinuria which usually occurs in the last trimester of pregnancy or the early puerperium. The term **eclamptogenic toxemia** encompasses both **preeclampsia** and eclampsia. Preeclampsia denotes the nonconvulsive form; with the development of convulsions and coma, the disorder is termed **eclampsia**. Chronic hypertensive and renal disease, although associated with and predisposing to toxemia of pregnancy, and hyperemesis gravidarum are no longer considered as toxemias of pregnancy.

Primigravidas of all ages are most commonly affected. Toxemia of pregnancy is more prevalent among the colored races, but this is probably due to economic factors and dietary deficiencies rather than racial susceptibility.

The importance of early recognition of toxemia of pregnancy cannot be overemphasized, especially since the patient is initially asymptomatic. Uncontrolled toxemia causes permanent disability or death, and is a major cause (with hemorrhage and infection) of maternal mortality. Six to 7% of all pregnant women in the USA develop toxemia. About 5% of these have eclampsia; almost 15% of eclamptics die of the disease.

The cause of toxemia of pregnancy is not known. Speculation about the probable cause or causes has been so extensive that this disorder has been called a "disease of theories." Predisposing factors include vascular and renal disease, malnutrition, and sodium retention, which seems to "sensitize" an otherwise healthy pregnant woman. Precipitating factors, if any, are probably present in the placenta and perhaps the decidua, inasmuch as a fetus is not essential for the development of toxemia (which may occur in hydatidiform mole or after delivery). Uterine distention is not essential either, since toxemia has been reported as a complication of extrauterine pregnancy. Proximal factors have traditionally included a postulated "toxic" substance of some type, derived from the pregnancy, which is presumably transported in the blood to neighboring and distant structures. The theory of primary neurologic mediation (uterus to kidney) has not met with wide acceptance.

One popular and plausible theory is that of E. W. Page, which may be summarized as follows: Impairment of the circulation and nutrition of the placenta by extrinsic (reduced uterine blood supply) or intrinsic (placental degeneration) factors leads to disordered metabolism of the placenta and decidua, which in turn provokes the secretion of substances such as sodium-retaining corticoids and histaminoids into the maternal circulation from the placental site, and the development of toxemia in susceptible, sensitized pregnant women.

Pathology.

In preeclampsia there are no characteristic anatomic lesions; in eclampsia, definite gross and microscopic abnormalities are often seen. Although striking, the organic lesions generally are not sufficiently extensive to cause death. If the patient recovers from eclampsia, most (perhaps all) of the morphologic abnormalities are reversible.

A. Brain: Edema with slight flattening of the convolutions. On section, scattered focal hemorrhages may be discovered.

B. Lungs: "Wet" (edematous) congested lungs with multiple minute thrombi are commonly reported.

C. Liver: Usually pale, mottled, and firm, with small subcapsular hemorrhages. The capillaries around the portal spaces are dilated. Periportal hemorrhage, thrombosis, and necrosis are characteristic. The right lobe is usually more severely affected than the left.

D. Kidneys: The kidneys are most often slightly enlarged and pale. On section, the cortex is pale, and numerous small hemorrhagic points are seen. The glomerular vascular loop actually fills Bowman's capsule with large ischemic capillaries coiled in simplified loops having ballooned tufts. The glomerular cells are swollen and prominent, but no evidence of proliferation is present. Adhesions between the thickened, wrinkled basement membrane and capillary rosette are typical. Vacuolization develops in the cells of the intercapillary space beneath the glomerular basement membrane. The tubules are often dilated with protein-containing urine. Few intraluminal red and white blood cells are seen. Hyaline degeneration and fatty infiltration of tubule cells are often described.

E. Placenta: No specific placental lesions are typical of toxemia of pregnancy. The placenta is often smaller than normal, however, and "red infarcts" are common. Premature aging or dysmaturity frequently occurs, as shown by increased and more severe endarteritis and periarteritis, a thinned and broken syncytium, and calcium and intervillous fibrin deposition.

Pathologic Physiology.
A. Arteriolar spasm, consistently observed in the retinas, kidneys, and the splanchnic region, promotes hypertension. A heightened pressor (and depressor) response indicates the lability of the vascular system.
B. Sodium and Water Retention:
  1. Reduced glomerular filtration - A small volume of urine permits more efficient sodium reabsorption by the kidney tubules.
  2. Reduced serum albumin and globulin due to proteinuria account for diminished osmotic pressure of the blood, despite hemoconcentration.
  3. In certain patients, increased excretion of corticoids (including aldosterone) and antidiuretic hormone suggest larger tissue concentrations of these substances, which encourages sodium and water retention.
C. Proteinuria: Degenerative changes in the glomeruli permit the loss of serum protein via the urine. The albumin:globulin ratio in the urine of toxemic patients is approximately 3:1 (in contrast with 6:7 in nephritis). Tubular disease contributes only slightly to the leakage of protein. When the volume of urine is small, the concentration of protein is high: excretion of less than 500 ml of urine per day is associated with a urine protein of 1-4 gm/100 ml (3-4+).
D. Abnormal Blood Chemistry:
  1. Elevations of serum uric acid, urea nitrogen, and creatinine are due to impaired renal clearance of these catabolites.
  2. Serum albumin and serum globulin are reduced because of increased permeability of the glomeruli. This accounts for some of the proteinuria. Loss or destruction of blood proteins must also occur due to other causes, however, because proteinuria alone is not sufficient to explain abnormally low levels in severe cases.
  3. Low CO_2 combining power, especially after convulsions, is due to increased serum lactic acid and acidosis.

Clinical Findings.
A. Symptoms and Signs:
  1. Preeclampsia - As defined by Tatum and Mulé, preeclampsia is a disease peculiar to pregnant women which is characterized by hypertension, proteinuria, and generalized edema. The manifestations develop from the 24th week of pregnancy through the second week after delivery. Severe, persistent, generalized headache, vertigo, malaise, and nervous irritability are prominent symptoms which are due in part to cerebral edema. Scintillating scotomas and partial or

complete blindness are due to edema of the retina, retinal hemorrhage, and retinal detachment. Epigastric pain, nausea, and liver tenderness are the result of congestion, thrombosis of the periportal system, and subcapsular hepatic hemorrhages.

Preeclampsia is diagnosed by observing persistent hypertension or a sudden rise of blood pressure plus generalized edema and proteinuria during the last 3 months of pregnancy. Ninety-five per cent of cases occur after the 32nd week, and 75% of these patients are primigravidas. The incidence is at least doubled with multiple pregnancy, hydatidiform mole, and polyhydramnios.

Hypertension is determined by reference to the patient's age and the usual rise of blood pressure with the passing years: In patients under 40 years of age, hypertension is said to be present when there is an elevation of resting blood pressure above 145/90 (over age 40: 150/90) or when there is a rise of 30 or more mm Hg systolic or 15 or more mm Hg diastolic pressure (for 2 or more days) above the average of recordings taken during the pregravid period or prior to the 6th month of pregnancy, excluding the first 2 weeks of the puerperium in the previous pregnancy. Hypertonicity of the vasculature is responsible.

The generalized edema of preeclampsia must be apparent above the waist. Such patients usually have a weight gain of 4 lb (1.8 kg) or more during any two-week period from the 24th through the 35th week of pregnancy, or a gain of 2 lb (0.9 kg) or more per week from the 35th week to term.

Edema involving the upper part of the body is always a pathologic finding; it may be an early indication of toxemia. Swelling due to fluid accumulation begins in the lower extremities and progresses upward. Tightness of finger rings and puffiness of the face are danger signs. Oliguria accompanies edema in many patients; anuria is a grave sign.

Any grossly detectable protein in a catheterized or clean-catch urine specimen is abnormal. Proteinuria implies a 1+ qualitative test or greater, or a minimum of 100 mg/100 ml on quantitative urinalysis of a 24-hour collection, assuming normal urine output. Glomerular permeability is the cause. (Pyuria or hematuria is due to other causes.)

Note: We no longer distinguish between mild and severe preeclampsia. Such a designation detracts from a proper appreciation of the seriousness of the disorder.

2. Eclampsia - A patient with signs of preeclampsia who has at least one convulsion or episode of coma between

the 24th week of pregnancy and the end of the second week after delivery (including the third stage of labor) must be presumed to have eclampsia if other causes can be excluded. Eclampsia is classified according to the time of occurrence of the first convulsion with respect to the time of delivery: (1) Prepartal eclampsia denotes convulsions prior to delivery. In intercurrent eclampsia, the patient is free of convulsions for at least 24 hours during the antenatal period; this designation is continued until the patient is delivered or has another convulsion. Patients in this group tolerate labor much better and can be delivered with greater safety than most intrapartal eclamptics. (2) Intrapartal eclampsia denotes one or more convulsions during labor or delivery. (3) Postpartal eclampsia denotes one or more convulsions after the third stage of labor and up to 2 weeks after delivery. Almost 90% of convulsions during the early puerperium occur on the first day.

Example: A patient who has convulsions before labor, during delivery, and on the 10th postpartal day is diagnosed as having had prepartal eclampsia with additional intrapartal and postpartal convulsions.

Preconvulsive symptoms are those of severe preeclampsia. Eclampsia is further characterized by generalized tonic-clonic convulsions; coma after convulsions followed by amnesia and confusion; marked hypertension preceding a convulsion, and hypotension thereafter (during coma or vascular collapse); stertorous breathing, rhonchi, and frothing at the mouth; twitching of muscle groups (face, arms, etc); nystagmus; and oliguria or anuria.

B. Laboratory Findings:
  1. Preeclampsia - Only the urinalysis (revealing proteinuria without hematuria or pyuria) is helpful in diagnosis. The hematocrit rises in proportion to the severity of toxemia. Blood chemistry findings are usually slightly elevated. Repeated BUN and serum uric acid studies often show a gradual increase concomitant with reduction of creatinine clearance as toxemia becomes more severe.
  2. Eclampsia is associated with proteinuria (3-4+), hemoconcentration, a greatly reduced blood CO_2 combining power, and increased serum uric acid and blood NPN and BUN.

C. Special Examinations: Ophthalmoscopic examination may reveal papilledema, retinal edema, retinal detachment, vascular spasm, arteriovenous "nicking," and hemorrhages. Repeated examination is helpful in determining improvement or failure of treatment in toxemia of pregnancy.

Differential Diagnosis.

Hypertensive disease and renal disease are discussed here because it is important to differentiate them from preeclampsia and because eclamptogenic toxemia is frequently superimposed upon them. Atypical disorders associated with hypertension or proteinuria should be reevaluated 4-6 months after delivery.

A. "Essential Hypertension": Hypertension is a significant sign in essential hypertension, glomerulonephritis, pyelonephritis, and toxemia of pregnancy. A history of persistent blood pressure elevation before pregnancy is the most valuable clue to the diagnosis; but if hypertension is recorded before the 5th month (when normotension or hypotension is the rule), one is safe in concluding that it was present before pregnancy. Preeclampsia and eclampsia occur before the 6th month only in hydatidiform mole.

Essential hypertension may be graded as (1) mild (slight to moderate hypertension; blood pressure 140-180/90-100 mm Hg, proteinuria 0-trace); or (2) severe (blood pressure over 180/100 mm Hg and 1+ proteinuria or more, almost always with ocular, cardiac, and renal damage). This disorder complicates 10-15% of all pregnancies. A family history of hypertension is recognized in 75% of all pregnant women with essential hypertension. Multiparas or women over 35 years of age are most commonly affected. The blood pressure is labile to activity, heat and cold, sedation, and emotional stress. Blood chemistry and renal function studies are normal unless the disease is severe. A clean-catch or catheterized specimen rarely contains more than a trace to 1+ protein (in the absence of other complications). The extent of the changes in the retinal arterioles (e.g., narrowing), cardiac enlargement, electrocardiographic changes, arrhythmias, and other findings are in proportion to the severity of the disease. Sudden, excessive weight gain and generalized edema are not present unless toxemia is superimposed.

The amobarbital (Amytal®) test causes a marked fall of blood pressure in essential hypertension; moderate depression in severe preeclampsia; and little change in renal disease.

B. Primary Renal Disease: Chronic glomerulonephritis, chronic pyelonephritis, and polycystic kidney disease account for only about 5% of all instances of hypertension during pregnancy, but are accompanied by preeclampsia in almost 50% of cases. Renal disease almost invariably antedates the pregnancy. A history of glomerulonephritis after scarlet fever, pyelonephritis after "honeymoon cystitis," and similar disorders—or a family history of polycystic kidney disease—is of great value in the diagnosis. Gross proteinuria and cellular elements and casts in the centrifuged sediment (with or without hypertension) are usually noted at first visit. The specific gravity of the urine is of narrowed range or fixed. Retinal damage may be present.

The Addis test is not diagnostic but gives a quantitative estimate of the severity of renal disease. It may reveal marked impairment of the kidney in primary renal disease; moderate impairment in severe preeclampsia; and only slight renal impairment in most cases of hypertensive disease complicating pregnancy.

C. Convulsive Disorders: Convulsions may be due to hypertensive encephalopathy, epilepsy, hypoglycemia, hypocalcemia (of parathyroid or renal origin), hemolytic crisis of sickle cell anemia, and the tetany of alkalosis as well as eclampsia.

Complications.

A. Early: About 5% of preeclamptic patients develop eclampsia. The more marked the symptomatology, the greater the likelihood of convulsions and coma and the higher the fetal and maternal mortality and morbidity rates. Convulsions increase maternal mortality ten-fold and fetal mortality forty-fold. The causes of maternal death due to eclampsia are (in order of incidence) circulatory collapse (cardiac arrest, pulmonary edema, shock), cerebral hemorrhage, and renal failure. The fetus dies in the uterus, usually of hypoxia or acidosis.

Blindness due to retinal detachment or intracranial hemorrhage, or paralysis due to cerebrovascular accident, may persist in patients who survive eclampsia.

Thirty per cent of patients who develop premature separation of the placenta have one of the hypertensive disorders. One-half of these will be found to have hypertensive disease and one-fourth eclamptogenic toxemia. So-called "toxic separation of the placenta" (abruptio placentae) is almost always associated with severe preeclampsia or eclampsia.

Postpartal hemorrhage is common in patients with hypertensive syndromes during pregnancy.

Toxic delirium in patients with eclampsia, either before or after delivery, poses serious medical and nursing problems.

Injuries incurred during convulsions include lacerations of lips and tongue and fractures of the vertebrae. Aspiration pneumonia may also occur.

B. Late: Fifteen to 20% of patients with severe preeclampsia or eclampsia (without known preexisting hypertensive or renal disease) suffer a recurrence of eclamptogenic toxemia with subsequent pregnancies. This is probably due to the same pattern of faulty diet (hypovitaminosis, deficient protein intake, excessive sodium ingestion), poor hygiene, and exaggerated physiologic changes of pregnancy which were responsible for the first attack.

Permanent hypertension, the result of vascular damage, may occur as a result of toxemia of pregnancy (see below).

Preeclampsia is superimposed upon mild essential hypertension in at least 30% of cases of toxemia; the seriousness of the toxemia is directly related to the severity of the essential hypertension. Fetal growth is retarded, probably because of placental dysmaturity (premature aging). The fetal mortality rate is much higher than that observed in normal pregnancies or in toxemia not associated with essential hypertension.

Preeclampsia will occur in about 50% of women with severe essential hypertension who become pregnant. However, repeated pregnancies in women with mild essential hypertension who do not develop preeclampsia will not cause a progression of the hypertensive disease.

It is usually impossible to determine the vascular and renal status of the patient before pregnancy. Therefore, some patients who are assumed to have post-toxemic hypertension probably have essential hypertension which was not apparent before pregnancy but which has progressed without relation to the pregnancy.

Prevention.

Patients with severe vascular and renal disease should be advised against becoming pregnant. (However, unless hypertension or infection supervenes, moderate impairment of renal function due to primary renal disease does not affect and is not affected by pregnancy.)

Treatment.

Treat nonconvulsive toxemia patients vigorously. Deliver by the most expeditious means available which is least harmful to the patient and fetus. Cesarean section after the 36th week may be indicated for patients who are not good candidates for induction of labor. Avoid delaying more than 3 weeks in preeclampsia for fear of permanent vascular damage.

Convulsive toxemia must be treated with appropriate palliative measures. Conservative treatment is indicated initially. Pregnancy should not be terminated until the patient has definitely recovered from the convulsive episode, as in intercurrent eclampsia; but should then be terminated as soon as possible (as in severe preeclampsia).

A. Preeclampsia: The objectives of treatment are to prevent eclampsia, permanent cardiovascular and renal damage, and vascular accidents; to preserve the pregnancy to certain viability; and to deliver a normal, living infant. A compromise is often necessary in severe cases during the early part of the third trimester; delivery may be postponed until the fetus is considered to be mature enough to survive.

Treatment consists of palliative measures and termination of pregnancy at the appropriate time. The patient should be placed at bed rest and must avoid all unnecessary contacts, tension, and activity. Sedatives are given to provide rest and relief from anxiety and to reduce hypertension. Excess extracellular fluid should be mobilized with diuretics. In addition to bed rest and sedatives, antihypertensive drugs should be given as indicated to reduce hypertension and vascular accidents. Delivery should be delayed, if possible, until the disease is under control or is improving. Although delivery of the fetus and placenta usually cures toxemia of pregnancy, hasty or forced delivery by any route is hazardous.

1. Home management - Most patients with preeclampsia can be managed at home, and the attempt should be made in all cases. The patient who has not responded to the following program of treatment after 48 hours must be hospitalized for more intensive care.
    a. General care - Place the patient at bed rest in a single room; allow only the husband to visit her for a brief period each day. (If she is in the hospital, discharge her 48 hours after the signs and symptoms of toxemia subside.)
    b. Examinations and procedures - Check blood pressure every 4 hours when awake; determine urine protein daily on a clean-catch voided morning specimen; and examine with the ophthalmoscope.
    c. Diet and fluids - Prescribe a low sodium diet (less than 3 gm salt per day) and withhold all foods and drugs containing sodium (e.g., baking soda, antacids). Record fluid intake and output. If urine output is within the normal range (1000 ml or more daily), encourage an intake of 2500 ml of salt-free fluid per day.
    d. Medications - Sedatives, e.g., phenobarbital, 30 mg ($1/2$ gr) orally 3 times daily; and diuretics, e.g., hydrochlorothiazide (Hydro-Diuril®), 50 mg orally daily in the morning.
2. Hospital care - Any patient who does not respond to home management (as above) after 48 hours must be hospitalized in a single room with no visitors (not even the husband); complete rest is mandatory.
    a. Examinations and procedures - If blood pressure rises above 170/110 mm Hg, give magnesium sul-

fate or other antihypertensive drug (see below). Perform daily quantitative measurement of protein on a 24-hour urine collection. If possible, obtain urine by the clean-catch method to avoid admixture with vaginal mucus. Determine serum concentrations of NPN and protein. Blood urea nitrogen and serum uric acid levels may be useful but are not essential. Perform daily ophthalmoscopic examination, noting in particular arteriolar spasm, edema, hemorrhages, and exudates.

b. Diet and fluids - Prescribe a very low sodium (less than 1 gm of salt per day), low fat, high carbohydrate, high protein diet (1800 Cal). Record fluid intake and output. If urine output exceeds 500 ml/day, give fluids to replace this amount. The author feels that it is desirable to give 500 ml/day of fluid from all sources in addition to the replacement of all visible (e.g., urine, vomitus) losses. Some clinicians feel that fluids should be neither specifically limited nor forced.

c. Sedatives and anticonvulsants - Give sedatives in adequate doses, e.g., phenobarbital, 60 mg (1 gr) orally 3 times daily, to calm the patient. Heavy sedation (e.g., morphine, thiopental) is undesirable since it impairs cerebral oxygenation and renal function and depresses fetal circulation and respiration. Diphenylhydantoin sodium (Dilantin®) may be injected I.V. at a rate not exceeding 50 mg/minute. A total dosage of 150-250 mg may be required.

Magnesium sulfate (an excellent anticonvulsant) may be given I.V., 20 ml of 10% aqueous solution injected slowly and repeated hourly to prevent or control seizures. Do not give more than 20-25 gm in 24 hours. Magnesium sulfate may also be given I.M., 10 ml of 50% solution injected slowly into each buttock followed by single injections of 10 ml every 6 hours. The recommended maximum dosage is 50 ml in 24 hours.

Magnesium sulfate also causes splanchnic vasodilatation, with resultant lowering of blood pressure. The flow of urine is augmented. (Do not repeat this drug if the urinary output is below 100 ml/hour, the respirations are less than 16/minute, or the knee jerk reflex is absent.) In cases of overdosage, give a calcium salt such as calcium gluconate, 20 ml of a 10% aqueous solution I.V. slowly, and repeat every hour until urinary, respiratory, and neurologic depression has cleared. (Do not give more than 8 injections of a calcium salt within 24 hours.)

278 Toxemia of Pregnancy

    d. Diuretics - Chlorothiazide (Diuril®), 250-500 mg orally daily, or hydrochlorothiazide (Hydro-Diuril®), 25-50 mg orally daily, may be given to promote diuresis and reduce blood pressure. There is recent evidence that parenteral administration of the thiazides may be more effective in the treatment of eclampsia than the oral preparations. Avoid hypokalemia by giving potassium chloride, orange juice, bananas, or other foods rich in potassium.

       Acetazolamide (Diamox®) acts as a sedative in convulsive disorders as well as a diuretic. Give 1-3 gm in divided doses, beginning with 0.25 gm 3 times a day. If drowsiness or paresthesias occur, reduce the dosage.

    e. Antihypertensive drugs - (See also Magnesium Sulfate, above.) Hydralazine (Apresoline®) causes vasodilatation and increases cerebral, coronary, and renal circulation and function. Give 20-40 mg in 250 ml of 5% dextrose in water slowly I.V. for a potent hypotensive effect. After the blood pressure has been reduced gradually to normal levels, 150 mg of the drug orally 4 times daily will often control the hypertension, although one-tenth of this dose administered in dilute solution I.V. 3-4 times daily may be more effective. The most common side effects are tachycardia, nausea, and vomiting.

       Alkavervir (Veriloid®), 20 mg in 250 ml of 5% dextrose in water slowly I.V., causes a gradual drop in blood pressure; a maximum is reached in less than one hour. The hypertension of toxemia can often be controlled with this drug given by slow daily intravenous drip. Side effects include bradycardia and nausea, but these can usually be prevented by slow administration.

       Cryptenamine (Unitensen®) causes bradycardia, but in toxemia patients results in gradual stabilization of the blood pressure at more normal levels. Give 2 mg slowly I.V. and maintain with 2 mg orally 3 times daily. A combination of hydralazine and cryptenamine (half the recommended dose of each) is quite effective.

B. Eclampsia:
  1. General care - Hospitalize the patient in a single, darkened, quiet room, at absolute bed rest with side rails for protection during convulsions, and provide special nurses around the clock. Allow no visitors (not even the husband).

      Do not disturb the patient for unnecessary procedures (e.g., enemas, douches), and leave the blood pressure cuff on the arm. Turn her on her side to prevent the inferior vena caval syndrome and aspiration of vomitus. A padded tongue blade should be kept at hand to be placed between her teeth during convulsions; a bulb syringe and catheter or suction machine to aspirate mucus or vomitus from the glottis or trachea; and an oxygen cone or tent (since masks and nasal catheters produce excessive stimulation). Typed and crossmatched whole blood must be available for immediate use because patients in eclampsia often develop premature separation of the placenta with hemorrhage and are susceptible to shock.

2. Laboratory procedures - Insert a retention catheter for accurate measurement of the quantity of urine passed. Determine the quantitative protein content of each 24-hour specimen until the 4th or 5th postpartal day. NPN, CO_2 combining power, and serum protein should be determined (for evidence of nitrogen retention and acidosis) as often as the severity and progression of the disease indicate. If serum protein is below 5 gm/100 ml, give salt-poor albumin, 25-50 ml, or plasma or serum, 250-500 ml, by transfusion. Since serum contains sodium, it should be used only if salt-poor albumin is not available.

3. Physical examination - Check blood pressure hourly during the acute phase and every 2-4 hours thereafter. Observe fetal heart tones every time the blood pressure is obtained. Perform ophthalmoscopic examination once a day. Examine the face, extremities, and especially the sacrum (which becomes dependent when the patient is in bed) for signs of edema.

4. Diet and fluids - If the patient is convulsing, give nothing by mouth. Measure and record fluid intake and output for each 24-hour period. If the patient can eat and drink, give a low salt (1 gm of salt per day), high carbohydrate, high protein, low fat diet (1500 Cal). Provide potassium chloride as a salt substitute. If the urine output exceeds 700 ml/day, replace the output plus invisible fluid loss (approximately 500 ml/day) with salt-free fluid (including parenteral fluids). Give 200-300 ml of a 20% solution of dextrose in water 2-3 times a day during the acute phase to protect the liver, to replace fluids, and to aid in nutrition. (Do not give 50% glucose; it will sclerose the veins.) Use no sodium-containing fluids (e.g., physiologic saline, Ringer's injection).

Give 25-50 ml of salt-poor albumin or 250-500 ml of plasma or serum if oliguria is present or if the serum protein is low.

5. Sedatives - Administer a sedative upon admission and maintain reasonable sedation thereafter. Any of the following may be used: (1) Magnesium sulfate, 10 ml

of a 25% solution I.V. when the patient enters the hospital and then one injection after each convulsion or every hour during the acute phase (depending upon toxic manifestations). Test knee jerks before each injection. Administer only one dose if the patient is markedly oliguric or anuric. (2) Amobarbital (Amytal®) sodium, 0.5 gm I.M. every 6-8 hours. (Sodium content is unimportant.) (3) Sodium phenobarbital, 0.25-0.5 gm I.M. every 6-8 hours. (Sodium content is insignificant.) (4) Paraldehyde, 8-12 ml I.M. or 15-30 ml in oil rectally every 4-6 hours. Use this drug carefully; do not over-sedate. (5) Diphenylhydantoin sodium (Dilantin®) I.V. at a rate not exceeding 50 mg/minute. A total dose of 150-250 mg usually is required.

6. Delivery - Because severe hypertensive disease, renal disease, and toxemia of pregnancy are usually aggravated by continuing pregnancy, the most direct method of treatment of any of these disorders is termination of pregnancy. Control eclampsia before attempting induction of labor or delivery. Induce labor, preferably by amniotomy alone, when the patient's condition permits. Use oxytocin to stimulate labor if necessary. Pituitary extract (pituitrin) is contraindicated because of its vasopressor and antidiuretic effects. Regional anesthesia (preferably pudendal block) is the technic of choice. Spinal anesthesia is contraindicated because it may cause sudden, severe hypotension. A mixture of nitrous oxide (70%) and oxygen (30%) may be given with contractions, but 100% oxygen should be administered between contractions. Do not use chloroform or ether since both may increase hepatic damage.

Vaginal delivery is preferred. If the patient is not at term, is not inducible, if she is bleeding, or if there is a question of disproportion, cesarean section may be necessary. If cesarean section is necessary use procaine, 0.5 or 1% (or its equivalent) for local infiltration of the abdominal wall. If well controlled, epidural or caudal anesthesia may be employed. After delivery, give thiopental anesthesia during abdominal closure.

When patients appear late in pregnancy with incomplete histories, it may be impossible to differentiate preeclampsia from hypertensive disease with preeclampsia or chronic renal disease with or without preeclampsia. Such patients should be treated as though they had preeclampsia requiring hospital management. If improvement is not satisfactory after a trial of medical management, consider termination of pregnancy at the optimal time. The decision about when and how to empty the uterus depends upon (1) the probable type and severity of hypertensive disorder involved; (2) the parity of the patient and the number of living children; (3) the duration of the pregnancy; and (4) the status of the cervix and the station of the presenting part. Do not temporize over 2-3 weeks.

Prognosis.

The hypertensive syndromes of pregnancy, including toxemia of pregnancy, rarely cause maternal death unless eclampsia occurs, but these toxic disorders are the largest maternal cause of fetal mortality (about 20% in the USA). The maternal mortality rate in eclampsia is 10-15%. The prognosis for the mother and fetus in toxemia of pregnancy depends upon the adequacy of prenatal care, the time of onset and duration of toxemia, the occurrence of eclampsia, the development of premature separation of the placenta, and the adequacy of treatment. Most patients with toxemia of pregnancy improve strikingly in 24-48 hours with modern therapy. However, because hypertension and proteinuria usually persist and very few patients are cured, early termination of pregnancy is usually required.

Conservative therapy will benefit the fetus more than delivery before the 35th week. After this time, if medical therapy is unsuccessful, induction should be attempted. If good labor does not ensue, cesarean section offers the best hope of delivering a live infant.

Although babies of mothers with toxemia of pregnancy are small for their gestational age (mainly because of placental malfunction), these infants fare better than prematures of the same weight born of nontoxemic mothers. If the duration of pregnancy can be accurately determined, the fact that the fetus is small is an added incentive to early delivery.

12...
Medical & Surgical Complications During Pregnancy

DERMATOLOGIC COMPLICATIONS

In general, pregnancy has a sparing effect on dermatoses; but with a few exceptions skin disorders during pregnancy and the puerperium are otherwise similar to those observed in nonpregnant women.

Dermatologic disorders induced by pregnancy include abnormalities of pigmentation (e.g., chloasma), herpes gestationis, noninflammatory pruritus of pregnancy, vascular spiders, and erythema palmare. Dermatologic disorders usually aggravated by pregnancy include candidal vulvovaginitis, acne vulgaris (early in pregnancy), erythema multiforme, dermatitis herpetiformis, granuloma inguinale, condylomata acuminata, pemphigus, and systemic lupus erythematosus. It is unlikely that malignant melanoma is aggravated by pregnancy.

Chloasma.

Chloasma consists of blotchy, petal-shaped, yellowish-brown macular patches symmetrically distributed over the forehead, nose, and malar prominences which become confluent to form the "mask of pregnancy." Chloasma usually fades soon after delivery. Cosmetic treatment is all that is required.

Herpes Gestationis.

This serious but rare disease, which occurs only during pregnancy, may be a variation of dermatitis herpetiformis. It is an intensely burning, itching, occasionally painful, urticarial, papulovesicular eruption. It involves the buttocks, legs, back, upper abdomen, and extensor surfaces, and rarely affects the mucosa. Grouped vesicles on inflammatory bases are noted. The lesions leave small pigmented scars on healing. This disease usually begins after the 5th month of pregnancy and disappears early in the puerperium. A high eosinophil count in the blood and in vesicle fluid is typical. Biopsy shows subepidermal bullae and high tissue eosinophilia. Herpes gestationis almost always disappears after pregnancy, but fetal death in utero frequently occurs despite the fact that the fetus never develops dermatologic lesions.

Treat first with sulfonamides, 1 gm orally 3 times daily for one week and then 0.5-1 gm daily. If this is unsuccessful, give corticotropin repository injection (gel), 50 units I.M. daily for 3 days, followed by prednisone (or equivalent), 20-30 mg orally daily in divided doses for 10-14 days. If improvement occurs, reduce the dose of prednisone to the lowest amount which will control the disorder.

Termination of pregnancy, without sterilization, may be justified in severe, unresponsive cases of herpes gestationis.

Herpes gestationis may recur in subsequent pregnancies.

Noninflammatory Pruritus of Pregnancy.

The cause is not known. No cutaneous lesions can be seen, but the patient experiences intense itching all over the body. Areas excoriated by scratching may become infected. Treatment is symptomatic.

A papular pruritic dermatosis of pregnancy has been described recently with a high fetal mortality rate. Abnormally elevated chorionic gonadotropin levels are reported with this dermatologic problem of unknown etiology. Symptomatic therapy is advised.

Erythema Palmare.

This benign disorder is a dusky thenar and hypothenar vascular engorgement of the skin of the hands noted 4-6 weeks after the onset of pregnancy. The erythema disappears during the early puerperium. It is based upon genetic predisposition, and provoked by hyperestrogenism (as are vascular spiders also; see below).

Vascular Spiders or Spider Angiomas.

These are small, red, pulsating (arteriolar) telangiectatic points in the skin over the face, neck, thorax, and arms. Most vascular spiders develop during the second and third trimesters of pregnancy and fade almost to invisibility after delivery. They reappear during later advanced pregnancies. In most instances, these angiomas have only minor, temporary cosmetic significance, but the possibility of cirrhosis and of hereditary hemorrhagic telangiectasia (and their complications) must be kept in mind.

HEART DISEASE

Rheumatic heart disease comprises 90-95% of cases of heart disease observed during pregnancy in the USA; about 3% are congenital anomalies. Syphilitic carditis still occurs, and "beriberi heart" may occur as a result of thiamine deficiency.

Reported incidences of heart disease vary from 0.5-2% of obstetric patients.

Heart disease is a major cause of maternal death, but maternal and infant mortality rates are only slightly increased if the disability is minimal. With marked degrees of cardiac disease, the maternal death rate is 1-3% and the infant mortality may reach 50% even in large medical centers.

Functional Classification of Heart Disease.*

For practical purposes, the functional capacity of the heart is the best single measurement of cardiopulmonary status.

Class I: Ordinary physical activity causes no discomfort.
Class II: Ordinary activity causes discomfort.
Class III: Less than ordinary activity causes discomfort.
Class IV: Any physical activity causes discomfort.

Eighty per cent of obstetric patients with heart disease have lesions which do not interfere seriously with their activities (classes I and II) and usually do well. About 85% of deaths ascribed to heart disease complicating pregnancy occur in patients with class III or IV lesions (20% of all pregnant patients with heart disease). Nevertheless, much can still be done to improve the prognosis for the mother and her baby in these unfavorable circumstances.

Pathologic Physiology.

The effects of pregnancy on circulatory and respiratory function are summarized in Table 12-1.

Three major burdens on the heart are associated with pregnancy: cardiac output is increased by more than one-third; the pulse rate is accelerated by 10 beats/minute; and blood volume expands by one-third. These unavoidable stresses must be considered in an appraisal of the patient's ability to undergo pregnancy, delivery, and the puerperium.

In addition to these unavoidable physiologic burdens, there are medical liabilities which are avoidable or can be treated; e.g., anemia, obesity, hyperthyroidism, myxedema, infection, and emotional and physical stresses.

Youth, adequate functional cardiac reserve, stability of the cardiac lesion, and an optimistic, cooperative attitude are important assets which do much to improve the cardiac patient's chances for a successful confinement. Good antenatal care and help at home are essential features of the total medical program. The physician must help the pregnant cardiac

---

*New York Heart Association, 1964.

patient to avoid overburdening the heart. Avoidable burdens and stresses must be eliminated or drastically curtailed so that the patient's assets will tip the scales favorably to preserve health and avoid cardiac disaster.

Labor, delivery, and the early puerperium impose the following specific physiologic burdens on the maternal heart:

A. During Labor and Delivery:
 1. A rise in pulse rate with the beginning of each contraction. This is the reaction of the heart to intermittent work.
 2. Slowing of the pulse at the end of each contraction.
 3. Return of the pulse to the resting level between contractions.
 4. Intermittent increase of oxygen consumption with uterine contractions, approaching that of moderate to severe exercise.
 5. Tachycardia during the second stage may result from distention of the right atrium and ventricle by blood from the uterus and from the effect of straining.

B. During the Puerperium:
 1. A slight increase in cardiac output occurs for about one week after delivery. Elimination of the placenta, contracture of the uterus, and reduction of the pelvic circulation suddenly makes more blood available to the heart.
 2. Decrease in the plasma volume (Hct increase) for 12 hours after delivery is due primarily to readjustments in venous pressure. A second marked decrease in plasma volume persists for 7-9 days together with a reduction in the amount of total body water during the same period. These changes are due to postpartal diuresis.

Treatment.

Determine the functional cardiac status (class I-IV) before the third month if possible and again at 7-8 months. Restrict physical activity to necessary duties only, using fatigue as a limiting factor. Make certain that the patient obtains assistance with essential household duties (child care, laundry, cleaning, and marketing). Help the patient and her family to understand the medical problem, and allay her fears, anxiety, and tension. Periods of maximal cardiac stress occur at 14-32 weeks, during labor, and, particularly, during the immediate postpartal period. Especially good rapport and medical control must be maintained at these times.

A. Medical Measures: Correct anemia, hyperthyroidism, and obesity as indicated. Treat cardiac complications such as congestive failure, pulmonary edema, bacterial endocarditis, and arrhythmia as in the nonpregnant patient. Treat all infections specifically, promptly, and

Table 12-1. Effect of pregnancy on maternal circulatory and respiratory functions.

Function	Change
Heart rate	Slow increase of 10 beats/minute from 14-30 weeks. Rate maintained at this level to 40 weeks.
Arterial BP	Systolic unchanged until the 30th week. Diastolic slightly reduced (period of maximal pulse pressure).
Venous BP	Arms: No change. Legs: Gradual marked increase between 8-40 weeks. 7-8 mo.
Cardiac output	Increase of 30-50% by the 32nd week; decline to 20% increase at 40 weeks.
Total body water	Increased between 10-40 weeks
Plasma and blood volume	Rise of 15% between 12-32 weeks; slight decline to 40 weeks.
Red cell mass	Augmented 10-15% between 8-40 weeks
Vital capacity	Rises 15% by the 20th week; decline of 5% by 40 weeks.
Oxygen consumption	Increased 15% between 16-40 weeks
Circulation time	Decreases 13-11 seconds by 32nd week, then returns to 13 seconds by 40th week.

vigorously. Intercurrent respiratory, gastrointestinal tract, or urinary tract infections can be serious. Restrict sodium intake and use diuretics, but not to the point of hyponatremia. Avoid hypokalemia.

B. Obstetric Measures:
1. Avoid complications in labor, delivery, and the puerperium.
2. Administer full doses of analgesics as necessary, but do not give scopolamine since it may cause excitement and overactivity.
3. Delivery should be under local or regional anesthesia if possible. Administer oxygen freely during labor and in the early puerperium, when tachycardia, dyspnea, and chest pain are most severe.
4. Shorten the terminal stage of labor by elective low forceps delivery to spare the patient the effort of bearing down in the second stage. Do not intervene too early, however, or lacerations, excessive blood loss, and shock may occur.
5. Manage the third stage of labor carefully to limit postpartal bleeding. Do not administer ergot preparations (to avoid a drug pressor effect), and give oxytocin only if necessary after delivery for uterine atony.

Heart Disease 287

6. Lower the patient's legs promptly after delivery to reduce drainage of blood into the general circulation.
7. Anticipate the possibility that some women, who have experienced no cardiac symptoms during pregnancy or labor, sometimes go into shock or acute failure immediately after delivery due to the sudden engorgement of the splanchnic vessels. Treat for hypovolemic shock and acute cardiac failure.
8. Permit the patient to nurse if she wishes to do so, but not if she has class IV functional disability.
9. Prescribe cautious, brief, early ambulation for patients with class I-III functional disability provided the medical course is otherwise uncomplicated. Class I patients may be sent home.
10. Patients with class II-IV functional disability should remain in the hospital at least 2 weeks after delivery until the cardiovascular function is stable. Class IV patients must remain in bed for as long as necessary to recover from the effects of labor and delivery.
11. Before discharge, make certain that the patient is returning to a controlled home situation where adequate rest in a nonstressful milieu will be possible. Recommend contraception, particularly for class II-IV patients, unless there are personal contraindications to its use.

C. Surgical Measures:
1. Therapeutic abortion - Therapeutic abortion may be indicated in 5-8% of cases of heart disease complicating pregnancy. The decision to abort is not based upon the presence of any specific lesion but on a thorough evaluation of the patient's total life situation, including the type and severity of the heart disease, other medical illnesses, and religious and emotional factors. Most candidates for abortion have class IV functional disability, and many are multiparas. Patients who have had cardiac failure in previous pregnancy will usually have failure again with another pregnancy, and so should be aborted. Abortion is seldom beneficial after the 4th month but may be considered. The patient's life must be seriously jeopardized to justify sacrifice of the pregnancy.
2. If the cardiac lesion is severe enough to warrant abortion and if surgical treatment is not available and there is little prospect that therapeutic advances will alter the situation favorably, sterilization may be indicated. If the patient is not sterilized, contraception should be employed.
3. Mitral valvulotomy is indicated only in patients with severe stenosis of the mitral valve who have insufficient cardiac reserve, even with ideal supportive

therapy, to sustain the burden of pregnancy. In general, such patients will have had cardiac decompensation in a previous pregnancy despite the best care.
4. Cesarean section is not recommended for the pregnant cardiac patient unless it is performed for primarily obstetric reasons. The woman who can withstand a major operation almost always can undergo vaginal delivery.

Prognosis.

The prognosis in heart disease complicating pregnancy depends upon the severity of the heart disorder, the availability of medical and obstetric care, medical and surgical complications, the patient's emotional, socioeconomic, and environmental status, and local policy regarding therapeutic abortion and sterilization. Although rheumatic heart disease is not exacerbated by successive pregnancies, the increased load of pregnancy and the care of an infant by a rheumatic patient frequently will cause a downhill course. Data are not available regarding the long-range prognosis for other types of heart disease.

The maternal mortality for all types of heart disease is 0.5-3% in large medical centers in the USA, and heart disease accounts for 5-10% of all maternal deaths.

Perinatal mortality (including fetal deaths due to therapeutic abortion) largely depends upon the functional severity of the mother's heart disease:

Mother's Functional Disability	Infant Mortality
Class I	About 5%
Class II	10-15%
Class III	About 35%
Class IV	Over 50%

The incidence of congenital defects is greater among infants delivered of women with congenital and syphilitic heart disease than among those delivered of women with normal hearts, but rheumatic and other types of heart disease do not increase the incidence of fetal anomalies.

CARDIAC ARREST

Cardiac arrest is cessation of heart action as a result of acute myocardial hypoxia or alteration in conduction. Ventricular standstill (asystole) and ventricular fibrillation are the immediate causes. Cardiac arrest occurs most commonly during induction of anesthesia and during operative surgery or obstetric delivery. Cardiovascular disease increases the risk of cardiac arrest; hypoxia and hypertension are contributory causes. Cardiac arrest may follow shock, hypoventilation, airway obstruction, excessive anesthesia, drug administration or drug sensitivity, vagovagal reflex activity, myocardial infarction, air and amniotic fluid embolism, and heart block.

Cardiac arrest occurs about once in 800-1000 operations, and is apt to occur during minor surgical procedures as well as during major surgery. It occurs about once in 8000 obstetric deliveries—usually operative, complicated cases. Fortunately, it is possible to save up to 75% of patients when cardiac arrest occurs in the operating or delivery room.

Clinical Findings.

Premonitory signs (especially during induction of anesthesia, intubation or extubation, moving the patient, deep or prolonged anesthesia, hypoxia or hypotension with vagotonal effect) consist of irregular cardiac rhythm, bradycardia, and sudden or marked hypertension. Absence of a palpable pulse in a major artery (aorta, carotid, femoral), absence of heart sounds over the precordium, and dilatation of the pupils are diagnostic of cardiac arrest. Emergency treatment should not be withheld for electrocardiographic confirmation of the diagnosis.

Prevention.

Ensure a constant, generous oxygen supply during induction of anesthesia and throughout surgery and delivery.

Avoid undesirable vagal effects: (1) Give atropine before surgery or delivery. (2) Give atropine sulfate, 0.4-0.6 mg ($1/150$-$1/100$ gr) I.V., for bradycardia, AV dissociation, or AV nodal rhythm. (3) Avoid placing excessive traction on the viscera during surgery or on the fetus during delivery. (4) Do not administer vasopressors such as epinephrine or ephedrine during cyclopropane, trichloroethylene, or chloroform anesthesia.

Prevent and treat hypotension promptly and effectively.

Heart-Lung Resuscitation. * (For treatment of asphyxia or cardiac arrest.)

Phase I: First Aid (Emergency Oxygenation of the Brain).

Must be instituted within 3-4 minutes for optimal effectiveness and to minimize permanent brain damage. **Do not wait for confirmation of suspected cardiac arrest.**

Step 1: Place patient in a supine position on a firm surface (not a bed). (A 4 × 6 foot plywood board should be available in emergency aid stations.)

---

*Modified after Safar.

Step 2: Tilt head backward and maintain in this hyperextended position. Keep mandible displaced forward by pulling strongly at the angle of the jaw.

If Victim Is Not Breathing:

Step 3: Clear mouth and pharynx of mucus, blood, vomitus, or foreign material.
Step 4: Separate lips and teeth to open oral airway.
Step 5: If steps 2-4 fail to open airway, forcibly blow air through mouth (keeping nose closed) or nose (keeping mouth closed) and inflate the lungs 3-5 times. Watch for chest movement. If chest movement does not occur immediately and if pharyngeal or tracheal tubes are available, use them without delay. Tracheostomy may be necessary.
Step 6: Feel the carotid artery for pulsations.

a. If Carotid Pulsations Are Present:

Give lung inflation by mouth to mouth breathing (keeping patient's nostrils closed) or mouth to nose breathing (keeping patient's mouth closed) 12-15 times per minute—allowing about 2 seconds for inspiration and 3 seconds for expiration—until spontaneous respirations return. Continue as long as the pulses remain palpable and previously dilated pupils remain constricted. Bag-mask technics for lung inflation should be reserved for experts. If pulsations cease, follow directions as in 6b, below.

b. If Carotid Pulsations Are Absent:

Alternate cardiac compression (closed chest cardiac massage) and pulmonary ventilation as in 6a, above. Place the heel of one hand on the sternum just above the xiphoid. With the heel of the other hand on top of it, apply firm vertical pressure sufficient to force the sternum about 2 inches downward (less in children) about once every second. After 15 sternal compressions, alternate with 3-5 deep lung inflations. Repeat and continue this alternating procedure until it is possible to obtain additional assistance and more definitive care. Resuscitation must be continuous during transportation to the hospital. Open heart massage should be attempted only in a hospital. When possible, obtain an ECG, but do not interrupt resuscitation to do so.

Phase II: Restoration of Spontaneous Circulation.

Until spontaneous respiration and circulation are restored there must be no interruption of artificial ventilation and cardiac massage while steps 7-13 (below) are being carried out. Three basic questions must be considered at this point:

(1) What is the underlying cause, and is it correctable?
(2) What is the nature of the cardiac arrest?
(3) What further measures will be necessary? The physician must make plans for the assistance of trained hospital personnel, an ECG, a defibrillator, and emergency drugs.

Step 7: If a spontaneous effective heartbeat is not restored after 1-2 minutes of cardiac compression, have an assistant give epinephrine (adrenaline), 1 mg (1 ml of 1:1000 or 10 ml of 1:10,000 aqueous solution) I.V. **or** 0.5 mg (0.5 ml of 1:1000 aqueous solution) by the intracardiac route. Repeat larger dose at 5-10 minute intervals if necessary. The intracardiac method is not without hazard.

Step 8: Promote venous return and combat shock by elevating legs, and give I.V. fluids as available and indicated. The use of firmly applied tourniquets on the extremities to occlude arteries in order to reduce the circulating bed may be of value.

Step 9: If the victim is pulseless for more than 5 minutes, give sodium bicarbonate solution, 3-4 gm/50 ml (1.5-2 gm/50 ml in children) I.V. to combat impending metabolic acidosis. Repeat every 5-10 minutes as indicated.

Step 10: If pulsations still do not return, suspect ventricular fibrillation. Obtain ECG.

Step 11: If ECG demonstrates ventricular fibrillation, maintain cardiac massage until just before giving an external defibrillating shock of 440-1000 volts AC for 0.25 second with one electrode firmly applied to the skin over the apex of the heart and the other over the sternal notch. Monitor with ECG. (A 50-400 watt-second DC shock is superior if a DC defibrillator is available.) If cardiac function is not restored, resume massage and repeat 3 shocks at intervals of 1-3 minutes. If cardiac action is re-established but remains weak, give calcium chloride or calcium gluconate, 5-10 ml (0.5-1 gm) of 10% solution I.V.; it probably should not be used in patients who have been taking digitalis.

292 Cardiac Arrest

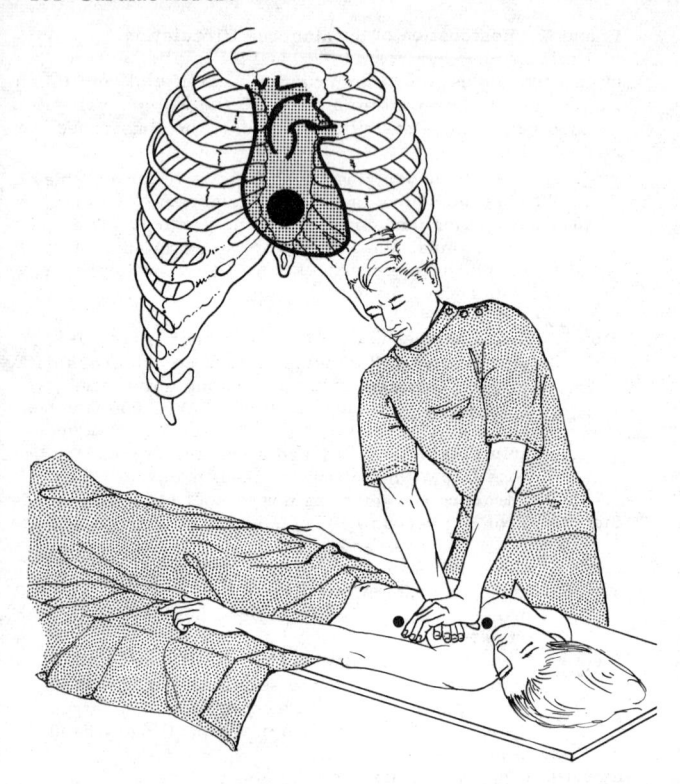

Fig 12-1. Technic of closed chest cardiac massage. Heavy circle in heart drawing shows area of application of force. Circles on supine figure show points of application of electrodes for defibrillation.

Step 12: Thoracotomy and open heart massage may be considered (but only in a hospital) if cardiac function fails to return after all of the above measures have been used.

Step 13: If cardiac, pulmonary, and CNS functions are restored, the patient should be carefully observed for shock and complications of the precipitating cause.

Phase III: Follow-up Measures.

When cardiac and pulmonary function have been re-

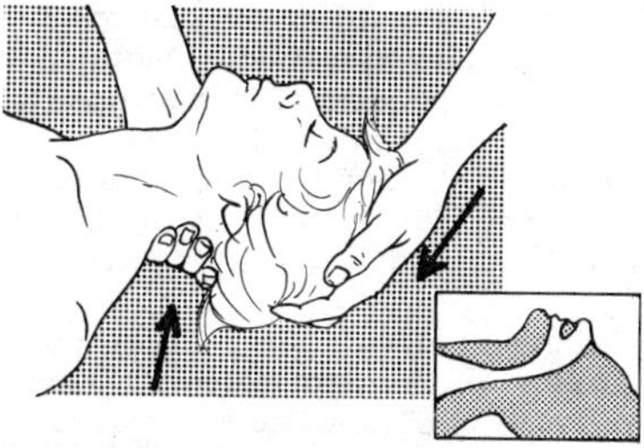

Cardiac Arrest 293

(1)

The operator takes his position at the patient's head.

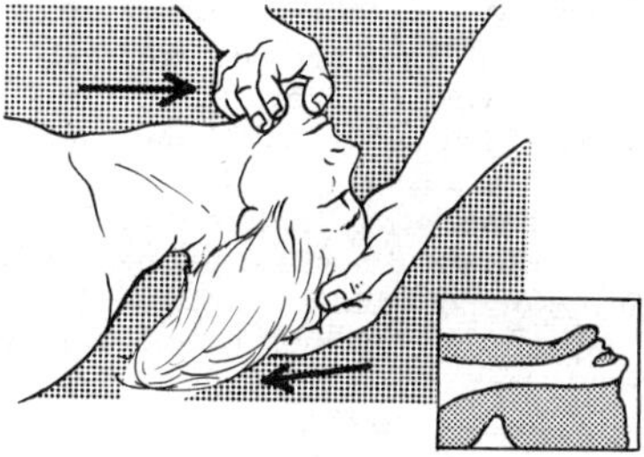

(2)

With the right thumb and index finger he displaces the mandible forward by pressing at its central portion, at the same time lifting the neck and tilting the head as far back as possible.

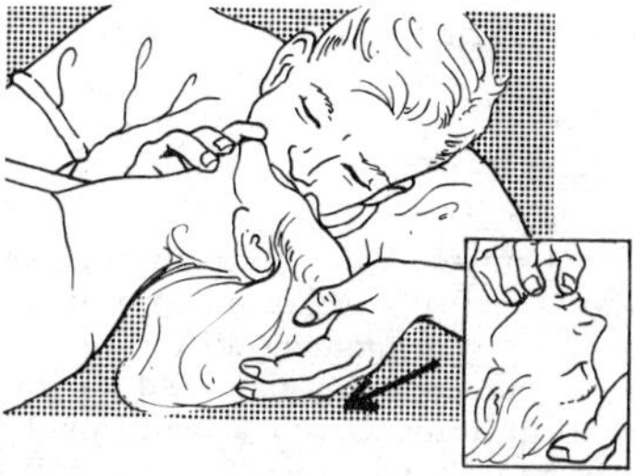

(3)

After taking a deep breath, the operator immediately seals his mouth around the mouth (or nose) of the victim and exhales until the chest of the victim rises.

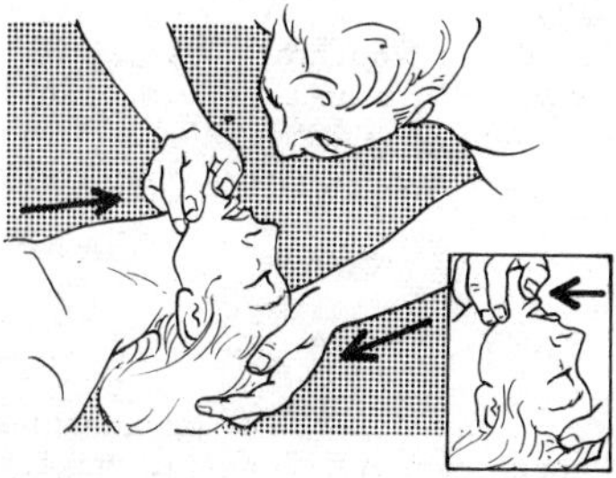

(4)

The victim's mouth is opened by downward and forward traction on the lower jaw or by pulling down the lower lip.

Fig 12-2. Technic of mouth to mouth insufflation.

established and satisfactorily maintained, evaluation of CNS function deserves careful consideration. Decision as to the nature and duration of subsequent treatment must be individualized. The physician must decide if he is "prolonging life" or simply "prolonging dying." Apparent CNS recovery has been reported in a few patients unconscious up to a week after appropriate treatment.

Step 14: Support ventilation and circulation. Treat any other complications which might arise. Do not overlook the possibility of complications of external cardiac massage (e.g., broken ribs, ruptured viscera).

Step 15: If circulation and respiration are restored but there are no signs of CNS recovery within 30 minutes, hypothermia at 30°C for 2-3 days may lessen the degree of brain damage.

Step 16: Meticulous post-resuscitation care is required, particularly for the first 48 hours after recovery. Observe carefully for possible multiple cardiac arrhythmias, especially recurrent fibrillation or cardiac standstill.

HEMATOLOGIC DISORDERS

Anemia

Physiologic and pathologic changes in the maternal organism during pregnancy make the determination of anemia difficult. Not only do blood values during pregnancy differ from those in the nonpregnant patient, but these factors also vary with the course of pregnancy. If deficiencies of a significant degree are noted, the patient is anemic and specific therapy is indicated.

In every evaluation of clinical and laboratory data, the following questions must be answered: (1) Is anemia present? (2) Is there evidence of iron deficiency? (3) Are megaloblasts present in the blood smear? (4) Are there signs of hemolysis? (5) Is there bone marrow deficiency?

IRON DEFICIENCY ANEMIA

Iron deficiency anemia occurs in about 20% of pregnancies in the USA. About 95% of pregnant women with anemia have the iron deficiency type. Pregnancy increases the body's iron requirement. Many nonpregnant women are iron deficient because of excessive menstrual blood loss, dysfunctional uterine bleeding, or postpartal hemorrhage or as a result of iron deprivation from previous pregnancies and inadequate diet. Many women, anemic before pregnancy, never "catch up" during or after pregnancy. Iron deficiency anemia often develops or increases as pregnancy progresses.

Fetal and maternal morbidity are usually increased in proportion to the severity of the anemia, although at times marked maternal anemia has no effect on the offspring. Most obstetric problems involving anemia relate to premature delivery. Oral iron supplements (e.g., ferrous sulfate, 200 mg 3 times daily after meals) are desirable during pregnancy; if iron deficiency anemia is marked, intramuscular or intravenous iron therapy may be required late in pregnancy.

MEGALOBLASTIC ANEMIA OF PREGNANCY
(Pernicious Anemia of Pregnancy)

Megaloblastic anemia occurring during pregnancy is caused by deficiency of folic acid. This disorder may involve women of any age and parity, but it is most common in multiparas over 30. The reported incidence varies from 1:40-1:200 deliveries. Although this type of anemia is more common among nutritionally deprived populations, it is often described in patients on apparently adequate diets.

Clinical Findings.

Lassitude, progressive anorexia, mental depression, and nausea are the principal complaints. Pallor is often not marked. Glossitis, gingivitis, vomiting, and diarrhea are frequently troublesome. There are no abnormal neurologic findings. The Hgb may be as low as 4-6 gm/100 ml. The red cell count may be under 2 million in severe cases. Extreme anemia is often associated with leukopenia and thrombocytopenia. The MCV is usually normal or increased. The MCH is normal or increased above 30%. The peripheral white blood cells are hypersegmented. The bone marrow is hyperplastic and megaloblastic. Free gastric hydrochloric acid is present in normal amounts. Serum iron values are high, and serum vitamin B_{12} levels are normal. Spontaneous remissions usually occur after delivery.

Secondary infection, hemorrhage, fetal death in utero, and maternal death may occur. The fetus does surprisingly well even when the mother's anemia is severe.

Treatment.

Give folic acid, 5-10 mg/day orally or parenterally, until a hematologic remission is achieved. Megaloblastic anemia of pregnancy does not usually respond to vitamin B_{12} even in large doses. Administer iron orally or parenterally (or both) as indicated. Prescribe a high vitamin, high protein diet. Transfusions are rarely necessary except when anemia is extreme, especially if the patient is near term.

Employ appropriate antibiotics for infection.

Therapeutic abortion and sterilization are not indicated for megaloblastic anemia.

Prognosis.

Megaloblastic anemia during pregnancy is not apt to be severe unless it is associated with systemic infection or toxemia. If the diagnosis is made at least 4 weeks before term, treatment can often raise the Hgb to normal or nearly normal levels. The outlook for mother and baby are good if there is adequate time for treatment. Anemia usually recurs only when the patient becomes pregnant again.

REFRACTORY ANEMIA

Anemia refractory to adequate dosage of all known hematinics during pregnancy is of undetermined cause, but it may be due to an unrecognized infection, e.g., of the urinary tract. Most patients are multiparas. The disorder is relatively common, but is usually not a serious problem for the mother or her offspring. The diagnosis is based upon careful exclusion of all other known causes of anemia and thrombocytopenia. Anemia is usually of the normocytic, normochromic, or hypochromic type. Slight leukocytosis, low serum iron levels, toxic granulocytosis, and the demonstration of storage iron present in the bone marrow are typical. Red cell survival is normal.

Remission sometimes follows appropriate antibiotic therapy. Blood transfusion may be necessary. The condition usually clears spontaneously after delivery.

SICKLE CELL ANEMIA

Sickle cell anemia, a chronic hereditary hemolytic anemia limited almost exclusively to Negroes, may complicate pregnancy in several respects. In severe cases the perinatal mortality may be 50% and the maternal mortality 10%. The most common complications during and immediately after pregnancy (in order of frequency) are urinary tract, pelvic, and respiratory infections. The incidence of toxemia of pregnancy is increased. Differentiation of a hemolytic crisis from eclamptogenic toxemia of a fulminating type may be difficult. Faulty development of the pelvis due to sclerosis of bone may cause dystocia.

Blood transfusions may be lifesaving during a hemolytic crisis and may be given in the last trimester to dilute sickle cells and prevent crisis. Otherwise the treatment is symptomatic and supportive. Await the onset of spontaneous labor, and avoid surgery and instrumentation if possible. Therapeutic abortion is not usually indicated, but subsequent sterilization may be necessary in severe cases.

HEREDITARY LEPTOCYTOSIS
(Thalassemia, Mediterranean Anemia)

Hereditary leptocytosis is a type of hypochromic microcytic anemia which is not due to dietary deficiency, fails to respond to iron therapy, and is caused by a genetic defect. The term leptocytosis is descriptive of the thin, target-shaped mature red cells. Hgb electrophoretic studies may be necessary to establish the diagnosis, especially in the heterozygous form of the disorder (thalassemia minor) wherein the trait is present but the anemia is mild and usually asymptomatic. There are no obstetric complications peculiar to thalassemia other than those due to anemia, and patients carrying the trait tolerate pregnancy and delivery without difficulty. The diagnosis of hereditary leptocytosis in women of the childbearing age is important for genetic counseling to assess the risk of transmitting the trait or homozygous disease (thalassemia major) to progeny and to avoid hazardous treatment.

There is no need for transfusions unless hemorrhage occurs or the Hgb level falls below 9 gm/100 ml.

Marriage between individuals with family histories of homo- or heterozygous leptocytosis should be discouraged.

HEMORRHAGIC DISORDERS

The incidence, types, diagnosis, and treatment of hemorrhagic disorders complicating pregnancy are in most respects the same as in nonpregnant women. Anemia due to blood loss, postpartal hemorrhage, and development of bleeding diseases in the infant may at times have a significant influence on the morbidity and mortality rates of both mother and infant.

Idiopathic thrombocytopenic purpura, when it has its onset during pregnancy, may be very serious. The maternal death rate in this condition is 1-2%, but the fetal death rate may be as high as 20%. If the mother fails to respond adequately to medical measures, including corticosteroids and blood transfusions, it may be necessary to perform a splenectomy. In early pregnancy, surgery may produce abortion. Cesarian section must also be considered in such cases.

Hypofibrinogenemia may occur in cases of abruptio placentae, amniotic fluid embolism, and intrauterine retention of a dead fetus. Bleeding in such instances may be very severe and requires emergency administration of fresh whole blood and Fibrinogen, U.S.P., 5-20 gm.

Circulating anticoagulants of unknown origin, presumably immunologic, may cause hemorrhagic manifestations some time after delivery. Treatment is symptomatic and supportive.

LEUKEMIAS & LYMPHOMAS

Leukemias and lymphomas complicating pregnancy have the same clinical characteristics as in nonpregnant women. Treatment must be modified, however, because of potential harmful effects to the fetus. Chemotherapy should be avoided during the first trimester of pregnancy because the drugs required have abortifacient and teratogenic properties, but they have been used during the second and third trimesters without apparent fetal injury. Radioisotopes must be avoided during pregnancy, but local x-ray therapy to the liver, spleen, or lymphatic masses may be given provided the uterus is shielded from radiation. Therapeutic abortion is seldom indicated.

GASTROINTESTINAL DISORDERS

PEPTIC ULCER

Although pregnancy generally exerts an ameliorating effect on peptic ulcer, hemorrhage or perforation may occur during or shortly after pregnancy. During late pregnancy, a flare-up of peptic ulcer may be due to aggravation by anxiety. Exacerbation of peptic ulcer may occur in the puerperium in response to the stress of labor and delivery or as a result of a rise in gastric acidity during lactation and the anxieties and obligations of motherhood.

Medical treatment is the same as that in the nonpregnant woman. Surgery should be reserved for emergencies.

HIATUS HERNIA

Hiatus hernia, or partial rupture of the stomach or esophagus (or both) through the diaphragm, develops in patients with a weakened or congenitally widened diaphragmatic crux because of increased intra-abdominal pressure during pregnancy and progressive enlargement of the uterus with elevation of the stomach by the uterine fundus. It occurs more frequently in multiparas and in older or obese gravidas. About 15% of all pregnant women develop hiatus hernia.

Persistence of nausea and vomiting beyond mid-pregnancy and progressive pyrosis, eructation, and regurgitation of food and acid contents during recumbency are typical findings. The sensation of substernal pressure may be quite severe, and is relieved by erect posture but is aggravated by recumbency.

Conservative treatment is usually adequate to carry the patient through pregnancy and delivery. Prescribe a bland diet, antispasmodics, antacids, and sedatives, and caution the patient against lying down or exercising immediately after eating or drinking. Prevent unnecessary increases in intra-abdominal pressure by prescribing laxatives for constipation, by restricting lifting and straining, and by the use of low forceps delivery so that the patient will not have to bear down during the second stage of labor. The patient should sleep in a semi-reclining position. Obese women should be encouraged to reduce.

Postpartal surgery should be considered only if the symptoms are persistent and marked. Excessive blood loss should be replaced by means of transfusions, and iron given for chronic anemia.

The great majority of hiatus hernias disappear soon after delivery, and the relief of symptoms is usually dramatic.

DYNAMIC ILEUS

Mechanical obstruction of the intestine (most frequently the small bowel) occurs about once in 6000 pregnancies. About half of cases occur during the mid-trimester, when the enlarging uterus displaces the bowel sufficiently to stretch adhesions. Mechanical obstruction is often due to adherence of an ileal loop and the cecum after appendectomy or of the small intestine and uterus or broad ligament after myomectomy, uterine suspension, or adnexectomy. Mechanical obstruction should be considered as a cause of ileus in women with one or more abdominal scars. Other causes of obstruction include incarceration of a loop of intestine in an external or internal hernia, volvulus, or intussusception.

Surgical relief of the obstruction is indicated without delay. Pre- and postoperative gastric suction is required. Fluid and electrolyte imbalance must be corrected early. **(Note:** Hypokalemic alkalosis can cause convulsions which may be confused with eclamptic seizures.) Broad-spectrum antibiotics should be given parenterally if infection occurs.

The maternal mortality rate may be as high as 20% if treatment of septic, closed-loop obstruction is delayed.

ADYNAMIC ILEUS

Adynamic (paralytic) ileus, diminished or absent contractility of the bowel, is a cause of intestinal obstruction. Mild adynamic ileus is present for 1-3 days even after normal delivery; brief moderate paralysis of the bowel is a secondary consequence to laparotomy, including cesarean section. Other obstetric and gynecologic conditions which may cause paralytic ileus are intra- and retroperitoneal hemorrhage and infection, pyelonephritis, nephro-ureterolithiasis, torsion of the adnexa, bladder atony, and hypokalemic acidosis. Older women seem more prone to paralytic ileus than young ones.

Paralytic ileus in obstetric and gynecologic patients almost always responds to withholding oral food and fluids, correction of fluid and electrolyte imbalance by means of parenteral fluids, intestinal decompression, and evacuation of the rectosigmoid by means of enemas. If mechanical obstruction can be ruled out, vasopressin (Pitressin®), 1-2 units subcut. or I.M. (**not** intravenously) every 30 minutes for 6-8 injections, may be helpful. (**Caution:** Vasopressin is contraindicated in toxemia of pregnancy, epilepsy, and cardiac and renal disease.) Gastric suction usually will suffice. If ileus is marked, a long intestinal tube (Werner, Miller-Abbott) should be inserted to decompress the small bowel.

In the rare event of failure to respond to conservative measures, abdominal exploration may be necessary if the patient's condition is deteriorating.

APPENDICITIS

Appendicitis occurs about once in 1200 pregnancies. Management is more difficult than when the disease occurs in nonpregnant persons since the appendix is carried high and to the right, away from McBurney's point, and the traditional localization of the pain does not usually occur. The distended uterus displaces the colon and small bowel; uterine contractions prevent abscess formation and walling-off; and the intestinal relationships are disturbed. In at least 20% of obstetric patients, the correct diagnosis is not made until the appendix has ruptured and peritonitis has become established. Delay may lead to premature labor or abortion.

Early appendectomy is indicated. If the diagnosis is made during labor at or near term, extraperitoneal cesarean section and appendectomy should be done to minimize peritonitis. Therapeutic abortion is never indicated. If drains are necessary, they should be transabdominal, not transvaginal.

With early diagnosis and appendectomy, the prognosis is good for the mother and her baby.

ULCERATIVE COLITIS
(Nonspecific or Idiopathic Colitis)

The cause of ulcerative colitis is not known. Young women are most commonly affected, and the peak incidence is in the second and third decades. Girls occasionally develop the disorder prior to adolescence, and sexual development is either delayed or arrested.

In severe, fulminating cases, colitis induces intractable bloody diarrhea, fever, fluid and electrolyte imbalance, collapse, toxicosis, and death. When the disease becomes chronic, malnutrition and invalidism are associated with remissions and exacerbations of diarrhea.

Ulcerative colitis in mature women has little or no effect upon fertility or pregnancy, but pregnancy may have a profound effect on this disease under certain circumstances. When pregnancy occurs while the colitis is inactive, an exacerbation is unlikely; but when conception coincides with active ulcerative colitis, one-half to three-fourths of patients will suffer a severe relapse during pregnancy and in the puerperium. When colitis has its onset during pregnancy, more than half of the patients will suffer a hectic course and a few will die. When colitis has its onset during the puerperium, most patients will have a very severe, often protracted course. Pregnancy almost never exerts a favorable effect on the course of ulcerative colitis.

There is no specific treatment. Symptomatic and supportive medical measures, adrenal steroids, and the sulfonamide and antibiotic drugs are usually employed during pregnancy, and ileostomy may occasionally be used in emergencies.

Therapeutic abortion is justified only in rare cases of acute, fulminating, treatment-resistant colitis which are exacerbated by pregnancy or when uncontrollable colitis is first noted during pregnancy.

COLON & RECTAL CARCINOMA

Pregnancy increases the likelihood of spread of carcinoma of the colon or rectum. Malignant tumors of the lower bowel are often neglected or treated palliatively during pregnancy with tragic results. The prognosis is extremely poor for the pregnant carcinoma patient unless prompt radical surgery is possible.

The symptoms of rectal and colon carcinoma include constipation of increasing severity, often alternating with transient diarrhea, and rectal bleeding or blood-streaked stools. Anemia and weight loss are late signs.

In almost two-thirds of cases the lesion can be reached by the examining finger and biopsied through the sigmoidoscope even during pregnancy. Barium x-ray studies may reveal the site and extent of the lesion.

The treatment of apparently resectable carcinoma of the rectum and colon during pregnancy depends upon the duration of the pregnancy at the time of the diagnosis as well as the extent of the malignancy. From the 4th-20th weeks, radical resection and colostomy via the abdominoperineal approach is indicated, avoiding the pregnant uterus. In the absence of obstetric contraindications, vaginal delivery at term should be permitted. From the 21st-28th weeks, the pregnancy should be sacrificed by hysterectomy and abdominoperineal resection and colostomy performed. After the 28th week, cesarean section should be done as soon as fetal viability seems likely. The cancerous bowel is then resected and a colostomy constructed 3-4 weeks after delivery.

For incurable cases, cesarean delivery is indicated as soon as the fetus is viable. Palliative resection should be done at delivery or afterward to prevent intestinal obstruction.

CHOLEDOCHOLITHIASIS & CHOLECYSTITIS

Severe choledocholithiasis and cholecystitis are uncommon during pregnancy despite the fact that women have an increased tendency to form gallstones (one-third of all women over 40 have gallstones). When acute gallbladder inflammation or biliary colic does occur, it is usually in late pregnancy or, more often, in the puerperium. Pregnancy is considered to be a predisposing cause of gallstones; and although mechanical stasis and altered blood cholesterol have been mentioned as contributing factors, the true relationship remains unknown. About 90% of patients with cholecystitis have stones.

Symptomatic relief may be all that is required. Meperidine (Demerol®) and atropine are effective in alleviating pain and ductal spasm. Morphine is contraindicated in choledocholithiasis or cholecystitis because it may induce spasm of the sphincter of Oddi.

Gallbladder surgery in pregnant women should be attempted only in extreme cases (e.g., obstruction) because it greatly increases the fetal mortality rate (up to about 15%). Cholecystostomy and lithotomy may be all that is feasible during advanced pregnancy, deferring cholecystectomy until after delivery. On the other hand, withholding surgery when it is definitely needed may result in necrosis and perforation of the gallbladder and peritonitis. Intermittent high fever, jaundice, and right upper quadrant pain may indicate cholangitis due to impacted common duct stone. Surgical removal of gallstones and establishment of biliary drainage are then essential.

Therapeutic abortion or early delivery (by induction or cesarean section) is not warranted.

INTRA-ABDOMINAL SURGERY

Elective major surgery should be avoided during pregnancy. However, normal, uncomplicated pregnancy has no debilitating effect and does not alter operative risk except as it may interfere with the diagnosis of abdominal disorders and increase the technical problems of intra-abdominal surgery. Abortion is not a serious hazard after operation unless peritoneal sepsis or other significant complications occur.

During the first trimester, congenital anomalies may be induced in the developing fetus by hypoxia. It is preferable to avoid surgical intervention during this period; if surgery does become necessary, the greatest precautions must be taken to prevent hypoxia and hypotension.

The second trimester is usually the optimal time for operative procedures.

VIRAL HEPATITIS
(Infectious or Epidemic Hepatitis)

Infectious hepatitis affects females of all ages. Pregnancy has been said to increase resistance to epidemic hepatitis, but, paradoxically, the manifestations may be more severe and prolonged when the disease occurs in advanced pregnancy. When infectious hepatitis develops during the first trimester, the likelihood of fetal anomalies is increased about two-fold. The incidence of abortion is not increased, but the frequency of premature delivery is.

Treatment consists of supportive medical measures as for the nonpregnant patient. Avoid operative obstetric intervention. Anesthetics, analgesics, and sedatives may be hepatotoxic. A diminished prothrombin concentration may cause hemorrhage which should be treated with oral or parenteral vitamin K. No major surgical procedures should be performed unless the need is great. Therapeutic abortion is almost never advisable. The maternal and fetal risks are low if adequate nutrition is maintained.

Terminate pregnancy only in case of hepatic coma. Deterioration may justify cesarean section if the infant is viable.

Administer gamma globulin, 0.02-0.06 ml/lb body weight I.M., to all contacts to prevent or reduce the severity of viral hepatitis. Unnecessary transfusions increase the risk of viral hepatitis. Do not allow a pregnant patient to lose too much weight during periods when hepatitis is prevalent in the community (usually in the winter). Malnutrition may make the patient more susceptible to viral hepatitis.

Assuming good obstetric care and nutrition, the maternal mortality is approximately that of nonpregnant women with viral hepatitis.

It is wise to allow 1-2 years to elapse between hepatitis and subsequent pregnancy. During this interval there must be no clinical abnormality related to liver dysfunction and no alterations in the BSP excretion, total blood proteins, serum albumin and globulin, A/G ratio, cephalin flocculation, thymol turbidity, alkaline phosphatase, and serum transaminase. All tests should be done in the same laboratory and repeated at 3 months, 6 months, and 9 months after delivery and early during the next pregnancy.

Liver Function Test Values in Pregnancy.

Liver function test values in pregnancy are the same as in the nonpregnant state with the following exceptions:
  A. Serum Albumin: Decreased during pregnancy.
  B. Serum Globulins: Alpha and beta, increased; gamma, no change.
  C. Cephalin Flocculation: Elevated in 25% of pregnancies.
  D. Serum Alkaline Phosphatase: Increases gradually during pregnancy; at term, average values are 6.3 units Bodansky and 19 units King-Armstrong.

ABDOMINAL HERNIAS
(Intestinal)

As pregnancy advances, the enlarging uterus tends to fill the abdomen and displace the intestines, so that nonadherent bowel may be drawn out of an inguinal aperture. The uterus also shields incisional and other "weak points" from herniation. Hence, many abdominal hernias reduce spontaneously during pregnancy. A few irreducible (adherent) ones become incarcerated. Pregnancy permanently enlarges umbilical and incisional hernial rings. Femoral and pelvic hernias are uncommon, but are important because they are often overlooked in the obstetric patient.

The patient must not be permitted to strain in the second stage of delivery; low forceps are employed after full dilatation of the cervix.

Emergency operation for the relief and correction of an incarcerated hernia may be required during pregnancy. Elective surgery for the repair of an abdominal hernia should be delayed until after delivery because the need for herniorrhaphy is not an indication for cesarean section.

CARCINOMA OF THE BREAST

Cancer of the breast is diagnosed in about one in 3500 pregnancies, and 2.5% of breast cancers occur in pregnant women. Pregnancy accelerates the spread of cancer of the breast. About three-fourths of breast cancers are adenocarcinomas. Inflammatory carcinoma is an extremely vicious type of breast cancer which occurs most commonly during lactation in young, obese women with pendulous breasts.

If breast biopsy confirms the diagnosis of cancer, radical mastectomy should be done (except for inflammatory carcinoma) regardless of the stage of the pregnancy. If spread to

the regional glands has occurred, x-ray therapy should be
given also. Therapeutic abortion is usually of no value.
Cesarean section should be performed only upon obstetric
indications. After delivery, oophorectomy, androgen therapy,
adrenalectomy, and hypophysectomy may be considered for
palliation of advanced breast cancer.

The five-year survival rate in patients with stage I cancer
of the breast diagnosed during pregnancy and treated by radical
surgery is 60-70%; with stage II breast cancer, the survival
rate drops to less than 10% even with radical surgery and x-ray
therapy.

RHEUMATIC DISORDERS

RELAXATION OF THE PELVIC JOINTS
(Pregnancy Pelvic Arthropathy)

Slight relaxation of the pelvic joints, the result of increased circulating steroid sex hormones and relaxin, is
normal during pregnancy. The degree of relaxation is variable, but considerable separation of the pubis and instability
of the sacro-iliac joint, causing pain and difficulty in walking,
occur occasionally. Obesity and multiple pregnancy contribute to the disability of pregnancy pelvic arthropathy. About
one patient in 150 suffers from pelvic joint pain; about one in
1500 is seriously incapacitated.

Joint relaxation is progressive in most obstetric patients
during the second and early part of the third trimester. Undue mobility persists until after delivery. Return to normal
joint stability following parturition may require several
months.

An exaggerated elasticity of connective and collagen tissue in response to the hormones of pregnancy is presumed to
occur in pelvic arthropathy. However, the extent of disability
is not always directly related to the degree of play in the
joints concerned.

Pain in the sacro-iliac and pubic joints on standing, walking, and turning may be extreme. With the index finger in the
vagina and the thumb above the symphysis, the examiner can
feel abnormal movement of the pubic bone when traction is
placed on one of the patient's legs while the other thigh is held
firmly. X-ray evidence of separation of the pubic bone of
more than 2 cm is abnormal. X-rays of the patient's pelvis,
one taken while she is standing on the right leg and another
while she is supported by the left, will usually reveal the
magnitude of pelvic joint relaxation.

Prolonged sacro-iliac backache may be a sequel to sacro-
iliac arthropathy of pregnancy.

The treatment consists of limitation of activities, analgesics, and a sturdy, fitted girdle which gives support by snug encirclement of the sacrum, symphysis, and greater trochanters.

To prevent prolonged disability, avoid exaggerated positions, marked traction, and sudden movement of the patient while she is under general anesthesia during delivery.

RHEUMATOID ARTHRITIS

Rheumatoid arthritis occurs rarely during pregnancy, but it may be extremely serious, especially during the puerperium.

Pregnancy suppresses rheumatoid arthritis. In general, patients with this disease are considerably improved during the last trimester, presumably because of an elevated titer of corticosteroids. Following delivery, however, and for as long as 2-4 months thereafter, there is a likelihood of serious relapse and rapid progression of the disease. Lactation appears to prolong the remission. The fetus is never adversely affected.

Treatment is directed toward reduction of inflammation and pain, preservation of joint function, and prevention of deformity. Adequate diet, rest, analgesic drugs, and physical therapy are the mainstays of treatment. Pregnancy is not a contraindication to corticosteroids and other drugs used in the treatment of rheumatoid arthritis, although they should be employed with due caution during the first trimester.

The prognosis is unpredictable but generally discouraging.

SYSTEMIC LUPUS ERYTHEMATOSUS (LE)

Systemic lupus erythematosus affects principally females and develops most frequently during the childbearing years. It is a rare but often extremely serious complication of pregnancy. About 500 cases of LE during pregnancy have been reported in the medical literature in the past 10 years.

Pregnancy does not consistently influence the course of this disorder. In over half of patients with LE, the disease remains unchanged, and in a few cases it improves during pregnancy; but increase in the number and severity of exacerbations may occur during pregnancy and the puerperium. In contrast with nonpregnant patients with acute LE, the probability of an exacerbation is 1-3 times greater in the first half of pregnancy and 1-2 times greater in the second half of pregnancy. The probability of a flare-up during the puerperium is 6-7 times that during the nonpregnant period.

Neither the disease itself nor its treatment with corticosteroids commonly reduces the incidence of conception. Spontaneous abortion, usually before the 14th week, occurs in about 20% of patients with acute LE. The incidence of premature labor and delivery and of toxemia is also increased.

Cardiac insufficiency is often a critical problem, but progressive renal failure is the most frequent contributory cause of death in pregnant women with systemic LE.

Fetal anomalies and growth retardation of the fetus are not increased because of LE or corticosteroid therapy. Fetal adrenal insufficiency due to maternal corticosteroid therapy is rarely a problem.

Corticotropin and the corticosteroids usually relieve the symptoms and reduce the number and intensity of the acute exacerbations. There is no agreement about whether the corticosteroids should be given only to treat acute attacks or whether they should be administered for maintenance therapy also.

Prednisone, 30-50 mg (or equivalent) daily orally in 4 divided doses, may be required for the treatment of an acute attack. After improvement has occurred, gradual reduction to withdrawal or to a maintenance dose of about 10 mg/day may be employed for a prolonged period during pregnancy and the puerperium.

Admit the patient to a hospital promptly for treatment if acute LE is likely. Patients must avoid overactivity and exposure to sunlight and other sources of ultraviolet light. Pigmented, emollient cosmetic lotions which are opaque to ultraviolet light may be applied over the face lesions. Analgesics and physical therapy may be given for musculoskeletal discomfort.

Pregnancy rarely exacerbates LE so severely that therapeutic abortion is justified. Employ cesarean section for clear-cut obstetric indications only.

The maternal mortality is approximately 20% and the perinatal mortality is about 30% in acute disseminated LE. The mortality rates in chronic systemic LE depend upon the duration and severity of the disease.

Adrenocorticosteroid therapy before or during pregnancy probably does not influence the number of patients going to term nor the fetal outcome, but it does limit the number of exacerbations and their severity.

GOUT

Only 5% of patients with gout are women, and many of these are postmenopausal. Moreover, gout is exceedingly rare during pregnancy. Nevertheless, gouty arthritis is mentioned because of the importance of a positive family history of the abnormality, the hereditary nature of the disease, and the marked remission of symptoms and signs during pregnancy. One must recognize the teratogenic properties of colchicine and phenylbutazone (Butazolidin®)—the most

RENAL DISEASES

URINARY TRACT INFECTION

The urinary tract is especially vulnerable to infections during pregnancy because the altered secretions of steroid sex hormones and the pressure exerted by the gravid uterus upon the ureters and bladder cause hypotonia and congestion and predispose to ureterovesical reflux and urinary stasis. Cervicitis and vaginitis also predispose to urinary infection. The trauma of labor and delivery and urinary retention after delivery may initiate or aggravate infection in the urinary system. Escherichia coli is the offending organism in over one-third of cases.

Almost 10% of pregnant women suffer from urinary tract infection. Serious antepartal infection occurs in 5-8% of pregnant women. An additional 5% develop urinary tract infections after delivery. Chronic pyelonephritis, a major cause of death in older women, often follows recurrent acute urinary tract infections during successive pregnancies. Urinary tract infection increases the likelihood of premature delivery and the incidence of perinatal mortality.

The diagnosis should be based upon stained smear and culture of a catheterized or clean-catch specimen of urine. An acid-fast stain of the urinary sediment should be performed if tuberculosis is suspected. Sensitivity tests to determine response to the various anti-infective agents are desirable. Bacillary infection should be treated initially with sulfisoxazole (Gantrisin®), 2 gm orally stat. and then 1 gm 4 times daily; or nitrofurantoin (Furadantin®), 100 mg orally 4 times daily. If cocci are present, give procaine penicillin G, 1 million units I.M. stat. and then 600,000 units I.M. twice daily. Mixed infections should be treated with streptomycin, 1 gm I.M., and procaine penicillin G, 600,000 units I.M. stat., and then 0.5 gm of streptomycin and 600,000 units of penicillin twice daily. Change to other drugs as dictated by the results of laboratory studies. Do not give tetracyclines to pregnant women. Children are apt to develop yellow deciduous teeth of poor quality.

For urgency and frequency give one Levamine® (butabarbital and hyoscyamine) capsule every 2 hours as necessary.

Force fluids (if indicated) and alkalinize the urine. Give analgesics, laxatives, and antipyretic drugs as indicated.

Three successive, negative urine cultures taken at weekly intervals are necessary before the patient can be considered to be "cured."

If urine cultures are not available, a stained smear of the centrifuged sediment of a catheterized or "clean catch" specimen may be examined for bacteria each week for 3 weeks. If no bacteria or pus cells are seen and the patient is asymptomatic, she is presumed to be cured.

If obstruction is present it may be necessary to employ urethral or ureteral catheterization. Ureteral obstruction usually resolves after delivery, but if it is permanent surgical repair may be required. If response to chemotherapy and ureteral catheterization is inadequate, nephrostomy is indicated, particularly during the second trimester and prior to fetal viability. Induce labor at term by amniotomy. Consider therapeutic abortion if there is no response to medical and surgical therapy when the mother's life is in jeopardy.

Routine urinalysis during pregnancy must include microscopic examination and stain for bacteria (and cultures) to discover asymptomatic bacteriuria.

Avoid catheterization whenever possible; when catheterization is necessary, sterile technic is essential. Eradicate genital and urinary tract infections promptly. Study and treat patients before or early in pregnancy when there is evidence or a history of a previous urinary tract infection, especially during gestation. Even if a "cure" is achieved, suppressive long-term antibiotic therapy continued throughout pregnancy and the puerperium is mandatory.

If initial treatment proves ineffective the patient should be thoroughly studied by a urologist.

GLOMERULONEPHRITIS

An initial attack of acute glomerulonephritis is rare during pregnancy; most obstetric problems relating to glomerulonephritis involve transitional chronic forms of the disease. There is no evidence that pregnancy aggravates glomerulonephritis.

Infertility, abortion, premature delivery, fetal death in utero, premature separation of the normally implanted placenta, and placental dysmaturity occur with greater frequency in women with glomerulonephritis than in normal women. Nephritis causes hypertension, predisposes to eclamptogenic toxemia, and is associated with a high incidence of perinatal mortality and morbidity.

The medical treatment of glomerulonephritis in pregnancy is the same as that of the nonpregnant patient. Adrenocortical steroids may be harmful, and antibiotics are ineffective. Therapeutic abortion may be justified for acute, severe exacerbation of glomerulonephritis with renal insufficiency.

Glomerulonephritis may be an indication for cesarean section when placental dysmaturity or eclamptogenic toxemia occurs.

URETERAL STONE

Ureteral stone is more common during pregnancy than otherwise because of the hypercalciuria which occurs during pregnancy and the calcium and vitamin D which are prescribed; because of the dilatation of the renal pelvis and ureter which occurs in response to high titers of steroid sex hormones; and because of the minor (physiologic) obstructive uropathy characteristic of pregnancy. Small stones, previously retained, are thus permitted to enter the proximal ureter. Most ureteral stones are passed in the urine, albeit painfully; others become impacted. Sudden, agonizing pain in the costovertebral angle and flank with radiation to the lower quadrant and vulva, urinary urgency, and hematuria without (initially) pyuria or fever are characteristic of ureteral stone. Intravenous urography may demonstrate partial obstruction and the stone.

Symptomatic therapy with analgesics and antispasmodics is always indicated, and may be best given parenterally. Retrograde catheter manipulation may dislodge the stone and permit it to pass, or the stone may be extracted transurethrally. If such efforts are unsuccessful and if severe pain persists and progressive hydronephrosis develops, remove the stone by extraperitoneal ureterolithotomy irrespective of the patient's obstetric status.

NEUROLOGIC DISEASES

The effect of neurologic diseases on pregnancy is rarely critical. Certain neurologic diseases may be aggravated by pregnancy (e.g., chorea gravidarum [Sydenham's chorea], severe nonspecific polyneuritis, and herniation of an intervertebral disk).

HEADACHES

The patient with a constant, throbbing, "splitting" headache, usually of the bilateral type, either frontal, sincipital, or occipital, should be examined for generalized edema, hypertension, and proteinuria, which may indicate eclamptogenic toxemia. Tension headaches, functional in origin, are likely to occur for the first time or in severe exacerbation during pregnancy. Tension headaches are much more common than vascular (migraine) type headaches.

VERTIGO & SYNCOPE

Vertigo and syncope occur occasionally during pregnancy. Such patients note dizziness or "blackout" on sudden change of position or station (standing up quickly, rapid turns, acceleration or deceleration in a car or elevator). Weakness due to low blood glucose, postural hypotension, or cerebrovascular insufficiency may be interpreted as "unsteadiness." Dizziness and faintness during pregnancy are usually brief sensations; the patient rarely falls, but frequently slides to the floor or a chair; she almost never injures herself nor soils her clothing.

EPILEPSY

Idiopathic or symptomatic (e.g., brain tumor, focal scar) epilepsy may be activated or intensified during pregnancy. The attacks almost always occur during the last trimester in women who are hypertensive, proteinuric, and edematous. Abnormal fluid retention may increase the frequency of seizures and make them more difficult to control just prior to delivery and immediately afterward. It is important to keep epileptic patients on adequate anticonvulsant therapy during pregnancy and after labor.

Prevent aspiration of gastric contents by placing the patient on her side (never on her back). Extend the head and hold the tongue out to ensure a clear air passage. Restrain the patient gently to prevent injury. Slip a soft mouth gag between her jaws so that she will not bite her tongue. If convulsions are prolonged or severe, give secobarbital sodium (Seconal®), 0.1-0.2 gm slowly I.V. or I.M., or diphenylhydantoin sodium (Dilantin®), 150-250 mg I.V. at a rate not exceeding 50 mg/minute. (**Caution:** Because of their depressive central nervous system effects, do not administer narcotics or general anesthetics unless absolutely necessary to control repeated seizures.) When seizures occur for the first time in a woman during pregnancy, careful neurologic examination, including special studies, is indicated.

POLYNEURITIS OF PREGNANCY

Polyneuritis of pregnancy is largely, if not completely, due to vitamin B complex deficiency; more specifically, to a lack of thiamine (vitamin B_1). Polyneuritis is rare where the socioeconomic level of the population is high. In the USA, the disorder is generally the result of pernicious vomiting or chronic alcoholism in early pregnancy. After 2-3 months of hyperemesis gravidarum or inadequate thiamine intake, signs and symptoms of polyneuritis develop, first in the lower and then in the upper extremities. Cardiorespiratory and central nervous system problems follow.

Treatment consists of thiamine hydrochloride, 20-50 mg orally, I.M., or I.V. daily in divided doses for 2 weeks, and then 10 mg orally daily. A high caloric, well balanced diet should be given when tolerated.

With early and adequate treatment, the prognosis is favorable.

CEREBROVASCULAR ACCIDENTS

The higher incidence of vascular accidents during pregnancy than in the nonpregnant state may be partially explained by collagen changes in the blood vessels during pregnancy. Subarachnoid hemorrhage from all causes is more common during pregnancy. Recurrent subarachnoid hemorrhage may be an indication for cesarean section. Hypertension of eclamptogenic toxemia, the intravenous administration of ergot (pressor) preparations, and increased intracranial pressure with straining during the second stage of labor may account for rupture of congenital cerebral aneurysms, arteriovenous malformations, thrombosed cerebral veins, or weakened vessels of any organ.

MULTIPLE SCLEROSIS

Multiple sclerosis may be aggravated by pregnancy when the disorder is in a stage of active progression or when the patient is critically disabled by the disease. The question of aggravation of multiple sclerosis by pregnancy is still in doubt.

CHOREA GRAVIDARUM

Sydenham's chorea which recurs or develops for the first time in young women during pregnancy is believed by many to be a form of encephalitis. Although very rare, it may be a serious complication of pregnancy. It usually appears early after the first missed period and, curiously, it vanishes following termination of pregnancy. Treatment is similar to that of Sydenham's chorea in the nonpregnant patient.

MYASTHENIA GRAVIS

Many obstetric patients with myasthenia gravis require increasingly large doses of neostigmine to remain at normal activity. Edrophonium chloride (Tensilon®), 2-3 mg I.V., may be used as a test dose for patients under treatment to distinguish between myasthenic crisis (improves) and overtreatment (no change). Certain patients, however, are better during pregnancy and require much less medication or go into remission for the duration of pregnancy. Most myasthenic patients complete pregnancy without complications. An occasional infant born of a mother with severe myasthenia gravis may also show myasthenic signs. This weakness may be sufficient to require neostigmine treatment for 1-2 months. Complete recovery of the infant is the rule.

HERNIATED INTERVERTEBRAL DISK

Herniation of the nucleus pulposus of an intervertebral disk in the lumbar region is prone to occur during pregnancy. The estrogens, progestogens, and relaxin cause weakening of the fibrous rings of the intervertebral disks and swelling of the nuclei pulposi. Hypervascularization of the nonosseous tissue of the back and pelvis contributes to the relaxation of back support. Moreover, disturbed equilibrium of the lumbosacral joint develops during pregnancy because of an increase in the volume and weight of the abdominal contents.

There are no obstetric complications due to disk hernia, but disability and even paralysis may occur in extreme, neglected cases.

Prescribe bed rest and traction. Sedatives and analgesics are beneficial. Correct obesity and avoid back strain or injury during pregnancy and the puerperium. Temporary or permanent relief usually follows medical management. Severe, recurrent, or progressive pain and incapacity may require surgery, but this is rarely necessary during pregnancy.

GENERAL COMMENTS REGARDING NEUROLOGIC DISEASE DURING PREGNANCY

Pregnancy is not an absolute contraindication to urgent neurosurgery for the evacuation of a subdural hematoma, removal of an intracranial tumor, or treatment of an intracranial aneurysm.

Only rarely are neurologic disorders so disturbing as to require interruption of pregnancy.

Consider sterilization only when the woman's future life and health will be jeopardized by subsequent pregnancy or when there is a significant likelihood of transmission of serious hereditary disorders.

Marriage or childbearing by individuals with serious hereditary neurologic diseases should be discouraged.

ENDOCRINE & METABOLIC DISEASES

THYROTOXICOSIS

Toxic goiter is extremely serious for the pregnant patient and, indirectly, for her offspring. Overtreatment of thyrotoxicosis during pregnancy may result in maternal and fetal hypothyroidism and may cause maldevelopment and goiter in the child.

Toxic goiter does not increase the hazard of spontaneous abortion or fetal anomalies, but does increase the incidence of premature delivery, postpartal hemorrhage, cardiovascular complications secondary to myocardial strain, psychosis, liver damage, and thyroid "storm." Toxemia of pregnancy may be slightly more frequent in women with toxic goiter.

Most of the complications and sequelae relate to overtreatment, particularly the development of hypothyroidism during pregnancy. Thyroid lack increases the frequency of abortion, fetal abnormalities, and premature labor and delivery. A critical reduction in the level of circulating thyroid hormone following surgery or the administration of antithyroid drugs, particularly during the first and early second trimester, may result in fetal maldevelopment, cretinism, or goiter.

Treatment.
A. Emergency Measures: All pregnant patients with moderate or marked thyrotoxicosis should be hospitalized at bed rest and given sedatives.
B. Specific Measures: Individualize therapy in accordance with the degree of toxicity and duration of the pregnancy. Subtotal thyroidectomy must not be attempted until the patient has become euthyroid following medical treatment with rest, sedation, and iodine. Premature termination of pregnancy is less likely to occur if surgery can be deferred until after the first trimester.

Therapeutic abortion is almost never required, but might be indicated (1) for the patient who does not respond to medical treatment and who has already had surgery with a poor result (in which case I^{131} might be considered after therapeutic abortion) or (2) for the pregnant woman suffering from functional thyroid carcinoma for whom I^{131} therapy is prescribed after therapeutic abortion.

Toxic goiter is not an indication for induction of labor or cesarean section. These procedures are ordered only on obstetric indications.
C. Treatment of Complications: The physician should anticipate a significant reduction in the patient's thyroid function and must treat hypothyroidism promptly to pro-

tect the fetus, especially during the first and second trimesters. Thyroid, levothyroxine sodium (Synthroid®), or triiodothyronine (T_3) should be administered whenever hypothyroidism exists: immediately before and for several weeks after thyroidectomy, or when the patient receives excessive doses of a thiourea compound.

Normal childhood development, particularly mental, cannot be expected if a congenital athyreotic or markedly hypothyroid infant does not receive thyroid or one of its analogues promptly followed by continuation of the maintenance dose to ensure euthyroidism.

Prognosis.

The prognosis is excellent for mother and fetus if normal thyroid function can be achieved promptly and then maintained.

HYPOTHYROIDISM

Slight thyroid deficiency is common among obstetric patients, and replacement therapy is indicated to maintain optimal physical status of the mother and to ensure uneventful continuance of pregnancy. More severe deficiency causes abortion, premature labor, and congenital fetal anomalies. Women with moderate to severe degrees of hypothyroidism are relatively infertile, and sterility is the rule in myxedema.

Maternal hypothyroidism may improve slightly during pregnancy in response to fetal thyroid function.

Treatment.
A. The Mother: Initial treatment of pregnant women with early hypothyroidism may be with relatively large doses of thyroid supplement. Levothyroxine sodium (Synthroid®), 0.05-0.3 mg/day, probably is better than desiccated thyroid because its action is more rapid and more predictable than that of crude thyroid. Begin with 0.05-0.1 mg/day and increase the dose weekly to the limit of tolerance, adjusting the dosage to maintain optimal effect. Desiccated thyroid may be given in doses of 30 mg (1/2 gr)/day initially, increasing the dosage weekly to 60-200 mg (1-3 gr) daily for maintenance. The optimal dosage may be estimated on the basis of the PBI or BEI, but clinical judgment is often the best guide. Thyroid overdosage causes nervousness, tremors, tachycardia, insomnia, sweating, vomiting, diarrhea, and weight loss.

The nonspecific use of thyroid is to be condemned.

B. The Infant: Give levothyroxine sodium (Synthroid®), 0.025-0.05 mg (or equivalent of desiccated thyroid) orally daily for 1-2 weeks, and then increase the dose gradually to 0.1 mg/day or more depending upon response. Reduce dosage if irritability, tachycardia, fever, or diarrhea occurs.

Prognosis.

With prompt, adequate, and continued thyroid replacement, the prognosis is excellent for the mother and infant. If the hypothyroid infant does not receive prompt replacement therapy, irreversible mental and physical retardation is to be expected.

DIABETES MELLITUS

Diabetes mellitus occurs as a complication of one in every 325-350 pregnancies and is an important cause of maternal and fetal morbidity. Although maternal death is rare with modern treatment, the fetal mortality is 10-30%.

Pregnancy places an additional strain on carbohydrate metabolism even in a healthy woman, and the insulin requirements may be expected to increase; it may unmask the prediabetic state or may convert asymptomatic subclinical diabetes into frank clinical (gestational) diabetes.

Classification of Pregnant Diabetics. (After White & others.)
 Group A: Diabetic status based only on an abnormal glucose tolerance curve.
 Group B: Onset of diabetes after age 20; duration of diabetes 10-19 years; no vascular disease.
 Group C: Onset of diabetes between age 10-19; duration of diabetes 10-19 years; no vascular disease.
 Group D: Onset of diabetes under age 10; duration of diabetes 20 or more years; vascular disease, including calcification of leg vessels; diabetic retinopathy.
 Group E: Same as group D, plus calcification of pelvic vessels.
 Group F: Same as group E, plus nephropathy (often Kimmelstiel-Wilson intercapillary nephrosclerosis).

Effect of Diabetes Mellitus on Pregnancy & Delivery.

Infertility and abortion are increased in poorly controlled diabetes only. Fetal and maternal fluid and electrolyte balance are easily disrupted. Edema is to be expected in both the mother and the infant. The incidence of polyhydramnios is 10 times the general incidence. Eclamptogenic toxemia is much more frequent (30-50%), especially with prepregnancy vascular sclerosis and hypertension. Congenital anomalies of all types are 5-6 times more frequent. The risk of fetal death in utero is heightened, particularly after the 36th week, because of maternal acidosis and "placental insufficiency." Premature labor and delivery are common. The likelihood of an excessively large fetus (> 4000 gm) is greater. Dystocia and operative delivery are more frequent, and fetal mortality and morbidity are consequently increased.

The incidence of early neonatal death because of respiratory distress syndrome or hypoglycemia (due to hyperplasia of fetal islets of Langerhans) is increased.

Clinical Findings.

The diagnosis of diabetes mellitus is based upon the symptoms and signs but is largely dependent upon laboratory tests. The principal laboratory signs of this disease during pregnancy are persistent glycosuria, hyperglycemia, and a reduced tolerance for glucose.

Glycosuria noted in the fasting specimen is a presumptive sign of diabetes. This test is less reliable during pregnancy because many patients have a lowered renal threshold for glucose after the first trimester. Moreover, other substances—notably galactose—which may give false positive tests for glucose, may be excreted in the urine during the last 4-6 weeks and particularly during the postpartal period. For those reasons, glycosuria is not always a cause of great concern unless there is significant hyperglycemia, especially if ketosis is also present.

A normal fasting blood glucose level does not rule out diabetes. Moreover, slightly elevated fasting blood glucose levels may be noted, or the postprandial blood glucose may be elevated in other diseases besides diabetes (e.g., liver disease). For these reasons, glucose tolerance tests usually are required.

In pregnancy, the fasting blood glucose is often slightly decreased, yet the oral glucose tolerance curve may be of the diabetic type. These changes are most marked after the 6th month. However, blood glucose levels following intravenous injection of glucose do not rise as high during as after pregnancy.

Immediately after delivery, most normal patients' glucose tolerance test curves begin to approach nonpregnant levels. Many return to normal in 48-72 hours, and all readjust during the early puerperium.

Prior to glucose tolerance testing, place the patient on a high carbohydrate intake for at least 48-72 hours because carbohydrate restriction decreases tolerance.

Caution: It is unnecessary and possibly harmful to perform a glucose tolerance test on a patient whose initial fasting blood glucose level is 200 mg/100 ml or more.

Obtain x-ray pelvimetry (and cephalometry) in the last trimester on every diabetic patient who is a candidate for vaginal delivery to rule out fetal disproportion.

An AP film of the uterus should be taken at 36-37 weeks to disclose fetal abnormalities and the presence or absence of

318 Diabetes Mellitus

distal femoral epiphyses (80% will be present by 37 weeks). Repeat again in 1-2 weeks. Distal femoral ossification centers indicate adequate maturity and probable survival if delivery occurs and there are no complications.

Treatment.
   A. Emergency Measures:
      1. Diabetic acidosis and coma - Admit the patient to a hospital and obtain medical consultation. Determine blood glucose, CO_2 combining power, and, if possible, serum sodium and serum potassium levels. Treat as any patient with diabetic acidosis or coma.
      2. Insulin shock - If the patient is comatose and it is not possible to rapidly differentiate between diabetic coma and insulin shock, treat first for insulin shock by giving 20-40 ml of 50% glucose in water slowly I.V. Determine the cause and make the necessary adjustments of insulin or food.
   B. General Measures:
      1. Antenatal care - Evaluate the patient as a candidate for pregnancy before conception, if possible.
         a. Take blood for fasting and two-hour glucose tolerance test on all obstetric patients with glycosuria, and obtain a record of any previous fetal deaths in utero, previous large babies at birth, or fetal disproportion. If the patient is shown to have diabetes or is a diabetes suspect or asymptomatic subclinical diabetic, obtain consultation with an internist. The patient, internist, and obstetrician should work in close cooperation, but the obstetrician must assume primary responsibility. Admit the patient to the hospital if necessary.
         b. Adjust diet to the ideal nutritional state depending upon the patient's height, weight, and build. Restrict salt intake to 1 gm/day in the absence of fluid retention; reduce to 400 mg/day if she is edematous. Prescribe vitamin and mineral supplements as indicated.
         c. Overt diabetics usually require insulin, and the insulin requirement is usually greater during pregnancy. Utilize blood glucose determinations (never urine glucose) for regulation of diet and insulin. Check urine frequently for ketosis. It is rarely possible or advisable to control diabetes in a pregnant woman with oral hypoglycemic agents.
         d. The patient must be seen by both the obstetrician and the internist at least every 2 weeks to maintain control of diabetes and weight gain and to prevent toxemia and infection. Avoid hyperglycemia and glycosuria. The fasting blood glucose should remain

at 110-150 mg/100 ml and the 24-hour urine glucose should be about 10-15 gm. Prevent acidosis and ketosis or sustained hypoglycemia. Check carefully for the possibility of urinary tract infection.
  e. Admit the patient to the hospital in midpregnancy for re-evaluation unless the diabetes is mild and the course completely uncomplicated. About 75% of patients taking insulin will require more insulin in the second or third trimester.
 2. Delivery (timing and procedure) - Readmit the patient to the hospital at the 36th-37th week (or earlier if polyhydramnios, toxemia, or other potentially serious complications indicate the need for study and treatment).
  a. If the patient is difficult to control, maintain on crystalline zinc insulin alone or reduce the dosage of long-acting insulin by half and use crystalline zinc insulin to complete the daily requirement. This may help to stabilize the diabetes during labor, cesarean section, or premature delivery.
  b. Estrogen therapy has been recommended in case of threatened abortion if the FSH is high. The value of this is still uncertain.
  c. Decide when and how to deliver the infant. Fetal death in utero occurs frequently after the 37th week, so it is well to plan to deliver the patient at about this time. Current practice is to attempt to deliver vaginally if induction is likely to result in good labor and delivery within approximately 12 hours. If this is not possible, cesarean section is indicated.
   (1) Perform a sterile vaginal examination. If the cervix is 50% effaced and 1-2 cm dilated and the vertex is at the spines and the fetus is estimated to weigh 3400 gm or less (disproportion unlikely), rupture the membranes. If labor does not ensue in 4 hours, begin an intravenous oxytocin drip (1 ml in 1 liter of saline). If delivery is not likely to occur within about 12 hours, perform cesarean section, preferably under regional anesthesia.
   (2) Perform cesarean section if the cervix is unfavorable for delivery from below, if the vertex is floating, if a breech is presenting, if the fetus is estimated to weigh more than 3400 gm, if complications (e.g., toxemia) ensue, or if labor is likely to continue longer than 12 hours.
C. Obstetric Measures: Therapeutic abortion may be justified in certain instances of diabetic retinitis or retinitis proliferans, or in Kimmelstiel-Wilson disease.

320 Diabetes Mellitus

Neonatal Care.

A pediatrician should be present at delivery. Engage special nurses for 24-hour care of diabetic babies in the premature nursery, if possible.

A. At Delivery:
1. Clamp the cord immediately after delivery to avoid hypervolemia.
2. Obtain blood for glucose determination at birth and every 3 hours for 12 hours. If the level is less than 30 mg/100 ml, give glucose, 65 mg/kg, in 0.25 N saline I.V. slowly. After resuscitation, instill 10 ml of 20% glucose into the stomach and remove the tube.

B. In the Nursery:
1. Give 4 ml of 20% glucose in water orally through a rubber-tipped medicine dropper every hour for at least 12 hours; then start a feeding of 5% glucose in water followed in 12 hours by milk formula.
2. Administer phytonadione (vitamin K_1), 1 mg I.M.
3. Observe for tremor and convulsive movements. These may be due to hypocalcemia, in which case give calcium gluconate, 5 ml of 10% solution I.V., after a blood specimen is drawn for calcium and glucose determinations.
4. Keep warm in a heated Isolette® or crib.
5. Administer oxygen, 30-40% concentration, 55% humidity, at a temperature of 80-85° F.
6. Observe respirations; turn the child frequently; stimulate to breathe when necessary.
7. If signs of the respiratory distress syndrome develop, give glucose solution intravenously (as above) whether the blood glucose level is low or not. Give a broad-spectrum antibiotic (but avoid the tetracyclines because of the dental dysplasia which results from their use). Discontinue oral feedings temporarily.

Postpartal Management.

Carefully evaluate the mother's diabetic status during the puerperium since persistent changes may occur.

Prognosis.

Joint management by an internist, obstetrician, and pediatrician will result in lower maternal and fetal mortality and morbidity rates. Maternal mortality with modern therapy should be less than 0.2%. Deaths are due to diabetic coma, toxemia, infection, nephropathy, cardiac complications, dystocia, and embolism. Neglect and improper treatment are the main contributory causes of virtually all maternal deaths. An irreversible increase of diabetic retinopathy and nephropathy during pregnancy occurs in most patients.

Factors which bear upon fetal survival are the severity of diabetes, control of diabetes during pregnancy, placental bleeding, toxemia of pregnancy, polyhydramnios, and interruption of pregnancy before the 34th week or after the 39th week of gestation. Perinatal mortality even with modern therapy is 10-30%. Fetal anomalies occur in 5-6%, and are very frequent with polyhydramnios. Abnormalities cannot be correlated with the severity of the mother's diabetes, however.

In general, vaginal delivery is safer than cesarean section for the fetus.

OSTEOMALACIA

Osteomalacia is almost unknown in North America, but it may occur in Asia, North Africa, and Central Europe. In regions where osteomalacia is prevalent, one gravid woman in every 100 may have the disorder. The metabolic drain of pregnancy and lactation on women whose diets are severely deficient in calcium (particularly in the absence of sunshine) leads to demineralization of bone. The weight of the trunk and upper portions of the body applied to a yielding pelvis supported by relatively stronger femurs causes gross (often extreme) pelvic deformity. A normal gynecoid pelvic inlet may be changed into a compressed triradiate figure. The central cavity of the pelvis is greatly reduced in capacity, and the pubic arch becomes severely narrowed. The woman often "shrinks" 1-2 inches in height. Pseudofractures occur, and bowing of the bones is common. The capacity of the thoracic cavity is soon reduced. Exertional dyspnea and tachycardia develop. Despite these problems, osteomalacia patients remain fertile. Pains in the back, legs, and pelvis begin early and increase during pregnancy, often being confused with arthritis. Walking, bending, and lifting increase the discomfort. In severe cases the patient may be bedfast; walking is difficult for some, and the patient waddles or gets about haltingly with a cane or crutches.

Serum calcium is low or normal, serum phosphorus is low, and alkaline phosphatase is high (except in the early stages). X-rays of the pelvis and long bones reveal demineralization, bowing, and pseudofractures (Milkman's syndrome).

Dystocia is inevitable, even with slight to moderate pelvic contracture. Other complications of osteomalacia include crippling deformity and increased fetal and maternal morbidity and mortality.

Treatment consists of giving a diet rich in calcium, vitamins (especially A and D), and proteins as soon as possible to avoid deformities and dystocia. Vitamin D must be given in large doses, usually 25-100 thousand units/day. Give calcium and phosphorus supplements. If pancreatic insufficiency is present, replacement therapy is of the utmost importance. Correct acidosis if there is evidence of a renal tubular disorder. Prescribe analgesics and rest. Slow resumption of activity and a back support may be necessary to prevent gross deformity.

Cesarean section and sterilization may be considered for the individual patient.

Prophylaxis includes an adequate diet and, in severe cases, avoidance of pregnancy and lactation.

PARATHYROID DYSFUNCTION & TETANY

Pregnancy normally causes a slight (secondary) hyperparathyroidism. Severe, chronic hyperparathyroidism causing osteitis fibrosa cystica is rare during pregnancy except in patients with long-standing renal disease. The most serious problems relating to parathyroid dysfunction during pregnancy are hypoparathyroid tetany and muscle cramps. Tetany is usually associated with a deficiency of calcium or excess of phosphate (e.g., due to intake of calcium phosphate prenatal capsules), or lack of vitamin D and parathormone. In established hypoparathyroidism, hypocalcemia is observed during pregnancy as a dilutional phenomenon. The requirements for vitamin D and calcium may be greater than in nonpregnant women.

Tetany may follow infection or the hypocalcemia which sometimes occurs during lactation, or may be seen during the latter months of pregnancy if calcium supplements are inadequate. Hyperventilation during labor may precipitate tetany.

Tetany of the newborn is unusual in breast-fed infants, but it may occur transiently if phosphate intake of the infant is excessive (e.g., if too much cow's milk is given or as a result of relative hypoparathyroidism in the neonatal period).

INFECTIOUS DISEASES

All systemic infectious diseases of the mother, if severe enough, can complicate pregnancy by causing death of the embryo or fetus or premature labor and delivery. High fever, septicemia, and toxicosis are usually responsible. With the exceptions discussed in detail below, however, most maternal diseases such as pneumonia, scarlet fever, and typhoid fever are not responsible for fetal anomalies.

Table 12-2. Exanthematous diseases in pregnancy.

Disease	Effect of Disease on Pregnancy	Effect of Disease on Offspring
Variola (smallpox)	Abortion, premature delivery frequent; postpartal hemorrhage, maternal mortality increased.	May be born with pocks
Rubeola (measles)	Abortion; premature labor if disease is severe.	May be born with rash
Varicella (chickenpox)	Severe, disseminated epidemic type may be fatal to mother due to necrotizing angiitis.	Virulent infection may cause fetal death in utero. Neonate may be born with pocks.
Rubella (German measles)	Occasional early abortion	Congenital anomalies if disease occurs during first trimester.

EXANTHEMATOUS DISEASES

Most of the exanthematous diseases are caused by viruses which invariably gain access to the fetus via the placenta. The effect of these infective organisms on pregnancy and the fetus depends upon the virulence of the virus, the mother's resistance to the disease, and the stage of fetal development. Fetal immunity depends, in large measure, on maternal active immunity (e.g., smallpox) or passive immunity (e.g., measles vaccine administration). High fever or toxicosis may cause uterine contractility and loss of the pregnancy; viral placentitis and septicemia followed by fetal death in utero may lead to abortion or premature delivery.

Rubella (German Measles).

German measles virus is teratogenic. Many infants have been reported to be abnormal and maldeveloped if the mother contracted rubella during the first trimester of pregnancy. Excluding patients affected during epidemics, the risk of congenital anomalies occurring during the first 3 months of pregnancy varies from 50% (first month) down to 10%. After the first trimester, the danger of embryopathy is negligible.

Fetal defects include cataracts, congenital heart disease, dental defects, deafness, and mental retardation. It may take 1-2 years to be certain of the seriousness of infant defects. There is some evidence that an abnormal child may be born of a mother who has previously had the disease but contracts a subclinical form of the disease when re-exposed during pregnancy months or years after the first infection.

Although it is of doubtful value to either the mother or fetus, the intramuscular injection of 20 ml of pooled gamma globulin or 5 ml of convalescent gamma globulin may be tried.

In the event that a woman develops German measles in the first trimester of pregnancy, the question of whether or not to perform therapeutic abortion is invariably raised. Unfortunately, there is no unanimity of opinion. Despite the fact that there are no fetal indications for therapeutic abortion in the USA, many insist that even a 10-15% risk of a seriously damaged fetus is justification for a therapeutic abortion. On the other hand, one would have to ruthlessly sacrifice approximately 90% of fetuses in order to prevent the survival of 10% abnormal individuals. Moreover, the malformations may be so slight that good health is not precluded.

For prophylaxis, females may be inoculated with the virus or purposely exposed to rubella prior to pregnancy.

CYTOMEGALIC INCLUSION DISEASE

Cytomegalic inclusion disease is a rare but extremely serious viral disorder of the fetus usually acquired during early intrauterine life. A specific viral neutralizing and complement-fixing antibody reaction indicates that most women have sustained an asymptomatic infection by this virus. A carrier state probably exists and explains subsequent cases in the same family.

In the neonate, the disease produces erythroblastosis and thrombocytopenia which lead to scattered hemorrhages. Chorioretinitis, periventricular necrosis with calcification, microcephaly, and sclerosis of the bones are often noted at birth. Early jaundice, beginning on the first or second day, melena, hematemesis, and hematuria develop. The antemortem diagnosis can be made by the identification of cytomegalic inclusion cells in the gastric washings, cerebrospinal fluid, or fresh urine. Culture of the specific virus is proof of the diagnosis. The direct and indirect serum bilirubin are elevated, but the Coombs test is negative. Death usually occurs soon after birth as a result of interstitial pneumonitis, focal hepatitis, or adrenocortical failure. No specific therapy is known. Corticosteroids and supportive therapy together with gamma globulin may be helpful. Therapeutic abortion is not justified because there is no means of making the diagnosis prior to delivery. An occasional baby survives, but marked developmental and psychomotor deficiencies and hepatosplenomegaly are usually present.

POLIOMYELITIS

Poliomyelitis exerts an unfavorable effect on pregnancy and the puerperium. An increased incidence of poliomyelitis is reported in pregnant patients as compared with nonpregnant women of comparable ages. Approximately two-thirds of women who contract poliomyelitis during pregnancy are between the ages of 20-29, and about three-fourths are parous.

Pregnancy aggravates poliomyelitis, and the disease in turn increases the risk of abortion and fetal loss. Rare congenital anomalies are ascribed to poliomyelitis. The fetus may contract poliomyelitis during its passage through the birth canal.

The first stage of labor is normal in most instances. The failure of voluntary efforts to augment uterine contractions results in an increased frequency of obstetric operations in the second stage.

Most cases of nonparalytic and paralytic poliomyelitis occur between the third and the 5th months and between the 8th and 9th months of pregnancy. Bulbar poliomyelitis, most often observed in late pregnancy, carries the most serious prognosis. The danger of maternal and fetal loss is greatest in the third trimester.

The infant may show a growth retardation if the mother contracts poliomyelitis in the early months of pregnancy. The incidence of abortion is higher with poliomyelitis than with a comparable group of noninfected obstetric patients. If the fetus survives, it may display flaccid paralysis.

With paralysis of the intercostal, diaphragmatic, and abdominal muscles, the enlarged uterus reduces maternal ventilation when the patient is in a tank respirator. Therefore, early delivery, often by elective cesarean section at term, enhances mechanical ventilation by the tank and contributes to the survival of mother and infant.

Emergency treatment in acute bulbar poliomyelitis includes early tracheostomy, endotracheal suction, administration of oxygen and helium under positive pressure, and antibiotics.

Prepare tissue cultures from the infant's stools during the first day of life to distinguish between prenatal and postnatal poliomyelitis infections. Give gamma globulin to protect the infant against poliomyelitis.

Utilize Salk or Sabin vaccine immunization against poliomyelitis prior to or during pregnancy.

The maternal mortality rate in pregnancy which is complicated by poliomyelitis is 5-10% higher than in normal women. The morbidity and mortality rates increase the later in pregnancy the disease is contracted.

PULMONARY TUBERCULOSIS

Tuberculosis of the bronchi, lungs, and pleura is not directly affected by pregnancy. A pregnant tuberculous patient is slightly more prone to spontaneous abortion and premature delivery than other women. Tuberculous endometritis and placentitis occur in advanced cases, but congenital tuberculosis is rare. Interruption of pregnancy because of pulmonary tuberculosis is almost never justified since the advent of antituberculosis drugs. Pneumothorax, pneumoperitoneum, and thoracic surgery are not contraindicated. Babies born of tuberculous mothers are no more likely to develop the disease than others provided they are separated from the infected mother and unfavorable environment at birth.

However, it is important to discourage pregnancy in women with active tuberculosis and to maintain close medical supervision of those tuberculous women who do become pregnant. Institute a follow-up study of all women with a history of treated tuberculosis and be alert to the possibility of reactivation of tuberculosis during each pregnancy. Advise deferring pregnancy (and prescribe contraception, if acceptable) until tuberculosis has been inactive for at least 2 years, if minimal; 3 years, if moderately advanced; and 5 years, if far-advanced. Obtain chest x-rays of all obstetric patients as soon as pregnancy is diagnosed. In patients who have had tuberculosis, order chest x-rays during the third month, at term, and 6 months after delivery.

SYPHILIS

About two-thirds of pregnant patients with syphilis are between 20-30 years of age. Routine antepartal STS and early intensive antisyphilitic therapy have drastically reduced the incidence of congenital syphilis, hitherto a major cause of perinatal mortality, but the problem is still not solved.

Pregnancy appears to decrease the severity of syphilis in many pregnant women. The chancre is often unnoticed, insignificant, and asymptomatic; the nonpruritic rash may be transitory. Occasionally, the primary and secondary phases may be florid and complicated by secondary infection. Pregnancy will neither alter relapses after inadequate or ill-chosen therapy nor modify latent or late syphilis.

The effect of syphilis on pregnancy and the fetus depends largely upon whether the maternal infection occurs before pregnancy, at conception, or later. As the years pass from the time when the mother contracted syphilis, the likelihood of a fetus showing serologic or other evidence of syphilis diminishes despite lack of treatment. Untreated syphilis contracted more than a few months to several years prior to pregnancy usually causes midtrimester abortion or fetal death in utero. Abortion early in pregnancy is uncommon. When infection occurs at the time of conception or early in pregnancy and therapy is not given, the fetus, deformed by congenital syphilis, is often delivered prematurely. Syphilis contracted by the mother in the second half of pregnancy may or may not result in a syphilitic infant.

Diagnosis of Maternal Infection.

Single or multiple superficial ulcerative genital or oral lesions with nontender regional adenopathy or an unexplained rash should always raise the suspicion of syphilis. Treponema pallidum may be demonstrated by dark-field examination of genital, oral, or other suspicious lesions.

Obtain a STS at the first antenatal visit of all obstetric patients and preferably again late in pregnancy. Repeat STS in conflicting, equivocal cases and on admission to the hospital. A strongly positive STS or an increasing titer on repeated examination are strongly suggestive of syphilis. In the absence of a clear-cut explanation for a positive STS, it is extremely unwise to postpone treatment or to assume that the STS is a "false positive." Secure fluorescent treponemal antibody (FTA) and Treponema pallidum immobilization (TPI) tests during pregnancy to determine the specificity of repeatedly positive or uncertain STS when there is no historical or clinical evidence of syphilis or when the woman is not receiving antisyphilitic therapy.

A positive STS is not proof of syphilis nor is a negative STS an absolute refutation of the diagnosis. False positives occur in up to 10% of clinic patients and may be due to many disorders, including collagen diseases and viral, protozoal, or other spirochetal infections.

Prevention.

Reporting of all cases of syphilis is required in most public health jurisdictions.

Isolate any infant with stigmas of syphilis and the mother until a definite diagnosis can be made and treatment administered.

Require monthly physical examinations and quantitative blood STS of syphilitics until delivery and for one month afterward. If there is evidence of relapse or if the STS titer remains high, repeat penicillin therapy.

Examine the neonate for stigmas of syphilis at birth and repeat at intervals of 3 weeks to 4 months. If the mother's STS is positive at delivery, the neonate's will also be positive. Obtain serial quantitative STS of the infant's blood for 4 months. A rising titer indicates congenital syphilis, and treatment is indicated. For infants under 2 years, give 50,000 units of procaine penicillin G with 2% aluminum monostearate (PAM) per kg I.M. and repeat in 2 days.

Treatment.
A. Penicillin Therapy: For primary, secondary, or early latent syphilis during pregnancy, administer penicillin in any of the following ways: (1) Benzathine penicillin G, 1.2 million units in each buttock (2.4 million units total). If no spinal fluid examination is done, patients with latent syphilis should be re-treated with the same dosage in one week. (2) Procaine penicillin G with 2% aluminum monostearate (PAM), 4.8 million units total, usually given as 2.4 million units initially (as above) and then 1.2 million units at each of 2 subsequent injections 3 days apart. (3) Aqueous procaine penicillin G, 600,000 units I.M. daily for 8 days to a total of 4.8 million units.

If the patient is in labor, has syphilis, and has not had antisyphilitic treatment, give an initial 3 million units I.M. and 2 million units every other day for a total of 6 million units, and treat the neonate as above (see Prevention).

Repeat antisyphilitic therapy is not necessary when the woman has previously undergone sufficient treatment and the blood STS is negative. However, the United States Public Health Service recommends that when there is any doubt about the adequacy of previous treatment, every pregnant woman with a positive STS, regardless of titer, should be considered to require treatment. If the serology remains positive for three months after treatment, re-treat the patient.

B. Other Drugs: If the patient is sensitive to penicillin, give erythromycin, 20-30 gm orally over a period of 10-15 days. Insist upon a careful follow-up because of possible relapses.

MALARIA

Malaria may cause abortion or premature labor and delivery. The infants of mothers with malaria are often smaller than the average. Approximately 10% of infants born of women with demonstrable parasites in their blood will have plasmodia in cord blood films.

Malaria may cause infertility; it also complicates pregnancy. Malarial relapses often occur during pregnancy for unknown reasons. A renewal of attacks is common during the puerperium or after hemorrhage and infection.

Labor is frequently prolonged and hazardous for obstetric patients with malaria. These women become fatigued sooner, and operative delivery is required more often. The parasite is not transmitted in the milk, but lactation should be discouraged in women with clinical evidence of malaria. The severity of maternal malaria is reflected in the stillbirth rate, which rises as pregnancy approaches term, and the vitality of neonates which do survive is temporarily reduced.

Chloroquine (Aralen®), 1 gm orally stat. and 0.5 gm in 6 hours followed by 0.5 gm daily for 2 days is effective against all forms of malaria.

LISTERIOSIS

Maternal listeriosis may be responsible for abortion and fetal disease or death depending upon the severity of the infection and the duration of pregnancy. Encephalitis and granulomatosis of the newborn are described also. Pregnant women suffering from a septic form of this disease transmit the infection to the fetus either transplacentally or by exposure of the fetus to the organisms in the lower genital canal during the birth process.

In the mother, listeriosis causes slight temperature elevations and general malaise. The parasite may also be responsible for vaginitis, urinary tract infection or enteritis, and, rarely, meningitis.

A diagnosis of listeriosis during pregnancy can be made upon repeated clinical examination, complement fixation tests, and bacterial cultures of leukorrheic discharges or urine or stool specimens. A positive complement fixation test in high dilution is almost invariably present in an acute maternal infection. Gram-positive rods should be sought in the meconium of the newborn to diagnose listeriosis early.

Treat the mother and child with large doses of penicillin, erythromycin, or tetracyclines.

TOXOPLASMOSIS

Toxoplasmosis may be the cause of chronic abortion, premature delivery, and perinatal fetal death. Malformations are not ascribed to toxoplasmosis, however. The fetus probably becomes infected during a phase of parasitemia after placental invasion by Toxoplasmi gondii. The infant with toxoplasmosis often has septic meningitis or hydrocephalus.

A positive intradermal toxoplasmin skin test may indicate present or past infection. The diagnosis of active toxoplasmosis requires the use of the Sabin-Feldman serotest and the complement fixation reaction of Westphal. The tests should be performed in women with a history of frequent abortion, repeated premature delivery, and recurrent births of infants who succumb to obscure infections.

There is no effective treatment. Sulfadiazine with pyrimethamine (Daraprim®) therapy has shown promise. Toxoplasmosis is not an indication for therapeutic abortion or sterilization.

13...
Dystocia

PELVIC DYSTOCIA

Pelvic dystocia occurs when there is significant shortening of any of the internal dimensions of the bony pelvis. Unfavorable alterations in the structure and dimensions of the pelvis may be congenital or may be due to malnutrition, tumors, injuries, or disorders of the spine and lower extremities. About 15-20% of women in the USA have pelves which may cause complicated delivery.

Growth of the pelvic bones is complete in early adolescence, when the pelvic epiphyses fuse. The causes of abnormal human pelvic configuration generally relate to prepuberal disease, but fractures and neoplasms are also responsible:
  (1) Congenital and hereditary disorders: Congenital dislocation of the hips, chondrodystrophy.
  (2) Disease of the pelvic bones: Rickets, osteomalacia, fracture with misalignment, tumor.
  (3) Disorders of the spine: Lumbar kyphoscoliosis, causing abnormal transmission of force to the pelvis.
  (4) Abnormality of one extremity: Unilateral equinovarus or paralysis of one leg, causing unequal force to be transmitted to the sides of the pelvis.

The birth canal is a series of rigid spaces or areas bounded by bony walls or prominences which act as baffles. They limit or guide the presenting part largely by deflection. Descent and internal rotation are markedly influenced by the characteristics of the virtually unyielding bony pelvis.

The significant clinical pelvic measurements are as follows:*

External Pelvic Measurements. (See p. 81.)
  A. Intertuberous Diameter (TI): This is also known as the transverse diameter of the outlet or the intertrochanteric, biischial (BI), or bituberous diameter. It repre-

---

*The interspinous and intercristal diameters of the inlet and the intertrochanteric and external conjugate (Baudelocque) diameters have been abandoned as reliable guides to pelvic capacity.

sents the distance between the inner margins of the ischial tuberosities and is accessible to measurement above the anus or the hypotenuse of the anterior pudendal triangle. The actual distance between the bony margins is 11 cm or more, but when measured through the soft tissues the value is 8 cm or more for a normal pelvis. The fetal head (average biparietal diameter: 8 cm) impinges on the pubic rami during delivery or, in the case of an occiput anterior presentation, at the points where the intertuberous diameter is taken. Thoms's and Williams' outlet pelvimeters are useful for measuring the TI with accuracy. A rough estimate of this diameter may be obtained by pressing the closed fist against the pudendum beneath the arch and comparing the known width of the fist across the knuckles with the TI.
B. The Pubic Arch (90°+): The angle formed by the pubic arch is usually 110-120°. If the angle is narrow (< 90°), the TI may be considerably shortened. This is typical of a "funnel" type of pelvis.
C. Posterior Sagittal Diameter of the Outlet (PS) (8 cm + correction = direct): The PS is measured indirectly from the point corresponding to the midpoint of the TI to the base of the coccyx (sacrococcygeal joint) on its external (skin) surface. This measurement is usually 10.5-11 cm. One to 1.5 cm must be subtracted for bone and soft tissue. **Note:** When the sum of the posterior sagittal diameter and the intertuberous diameter is 15 cm or more, an infant of normal size will usually pass without difficulty (Thoms's or Klein's rule).
D. The Anterior Obstetric Sagittal Dimension (McDermott) (7-9 cm): This measurement provides important information regarding the forepelvis and the outlet since it is an estimation of the subpubic angle and the length of the symphysis. It is the distance from the midpoint of an 8 cm bar (the minimal intertuberous distance) placed beneath the pubic arch to the top of the symphysis. Descent of the head requires that it curve around the sacral promontory. Further descent and internal rotation demand that the head hug the inner aspect of the symphysis and then its lower surface. The longer the symphysis and the narrower the subpubic angle, the deeper the pelvis and the wider the retropubic curve must be for vaginal delivery. Prominent ischial spines and a narrow midpelvis may also cause dystocia. If the anterior obstetric sagittal dimension is 7-9 cm, midpelvic difficulties are not likely to occur. If the measurement is 9-10 cm, slight difficulty may be expected. Severe dystocia should be anticipated and cesarean section may be required when the measurement is more than 11.5 cm.

E. Anteroposterior Diameter of the Pelvic Outlet (AP)(11.9 cm or more): This is the distance from the inferior border of the symphysis to the posterior aspect of the tip of the sacrum. A Martin or Breisky pelvimeter is generally used. This is virtually as accurate as x-ray measurement even in the moderately obese patient.

A metal ring 8.5 cm in diameter (equivalent to the biparietal diameter of the average term infant's head) can also be fitted beneath the pelvic arch between the pelvic rami as an estimate of the available space at the pelvic outlet.

Internal Measurements. (See p. 81.)
A. The Diagonal Conjugate (DC): The DC is probably the most important single measurement of the pelvis. It is the distance from the midpoint of the promontory of the sacrum to the inferior border of the symphysis. To reach the promontory of the sacrum, the examiner must depress his elbow toward the floor. The DC is obtained for the purpose of approximating the true diameter of the pelvic inlet (conjugata vera, CV). The CV is estimated by subtracting 1.5 cm from the DC, and is the distance from the anterior midpoint of the promontory of the sacrum to the superior margin of the symphysis in the midline. The obstetric conjugate is measured from the sacral promontory to the nearest point on the symphysis, which usually is one-third of the distance below the superior margin. The obstetric conjugate is actually the shortest diameter of the pelvic inlet, normally at least 10 cm.

Measurements of DC of 11.5 cm or less or a CV of less than 10 cm indicate contracture of the pelvic inlet or superior strait; the likelihood of dystocia, assuming an average-sized infant, is inversely proportionate to this measurement.

B. Interspinous Diameter of the Midpelvis (10+ cm): This important measurement is usually obtained by x-ray, although with experience an accurate interspinous measurement (causing minor discomfort) can be taken with a Hanson pelvimeter. A DeLee or Breisky pelvimeter may be used, but these instruments are difficult to use transvaginally, especially in primigravidas, because of the pain caused by the rigidity of the narrow vault. The Hanson pelvimeter is used as follows: One blade of the instrument is passed into the rectum and the other is inserted into the vagina. The device is articulated so that the blades will spread to touch the ischial spines. The dimension is read on a centimeter scale.

C. The Posterior Sagittal Diameter of the Outlet (8-9.5 cm): This measurement is taken directly with the rectal finger touching the sacrococcygeal joint. The distance from the midpoint of a line marking the intertuberous diameter to the tip of the rectal finger is the posterior sagittal diameter of the outlet.

Dystocia occurs when any of the significant pelvic measurements are markedly shorter than normal unless other diameters are wider than normal. Relative disproportion will impede and absolute disproportion will prevent the safe vaginal delivery of a normal infant.

Obstruction may develop at the plane of the pelvic inlet, the midpelvis, or the pelvic outlet.

Actually, because the outlet is not truly a plane but a shallow space—an extension of the midplane of the pelvis—the midplane and the outlet should be considered as one in the management of the patient with a contracted pelvis.

Any pelvic measurement is important only in relation to fetal size. Disproportion may occur with "normal" or even spacious pelvic measurements if the child is relatively large. (See Fetal Dystocia.)

Clinical Classification.

The clinical classification of pelvic contraction shown in Table 13-1 is based principally upon pelvic measurements. It is used to establish an estimate of pelvic adequacy with reference to the present pregnancy.

Note: A pelvis is classified as contracted when the DC is measured at 11.5 cm or less or when the TI is measured at 8 cm or less. Pelvic contraction almost invariably causes narrowing of the subpubic angle and lack of roundness of the pubic arch. An intertuberous diameter of less than 8 cm and a posterior sagittal diameter of the outlet (direct) of less than 7 cm may cause difficulty in labor and delivery.

If small dimensions or gross distortions are recorded initially, repeat the pelvic measurements during the third trimester when greater muscular relaxation and patient cooperation may give more favorable results. Confirmed contracture usually requires x-ray pelvimetry and consultation regarding the management of labor and mode of delivery.

Three levels of pelvic dystocia are recognized: inlet, midpelvis, and outlet dystocia.

A. Inlet Dystocia: Inlet dystocia occurs in about 1-2% of patients at term. Lack of engagement of the vertex before or during early labor may indicate cephalopelvic disproportion. In addition to an adequate inlet (DC:10.5+ cm, etc), engagement depends upon the diameters and malleability of the fetal head, pseudo-overriding at the pelvic brim due to uterine anteversion, low-lying placenta, malpresentation of the fetus, and fetal anomalies. Inlet dystocia is suggested when attempts to maneuver the head

Table 13-1. Clinical classification of pelves.

	DC	TI	Remarks
Normal	> 11.5 cm	> 8 cm	(Exception: Robert's pelvis, i.e., abnormal narrowing of all transverse diameters.)
Simple flat (SF)	11.5 cm or less	> 8 cm	No stigmas of rickets
Funnel typical (FT)	> 11.5 cm	8 cm or less	No stigmas of rickets
Flat funnel (FF)	11.5 cm or less	8 cm or less	No stigmas of rickets
Generally contracted typical (GCT)	11.5 cm or less	> 8 cm	No stigmas of rickets
Generally contracted funnel (GCF)	11.5 cm or less	8 cm or less	No stigmas of rickets
Generally contracted rachitic (GCR)	11.5 cm or less (measured to false promontory if shorter than true)	> 8 cm	One of the following must be present: A rachitic sacrum, spines and crests within 2 cm, rachitic rosary, frontal bone bossae, bowed radii, bowed tibiae.
Flat rachitic (FR)	11.5 cm or less (false promontory if shorter)	> 8 cm	One sign of rickets as above

into the inlet by applying fundal pressure (DeLee-Hillis maneuver) are unsuccessful.

B. Midpelvis Dystocia: Midpelvic contraction alone is 3-4 times as frequent as isolated inlet contraction. Insufficient space in the midpelvis should be suspected, even before the head has engaged, in the presence of a contracted outlet, prominent or close spines, a male physique, a flattened or irregular sacrum, or premature rupture of the membranes or malposition of the fetus. Midpelvic dystocia may be due to funneling of the pelvis (convergence of the side walls and lateral bore, flattening of the sacral concavity) or abnormal projections into the pelvic canal by bony protuberances (prominent ischial spines or genital neoplasms).

Distortion of the birth canal at the midpelvis prevents rotation of the head and may even direct the vertex toward the sacrum rather than toward the outlet. In other instances, only rotation to the transverse may be permitted. The vertex is commonly deflected in this variety of pelvic contracture.

C. **Outlet Dystocia:** Isolated outlet dystocia is rare; it is almost always associated with midpelvis dystocia.

X-Ray Pelvimetry.

The internal pelvic architecture cannot be precisely evaluated by clinical examination alone since it is difficult to obtain reliable midpelvic measurements manually. X-ray visualization is necessary for complete appraisal. However, radiologic measurements are only ancillary guides and should not be used to forecast the outcome of delivery. Descent and rotation may not occur until the cervix is fully dilated and the membranes have ruptured. The final decision to resort to cesarean section should almost never rest on x-ray pelvimetry alone. The following is the obstetric classification of pelvic types developed by Caldwell and Malloy, adapted to American usage: (1) Gynecoid or human female type, with a circular or

Table 13-2. Pelvic types. (After Caldwell and Moloy.)

	Gynecoid	Android	Anthropoid	Platypelloid
Inlet	Rounded or slightly heart-shaped. Ample anterior and posterior segments.	Wedge-shaped or rounded triangle. Posterior segment wide, flat; anterior narrow, pointed.	Anteroposterior ovoid with length of anterior and posterior segments increased. Transverse diameter reduced.	Transverse ovoid; increased transverse AP diameter of both segments.
Sacrum	Curved, average length	Straight with forward inclination	Normally curved, but long and narrow	Curved, short
Sacrosciatic notch	Medium width	Narrow	Wide, shallow	Slightly narrowed
Side walls	Straight, divergent, or convergent	Usually convergent	Straight	Straight or slightly divergent
Lateral bore	Straight, divergent, or convergent	Usually convergent	Often straight	Straight or divergent
Interspinous diameter	Wide	Shortened	Shortened	Increased
Pubic arch	Curved	Straight	Slightly curved	Curved
Subpubic angle	Wide	Narrow	Narrow	Wide
Intertuberous diameter	Wide	Shortened	Often shortened	Wide

slightly heart-shaped inlet (40-45%). (2) Android type, which simulates the male pelvis including the rounded or triangular superior strait (15-20%). (3) Anthropoid, ape-like, or antero-posterior ovoid pelvis (20-30%). (4) Platypelloid or flat pelvis, having a transverse oval inlet (2-5%).

Among American Negro women android pelvis is only about half as frequent as in white women and platypelloid pelves are seen only occasionally, but anthropoid pelves account for almost half.

Great variations in the heredity and environment of foreign populations make other generalizations regarding pelvic configurations futile.

The important x-ray features of each pelvic type are shown in Table 13-2.

Most pelves are not pure types but incorporate features of 2 varieties. For example, a pelvic inlet with a rounded (gynecoid) posterior segment and an elongated and ovoid (anthropoid) anterior portion is classified as a gynecoid-anthropoid inlet. Other variations or combinations of the 4 types are possible in the configuration of the inlet. The midpelvis and outlet are not designated as gynecoid, android, etc. Nevertheless, significant distortion and contracture at these levels may prevent spontaneous or even safe operative vaginal delivery.

The major dimensions of the superior strait influence the diameter and ease of engagement of the presenting part. The mechanism of labor depends upon the relative size and shape of the midpelvis and outlet.

A. Indications: X-ray pelvimetry may be indicated at term in 5-8% of obstetric patients, particularly in the following cases:
  1. A high premium on the baby - First pregnancy late in childbearing years or a record of previous stillbirths, birth injury, dystocia, or midforceps delivery.
  2. Unusual physical findings - Short stature, especially with stigmas of rickets or the dystocia dystrophy build; marked lordosis or kyphosis; unusual gait.
  3. Obstetric abnormality before labor - Contracted inlet or outlet, or narrowing of the bispinous diameter; breech presentation or unengaged vertex at term in a primigravida; large infant (over 4000 gm), especially in a diabetic; fetal malpresentation.
  4. Complications of labor - Failure to progress in labor despite frequent strong, sustained contractions; primary uterine inertia before oxytocin stimulation.
B. Methods: The most popular methods include the following:
  1. Isometry or positional method (Thoms, Torpin) - Two films are required:
    a. A lateral view of the pelvis is obtained after placing a graduated, notched metal rod in the patient's gluteal fold. The pelvic dimensions may be ob-

tained directly from the film by using a centimeter rule.
  b. An anteroposterior film of the pelvic inlet is taken with the plane of the superior strait and the film parallel at a known separation distance. A second exposure of the film is made with a metal grid placed in the plane of the inlet after the patient leaves the x-ray table. Proportionate or isometric diameter values may be obtained directly from the film.
2. Parallax or precision stereoscopic method (Caldwell-Moloy) - An anteroposterior film is obtained, followed by another after a slight measured lateral tube-shift. Using a stereoscopic viewer, accurate dimensions of the virtual image may be procured with a centimeter rule held at the same span as the tube distance (infinity). A third-dimensional appreciation of the pelvic form and capacity is also afforded.
3. Orthometric method (Hodges) - Reproductions of the pelvic planes in either lateral or AP views are made as accurate scale tracings using a calibrated instrument similar to the camera lucida. Precise measurements of the pelvis at all levels may be made in this manner.
4. Triangulation method (Ball) - Exact measurements of the pelvic diameter can be calculated using pairs of AP pelvic roentgenograms taken at 90° angles to one another.

X-Ray Fetal Cephalometry.

X-ray fetal cephalometry requires a lateral and, usually, an AP view using one of the methods outlined above. The patient should be erect so that the fetus will drop as far as possible into the true pelvis. A comparison of the fetal head size and the diameters and contour of the birth canal is the aim of such studies.

The fetal biparietal and the slightly larger suboccipito-bregmatic diameters are the significant fetal measurements in engagement. The biparietal diameter has important implications for pelvic "fit" at all levels. The fetal occipito-frontal diameter is a good index of maturity.

Serious technical difficulties in cephalometry always occur when the fetal head is in abnormal presentation: (1) head in the uterine fundus, with breech presentation; (2) floating vertex presentation; and (3) obliquity of the fetal head at any level.

Clinical Implications of Pelvic Types. (See Fig 13-1.)
  A. Gynecoid Pelvis: The inlet is rounded with open anterior and posterior segments. Unless the pelvis is diminutive

338 Pelvic Dystocia

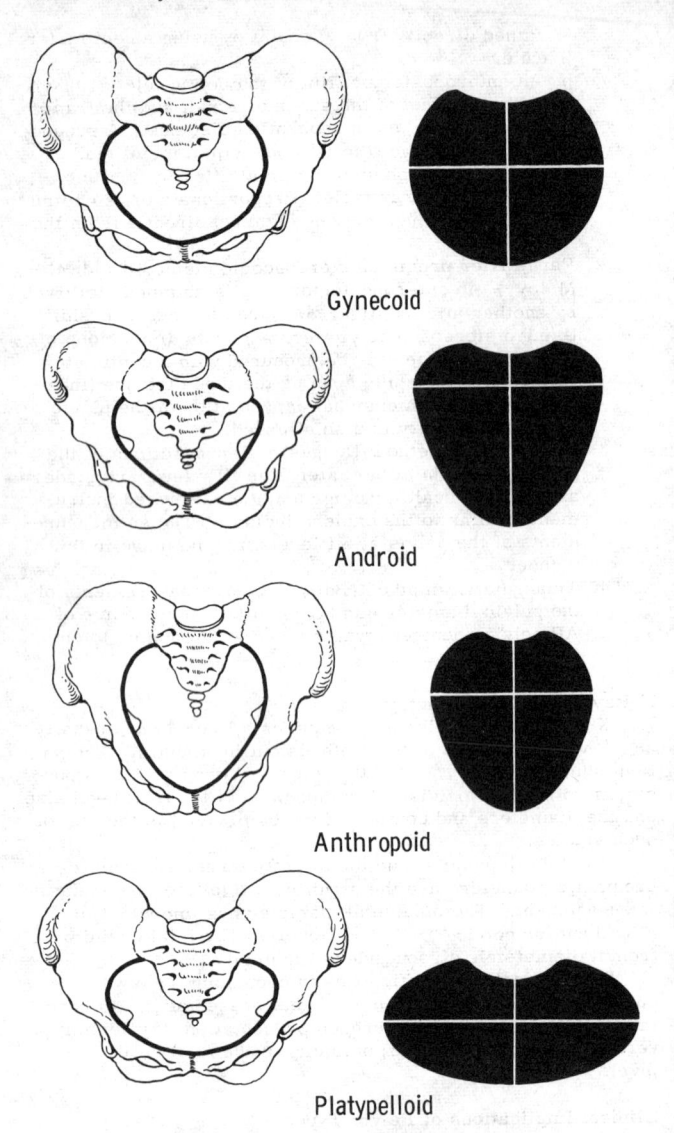

Gynecoid

Android

Anthropoid

Platypelloid

Fig 13-1. Types of pelves. White lines in the diagrams at right (after Steele) show the greatest diameters of the pelves at left.

(the generally contracted, so-called justo minor variety) or the fetus is large, a normal birth is likely.
1. Antepartum - Engagement of the vertex occurs at term or early in labor in the transverse diameter of the inlet in over two-thirds of patients.
2. Intrapartum - Normally, with good labor, descent of the vertex through the midplane of the pelvis is rapid, and internal rotation to an anterior occiput position takes place when the biparietal diameter of the head is at or slightly below the spines. Unless an extremely narrow pubic arch, anterior beaking of the sacrum, or other abnormality obstructs the outlet, further descent and extension of the head beneath the symphysis are unimpeded and the infant is delivered normally.

B. Android Pelvis:
1. Antepartum - Engagement is delayed by the encroachment of the sacral promontory into the posterior segment of the superior strait and the narrowness of the anterior segment of the inlet. Occiput transverse presentation occurs in almost three-fourths of cases.
2. Intrapartum - Convergent pelvic side walls and lateral bore, with contracted sacrosciatic notches and a narrow subpubic arch, predispose to a posterior position and require the descent of the vertex as a posterior practically to the pelvic floor. Funneling at the midpelvis wedges the presenting part and restricts its progress; and lack of space between the prominent spines and outlet contraction increase dystocia. Molding of the occiput often leads to its arrest in descent because it cannot rotate easily. Forceps delivery as an occiput posterior presentation may be required because of difficulty in rotation despite possible damage to the mother's soft tissues.

C. Anthropoid Pelvis:
1. Antepartum - This pelvic conformation is characterized by an elliptical inlet having a long AP and short transverse diameter. The sacral promontory is not prominent and does not impede engagement, and engagement is not usually delayed. The sacrosciatic notches are wide. The vertex usually enters the inlet in either the anterior or posterior position. The former occurs only slightly more often.
2. Intrapartum - Because the ischial spines are often prominent or close-set, the head descends in the position of engagement to the outlet. Rotation usually must be accomplished below the spines. If this is not possible, the head will have to be delivered as a posterior occiput presentation.

D. Platypelloid Pelvis: Rickets during childhood is often the cause of flat pelvis and sacral flattening with ridging or bossellation. This combination is extremely serious for the mother and child during labor. Nonrachitic pelves are often merely foreshortened in the AP dimensions; others are generally contracted. Each presents individual problems.

1. Antepartum - A contracted inlet causes malpresentation or delayed engagement of the vertex at term. A rachitic patient is often short in stature, and she may have a pendulous abdomen. The high, unengaged presenting part thus exaggerates the anteflexion of the uterus. Premature rupture of the membranes and prolapse of the cord are frequent complications of flat pelvis. If and when the vertex does enter the pelvis, it engages in the transverse position.

2. Intrapartum - Delivery may be difficult if the true conjugate is 8 cm or less even though the transverse diameter of the inlet is normal (13.5 cm).

   Engagement may occur in a flat pelvis with moderate extension of the head because the fetal bitemporal diameter is 1 cm less than the biparietal. Asynclitism (lateral flexion of the head) may aid engagement because the vertex must hug either the symphysis or the sacral promontory to enter the superior strait at all. Descent will be slow; the parietal bone may present with the sagittal suture far anterior or posterior depending upon whether anterior or posterior asynclitism (respectively) is present. Pelvic dystocia and failure of application of the presenting part to the cervix may result in secondary inertia; or poor labor may be observed from the start. Expect molding of the head with a large caput succedaneum.

   Fortunately, the flat pelvis is often a shallow one. However, the sacrum may be flattened and irregular, especially if it is rachitic. The arch is usually widened (unless the pelvis is generally contracted or has a funnel tendency). However, forceps application and downward traction in the transverse position with eventual rotation may bring the occiput beneath the symphysis for delivery.

Differential Diagnosis.

Lack of engagement may be due to abnormal fetal presentation or position, fetal anomaly, poor labor, placenta previa, pendulous abdomen with uterine anteflexion, or pelvic tumor rather than to fetopelvic disproportion. Failure of descent or rotation of the vertex may be due to ineffectual labor, bowel or bladder distention, or pelvic tumor.

Complications.

A. Maternal: Pelvic dystocia may cause prolonged labor (slow progress with relative disproportion), uterine in-

ertia (myometrial fatigue), contraction ring formation (exaggerated retraction), rupture of the uterus (dissipation of force), operative delivery (forceps, cesarean section), infection (premature rupture of membranes, long labor, trauma to the birth canal), hemorrhage (lacerations of the birth canal), separation of the symphysis (rupture of the symphysial ligament during forceps delivery or malrotated vertex), fistula formation (bladder, bowel), and levator or sphincter damage.
B. Common fetal injuries with any type of pelvic dystocia are intracranial hemorrhage, hypoxia, infection, depressed and other types of skull fracture, and cervical and brachial plexus damage.

Prevention.

The avoidance of pelvic dystocia requires accurate clinical pelvic measurement early in each pregnancy. If the findings are unusual or if obstructed labor ensues, x-ray pelvimetry and cephalometry are indicated.

Treatment: Inlet Dystocia.

A. Emergency Measures: Give oxygen for prolapse of the cord or fetal distress. Immediate cesarean section may be required for prolapse of the cord, marked fetal distress, or maternal exhaustion.
B. Specific Measures:
  1. The DC only helps to detect marked inlet contracture. However, if the DC is 5 inches or less in the average Caucasian patient at term, cesarean section will be required.
  2. Trial of labor* - A trial of labor permits observation for a reasonable period of time to determine the patient's progress. Observe the strength, frequency, and character of uterine contractions, effacement and dilatation of the cervix, and descent of the fetal head. A trial of labor should be undertaken only upon consultation with a radiologist. With rare exceptions, however, the radiologist cannot predict that a woman will or will not deliver vaginally because he cannot forecast the quality of labor nor how much the fetal head will mold. Nevertheless, if the CV is less than 8.5 cm, cesarean section is required. In vertex presentations, when the radiologist reports pelvimetry values below average with a "small" fetus (3000 gm), a trial of labor is indicated. If the values obtained by pelvimetry are above the mean and the infant is not excessively large, allow a trial of labor (even with slow progress) since pelvic dystocia will be unlikely.

---

*Cp. Test of Labor, below.

Await the onset of spontaneous labor and avoid heavy analgesia. Rupture the membranes artificially only when the cervix nears full dilatation. If advancement of the head does not occur within 4-6 hours of strong labor (or 6-8 hours of moderate labor), prepare for cesarean section.

The safety of a trial of labor is judged according to the maternal and fetal conditions before, during, and after labor, not by the number of hours.

There is no trial of labor (or test of labor; see below) for breech presentations because the fetal head presents the widest diameter of the passenger at term. With an average-sized or small infant, however, the decision to attempt vaginal delivery is based on the quality and intensity of labor and dilatation and effacement of the cervix as well as descent of the presenting part. X-ray pelvimetry and cephalometry should be done in questionable cases. The method of delivery should be decided before labor progresses too far.

3. "Test" of labor - The test of labor (not to be confused with trial of labor—see above) is an appraisal of the patient's ability to engage the fetal head with strong labor after complete dilatation of the cervix and rupture of the membranes. A test of labor is rarely performed today, since the decision to operate or continue labor should be made earlier.

C. Surgical Measures: If cesarean section is necessary, the low cervical type is preferred. (**Caution:** Never attempt vaginal delivery of a version or breech presentation or a high forceps delivery in cases of inlet disproportion. Death of the fetus—and perhaps the mother also—may occur. If the baby dies during labor, embryotomy and vaginal delivery are usually feasible.)

Treatment: Midpelvis Dystocia.
A. Emergency Measures: Give oxygen for fetal distress. Immediate cesarean section may be required for severe fetal distress or maternal exhaustion during labor.
B. Specific Measures:
 1. Obtain x-ray pelvimetry and cephalometry when an abnormal presentation (including breech) complicates midplane contracture. Determine the course of action before the onset of labor. Elective cesarean section is justified in the rare instance of marked midplane (or outlet) contraction.
 2. Excessive molding together with caput succedaneum may give the false impression that the head is engaged. If the fetal head obliterates the available retropubic space and the greatest diameter of the skull has passed through the inlet, engagement is certain.

3. Re-evaluate the midpelvis and outlet clinically when desultory labor (uterine inertia) or lack of satisfactory progress after good labor follow engagement. Consider the depth and regularity of the sacrum, the prominence of the ischial spines and the interspinous diameter, the width and depth of the sacrosciatic notches, and the intertuberous and posterior sagittal diameters of the outlet. If one or more of these indices are significantly abnormal in relation to the size of the fetus, x-ray pelvimetry and cephalometry are indicated. Permit a trial of labor when the interspinous diameter (observed by x-ray) is 9.5 cm or more and when the anteroposterior diameter of the midplane is 10.5 cm or more, assuming adequate outlet measurements and a small or average-sized fetus. When the Mengert index is less than 85%, perform cesarean section if a brief trial of labor is unsatisfactory. The product of the AP and tranverse diameters of the midplane has been calculated by Mengert as 125 (100%) for women in the USA.

   A trial forceps delivery—gentle traction or gradual rotation toward an anterior position (or both)—after a second stage of 1-2 hours may be elected by an experienced obstetrician when an infant of average size is arrested by a borderline midplane contraction in the absence of outlet contracture. If this is unsuccessful, cesarean section is required.
C. General Measures: Encourage the patient and avoid tension. Do not stimulate labor with oxytocics if disproportion is likely. Limit sedation; do not institute caudal or spinal block until the fetal biparietal diameter is well below the spines. Maintain fluid and electrolyte balance.
D. Treatment of Complications: Suture lacerations (especially cervical), replace excessive blood loss, and give appropriate antibiotics for infection. Consider laparotomy if rupture of the uterus is likely.

Treatment: Outlet Dystocia.
A. Emergency Measures: Give oxygen for fetal distress. Cesarean section is required if fetal distress complicates a severe but previously unrecognized outlet disproportion during labor.
B. Specific Measures:
  1. Perform elective cesarean section when the sum of the TI and PS of the outlet is appreciably less than 15 cm. (See Thoms's rule, p. 81.)
  2. A trial of labor is not possible in outlet dystocia because of the hazard to the fetus.
  3. If an incurved, ankylosed coccyx obstructs the presenting part, fracture it at the sacrococcygeal articu-

lation after induction of anesthesia and then deliver the fetus with forceps.
C. Supportive Measures: As for midpelvis dystocia.
D. Treatment of Complications: Suture birth canal lacerations, give blood by transfusion if blood loss is excessive, and prescribe broad-spectrum antibiotics for infection.

Prognosis.

In general, the size of the pelvis is more significant to the outcome of labor than its shape.

An experienced physician can accurately predict the course of labor in about two-thirds of patients before or early in labor. The remainder will require trials of labor and x-ray or other consultation.

The diagnosis of pelvic adequacy is generally easy and accurate; the diagnosis of pelvic inadequacy is difficult and inaccurate. The price of error in either case is increased fetal and maternal mortality and morbidity.

DYSTOCIA DUE TO UTERINE DYSFUNCTION

Dystocia may occur when the myometrial contractions are too weak or too strong, too frequent or too infrequent, too brief or too prolonged, or when they are irregular. The tone of the uterine wall is perhaps even more important than the character of the contractions to the progress of labor. When the uterus relaxes poorly between contractions and is unusually firm during contractions, it is hypertonic; when it is flaccid between contractions and not firm even at the height of contractions, it is hypotonic. Neither a "tight" nor a "loose" uterine wall is efficient during labor.

At least 90% of cases of uterine dystocia occur in primigravidas. This disorder complicates 2-3% of labors at term.

Cervical effacement and dilatation depend upon frequent strong, sustained, regular uterine contractions, with good relaxation between contractions. Hypotonicity or hypertonicity of the uterus results in poor labor and implies an unfavorable prognosis. Normally, a uterine contraction begins near one cornu and spreads over the uterus to the lower segment. When contractions are inefficient—especially in hypertonic uterine states—contraction begins in the lower segment and spreads upward. This is reversed polarity. The so-called colicky uterus is characterized by general irritability and many ectopic contractions, which result in inadequate cervical dilatation and effacement.

In many cases of uterine dystocia, minor degrees of fetopelvic disproportion or resistance of the soft parts within the pelvis appear to reduce the efficiency of contractions. When there is lack of engagement, labor is further compromised.

Any of the following may cause uterine dystocia: Uterine anomalies and tumors (e.g., bicornuate uterus, myomas), uterine distention (e.g., polyhydramnios), delayed or missed labor (e.g., fetal death in utero), cervical abnormalities (e.g., scarring, fibrosis, tumors), and maternal disease (e.g., ventral hernia, chronic illness). Some cases classed as idiopathic are perhaps due to psychogenic factors.

Uterine dysfunction may complicate all stages of labor. Prompt diagnosis and appropriate treatment are essential in order to avoid dire consequences for the mother and fetus. Even if delivery is accomplished eventually, postpartal atony of the uterus may cause exsanguinating hemorrage.

In most instances of dysfunction due to abnormality of the uterine forces hypotonic contractions prolong the acceleration phase of labor. Hypotonic contractions occasionally occur during the latent phase of labor also.

Hypertonic contractions are more serious for the mother and fetus. They usually occur during the active phase of labor and become more severe as labor progresses.

The term uterine inertia is synonymous with uterine dystocia and implies ineffectual labor. There are 2 types: primary and secondary: (1) Primary uterine inertia: Ineffectual contractions from the start of labor may be caused by induction of labor or spontaneous rupture of the membranes before the uterus is "ready" to contract normally; congenital anomalies of the uterus; unengaged presenting part, malpresentation, or malposition. (2) Secondary uterine inertia: Good contractions may give way to poor ones for any of the following reasons: Overdistention of the uterus (due to polyhydramnios, multiple pregnancy, or a large fetus), which stretches and thins the myometrium; excessive analgesia and anesthesia, which obliterates uterine contractions; emotional tension and release of catecholamines, which may reduce the stimulatory effect of oxytocin on the myometrium; fetopelvic disproportion, which causes uterine fatigue.

Infection and trauma are the principal dangers for both the patient and the fetus. Violent labor may result in precipitate delivery and injury to both.

Failure of the cervix to dilate and efface, coupled with inefficient labor, leads to prolonged labor. The incidence of infection during delivery is directly related to the length of labor, particularly when the membranes are ruptured. The necessity for operative delivery is increased in prolonged labor.

The quality of labor must be evaluated with regard to the presentation, position, and size of the fetus and the dimensions and configuration of the pelvis. The expulsive forces work against the resistance of the soft and firm tissues of the pelvis. Resistance is overcome slowly or not at all in dystocia due to faulty uterine action.

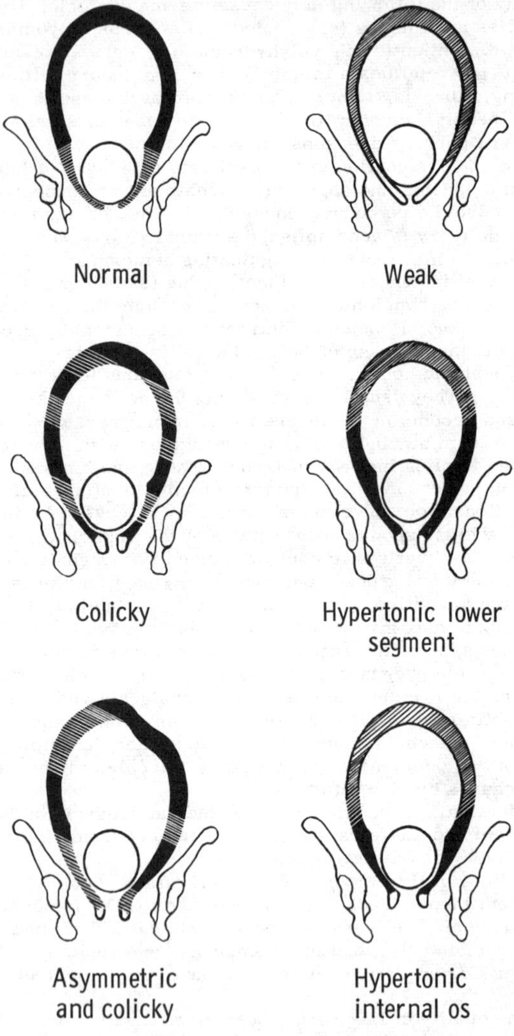

346 Dystocia Due to Uterine Dysfunction

Fig 13-2. Normal and dysfunctional uterine contraction types. (After Jeffcoate.) Black, strong contraction; shaded, slight contraction; white, atonic areas.

Clinical Findings. (See Fig 13-2.)
  A. Hypotonic Uterus: In flaccid uterus cervical dilatation and effacement are usually normal; pain is slight and complaints are minor, and contractions are weak but fundal dominance is maintained.
  B. Hypertonic Uterus: There are 2 types.
    1. The fundus and lower uterine segment are tense, and the cervix may be normal or spastic. Pain is extreme, and seems to the observer to be out of proportion to the force of the contractions. Backache is persistent. Ileus and urinary retention are often observed. Uterine polarity is reversed, with lower segment dominance. A contraction ring often forms with uterine fatigue.
    2. In "colicky uterus" (occasionally with a septate or bicornuate fundus) with a normal or spastic cervix, the uterus is irritable and prone to asynchronous action. The patient complains of almost constant pain which is worse with contractions. Restlessness and aerophagia are common. Variable polarity and incoordinate contractions are apparent. A contraction ring may form eventually.

Differential Diagnosis.

False labor is usually a sequence of irregular, slightly crampy uterine contractions which do not increase in frequency or intensity. The uterus is generally hypotonic. The cervix does not dilate or efface, and the presenting part does not descend. False labor actually consists of strong Braxton Hicks contractions.

Cervical dystocia is due either to scarring and stenosis of the cervix, usually as a result of surgery or infection; or functional spasm, in which case hypertonic uterine inertia is often an associated factor.

Retraction ring (Bandl's ring) is a narrow but vise-like, unyielding zone of myometrial contraction between the upper and lower uterine segments—an exaggerated, pathologic retraction ring. This disorder is always a complication of malpresentation or fetopelvic disproportion. Constant, agonizing uterine pain and tenderness precede inevitable rupture of the lower uterine segment. The markedly thickened uterine wall above the ring makes palpation of the fetus difficult. Immediate cesarean section may allow delivery of a living offspring. A fetal destructive operation and vaginal delivery may be the best course after death in utero occurs.

Constriction ring is a persistent contraction of all or part of a segment of the uterus around a narrowed portion of the fetus. The ring, the result of dysrhythmic uterine contractions, may occur at any level during any stage of labor. Constriction ring often is associated with extended (never obstructed) labor, especially after prolonged rupture of membranes. Characteristically, colicky pains persist well after the uterine contraction ceases. On examination, the flaccid cervix is observed to hang loosely, even during a contraction, so that the presenting part remains abnormally mobile. Vaginal palpation often reveals the ring considerably above the relaxed cervix compressing the fetus. Magnesium sulfate, 50 ml of 20% solution I.V., heavy sedation, or deep anesthesia may relax the ring; epinephrine, 1:1000, 2-5 minims I.M., usually relieves the constriction for a brief interval. The incidence of operative intervention is increased. The fetus is endangered by hypoxia, asphyxia, and delivery trauma.

Missed labor is very rare. Labor begins at or near term but soon ceases. The fetus, dead before or soon after failure of labor, is retained. Amniotic fluid is reabsorbed. Disintegration of the products of conception follows, often as a result of infection. Weeks or months may pass, however, before portions of the fetus pass through the cervix. Fetal bones occasionally perforate the uterus to precipitate an acute abdominal emergency.

Uterine anomalies are discussed on p. 500.

Prolonged labor (i.e., that which continues for 24 hours or more) may be due to failure of the expulsive forces, fetopelvic disproportion, abnormal presentation, or abnormal fetal position.

Precipitate labor (i.e., delivery which occurs in 3 hours or less) may be due to excessively strong, frequent contractions or reduced resistance of soft tissues in the pelvis.

Complications.

Prolonged labor, operative delivery (and possible injury), and intrapartal and postpartal infection are increased in uterine dystocia.

Prevention.

Prepartal conditioning of the patient does much to allay her fears and anxieties and seems to improve the quality of labor if other factors are favorable. Early recognition and proper treatment of dystocia due to abnormal uterine action will usually prevent serious complications.

Treatment.

A. Specific Measures:
　1. Hypotonic uterus - Unless fetopelvic disproportion is present, stimulate labor by amniotomy and by giving oxytocin (Pitocin®), 1 ml (10 units) in 1 liter of 5% glucose in water I.V. (20-30 drops/minute).
　2. Hypertonic uterus - In the absence of fetopelvic disproportion, give morphine sulfate, 15 mg ($1/4$ gr) I.M., to relieve pain, and phenobarbital, 60 mg (1 gr) I.M. for sedation. Catheterize as necessary to avoid painful bladder distention. Correct fluid and electrolyte

Dystocia Due to Uterine Dysfunction 349

   imbalance if indicated. When labor resumes (in 2-4 hours), apply an abdominal binder if the uterus is pendulous and the direction of force of the uterine contraction is not in the axis of the birth canal. This maldirection of force may be the basic cause of poor engagement and failure of descent.
   3. "Colicky uterus" - Treat as for hypertonic uterus (above). Scopolamine amnesia may be of value if psychic factors are inhibiting labor. Paracervical anesthesia may relax the cervix sufficiently to permit effacement and dilatation.
B. General Measures: Give reassurance and maintain fluid and electrolyte balance. Broad-spectrum antibiotics should be given to all patients with signs or symptoms of intrapartal infection and to those in prolonged labor
C. Surgical Measures:
   1. When impending death of the fetus necessitates prompt delivery, make Dührssen's incisions in the partially dilated cervix and extract the infant with forceps after desultory labor despite stimulation of the hypotonic uterus.
   2. Cesarean section is justified in the uncommon case of prolonged labor, especially when associated with borderline cephalopelvic disproportion or hypertonic uterus.
D. Treatment of Associated Problems:
   1. False labor - Reassure the patient and await the onset of true labor.
   2. Cervical dystocia -
      a. Due to scarring and stenosis of the cervix - Incise the cervix when it becomes effaced. Perform cesarean section only if incision and vaginal delivery are not feasible.
      b. Hypertonic cervix - Sedate the patient adequately during labor if cervical spasticity and hypertonic uterine inertia are present. Use regional anesthesia in the late first stage and during the second stage of labor. Dührssen's incisions should be used only when absolutely necessary. Cesarean section should be done only as a last resort.
   3. Contraction ring -
      a. In the first stage of labor - Give glucose, 10% in water, containing calcium gluconate, 0.5 gm, and magnesium sulfate, 2.5 gm (5 ml of 50% solution), I.V.
      b. In the second stage of labor - Give amyl nitrite, one pellet inhaled, or epinephrine, 1:1000 solution, 0.5 ml I.M., and ether anesthesia.
   4. Missed labor - Prevent cervico-uterine contamination (avoid artificial rupture of the membranes) and stimulate the refractory uterus repeatedly and persistently

with oxytocin, 1-2 ml (10-20 units) per liter of 10%
glucose in water, I.V. If intrauterine infection occurs
and attempts at evaluation of the uterine contents are
not successful, consider anterior vaginal hysterotomy.
Laparotomy is indicated only for treatment of perforation of the uterus and intraperitoneal complications.
5. Precipitate labor - Give analgesics in minimal doses
and use regional anesthesia (spinal or caudal) in an
attempt to slow labor. Consider elective induction of
labor at term when the patient gives a history of repeated episodes of precipitate labor.

E. Treatment of Complications:
1. Prolonged labor - Determine the cause and give appropriate treatment; give broad-spectrum antibiotics
in full doses; and maintain fluid and electrolyte balance.
2. Postpartal hemorrhage - See p. 175.
3. Postpartal infection - Administer broad-spectrum
antibiotics.

Prognosis.

The prognosis is good for both the mother and the fetus
if the diagnosis is made early and appropriate treatment is
given. Prolonged labor and intrapartal infection are particularly dangerous to the fetus.

DYSTOCIA OF FETAL ORIGIN

Anomalous fetal development, large fetal size, or abnormal fetal presentation or position often retards or obstructs
the process of labor and delivery. This occurs in approximately 0.5% of labors at term.

Dystocia due to fetal abnormalities is caused by nonengagement or arrest of the presenting part. In vertex presentations with disproportion due to a large or hydrocephalic
fetus, the head may never enter the pelvic inlet. Lack of
engagement is notable also in malpresentation. Deformity or
enlargement of the fetus may permit only the head to traverse
the superior strait, but the body may then obstruct to prevent
further descent. In breech presentations, engagement with
obstruction by the deformity may prevent or retard the birth
process.

The site of arrest will depend upon the presentation and
the severity and location of the fetal deformity in relation to
the maternal pelvic dimensions and architecture.

Previous uncomplicated pregnancy is no guarantee of
safe delivery in subsequent pregnancies. A woman who has
been delivered of one or more average sized babies without
difficulty may produce one no larger which may present abnormally and fail to engage or which may arrest deep in the
pelvis because of malposition.

Dystocia of Fetal Origin 351

Causes of Fetal Dystocia.
The size of the infant in relation to the mother's pelvis and the shape and consistency of the fetal presenting part determine the "fit" of the passenger in the birth canal.
- A. Large Size of Fetus: (> 4000 gm.) Heredity, maternal diabetes mellitus, parity of the mother (the size of infants tends to increase with parity).
- B. Anomalous Development of the Fetus: Monsters, hydrocephalus.
- C. Abnormal Girth of Fetus:
    1. Internal abnormality - Hydrops fetalis, ascites, abdominal tumor (congenital cystic disease of the kidney, teratoma).
    2. External abnormality - Myelomeningocele, sacral neoplasm.
- D. Malpresentation of Fetus: Transverse, oblique, shoulder, or compound presentation.

Clinical Findings.
- A. Symptoms and Signs: Assuming good labor, with adequate uterine tone and strong, sustained, regular uterine contractions, slow progress may be due to fetal factors:

    When the head is abnormally large, one of the following may occur: Abnormal presentation, failure of the presenting part to engage, or unusual position. When the body is distended or deformed, engagement of the vertex may occur with arrest of descent after the thorax passes through the pelvic inlet. Hydrocephalus will occasionally deter engagement in vertex presentations, or there may be stoppage at the inlet if the infant presents by the breech. An unusual contour of the uterus may be noted on palpation in extreme cases of fetal anomaly near term.
- B. X-Ray Findings: X-ray films, if feasible during the first stage of labor, may disclose a skeletal anomaly.
- C. Special Examinations: Vaginal examination may reveal unusual cranial configuration (as with anencephaly, meningocele, etc).

Differential Diagnosis.
Malpresentation or faulty engagement may be due to a maternal disorder rather than a fetal anomaly. Abdominal or vaginal examination may disclose pelvic tumors or exostoses which arrest the presenting part after its engagement and partial descent. Abnormal position or even incomplete rotation of the fetus during the birth process may occur without obvious cause.

Complications.
Operative delivery may be necessary and maternal injury may occur. Fetal death usually follows cerebral or abdominal decompression upon delivery.

Dystocia of Fetal Origin

Prevention.

Early diagnosis of the fetal anomaly (preferably before labor begins) is important. Elective termination of pregnancy, usually by induction and vaginal delivery, is recommended when the fetus obviously cannot survive (e.g., anencephaly).

Treatment.
- A. Emergency Measures: Immediate sterile vaginal examination under deep inhalation anesthesia may be required when delivery is difficult or impossible after the birth of a part of its body. Rotate the fetus so that its shoulders are in the AP diameter of the pelvis; this may allow palpation of an anomaly or may facilitate delivery in shoulder dystocia.
- B. General Measures: Try to deliver the patient vaginally, but avoid heavy analgesia until the cause of the dystocia is known. If the hazard to the mother seems too great, perform cesarean section after first informing the husband or closest adult relative about the fetal deformity and the chances of its survival.
- C. Surgical Measures: Operative intervention is almost always required. Drainage of cerebrospinal fluid from a hydrocephalic infant or paracentesis for abdominal decompression may be required for delivery. Embryotomy may be necessary for the delivery of a dead fetus. Cesarean section may be justified in the rare instance of living conjoined twins or for other gross abnormality when vaginal delivery might jeopardize the mother's life or health.
- D. Treatment of Complications: Birth canal injury, postpartal hemorrhage, and puerperal infection are common consequences of delivery of malformed fetuses.

Prognosis.

If a complicated, traumatic delivery can be avoided, the prognosis for the mother is good. The prognosis for the fetus with developmental anomalies ranges from guarded to very poor depending upon the seriousness of the anomaly. A large infant safely delivered does just as well as an infant of normal size, although large infants born of diabetic mothers require special care (see p. 320).

14...
Operative Delivery

FORCEPS OPERATIONS

Forceps operations, providing traction or rotation of the fetal head (or both), are employed to expedite labor or to actually deliver the fetus in complicated labors. The use of obstetric forceps has both fetal and maternal indications; today, forceps are occasionally mandatory but are more often elective. Forceps procedures are classified principally according to the situation of the head within the bony pelvis (see p. 359). Some type of forceps operation is used in 40-60% of births in most large hospitals in the USA.

Properly performed forceps operations will frequently save the life of the mother and the baby; when improperly performed, forceps operations often cause serious permanent injury or death of one or both.

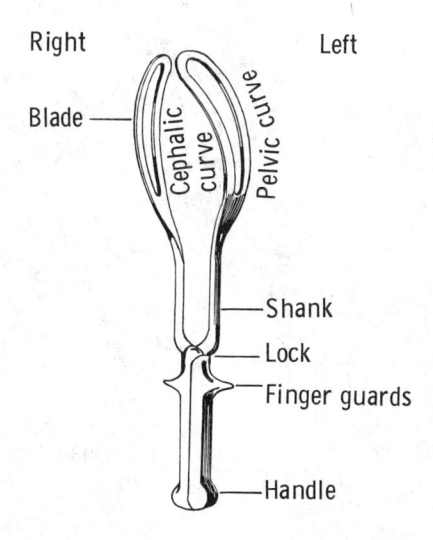

Fig 14-1. Simpson forceps.

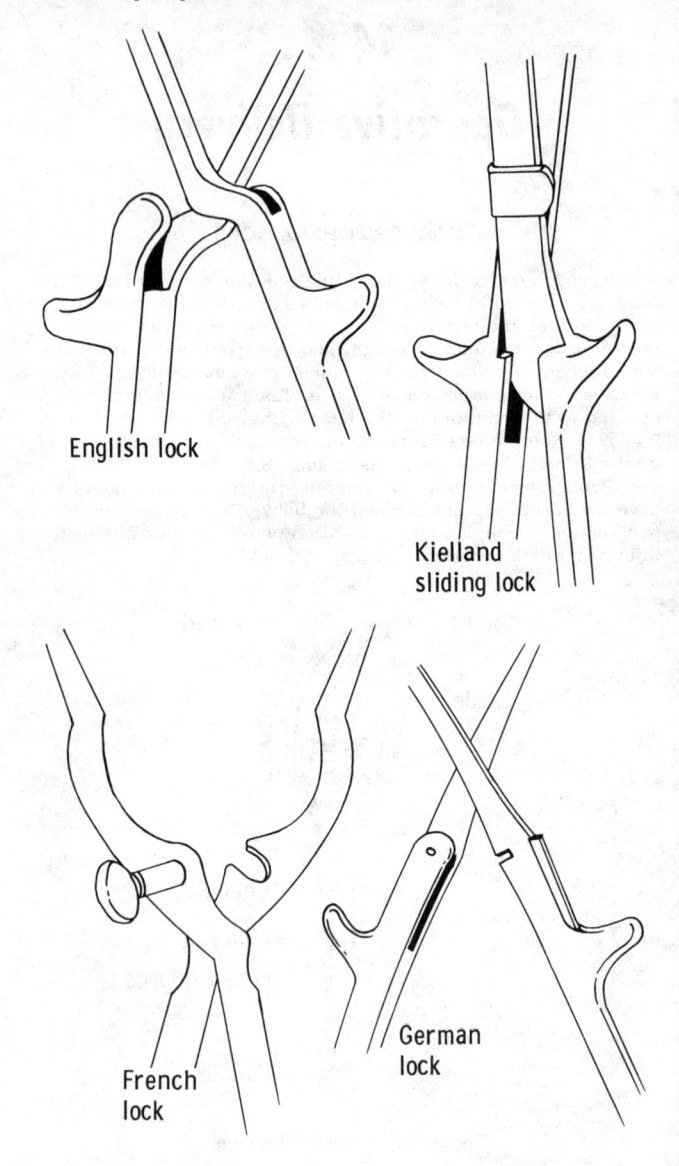

Fig 14-2. Types of forceps locks.

Forceps Operations 355

Simpson forceps

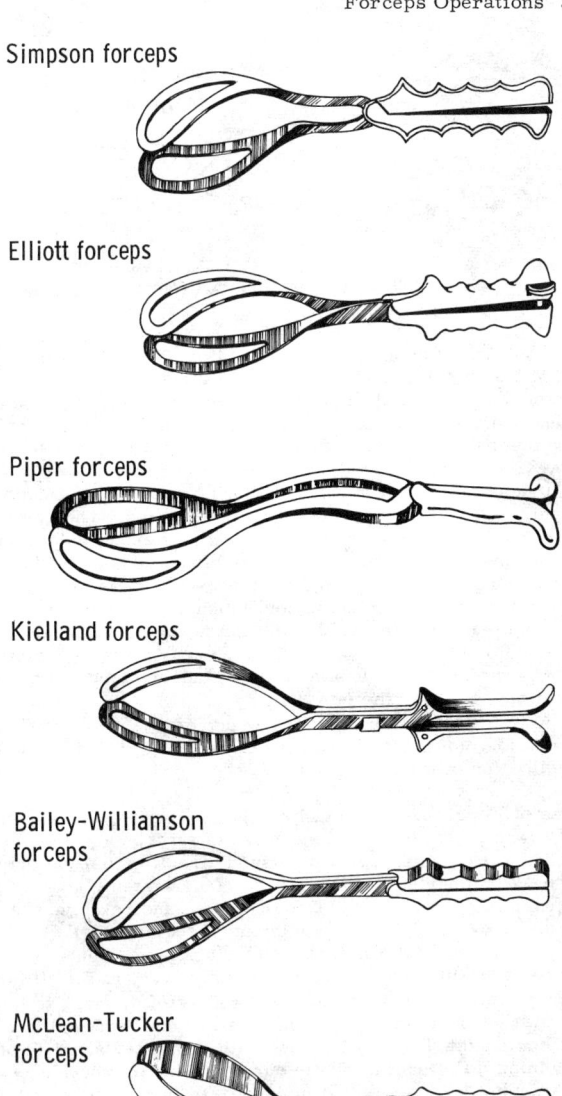

Elliott forceps

Piper forceps

Kielland forceps

Bailey-Williamson forceps

McLean-Tucker forceps

Fig 14-3. Types of forceps.

356　Forceps Operations

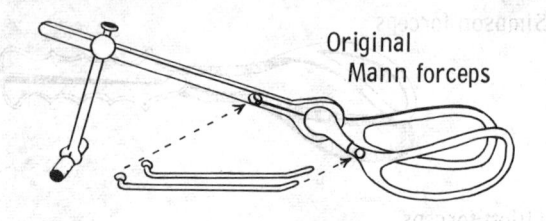

Fig 14-3. Types of forceps (cont'd.).

The Obstetric Forceps. (See Figs 14-1, 14-2, and 14-3.)
　　The obstetric forceps consists of a pair of metal blades each connected to a shank and the shank to a handle. The blades are crossed, like scissors, and lock by a flange arrangement (English lock), a screw (French lock), a sliding device (Kielland lock), or a notch and pin coupling (German lock). The blades are named right or left according to the side of the patient's pelvis toward which they are directed. They may be fenestrated, solid, or hollowed. The tip of each blade is called the toe; and the inferior curve of the blade, toward its juncture with the shank, is termed the heel. Most forceps blades are fixed to the shank at an angle corresponding to the pelvic axis when applied to the fetal head. Thus, in the classical forceps, the dorsal contour describes a pelvic curve. The cephalic curve is the lateral rounding of each blade designed to permit the forceps to "fit" the fetal head.

　　Axis traction is the correct forceps guidance of the head through the most favorable areas of the pelvis. It is actually a duplication of the mechanism of labor.

Types of Forceps. (See Fig 14-3.)
　　There are at least 6 basic types of forceps.
A. The classical forceps is derived directly from the original Chamberlen forceps. It has fenestrated blades and usually a flange lock. Good cephalic and pelvic curves are provided. Two subdivisions of the classical type are recognized: (1.) Forceps with overlapping shanks and considerably rounded cephalic curves. (The Elliott forceps is the prototype, and is considered by many to be a multipurpose forceps.) This instrument is ideal for the unmolded head. (2) Forceps with separated shanks, providing a flattened cephalic curve. (The Simpson forceps is the prime example.) A molded head is well accepted by this instrument. Modifications of both of these subtypes are now available with solid blades.
B. The Tarnier forceps, the first practical axis traction instrument, has fenestrated blades, partially closed shanks

Forceps Operations 357

Barton forceps and traction handle

Muirless head extractor (a vectis) for cesarean section

Tarnier forceps and axis traction

Bill traction handle

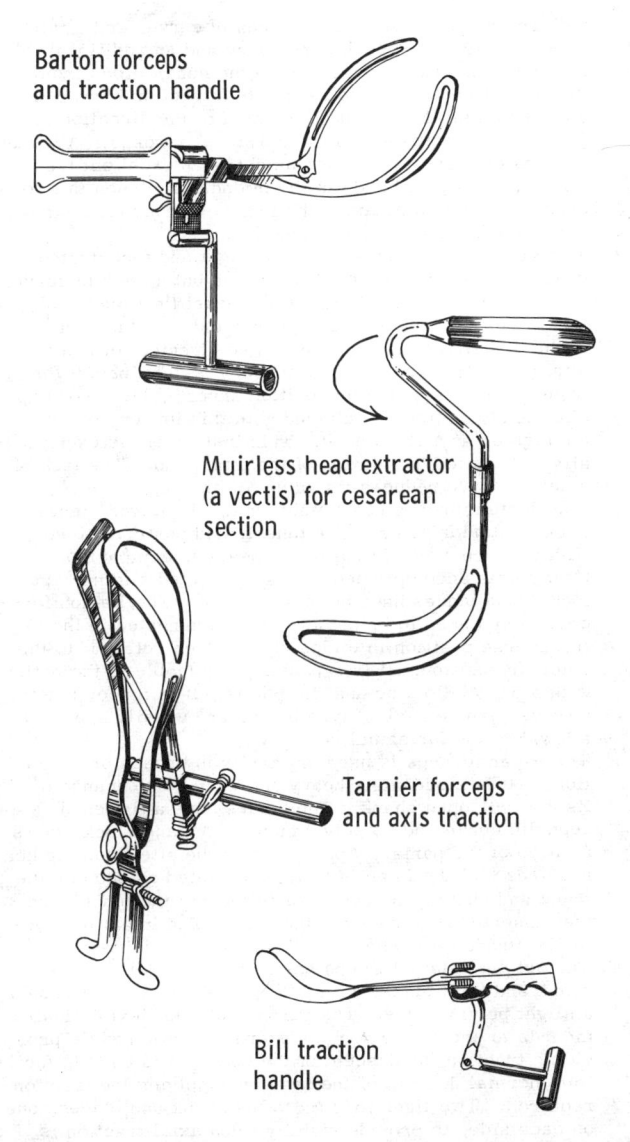

Fig 14-4. Types of forceps with traction handles and head extractor for cesarean section.

with an extended but shallow cephalic curve, and a fair pelvic curve. A French screw lock and an additional screw clamp ensure purchase on the head. Rods from the heel of each blade connect with a traction bar via 2 swivel joints. Excellent adjustment of the direction of force is accomplished with the Tarnier forceps. Although moderately heavy, this instrument is an excellent tractor for large, molded heads in the midpelvis. When this forceps is used as a rotator, the long, extended blades are dangerous to maternal soft parts.

C. The Kielland forceps is light in weight and fenestrated. It has an intermediate cephalic curve but no pelvic curve, a long shank, and a sliding lock bracket (left blade only). Buttons on the handle finger guards indicate the backs of the blades (which must always be directed toward the fetal occiput). The Kielland forceps is most useful for transverse and posterior position arrests, but a good application can often be obtained with this forceps on even the high or asynclitic head. This instrument is exceptionally well suited to rotation of the fetal head. The lack of a pelvic curve reduces its value for traction.

D. The Barton forceps has a light, uniquely hinged, fenestrated anterior blade. The fenestrated posterior blade, with its deep cephalic curve, is heavy in comparison. Coupling is accomplished with a restricted sliding-type lock. The blades have no pelvic curve. The Barton forceps is designed to bring down a head arrested in the transverse position in midpelvis and then rotate it to the anterior position. It is especially applicable to the patient with a platypelloid or android pelvis. It is a poor tractor, however, and classical type blades are usually applied as a low forceps for actual delivery.

E. The Piper forceps is used primarily in breech presentations. It is moderately heavy and very long because of its curved, open shank. The blades have a flattened cephalic curve and no pelvic curve. A flange lock allows fixation of the parts. Application to the after-coming head requires that the infant's body be elevated as soon as the trunk and shoulders have been delivered; the blades are then inserted from beneath the body. The infant may actually straddle the shanks until his head is delivered.

F. The original Mann forceps has a universal joint in the shank and light blades with a deep cephalic curve but only a slight pelvic curve. The purpose of this flexible instrument is to encourage normal internal rotation while providing traction for descent of the head. It is used to facilitate normal descent of the head by supplying the traction required. Two light rods fix to the shank and blades, one on each side, to provide rigidity when axial traction is required.

Hundreds of modifications of these and other forceps have been designed, and all have their advantages and disadvantages. The choice of whether to use forceps or not—and which forceps to use—always depends on the specific problem the physician faces and his experience with obstetric instruments.

Indications for Forceps Delivery.
A. Obstetric Complications of Labor:
 1. Dystocia - Ineffectual uterine contractions account for about three-fourths of indicated forceps operations. Prolonged or desultory labor may also be due to slight or relative fetopelvic disproportion. Although inadequate dimensions of the bony pelvis are a more important cause of disproportion, rigidity of the soft parts also impedes passage of the infant. Poor flexion or malrotation of the presenting part may also prevent progress in labor.
 2. Prophylactic forceps delivery (elective).
B. Medical and Surgical Complications of Labor: These include disorders such as heart disease (class III or IV), appendicitis complicating labor, and intracranial hemorrhage at term.
C. Fetal Complications of Labor: Marked irregularity of the fetal heartbeat, tachycardia (> 160/minute), or bradycardia (< 100/minute) may be indicative of hypoxia, intracranial injury, or infection.

Requirements for Forceps Application.
 1. Appropriate presentation (vertex presentation or for the aftercoming head in breech presentation).
 2. No demonstrable clinical cephalopelvic disproportion.
 3. Dilatation and effacement of the cervix.
 4. Ruptured membranes.
 5. Engagement of the head.
 6. Empty bladder and rectum.
 7. Episiotomy (generally a mediolateral incision for forceps operations other than outlet).
 8. Maternal or fetal indication (see above).

Classification of Forceps Deliveries. (After Weinberg.)
A. An outlet forceps delivery is described when the vertex distends the introitus or is visible at the introitus.
B. A low forceps delivery is one in which the presenting bony skull lies below the tuberosities of the ischium (deeply engaged).
C. A midforceps delivery refers to the application of the forceps when the vertex is between the planes of the ischial spines and tuberosities (well engaged).
D. A high forceps delivery is effected when the leading bony point of the vertex lies between the inlet and the ischial spines but with the greatest diameter of the head above the inlet (unengaged).

E. A floating forceps delivery is accomplished by applying the blades to a high, floating (unengaged) head.
F. A trial forceps is the application of cautious traction after apparently satisfactory midforceps application, with the intention of abandoning attempts at forceps delivery if resistance seems too formidable.
G. A failed forceps is the determined but unsuccessful attempt at forceps delivery (usually high or midforceps).
H. "Prophylactic forceps" (DeLee) is the principle of elective, early delivery by low forceps in order to (1) reduce maternal physical and emotional stress by shortening the second stage of labor; (2) protect the pelvic floor and viscera from laceration and overdistention; (3) limit blood loss; and (4) protect the fetus from cerebral damage.

Only experienced operators should be permitted to perform prophylactic forceps operations. For the inexperienced physician, prophylactic forceps delivery is meddlesome midwifery.

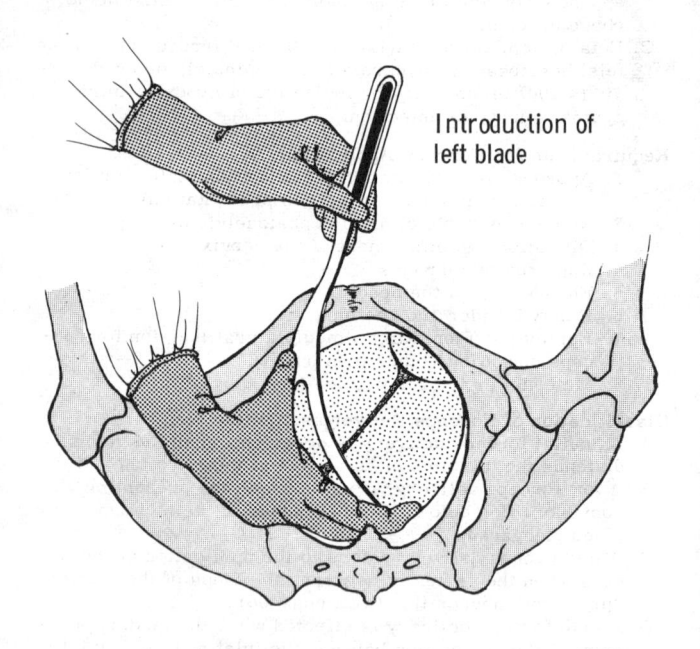

Introduction of left blade

Fig 14-5. Forceps application.

Forceps Operations 361

Left blade brought into position

Insertion of right blade

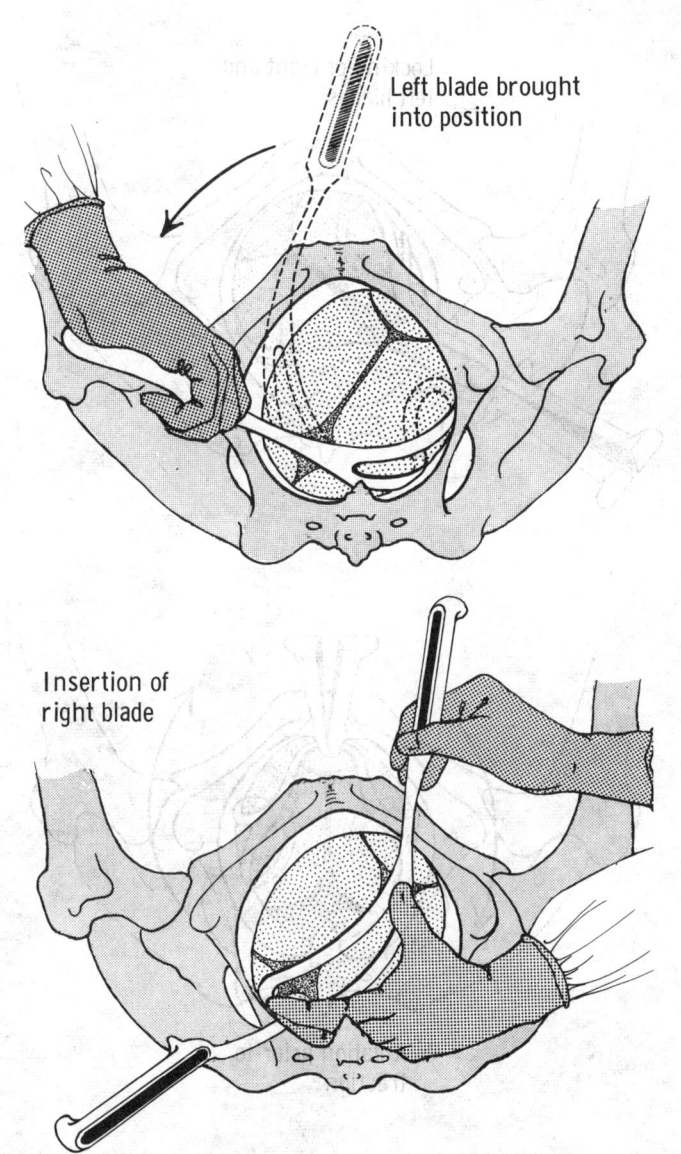

Fig 14-5. Forceps application (cont'd.).

362 Forceps Operations

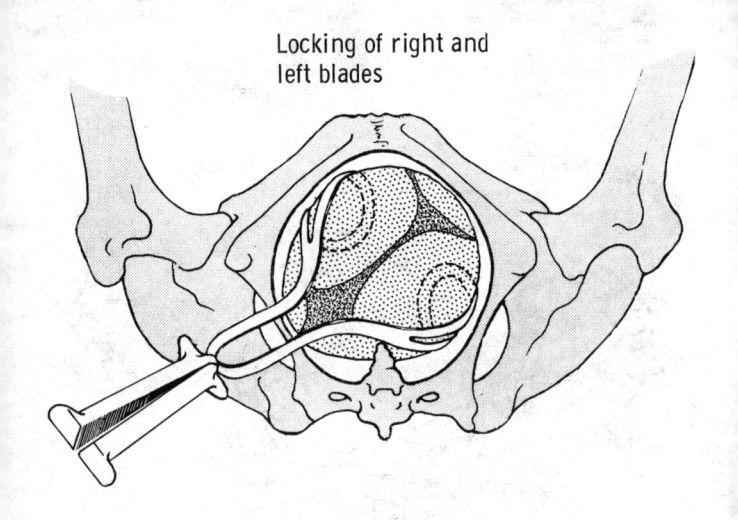

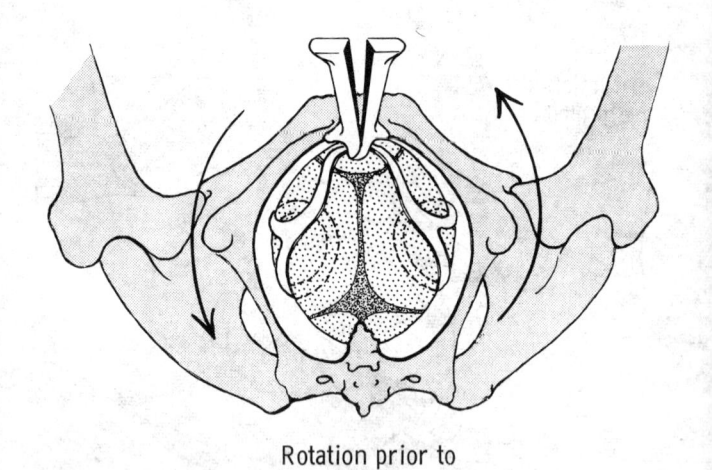

Locking of right and left blades

Rotation prior to traction

Fig 14-5. Forceps application (cont'd.).

Forceps Operations 363

The Technic of Use of Obstetric Forceps. (See Fig 14-5, pp. 360-3.)

The use of the obstetric forceps proceeds in the following steps:

A. Insertion: Classically, the left forceps handle is held in the operator's left hand, like a violin bow, and the blade is directed toward the left side of the patient's pelvis and to the left side of the fetal head. The right forceps handle is held in the right hand, and a similar procedure is followed on the opposite side.

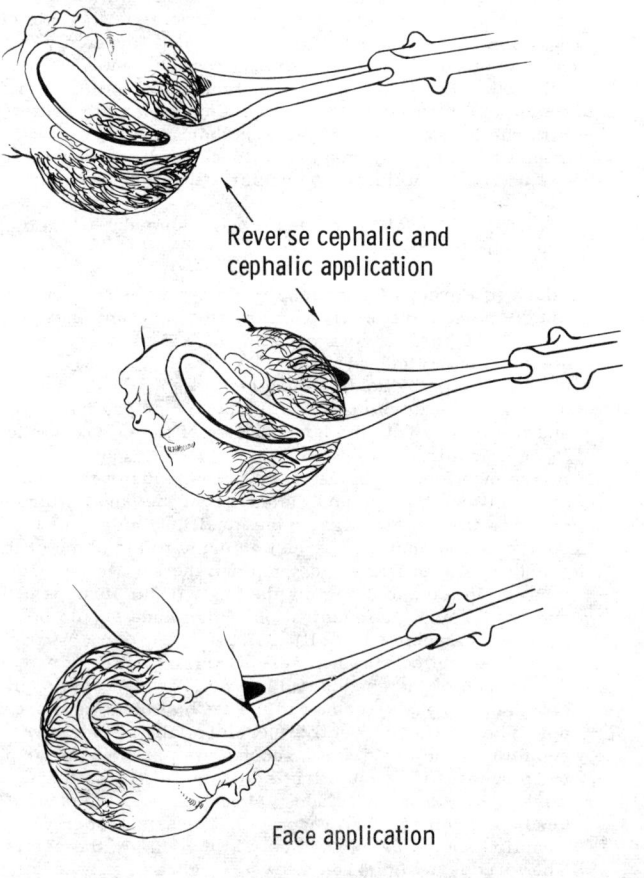

Reverse cephalic and cephalic application

Face application

Fig 14-5. Forceps application (cont'd.).

B. Application: Holding the left handle with the left hand, insert 2 or 3 fingers of the right hand into the vagina and guide the blade to its optimal position alongside the fetal head. Repeat with the right blade, using the left hand to guide the blade.

C. Articulation: Couple the blades at the shank only if this can be done without the use of force. Feel for an ear to establish the correct position. Revise the application as necessary, and depress the handles to secure a proper "fit."

D. Rotation and Traction: Turn the fetal head with the forceps or draw it outward, simulating the mechanism of labor in that particular pelvis. Apply traction only in the axis of the pelvis. Use steady traction with arm force only (never body weight). Simulate labor contractions: pull, relax, pull, etc. Extraction of the head may be possible with the same pair of forceps, or it may be necessary to rotate with one pair and deliver with another.

E. Disarticulation: Disengage the forceps when its purpose has been accomplished, or desist if this cannot be done easily and safely.

F. Removal: Extract the blades in reverse order of their insertion.

Procedure in Forceps Operations in Vertex Presentations.

A. Kneel on one knee or sit on a low stool in front of the patient. Be braced to avoid slipping and to maintain steady, controlled traction.

B. Insert forceps by holding each blade lightly. Slip each blade into the introitus along the posterior vaginal wall and then carry it to the correct side of the pelvis as the forceps is advanced.

C. Apply each forceps blade to the proper side of the fetal head between the eye and the ear from the parietal prominence to the malar ridge or the maxillary ridge. The posterior fontanel will be just anterior to the plane of the shanks. The posterior fontanel and the sagittal suture must be in a plane bisecting the angle of the forceps blade and shank, and the fenestration of the blade should be scarcely palpable (if at all).

D. Articulate or lock the forceps. If this is not easy and divergence of the shanks and handles is noted, malapplication has probably occurred. The first blade is more apt to be applied correctly; therefore, the second blade should be readjusted and a second attempt made to couple the forceps. If articulation is still not easily accomplished, remove both blades, check the position of the head, and reinsert and reapply the forceps properly.

E. Traction should be exerted only in the axis of the pelvis. The forceps design often allows a degree of axis traction

(Piper and Hawks-Dennen forceps). However, an axis traction arrangement built into the forceps (Tarnier, DeWeese) or an attachment to the shank of the forceps (Bill traction bar) will provide much more effective direction of force. Grasp the handles with the right hand, holding the palm upward, and insert the index or second finger between the shanks. Hold the shank near the blades with the left hand and gradually exert downward force toward the region of least resistance. Apply traction outward with the right hand, using the handles, but avoid compressing the head. This combined effort (Pajot's maneuver), which simulates axis traction, will generally draw the head away from the symphysis and downward. Alter the degree and direction of traction as the head descends in the birth canal. Avoid excessive force. Simulate labor contractions by brief pulls with a period of relaxation between each pull. It may be necessary to rotate the head back to an oblique position to bring it past an angulated, ankylosed coccyx. Check the fetal heart rate and rhythm after each pull.

F. Rotation:
  1. Oblique position to the anterior (ROA or LOA to OA) - Apply the classical forceps without the axis traction attachment in the usual manner. After forceps articulation, rotate the occiput to the anterior and apply traction downward in the axis of the pelvis.
  2. Transverse position to the anterior (ROT or LOT to OA) - Digitally or manually rotate the head to the oblique or anterior position if possible. Do this in the midpelvis where the pelvic diameters are greatest. Rotate left-sided positions with the right hand and vice versa. After rotation, exert counterpressure on the uterine fundus to hold the head in its new position.
     a. Digital rotation - Gently insert the tips of the first 2 fingers of one hand into the posterior fontanel. By lifting the head slightly toward the side of the occiput, it will generally turn to the anterior position. Fix by fundal pressure.
     b. Manual rotation - Insert the fingers and the thumb of one hand into the vagina with the palm up. Grasp the head with the tips of the fingers behind the posterior parietal bone and the thumb over the anterior malar bone. Flex the head and rotate it to the transverse position or farther, but do not let it disengage. Retain the vertex in its new position by fundal pressure.
     c. Forceps rotation using classical forceps - Introduce the anterior blade first. Do not insert the blade too far posteriorly into the vagina, but move it gently

366 Forceps Operations

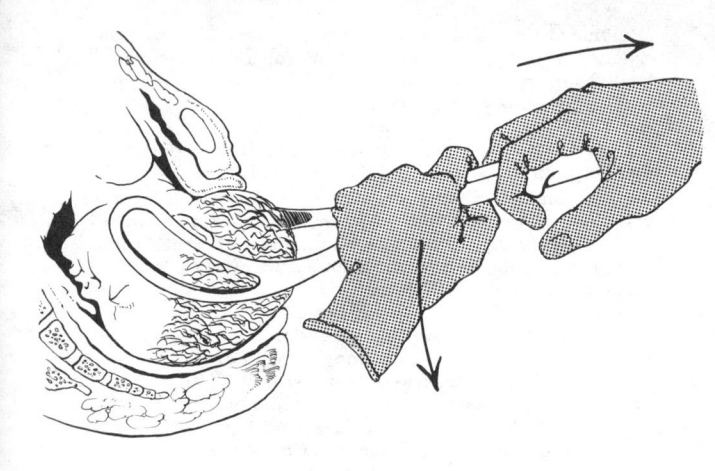

Fig 14-6. Axis traction (Pajot's maneuver).

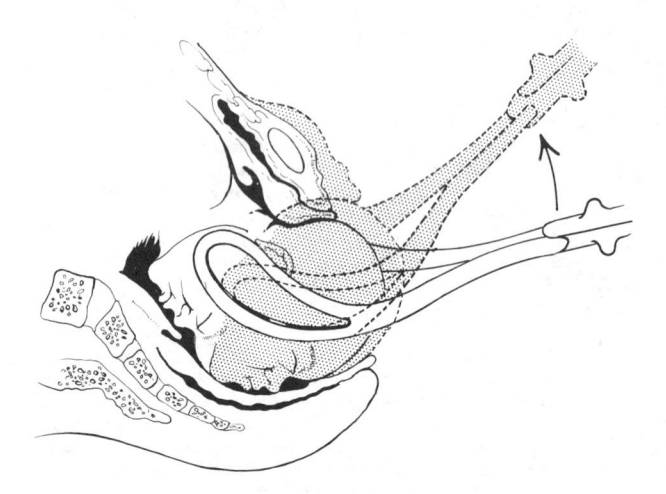

Fig 14-7. Upward traction with low forceps.

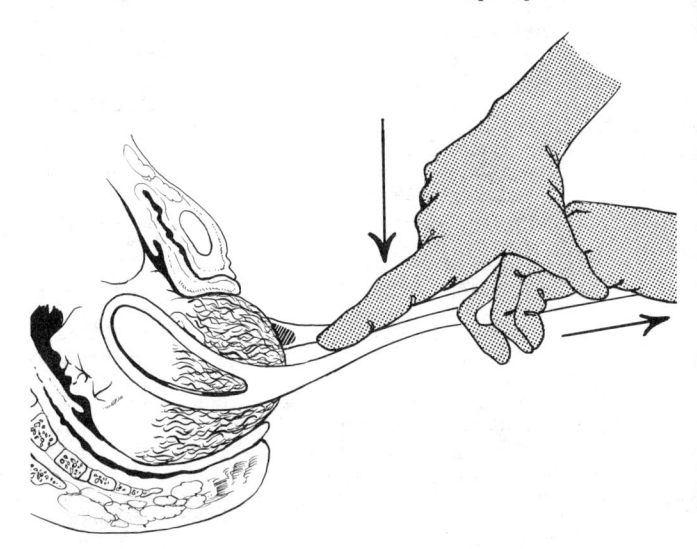

Fig 14-8. Modified Pajot's maneuver.

over the face to the anterior ear beneath the symphysis. Insert the posterior blade and adjust the application so that locking of the forceps is accomplished readily. Compress the blades to hold the head and bring the vertex anteriorly. Rotate the forceps handles in a wide arc, almost sweeping the thigh, to avoid gouging the fornices with the toe of the forceps. Deliver the infant by traction applied in the axis of the pelvis.

d. Forceps rotation using the Kielland forceps (ROT or LOT to OA) -
  (1) Classical application - Insert the first 2 fingers of the free hand into the vagina anterior to the head. Select the anterior blade and cautiously insert it into the vaginal canal along the hand, past the symphysis and cervix and into the cavity of the uterus, until only the handle and shank distal to the lock are visible. Depress the handle gently so that the toe of the blade can be seen or felt above the symphysis. "Flip" or quickly turn the blade over so that the button is directed toward the occiput. This can be done with remarkable ease. Insert and apply the posterior blade and lock the forceps, at this point with LOT or ROT. (Disregard asynclitism because this will

correct itself with rotation due to the sliding lock.) Rotate at the optimal level while applying slight downward traction. Recheck the application after rotation. Correct for asynclitism and deflection before continuing traction.

(2) Wandering method of application - Insertion, application, and articulation are approximately as described for the classical forceps rotation (see para. [c], p. 365). The buttons on the handles of the Kielland forceps aid in orientation.

e. Forceps rotation using the Barton forceps (ROT or LOT to OA) - Insert the hinged anterior blade posterior to the head with the fingers of the opposite hand within the vagina as a guide. Move the blade over the face (or occiput) to apply the forceps to the anterior aspect of the head behind the symphysis. While an assistant holds the handle of the anterior blade upward, insert the heavier, curved posterior blade along the head in the midline. Draw the handle of the posterior blade upward and lock it with the anterior blade. Apply downward traction in the axis of the pelvis (not in the axis of the forceps). Once the head is below the point of arrest, rotate it to the anterior position. Sweep the handles toward the opposite thigh to facilitate rotation, or use the axis traction bar attachment to turn the head in the proper arc. Disarticulate and remove the blades. Apply classical forceps for delivery.

3. Forceps rotation of posterior to anterior position (LOP or ROP to OA) -
  a. Manual rotation of a posterior position to a transverse should usually be attempted first, whereupon a classical or Kielland forceps (or even the Barton forceps in unusual cases) may be applied for further rotation to the anterior position.
  b. Scanzoni maneuver (double application of forceps) - Apply the blades as for an LOA, even though the true position is ROP. Move the more anterior blade into position; insert the posterior blade more directly. Rotate the head clockwise to an anterior position for an ROP and counterclockwise for an LOP. Rotation is best made in the shortest arc provided the turning process goes easily; otherwise, attempt rotation in the opposite direction. An axis traction bar will usually aid in rotation and extraction. Remove the blades and then reapply them for an anterior position (now achieved) and accomplish delivery by gradual traction.
  c. The DeLee "key-and-lock" maneuver is ideal for the rotation of posterior occiput positions. This is actually a stepwise rotation by simple multiple re-

adjustments of the forceps, preferably of the Simpson type.
   d. Kielland forceps rotation (single application of forceps) - If the position is ROP, apply the Kielland forceps "upside down" (buttons down, i.e., toward the occiput). After locking, rotate the head through the shorter arc and recheck the position of the blades but do not remove them. Correct the application, if necessary, and proceed to deliver the fetus by traction in the pelvic axis.
   e. Occasionally, it is safer for mother and baby to slowly deliver a large, markedly molded head which has been brought down to low forceps level by natural forces as a posterior presentation. Use a classical forceps applied for an anterior position and a generous mediolateral episiotomy.
G. Disarticulate and remove the forceps by reversing the motions used in applying and articulating the blades. Unlock the forceps gently, and carry the handle of the top blade over the symphysis toward the opposite flank. Repeat the process with the other blade. The blades disengage easily because they follow the cephalic curve of the head. If there is resistance to removal of the blades, deliver the head with one or both blades still applied.

Forceps Operations in Face Presentations.

Delivery is impossible when the chin is posterior unless the fetus is extremely small, and delivery as a posterior should be avoided even then. Regard the chin as a point of reference in face presentations (like the occiput in vertex presentations).
A. The Kielland forceps is most effective in the rotation and delivery of a face presentation. If the position is a mentum posterior, the Kielland forceps should be applied with the buttons down. After articulation, rotate to the anterior position, check the application, and apply downward traction. When the chin is beneath the symphysis, begin upward traction for delivery of the face.
B. The classical and Tarnier forceps are frequently employed for delivery of face presentations. Assuming the chin to be anterior, these blades are applied as for an occiput anterior presentation. To increase the necessary extension of the head, hold the forceps loosely after articulation; raise the handles and lock the blades tightly; and then apply axis traction.

Forceps Operations in Brow Presentations.

In brow presentation the use of forceps is similar to that employed for occiput or face presentations, but the procedure is far more difficult and dangerous. Try to convert the brow presentation to an occiput or face presentation manually, and then apply the forceps for rotation and traction.

Complications of Forceps Operations.
A. Maternal: Perforation of uterus, separation of symphysis, fistula formation, tearing of the cervix and sulcus, third degree lacerations, and uterine prolapse.
B. Fetal: Skull fracture, intracranial injury.

THE VACUUM EXTRACTOR

The vacuum extractor or ventouse is an effective device for use instead of the obstetric forceps in expediting delivery of the fetus in vertex presentation. The indications for the use of the vacuum extractor are the same as for forceps delivery. It is essentially a suction cup which is applied to the infant's scalp for traction. A controlled negative pressure of 0.7-0.8 kg can be developed with the Malmström extractor.

Advantages.
(1) Combines uterine propulsion with synchronous ventouse traction.

(2) Often obviates hazardous forceps operations; may reduce incidence of cesarean section.

(3) Volume of presenting part is not increased; compression of the head is avoided; tentorial tears and cerebral hemorrhage in offspring are less common.

(4) Birth canal lacerations are infrequent; cervical incision is rarely necessary.

(5) Neither particular skill nor anesthesia is required. Patient cooperation is retained.

(6) May be applied early (cervix > 4-5 cm) at any station. Occasional "high" extraction is feasible.

(7) Frequently accelerates and shortens labor, especially when complicated by uterine inertia and cervical dystocia.

(8) Encourages "autorotation" and may correct minor degrees of malposition.

(9) Replaces more dangerous Voorhees bag or Willett forceps, as in treatment of partial placenta previa.

Disadvantages.
(1) Can never completely replace forceps: rotation is difficult; axis traction cannot be exerted.

(2) Scalp suffusion ecchymosis is usual; lacerations and cephalhematomas are frequent and intracranial injury occurs occasionally.

(3) If extraction time is > 35 minutes, fetal subgaleal hematoma or severe scalp damage is likely.

(4) Rarely applicable in acute fetal distress: very rapid

Vacuum Extractor 371

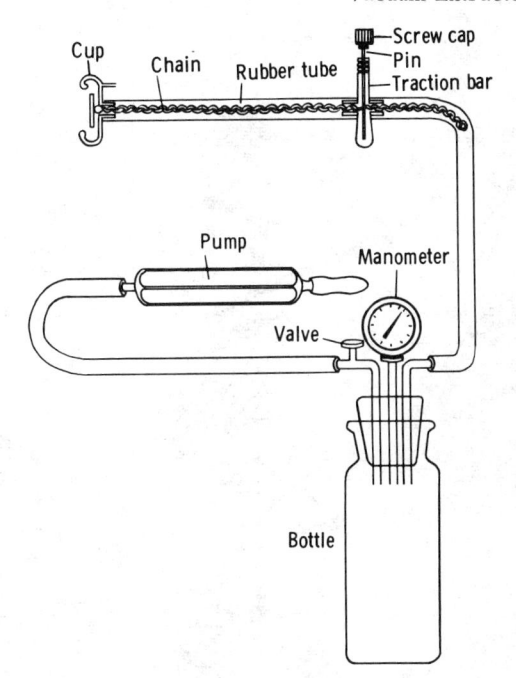

Fig 14-9. Modified Malmström vacuum extractor.

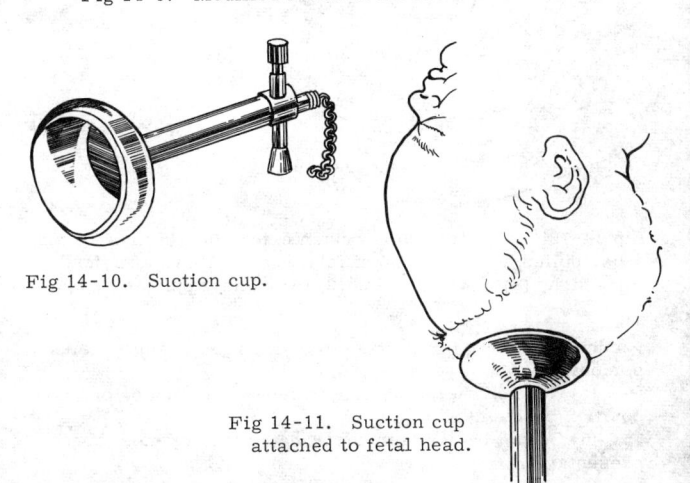

Fig 14-10. Suction cup.

Fig 14-11. Suction cup attached to fetal head.

372 Vacuum Extractor

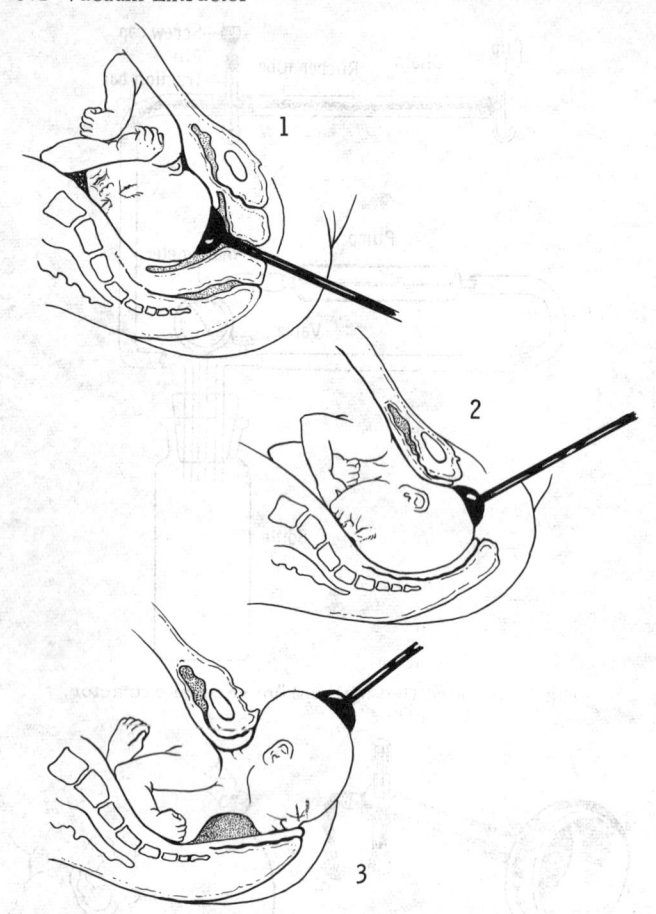

Fig 14-12. Application of vacuum extractor. Extractor may be applied at any station of fetal head. Above are shown (1) high, (2) mid-high, and (3) low outlet application.

vacuum sufficient for hurried extraction may damage fetus seriously.

(5) Not well suited for major cephalic deflexion or malposition problems.

(6) Cannot be used for uncorrected face or most breech presentations.

(7) Equipment is expensive.

VERSION

Version is a maneuver or operation by which the fetus is turned within the uterus from an unfavorable position or presentation to one more favorable for delivery. It is most often used to convert a transverse lie to a breech (podalic version) or vertex (cephalic version) presentation. Version "by the head" or "by the breech" refers to the polarity after turning.

Version may be accomplished by maternal postural change, by external or internal manipulation, or by a combination of external and internal manipulation. Version was used in at least 2% of deliveries a generation ago. Cesarean section has largely supplanted version today because it is safer for both the mother and the baby.

For the average physician, internal podalic version is a formidable procedure and should be undertaken only when strictly indicated. Prophylactic internal version is too dangerous even for the obstetrician. External version should be attempted only by physicians trained in this procedure.

Indications for Version.

In general, the various types of version are used for transverse lies and breech presentations.

A. Postural and External Version: Because the fetal death rate (including premature, term, and neonatal deaths) following breech delivery is about 15% as compared with 3% for vertex deliveries, postural and, especially, external version have great theoretical advantages. External version is successful on the first attempt in 70% of cases after the 32nd week. However, spontaneous verion does occur during the last trimester, and the manipulation required is associated with a fetal death rate of about 1% due to placental and cord accidents. The risk to the mother is negligible.

External version with anesthesia is successful in 90% of cases, and the incidence of breech presentations may be reduced from 3-4% to 1.5-2%. However, the fetal death rate attributable to the procedure usually rises to 2% or more, and maternal death occasionally occurs. Anesthesia for external version is rarely employed in the USA because of the danger of using too much force.

B. Internal Version: The indications for internal podalic version are relatively few, and the cervix must be almost completely or completely dilated. Internal version is indicated in the management of prolapsed cord, prolapse of one or both arms, and severe abruptio placentae; for delivery of a dead infant in transverse lie; and for delivery of the second twin in vertex or transverse presentation when hemorrhage, fetal distress, or long delay complicate the birth of the fetus.

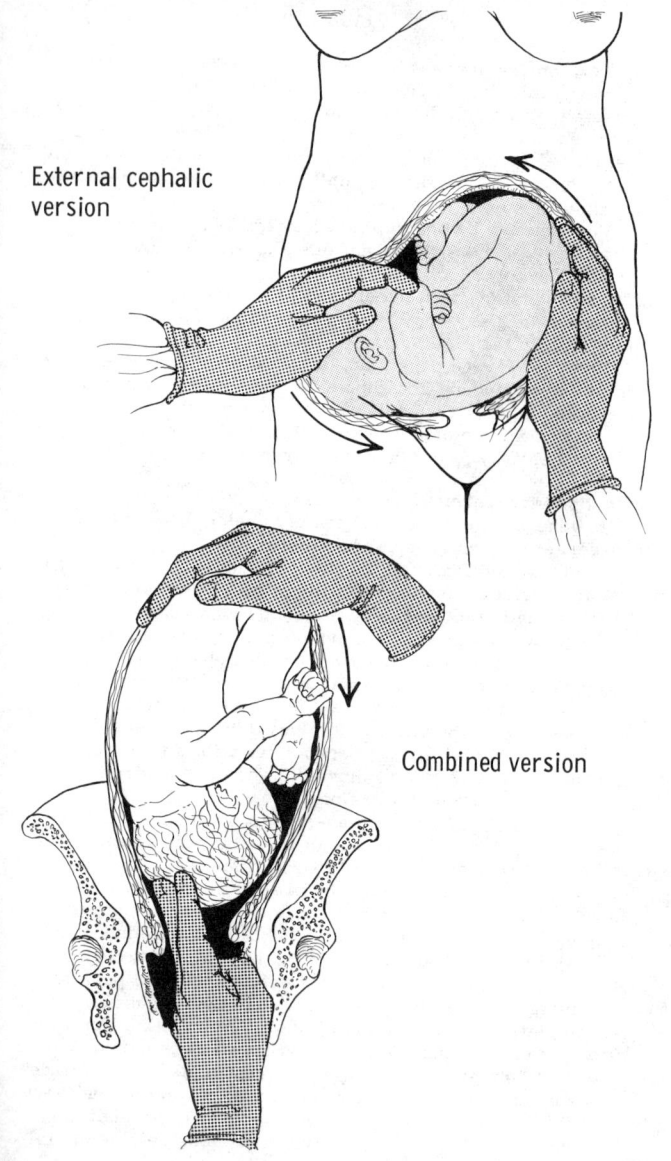

Fig 14-13. External and combined version.

C. Combined Version: Indications for combined version usually are a transverse lie or oblique presentation in the multiparous patient.

Contraindications to Internal & External Version.
A. Absolute Contraindications: Low engagement of the presenting part; threatened rupture of the lower uterine segment by a tight, high uterine contraction ring; uterine tetany, marked fetopelvic disproportion, previous cesarean section or an extensive myomectomy scar, first deliveries in multiple pregnancy, and large pelvic tumors complicating pregnancy.
B. Relative Contraindications: Placenta previa, eclampsia, undilated cervix, dry uterus, contracted vagina, obesity, poor (light) anesthesia, and insufficient assistance.

Methods of Accomplishing Version.
A. Postural Version: This may be done before or during early labor without anesthesia. The mother is placed in the knee-chest position or on one side with her head and thorax lower than her pelvis. The uterus is thereby raised out of the true pelvis, and more room is thus available for the fetus to shift. Postural version is most often used to correct position rather than presentation. However, in brow presentations, if the patient is placed on the side to which the fetal back is directed, the breech may gravitate to that side, bringing the occiput over the pelvic inlet. If the patient is cautiously returned to the supine position and rolled towels are applied to the sides of the abdomen and held by a binder, the fetus may be retained in the better presentation thus achieved. Unfortunately, postural version is rarely successful in completely correcting an unsatisfactory fetal lie.
B. External Version: This type of version is usually attempted before labor without anesthesia. By manipulation through the abdominal and uterine walls, a change in the polarity of the fetus (usually breech to vertex presentation) is often possible.

The patient's abdomen may be powdered so that the hands will move easily over it. The patient lies in the deep Trendelenburg position. Without excessive force, try to bring the fetus around by pushing the breech upward while deflecting the vertex in the other direction. This helps to maintain flexion of the head. The fetus may turn in a somersault movement.

The uterus must be relaxed.

If the fetal heart tones indicate distress, terminate attempts at version; if they do not improve, return the fetus to its original presentation. A short cord or tightening of coils or loops of cord may embarrass fetal circulation during attempted version.

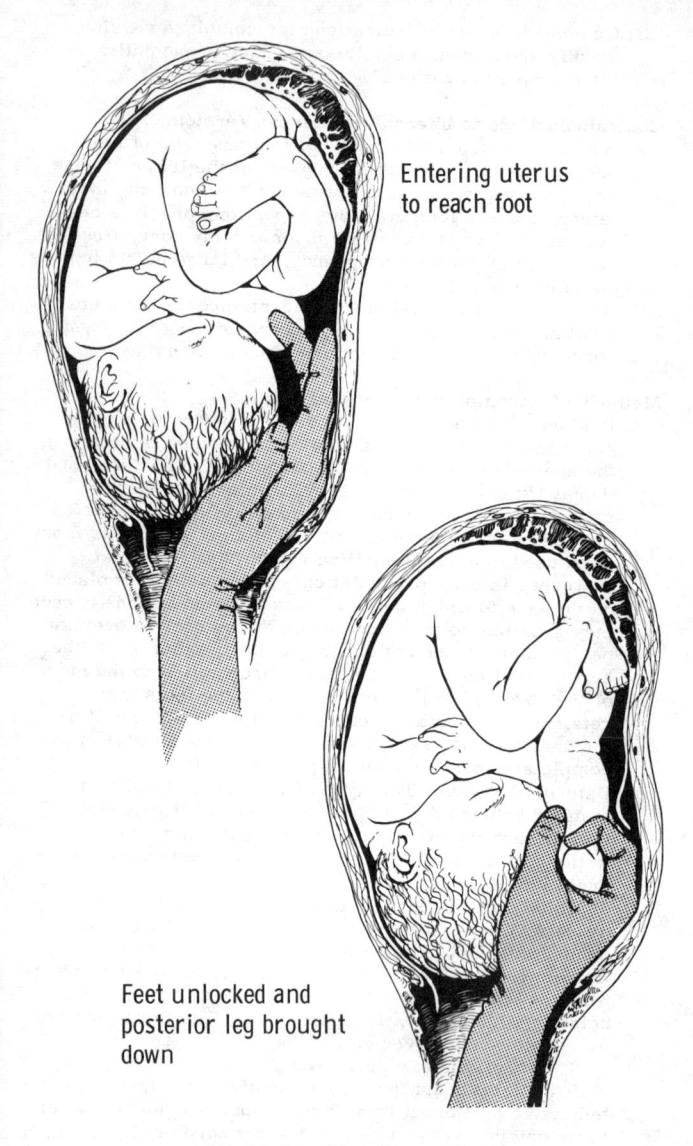

Fig 14-14. Podalic version.

Version 377

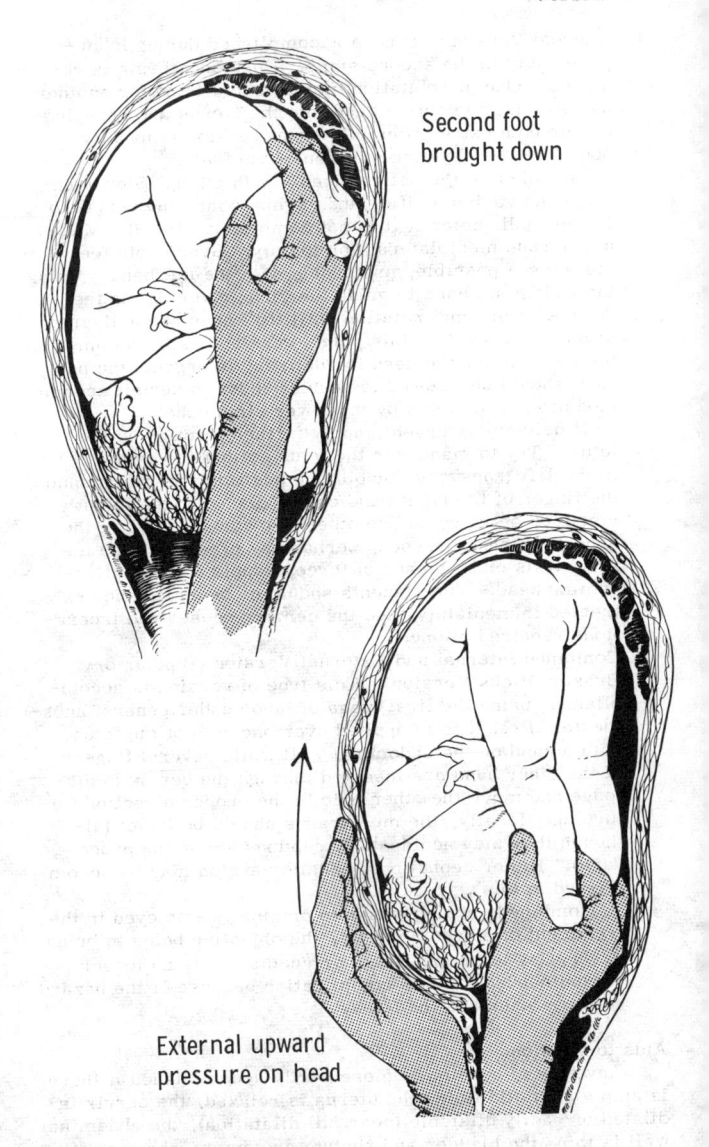

Second foot brought down

External upward pressure on head

Fig 14-14. Podalic version (cont'd.).

C. **Internal Version:** This is accomplished during labor—preferably in the second stage. Deep anesthesia is required. One presentation may be substituted for another by inserting the entire hand into the uterus and grasping one or both extremities. Internal version is usually podalic, i.e., by manipulation of the feet.

Anesthetize the patient deeply with ether. Slowly enlarge the vaginal orifice and vagina; widen the cervix to 10 cm in diameter if it is not completely dilated. Make a generous mediolateral episiotomy. Grasp both feet of the fetus if possible, preferably with the left hand. Using the abdominal hand to guide the turning, bring the feet down with internal rotation until the knees are delivered at the introitus. At this point, version has been completed. Unless the need for delivery is urgent, the patient should be allowed to resume labor to permit accommodation of the fetus by the lower birth canal.

If delivery is urgent, apply further traction on the fetus. Try to maneuver the fetus so that the chin will be in the left transverse or oblique position. In this manner, the finger of the right hand can be placed in the infant's mouth or delivery can be otherwise expedited while the head is being expressed, perhaps by pressure over the symphysis or by means of forceps applied to the aftercoming head. The placenta should be separated and extracted immediately, and the cervix exposed and lacerations repaired at once.

D. **Combined Internal and External Version (Bipolar or Braxton Hicks Version):** This type of version is accomplished during the first stage of labor under general anesthesia. Pressure is applied over one pole of the fetus with a hand on the abdominal wall while several fingers of the other hand are inserted through the cervix to dislodge and move the other pole in the proper direction for turning. Ideally, the membranes should be intact (although they may accidentally rupture during the procedure). Either cephalic or podalic version may be accomplished in this way.

Combined version was also originally employed in the treatment of placenta previa, the objective being to bring down a leg to tamponade the placenta. It is no longer recommended for this complication because of the hazard to the mother and the fetus.

Aids to Version.

Any type of version is more easily accomplished if there is ample amniotic fluid, the uterus is relaxed, the cervix is dilated or easily dilatable (near full dilatation), the abdominal wall is thin, the bladder and rectum are empty, the legs of the fetus are flexed, the physician has had adequate operative experience, and anesthesia is adequate.

Complications & Prognosis.

Internal version and breech extraction are associated with a 5-25% fetal death rate. Hemorrhage and asphyxia are the usual causes of death. Neural damage, fractures, dislocations, and epiphysial separation may complicate the course of survivors.

Maternal mortality in internal version is 1-2% in cases where indications are clear. Rupture of the uterus, hemorrhage, and shock are the most common causes of maternal death. Women who survive often sustain severe lacerations of the birth canal with excessive blood loss.

BREECH PRESENTATION

The presentation of the caudal pole of the fetus over the pelvic inlet or lower, within the birth canal, is called a breech presentation. There are 3 types—frank, complete, and incomplete (see Fig 14-15).

Fetal polarity is largely determined by the adaptation, attitude, and size of the fetus in relation to the volume and shape of the amniotic sac. Relatively more primaparas than multiparas deliver babies by the breech. Breech presentation is common until about the 32nd week of pregnancy, when the frequency declines. Only slightly over 2% of term infants are breech births. The perinatal mortality and morbidity and the maternal morbidity rates in breech delivery are much higher than with vertex (occipital) presentations. Breech presentation is therefore considered to be an unfavorable one and a cause of dystocia.

Contrary to former belief, the incidence of breech presentation is not increased in advanced multiparity, placenta previa, polyhydramnios, contracted pelvis, or pelvic tumor. The following factors are probable or possible causes of breech presentation:

(1) Accommodation: The implantation site is a major determinant of the shape of the amniotic sac. In most cases of breech presentation, the placenta occupies the cornual region of the uterus. In such instances, the breech seems to seek more commodious space (the lower portion of the uterine cavity); the head must then occupy the smaller, upper portion.

(2) Extension of the legs of the fetus: Flexion of the thighs on the abdomen and extension of the lower legs, as in frank breech presentation, discourages spontaneous or external version.

(3) The size of the fetus in relation to available intrauterine space: Children born by the breech at term are generally smaller than those delivered by the vertex.

(4) Fetal or maternal abnormality: Large congenital goiter, hydrocephalus, and uterus subseptus are frequently associated with breech presentation.

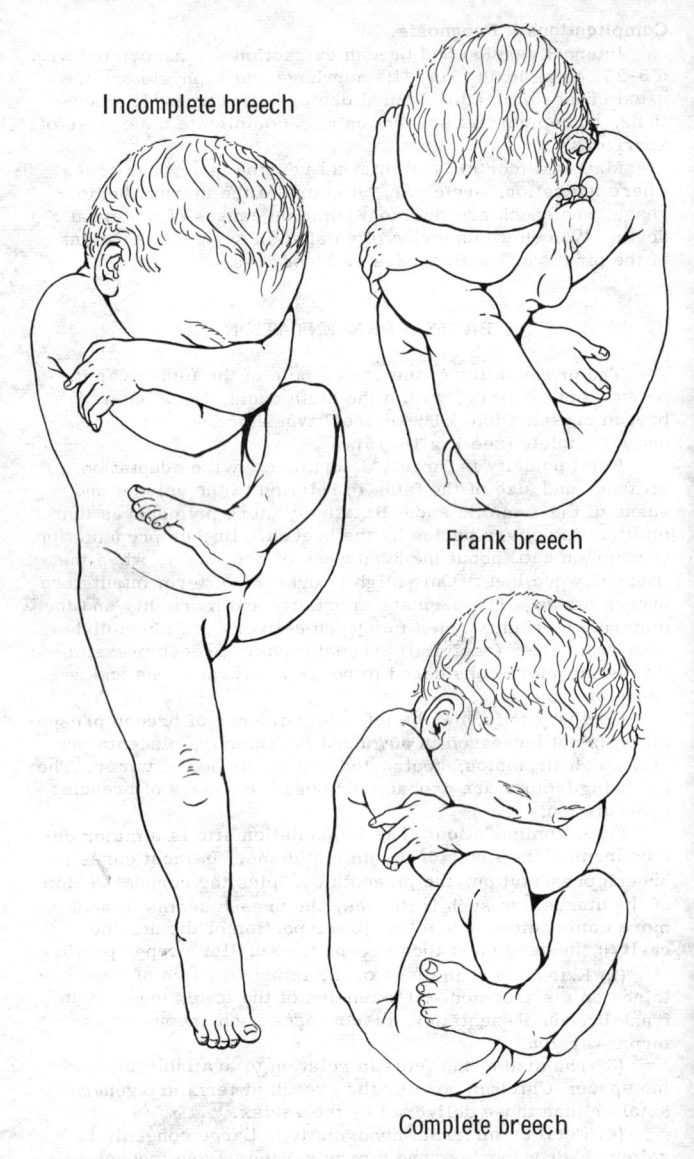

Fig 14-15. Types of breech presentation.

(5) Increased tone and firm contractions of the uterus: An original breech usually changes to a vertex presentation only once. In the last trimester, spontaneous version may be impeded when pronounced, early uterine activity occurs well before term. As a consequence, the uterine (and abdominal) wall may be tight when the amount of amniotic fluid is relatively small.

In breech presentations the presenting part does not fit or fill the pelvis as well as the vertex. Delayed engagement and premature rupture of the membranes may occur and may cause intrapartal and postpartal infection. Furthermore, the greater likelihood of operative intervention with breech presentation exposes the gravida to a greater risk of injury, hemorrhage, shock, and infection.

There is no significant difference between the length of the first stage of labor in breech and vertex presentations, nor does the position of the breech affect the length of most labors. Nevertheless, the percentage of abnormal labors is at least 3-5 times higher in breech presentations.

The second stage of labor is generally longer, especially in the frank breech. Labor is shorter with the footling than with other breech presentations, however. In the third stage of labor, blood loss is generally greater, especially in multiparas, because of uterine atony.

Breech Types.
A. Frank (Single) Breech: The legs are extended over the abdomen and thorax so that the feet lie lateral to the face.
B. Complete (Double) Breech: The so-called fetal position is maintained with the legs flexed and crossed.
C. Incomplete Breech: Prolapse of one or both lower legs and feet (or one or both knees) into the vagina may occur. The footling or knee (single or double) presentations are subdivisions of incomplete breech.

Breech Positions.
The relationship between the fetal sacrum and the side of the mother's pelvis toward which it is directed determines the position of the breech. The point of the sacrum and the genital crease are used for orientation. Six positions are possible, as shown in Fig 5-6, pp. 114 and 115.

Diagnosis.
A. Abdominal Palpation and Auscultation: (See Leopold's maneuvers, p. 107.) On abdominal examination the upper pole of the fetus is globular, firm, and ballottable (if the patient is not excessively obese and the uterus is not contractile, tender, or distorted by tumor) The fetal back or dorsum is identified on one side (RSA, LSA),

and the small parts are on the opposite side. Invariably, the lower fetal pole is less distinct, especially if engagement has occurred.

The fetal heart tones will be heard near the midline, slightly above and to one side of the umbilicus—usually higher in the abdomen than in vertex presentations.

B. Vaginal Examination: Vaginal examination may permit palpation of the presenting part, particularly when the cervix is slightly dilated and the membranes are ruptured. Specific identification of frank, complete, or incomplete breech presentation may also be possible.

When the breech presents, insert a finger through the cervix to feel a soft, smooth, irregularly-rounded surface (genitalia) with a dimpled depression (anus) nearby. The finger may be gently inserted into the anus and will be stained by meconium. The genital cleft or crease separates the pudendum from the sacrum (the point of reference for position) and the symphysis. Lateral to the anus it may be possible to palpate 2 rounded, bony landmarks (tuberosities of the ischium) for further orientation. One or both feet are usually felt opposite the sacrum in complete or incomplete breech.

C. X-Ray Examination: In case of poor patient cooperation or anxiety, roentgenography may provide the diagnosis in breech presentation. X-ray films are often the last resort in the diagnosis of breech in polyhydramnios, anencephaly, obesity, and pelvic tumor.

Fetometry in breech presentation is difficult, even with stereopelvimetry. However, it is possible to x-ray the fetal head in the fundus by the isometric technic if the metal centimeter ruler is placed externally beside the fetal head. Unless the skull is fixed in the oblique position, fairly accurate measurements may be made in this manner.

Differential Diagnosis.

Vaginal examination is essential. Do not depend upon rectal examination for more than an estimation of the station of the presenting breech. X-ray examination may be necessary for a positive diagnosis.

A. Face presentation is often difficult to distinguish from a breech. If breech presentation is suspected, palpate the mother's abdomen carefully to identify the head in the uterine fundus. On vaginal examination, note that the genital crease is midway between and perpendicular to a line joining the ischial tuberosities. In a face presentation, the mouth parallels the malar ridges. Further, the saddle of the nose and the alae of the nostrils are characteristic.

B. Fetal anomalies such as anencephaly presenting by the vertex may be confused with a breech or face. Virtually

no landmarks are felt through the cervix in anencephaly because the calvaria is missing. The soft, irregular vault may be particularly perplexing. Fetal inactivity, polyhydramnios, and postmaturity are signs of anencephaly.
C. A high shoulder presentation may be mistaken for a breech. Vaginal examination generally reveals the parallel ridges of the rib cage, the closed angle of the axilla at the shoulder, and the palpable characteristics of the face.
D. A hand or a foot (or both) may accompany an unengaged breech or vertex. The differentiation between a fetal hand and a foot is easy since the great toe parallels the others but the thumb is at an angle to the fingers. In addition, a line drawn across the tips of the fingers forms a curve, whereas a line across the tips of the toes is straight. Moreover, the foot has a raised heel and the hand does not; and, finally, the thumb is readily supinated across the palm but the great toe cannot be drawn over the sole.

Complications.

Lacerations of the birth canal, hemorrhage, shock, and subsequent infection commonly occur following breech delivery, particularly when surgical procedures such as complete breech extraction are required. Fetal complications include asphyxia and birth trauma.

Prolapse of the cord occurs in 5% of breech presentations (10 times the incidence in vertex presentations). Shoulder dystocia, single or double nuchal arm (also called nuchal hitch), and dystocia of the aftercoming head (extension, hyper-rotation) may be especially serious in breech presentations. However, the size and plasticity of the normal fetal cranium is not a cause of dystocia in breech presentation.

Fractures of the skull, clavicle, and humerus, dislocation of the hip, epiphysial separation, nerve damage due to hemorrhage, and spinal and nerve plexus traction occur much more often with breech than with vertex delivery. The optimal size for a breech baby is 2700-3400 gm (6-7 1/2 lb). Smaller or larger infants are exposed to a much greater risk of injury during delivery.

Aspiration pneumonia, omphalitis, and septicemia often result from premature rupture of the membranes or too frequent examinations in problem breech presentations.

Permanent wryneck may occur as a complication of breech delivery. In some cases, hemorrhage occurs into the sternocleidomastoid muscle with subsequent fibrosis and contracture.

Obstetric Management of Breech Delivery.

If possible, breech delivery should be performed in a well-equipped hospital by a specialist in obstetrics who is prepared to remain with the mother throughout labor and delivery.

An anesthesiologist and other professional assistants must also be available at all times.

Delivery may be accomplished in the following ways: Spontaneous breech delivery (15% of cases of breech presentation), assisted breech delivery (55%), partial breech extraction (extraction of the shoulders and head), forceps to the aftercoming head, complete breech extraction ("break-up" of the breech)(10%), or cesarean section (10%).

Avoid artificial rupture of the membranes, but examine the patient vaginally immediately after spontaneous rupture and at the onset of labor to rule out prolapse of the cord and to confirm the presentation and position. The fetal heart tones must be monitored during labor for signs of fetal distress.

A trial of labor is not possible with breech presentation. Therefore, it must be decided early in labor whether vaginal delivery is likely or whether cesarean section will be necessary. Four factors aid in the decision: (1) pelvic size, (2) pelvic architecture, (3) estimated fetal weight, and (4) quality of labor. X-ray studies (including pelvimetry) will serve for (1) and (2). If the true conjugate is less than 10 cm, vaginal delivery of an infant of average size or larger probably will not be possible. Fetal size can be estimated by McDonald's rule (see p. 48) and by averaging the estimates of several qualified examiners.

If labor is permitted, conservative management is indicated during the first stage. During the second stage, interfere as little and as late as possible.

A. Spontaneous Breech Delivery: Completely spontaneous (unassisted) breech delivery of a normal, living infant at term is rare, although prematures are often born unattended. Because of the many hazards involved, some aid to the fetus should be provided.

B. Assisted Breech Delivery: No matter how the remainder of the breech delivery is to be managed, a short loop of cord must be loosened and drawn down as soon as the umbilicus comes into view. This avoids later umbilical traction and injury and cord compression.

Bracht's method of assisted breech delivery is recommended. When the scapulas are visible, gently lift the infant's back toward the mother's abdomen. (Do not overextend the back, or spinal injury may result.) The arms will usually emerge spontaneously. Apply suprapubic pressure to force the head into the pelvis. The chin, mouth, nose, and brow emerge from the vagina spontaneously. The advantages of Bracht's method are that it involves no intravaginal manipulation, no traction on the infant's body or neck, and no forced rotation of the infant's thorax. The method is contraindicated by abnormal rotation of the fetus (back caudad), difficult position of the arms, abnormalities of the pelvis and soft parts (e.g., perineal rigidity), and weak uterine contractions, and cannot be successful unless the mother cooperates. Bracht's method should be abandoned in favor of extraction if the infant makes vigorous attempts to breathe before it is delivered.

C. Partial Breech Extraction: Nitrous oxide or trilene inhalation analgesia is permissible during the second stage, but regional anesthesia must be withheld (if possible) until the breech is crowning. A long mediolateral episiotomy incision is then made, preferably under pudendal block anesthesia. Do not give spinal anesthesia until a multipara is 8 cm dilated or a primigravida is fully dilated with the breech on the perineum.

Lubricate the vagina well with sterile vaginal jelly. Allow the fetus to deliver to the umbilicus spontaneously, and then proceed without delay.

Wrap a towel around the infant's thighs and trunk for better grasp during manipulation. Slowly draw the thighs downward (not outward); grasp the pelvis with the thumbs over the sacrum (not higher, or renal or adrenal injury may result); and apply traction and slight lateral rotation. When the scapulas are visible, complete the rotation of the infant laterally to bring the bisacromial diameter of its shoulders into the AP diameter of the mother's pelvis.

To deliver the first arm and shoulder, insert one or 2 fingers into the posterior vagina and sweep the posterior arm and shoulder out of the birth canal; then depress the trunk in the lateral position against the perineum while applying traction to the thighs. The anterior shoulder and arm will usually come beneath the symphysis for spontaneous delivery. Pressure applied medially over the angle of the exposed scapula may bring down the arm, or the arm may be swept out over the chest with the forefinger. The forefinger should be applied to the humerus in a parallel position, as a splint—not at a right angle, as a hook, in order to avoid fracturing the humerus.

Groin traction is then applied as follows: Hook one finger into the angle of the leg flexed on the abdomen of the frank breech if slight traction is needed. Apply force downward and slightly backward (as with traction forceps) during uterine contractions or combined with pressure over the fundus to dislodge an impacted breech, then rotate the infant slightly so the back will be upward when delivered.

Note: Never use more than one finger for fear of dislocating the hip. The anterior groin is usually the more accessible. It is usually not practical to hook fingers into both groins. Use a metal hook for traction only if the fetus is dead. Do not attempt to apply forceps to the breech; they will not hold.

386 Breech Presentation

Bringing down anterior foot

Delivery of anterior hip

Delivery of posterior foot

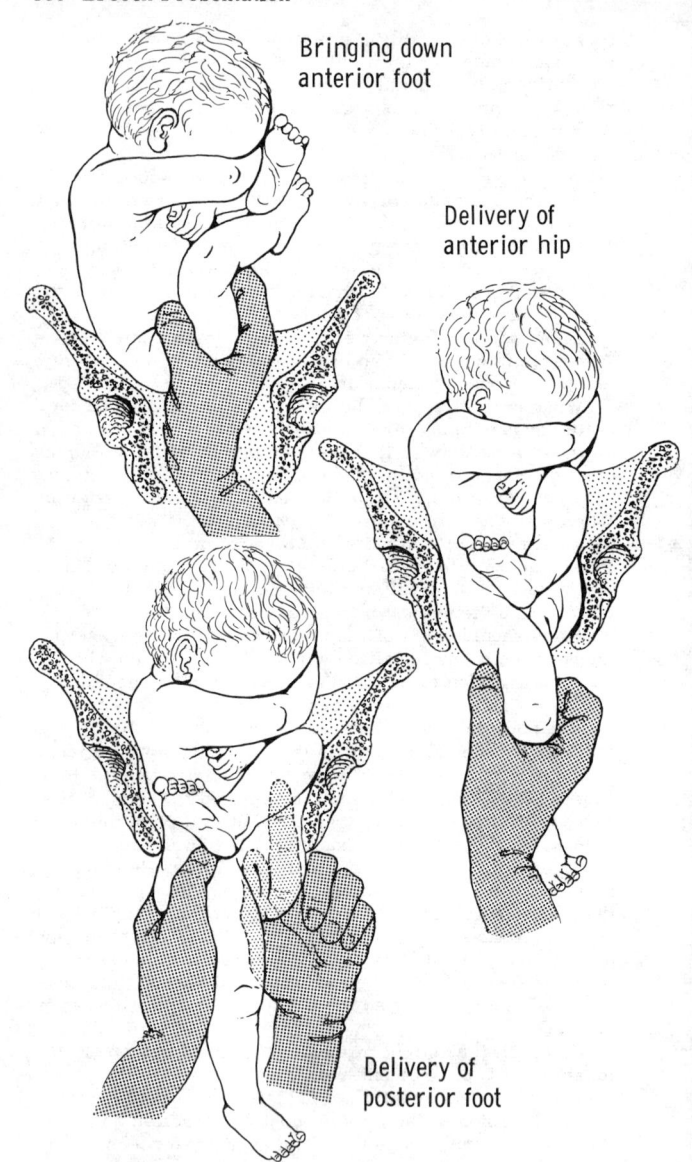

Fig 14-16. Breech delivery.

Breech Presentation 387

Descent and expulsion of breech

Delivery of posterior shoulder

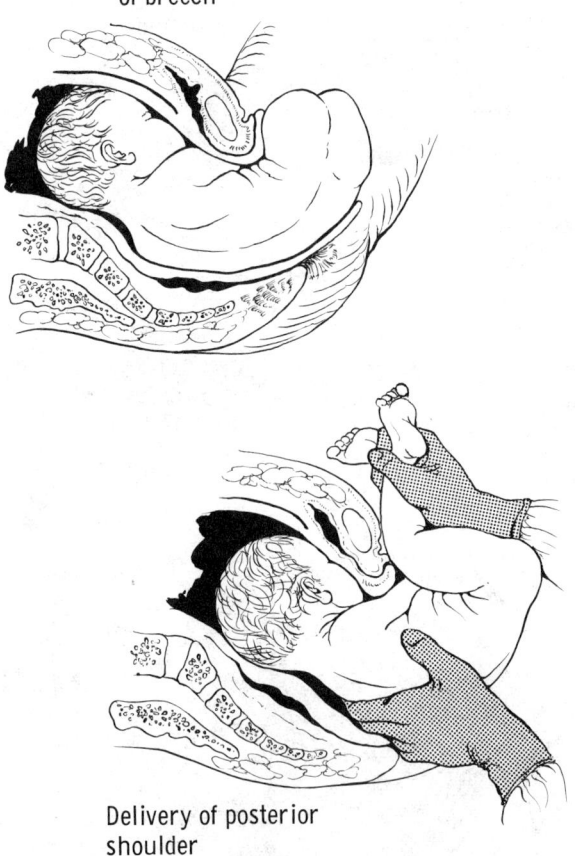

Fig 14-16. Breech delivery (cont'd.).

388 Breech Presentation

Delivery of anterior shoulder

Wigand

Mauriceau

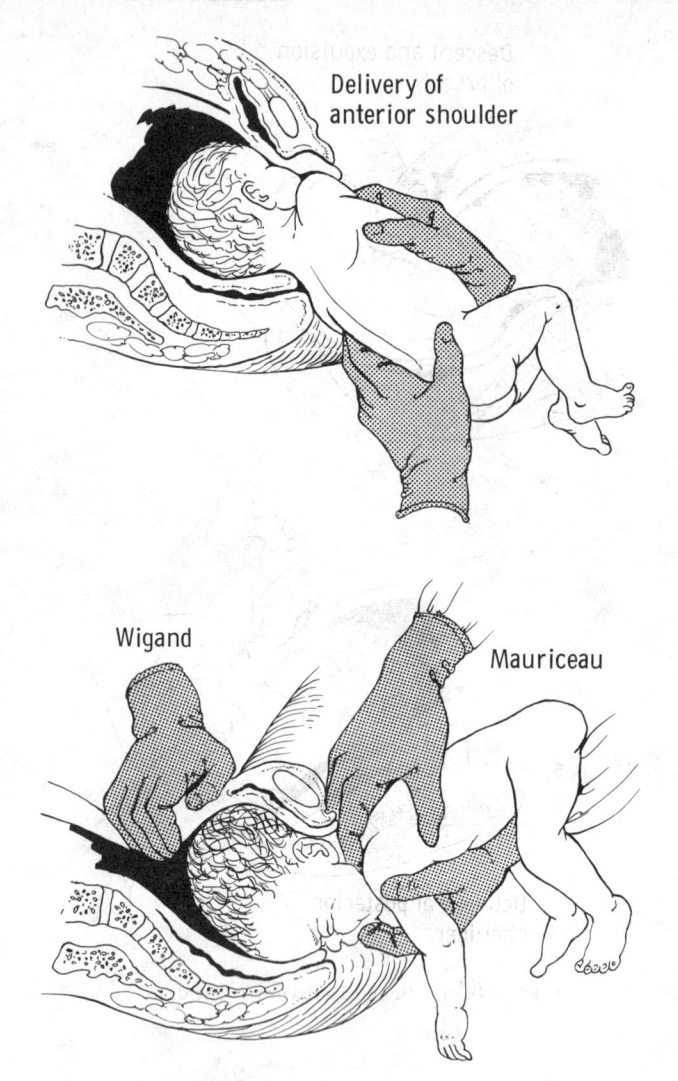

Fig 14-16. Breech delivery (cont'd.).

Delivery of the aftercoming head may be accomplished in several ways. **Wigand's method** is to hold the infant astride the left arm, insert 2 fingers of the left hand into the infant's mouth (or over the mandible) to direct the head to the pelvic AP or oblique diameter for delivery (also maintaining flexion of the head), and apply strong pressure with the right hand over the patient's symphysis to deliver the head. This avoids traction on the infant's shoulders. **Mauriceau's method** is to rotate the head to the OA position, support the infant on the left arm, insert the first 2 fingers of the left hand into the infant's mouth (or over the mandible) to flex the head, place the right hand over the infant's back with one or more fingers curved over the shoulders, and guide delivery with the right hand, using no traction, until the chin is born. An assistant then applies suprapubic pressure. The body is then elevated and delivery guided without using traction on the shoulders or excessive force. Holding the jaw to flex the head, the occiput is then delivered from beneath the symphysis.

The **Prague method** is applicable only when the occiput is directly posterior. This position is unusual and unfortunate. It is usually possible to rotate the fetus so that its occiput and back are anterior for delivery by the less traumatic Wigand or Mauriceau method. The procedure is to slip a finger into the infant's mouth before the head extends, and gently draw its jaw downward. This makes it possible to use the chin as a fulcrum for the head. The infant's body is then elevated, whereupon the face and brow should slowly come beneath the symphysis and the occiput should deliver over the perineum. If the head extends and the chin lodges behind the symphysis before the finger can be introduced into the infant's mouth, slip the left hand into the posterior vagina along the infant's back to its neck; hook the fingers over the infant's shoulders and apply gentle traction in the axis of the birth canal; elevate the infant's body in an arc high over the mother's lower abdomen; and ease the occiput out over the perineum.

D. Forceps to the Aftercoming Head: See p. 390.

E. Complete Breech Extraction: This operative procedure is employed for relief of dystocia due to a nuchal arm (or arms), delivery on an urgent indication after internal podalic version, fetal distress (heart rate less than 100/minute or very irregular), maternal exhaustion or failure to cooperate, and maternal complications such as heart disease (class III) or active pulmonary tuberculosis. Pelvic contraction, constriction of the vagina, or marked scarring of the pudendum are absolute contraindications to complete breech extraction. The procedure is relatively contraindicated if the fetus is over 4000 gm (8 lb 13 oz), the mother is an elderly primigravida, or if primary deflection of the head is present. Complete relaxation of

390 Breech Presentation

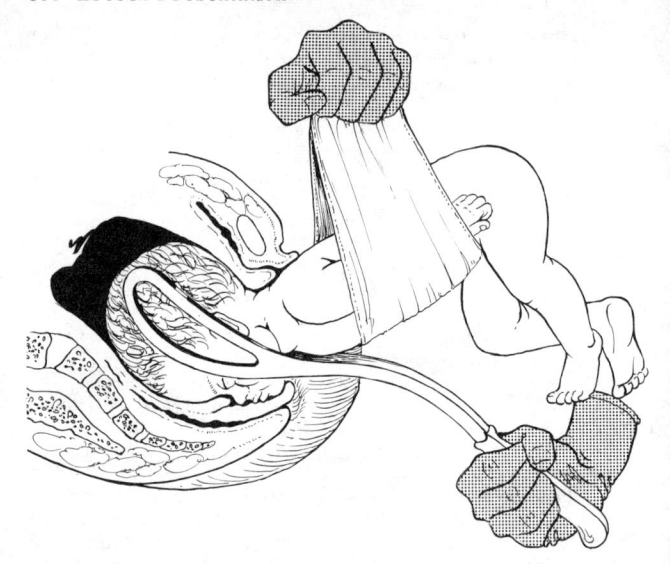

Fig 14-17. Application of Piper forceps and towel-sling support in breech delivery (Savage).

the uterus and cessation of uterine contractions are essential and require general anesthesia.

Dystocia due to persistent sacroanterior position of a frank breech is a serious problem. The legs of the fetus lie on opposite sides of the maternal spinal column. With a tight uterus, the fetus is held high before and during labor. Each contraction causes bowing of the fetal spine, and labor is relatively ineffective and engagement is delayed. Treatment entails early suspicion of the cause of dystocia, x-ray confirmation of the presentation and position, and complete breech extraction.

Pinard's maneuver to flex the extended legs in a frank breech is best done when the breech is not deeply engaged. Introduce a hand into the vagina (right hand if the fetal back is to the mother's right; left hand if the back is to the left); displace the breech out of the pelvis. Identify the anterior thigh of the fetus. Pass the fingers up along the inner aspect of the baby's thigh to the knee. Abduct the thigh, causing the leg to flex at the knee, and ensure adequate flexion with the index finger pressed into the popliteal space and the second finger triggered over the tibia and fibula. Grasp the foot and apply downward traction in the axis of the vagina. Try to get hold of the second foot in a similar manner if this is not too difficult.

F. Cesarean Section: Any significant complication of pregnancy or labor which constitutes an indication for cesarean section in the interest of the baby in vertex presentation is even more valid in the breech. Cesarean section is indicated for delivery of the fetus presenting by the breech in instances of definite fetopelvic disproportion; desultory, prolonged labor which does not progress despite stimulation; prolapse of the umbilical cord before the cervix is fully dilated or dilatable; severe premature separation of the placenta or placenta previa; or if an elderly primigravida must be delivered of a large term fetus.

Management of Special Problems.

A. Delivery of the Hydrocephalic Breech: **Danforth's method** of delivering a hydrocephalic infant in breech presentation is as follows: Deliver the breech and shoulders but do not engage the head too deeply. Rotate the back anteriorly. Visualize and palpate the 2 highest spinous processes, using a right-angled retractor beneath the urethra and bladder. Incise the skin over these spinous processes with a scalpel, and do a laminectomy. Introduce the tip of a uterine dressing forceps into the opening into the spinal canal; force the instrument up into the cranial cavity; and rotate the forceps to enlarge the tract. Apply pressure on the head from above to drain cerebrospinal fluid from the laminectomy site. Deliver the head when it decompresses.

An alternative is to deliver the breech, trunk, and shoulders and deeply engage the head; palpate the fetal foramen magnum with a long, large trochar; insert the trochar and allow steady decompression of the head; and deliver the head when its volume is adequately reduced.

B. Outlet Dystocia of the Aftercoming Head: Very rarely, miscalculation of the cephalopelvic relationships may lead to obstruction of a nonhydrocephalic aftercoming head at the outlet. When the Pinard and other methods fail, symphysiotomy may offer the only escape for the fetus from a desperate situation. The alternatives are a traumatic forceps extraction of a baby which will probably be too damaged to survive, or a craniotomy.

Prognosis.

If the mother is a primigravida, if the fetus is large, or if the presentation is complete breech, the prognosis for delivery of an undamaged infant is poor. The prognosis is improved if the mechanism of labor is normal, especially if rapid dilatation and effacement of the cervix occur. In most hospitals, the gross fetal mortality in breech deliveries is 10-20%. Excluding babies weighing less than 2500 gm (5 lb 8 oz), this figure is corrected to 5-6%.

Although the maternal mortality rate in breech presentation approximates that in vertex presentation, maternal morbidity is increased in proportion to the degree of operative intervention necessary.

Breech presentation recurs in 20% of cases.

CESAREAN SECTION

Cesarean section consists of delivery through an incision in the uterine wall. (The term does not include transabdominal recovery of a fetus extruded through a laceration or rupture of the uterus.) The surgical approach is usually abdominal, although vaginal cesarean section is also done. Five types of abdominal cesarean section are recognized: (1) classical (Sanger), (2) low cervical (laparotrachelotomy of Krönig and DeLee), (3) peritoneal exclusion (Hirst), (4) extraperitoneal (Physick), and (5) cesarean section followed by hysterectomy (Porro).

Cesarean section performed on valid indications will often preserve the life and health of the patient and the infant. However, no major operative procedure is without hazard, and cesarean delivery should not be employed without good reason.

The incidence of this operation varies from 2-10%, being highest in communities where deformed or contracted pelves are prevalent or where subsequent abdominal deliveries are done on the dictum of "once a cesarean, always a cesarean." Repeat cesarean sections account for 15-40% of all cesarean sections in large cities in the USA.

Indications.

The indications for cesarean section may be permanent or temporary. The indications should be single and clear. Combinations of factors, each of which separately would be insufficient to justify the operation, constitute a weak motive.
A. Maternal Indications:
 1. Fetopelvic disproportion, usually after a trial of labor in vertex presentations, is the most common indication for abdominal cesarean section.
 2. Potentially weak uterine scar after myomectomy, unification operation, or prior cesarean section. Dehiscence of the previous cesarean section uterine incision site occurs in 1-3% of cases.
 3. Placenta previa covering 30% or more of the cervix.
 4. Abruptio placentae with marked antepartal bleeding.
 5. Primary uterine inertia or desultory or prolonged labor despite stimulation.
 6. Ruptured uterus (an abdominal emergency).
 7. Pelvic tumors which obstruct the birth canal or weaken the uterine wall.
 8. Abnormal presentation (transverse, shoulder, posterior face).

9. Fulminating toxemia (progressive preeclampsia or eclampsia which recurs after temporary control).
10. Serious maternal problems such as previous vesicovaginal fistula or carcinoma of the cervix.

B. Fetal Indications: The fetal indications for cesarean section are only occasionally imperative.
  1. Fetal distress is recorded in 1-2% of maternity hospital admissions. The problem is generally hypoxia due to short cord, compression of the cord, premature separation of the placenta, or placenta previa.
  2. Diabetes mellitus - Cesarean section is now done to terminate pregnancy in 35-50% of cases involving diabetic women. Early delivery helps reduce the high incidence of intrapartal and postnatal death.
  3. Isoimmunization - Cesarean section is done in an effort to prevent possible fetal death in utero or irreparable damage to the infant from icterus gravis or hydrops fetalis in Rh and ABO sensitization of the mother.
  4. Prolapse of the cord in early labor, especially in the primigravida.
  5. High premium on the baby, e.g., elderly primigravida with complications, numerous advanced pregnancies without living children.

Types.

A. Classical: This operation is indicated in placenta previa (to avoid the vascular lower uterine segment and the placenta itself) and in obstetric emergencies such as abruptio placentae and prolapsed cord when speed of delivery is essential.

  A vertical incision is made through the visceral peritoneum and extended through the contractile portion of the corpus. The incidence should be less than 15%.

  1. Advantages - The classical operation is the simplest cesarean section to perform, and can be done under local infiltration anesthesia. Rapid entry and extraction of the fetus is possible.
  2. Disadvantages - Bleeding from the thick, vascular uterine wall is marked. Good peritonealization of the uterine scar is impossible; bowel adhesions to the corpus scar may cause intestinal obstruction. Faulty healing of the myometrium often occurs. Sinus formation and leakage of infected uterine cavity fluid into the peritoneal cavity is common. Rupture of the scar in subsequent pregnancies occurs in 1-2% of cases.

B. Low Cervical: The low segment operation is the best general purpose cesarean section. The visceral peritoneum over the uterus is incised at the bladder reflection. An upper and lower peritoneal flap is developed. The bladder is separated from its loose attachment to the anterior uterine wall and is displaced downward. A vertical or transverse incision is made through the thin lower uterine segment of the uterus several centimeters inferior to the initial entry through the visceral peritoneum. After delivery of the fetus, the uterine wall is closed in layers and the peritoneal flaps are secured. Thus, the bladder covers the uterine incision. This type of operation is chosen in over 70% of cases in modern hospitals. An even higher percentage is warranted.

1. Advantages - The danger of drainage of infected fluid from the uterine into the peritoneal cavity after delivery is minimized. The bladder wall and a peritoneal flap covers the uterine scar, so that the likelihood of secondary intraperitoneal drainage and peritonitis is reduced. Blood loss is lessened because the lower uterine segment is thinner and less vascular than the fundus. Omental and bowel adhesion to the uterine scar is prevented. Delivery is reasonably safe even if it must be delayed for 24 hours after rupture of the membranes (potential or subclinical intrauterine infection). The postoperative course is smoother than after classical cesarean section. Less packing-off of bowel and manipulation of the intestines are necessary.

2. Disadvantages - The operation is slightly more difficult and takes longer than the classical operation (especially in repeat cesarean sections). A placenta previa or low-lying placenta attached to the anterior uterine wall may be torn at entry. Marked maternal and fetal blood loss may occur. A low segment incision may extend to lacerate large vessels laterally (with a transverse incision), or may tear downward into the bladder and cervix (when the incision is vertical). A 10% occurrence of placenta previa over the lower segment scar must be anticipated (3 times the normal rate of low implantation). A retrovesical hematoma or abscess, or a rare vesicouterine or vesicoperitoneal fistula, may result. The scar will rupture in subsequent pregnancies in approximately 0.5-1% of cases.

C. Extraperitoneal: Extraperitoneal cesarean section may be employed in neglected frankly infected problem cases, although low cervical cesarean section and broad-spectrum antibiotics and blood replacement give results almost as good. A paravesical (Latzko or Norton) or retrovesical (Waters) incision into the uterus is made, avoiding the peritoneal cavity and bladder. The operation is best done after several hours or more of labor, so that definite planes of cleavage can be identified.

1. Advantages - Theoretically, extraperitoneal section is the ideal cesarean operation. Peritonitis secondary

to spill of infected amniotic fluid and blood into the peritoneal cavity is avoided. The operation is feasible even after dystocia associated with prolonged labor, prolonged rupture of the membranes, and frank amnionitis. Pneumoperitoneum never occurs, and ileus is rare. The postoperative course is often smoother than after a transperitoneal operation. The uterus need not be sacrificed.

2. Disadvantages - The operation is difficult, and peritoneal, bladder, and ureteral injury occasionally occur even when the surgeon is skilled in the technic. The operation is not practical before term, and peritonitis and thrombophlebitis may occur when an infected uterus is retained. Postoperative uterine bleeding may be difficult to control.

D. Peritoneal Exclusion: This operation may be chosen by the physician with inadequate experience in the extraperitoneal operation when cesarean section is required after the membranes have been ruptured for over 24 hours, or when intrauterine infection is known to be present. The operation has been infrequently used since the antibiotics and the extraperitoneal procedure became available.

Prior to incision of the uterus, the parietal and visceral peritoneal surfaces are sutured together in an attempt to prevent contamination of the peritoneal cavity with infected material from the uterus.

1. Advantages - Peritoneal exclusion is technically simple and usually restricts intrapartal infection to the uterus. If suppuration occurs, drainage will usually be extraperitoneal.

2. Disadvantages - Infection from the uterus may involve the peritoneal cavity despite suture closure since a peritoneal seal is virtually impossible to achieve. The procedure also requires more time than the other operations available. In spite of its theoretical advantages, peritoneal exclusion has not reduced maternal morbidity or mortality appreciably.

E. Cesarean Hysterectomy: Subtotal cesarean hysterectomy (removing only the uterus) and total hysterectomy (removing the cervix also) are usually done after classical or low segment cesarean section. In certain unusual cases such as those involving fetal death or intrapartal infection, the uterus containing the fetus may be excised unopened and the infant then delivered through an incision in the uterine wall. The operation may be done on urgent grounds, e.g., in the treatment of rupture of the uterus and placenta accreta; or electively, e.g., in the treatment of myomas and as a means of sterilization.

Cesarean hysterectomy is becoming a popular procedure, especially for sterilization. The majority of these operations are now done electively. Total cesarean hysterectomy is gradually supplanting the subtotal procedure because it eliminates the possibility of future carcinoma of the cervix, but at least two-thirds of cesarean hysterectomies are still subtotal.

The complications of cesarean hysterectomy are hemorrhage, shock, hypofibrinogenemia, and urinary tract injury. These problems are often referable to the original problem (e.g., rupture of the uterus) for which the operation was done.

Elective total cesarean hysterectomy carries a lower maternal mortality and morbidity than the urgently indicated operation, but only those surgeons who are skilled in performing this operation should undertake it. Tubal ligation is a far less formidable procedure.

1. Advantages - The operation removes the source of infection in intrapartal infection; eliminates the uterus and cervix as sources of abnormal bleeding, pain, and tumor formation; reduces risk of postoperative hemorrhage from an atonic uterus; prevents uterine pregnancy; and obviates a delayed second operation (hysterectomy).
2. Disadvantages - Cesarean hysterectomy is more complicated and more hazardous than cesarean section plus tubal ligation. Contamination of the peritoneal cavity may occur despite avoidance of gross spill and removal of the uterus. As with any type of hysterectomy, emotional crises may arise due to loss of menstrual function, and the elimination of menstrual function and fertility are of course irreversible.

F. Vaginal Cesarean Section: Vaginal cesarean section may be performed for early termination of pregnancy in cases of fetal death or anomaly before complete dilation of the cervix. The operation is actually an anterior vaginal hysterotomy done in late pregnancy. Abdominal surgery may be hazardous for the mother, and the recovery of a normal infant is a remote or impossible objective in such cases. The operation is often very difficult to accomplish after the 32nd week, and the fetal salvage is low. Vaginal cesarean section is almost never done in the USA today.

1. Advantages - The incision through the cervix and lower uterine segment is short, and blood loss is usually minimal.
2. Disadvantages - The operation is difficult to perform in the last trimester because exposure is poor and damage to the bladder may occur.

Healing of the Incision.

Theoretically, a uterine incision heals by regeneration of the muscle fibers with little or no fibroblastic response.

Unfortunately, about half of the incisions studied have healed imperfectly and have contained varying amounts of inelastic, weak scar tissue. The length and site of the incision, the accuracy of apposition of the wound edges in suturing, and the occurrence of exudation and infection all determine the quality of healing.

The strength of a uterine incision during pregnancy and labor following a previous cesarean section is commonly (but inadequately) appraised in the following ways: (1) Inquiry about the type of cesarean section performed. (A low segment operation is assumed to leave a stronger uterine wall than the classical procedure.) (2) A history of postoperative fever or the absence of fever. (Fever is presumed to relate to uterine and incisional infection. Successful primary healing is not guaranteed by a normal temperature course, however.) Tenderness over the incision and pain in the region of the surgical site may indicate dehiscence.

Actually, there is no accurate method of appraising the integrity or tensile strength of the uterine wall before or during labor. One-third to one-half of all disruptions of uterine scars occur before labor; the remainder occur during labor. Following delivery, manual exploration may disclose a definite defect, but serious damage may have already occurred.

About 1-2% of classical and 0.5-1% of low segment incisions rupture in subsequent pregnancies. The classical operation scar generally disrupts suddenly, violently, and often totally. The fetus almost always succumbs to asphyxia, and the mother may die of hemorrhage. The low segment scar usually ruptures subtly, silently, and often incompletely. In many cases a "window" is formed in the thin, scarred lower uterine segment, but the visceral peritoneum generally remains intact and bleeding is not extensive. Few babies and fewer mothers die. The rupture is discovered either at repeat cesarean section or subsequent laparotomy; after delivery at uterine exploration; or following a lateral hysterogram taken several months following delivery.

Maternal Morbidity & Mortality.

Maternal morbidity and mortality rates vary depending upon the reason for the operation; the duration of labor and the time between rupture of the membranes and surgery; the number of vaginal and rectal examinations; the effectiveness of antibiotic therapy; and the type of cesarean section chosen.

In many large hospitals in the USA, the death rate (all causes) following cesarean section is 0.1-0.2%. Maternal mortality exceeds 3% in some other areas.

Recent advances in obstetric care notwithstanding, there are still too many preventable maternal deaths following cesarean section. Many deaths occur as a result of deficient preoperative preparation, faulty surgical technic, the complications of anesthesia, errors in blood typing, inadequate blood replacement, and mismanagement of infection.

Perinatal Morbidity & Mortality.

Perinatal morbidity and mortality rates vary depending upon the status of the fetus prior to delivery, the difficulties encountered in the birth process, the development of post-delivery complications, and the quality of pediatric care.

Despite great improvements during the past decade, the perinatal mortality (including premature infants) following repeat, elective cesarean section is 2% in many hospitals. This is about twice as high as for vaginal delivery in the same institutions. Unfortunately, even in many well staffed hospitals, the perinatal mortality in all types of cesarean sections (including both first and repeat operations) is 5-6%.

A well-timed and properly executed cesarean section increases the fetal salvage rate, especially when the surgery is done for an obstetric emergency. Miscalculation of the duration of pregnancy, leading to the delivery of a premature or immature infant, is the most important single factor in perinatal death following cesarean delivery.

Cesarean section, like other obstetric operations, prolonged labor, and toxemia, reduces the fetal oxygen supply and thus contributes to fetal morbidity and mortality. However, the very complications of pregnancy and labor which make surgical delivery mandatory are themselves among the major causes of perinatal morbidity and mortality.

The causes of perinatal mortality (in order of frequency) are as follows: (1) Respiratory disorders (hypoxia, atelectasis, respiratory distress syndrome [hyaline membrane disease]). (2) Unknown causes (even after clinical and postmortem studies). (3) Fetal trauma (cerebral and other hemorrhage, neural injury, shock). (4) Infection (bacteremia, pneumonia, omphalitis). (5) Congenital anomalies incompatible with life.

Postcesarean Obstetrics.

If the problem for which the original cesarean section was done is still present (contracted pelvis, previous vesicovaginal fistula) and the fetus is of average term or larger, do a repeat (low segment) cesarean section. Because of the risk of rupture of classical incision scars, repeat elective cesarean section should be done at term or at the onset of labor during the last trimester.

If the indication for the first cesarean section no longer applies (e.g., placenta previa, prolapsed cord), a choice must be made between (1) a trial of labor, with the intention of delivering the baby vaginally if symptoms of uterine rupture do not appear; and (2) repeat cesarean section. The proponents of a trial of labor and vaginal delivery after low cervical cesarean section argue that most instances of disastrous uterine rupture occur before labor and that vaginal delivery may be safer for the mother than the complications which may occur following repeated cesarean section. It is observed that few women die of rupture of a low segment uterine scar if they receive careful observation during labor; that the maternal morbidity following repeat cesarean section is 5-10 times greater than following vaginal delivery; and that fetal morbidity and mortality rates are lower following vaginal delivery than following elective cesarean section.

A patient who has had an afebrile convalescence after a low cervical cesarean section done on a temporary indication; who has a normal pelvis; and who has had an uncomplicated subsequent pregnancy with an average sized fetus or smaller has a 70-80% likelihood of delivering successfully from below if the vertex is well engaged at term. Labor should not be induced. Low forceps extraction should be employed to avoid increased intra-abdominal pressure during the second stage of labor, and the interior of the uterus should be palpated after recovery of the placenta.

If labor is permitted after a previous cesarean section, the physician must remain in the hospital to observe his patient's progress and any indications of uterine rupture. An operating room should be ready and a full surgical team, including an anesthesiologist, must be in constant attendance. Blood for transfusion must be on hand. If these requirements cannot be met, elective repeat cesarean section is the only alternative. If signs of uterine dehiscence appear, do a classical cesarean section at once.

The proponents of repeat cesarean deliveries argue that the loss of one mother in 100-200 deliveries is a high price to pay for vaginal deliveries after cesarean section today. One may wonder whether a blind gamble on a potentially defective uterus is warranted.

Despite the fact that many women have had 6 or more cesarean sections without dehiscence of the closure, its integrity is theoretically weaker after each cesarean section. This is particularly true of the classical operation. It is therefore common practice to recommend termination of childbearing after the second section and to strongly urge tubal ligation or hysterectomy after the third.

Elective Appendectomy.

Elective appendectomy is generally a desirable and safe procedure at cesarean section unless the appendix is inaccessible or the patient's condition (hemorrhage, toxemia, infection) contraindicates the procedure. The operative time will be increased slightly, but significant complications attributable to appendectomy are rare. Not only may appendicitis be averted by this brief additional procedure, but carcinoid and other bowel problems may be reduced. The patient's consent must be obtained, and adequate anesthesia is necessary.

15...
Therapeutic Abortion & Sterilization

THERAPEUTIC ABORTION

Therapeutic abortion is the artificial termination of pregnancy during the first or second trimester. In the USA, abortion is permitted only to save the mother's life. In many instances, however, the operation is allowed to preserve her health (and ultimately, therefore, her life).

There are numerous medical and surgical indications for therapeutic abortion. The incidence varies widely; in many large medical centers it ranges from one in 75 to one in 175 deliveries. This is undoubtedly too many. Considering the advantages of modern therapy, therapeutic abortion is probably justified only about once in 500 pregnancies even in specialty practice.

Many physicians consider the laws relating to abortion (and sterilization) to be vague, inconsistent, and out-dated, and some disapprove of the omission of any fetal indication for therapeutic interruption of pregnancy. The law does not change overnight in response to the latest scientific opinion, but continues to reflect popular conceptions and prejudices even when they are clearly insupportable on logical grounds. Change, therefore, is gradual, and the physician must accommodate his practice to the legal restrictions of his community.

The assumption that interruption of a pregnancy will improve a seriously ill patient's prognosis for life is only occasionally justified. Well controlled experiments to study the effects of pregnancy on disease are not possible. Even the specialist's best judgment may therefore be only an opinion based on insufficient objective evidence.

Before contemplating therapeutic abortion, the physician must be reasonably certain that pregnancy is a threat to the mother's life and that the risks of therapeutic abortion will be less than continued pregnancy, labor, and delivery. Moreover, he must be prepared to defend his judgment before the appropriate hospital committee to whom he must apply for permission to proceed.

Unfortunately, it is difficult for a physician to be purely objective in his estimate of jeopardy to the patient by a pregnancy. Moreover, statistics are usually not helpful in establishing the prognosis in an individual case. The decision to abort a patient is always a difficult one.

In most instances, if therapeutic abortion is warranted, sterilization is indicated also. Thirty to 50% of women who are aborted become pregnant again, in many cases before resolution of the problem for which the abortion was done.

The physician should avoid mentioning therapeutic abortion to the patient or her husband until one or more expert opinions have led him to the conclusion that the pregnancy should be sacrificed. The alternatives should then be explained, whereupon the couple must decide whether to accept or reject their physician's advice. Neither the patient nor her husband should be energetically persuaded to agree to an abortion, and both should be assured of the physician's continued sympathetic care whatever their decision.

Indications.*

In the USA, therapeutic abortion is legal when, in the opinion of at least 2 licensed physicians, continuation of pregnancy jeopardizes the patient's life (or, in some states, health). Critical neuropsychiatric, renal, and cardiac disorders (in that order) are currently the most frequent indications. Hyperemesis gravidarum, epilepsy, and multiple sclerosis are no longer considered indications for therapeutic abortion.

There are no fetal indications for therapeutic abortion in the USA. It is rarely possible to predict a crippling abnormality in early pregnancy with certainty, and most severe maternal diseases have no effect upon the fetus. Abortion in these cases will undoubtedly destroy many normal fetuses merely to prevent the birth of a few abnormal or stillborn infants. Abortions done for eugenic reasons are either in defiance of the law or are "prophylactic" (to prevent the delivery of an abnormal fetus). Abortion to prevent the potentially disastrous impact of a monstrous birth on the life and health of the mother has not met with favor in the USA.

Socioeconomic factors cannot be used legally in the USA as indications for therapeutic abortion, although they often contribute to the patient's problem.

American statutes designed to limit the occurrence of medically unwarranted abortions usually do not include a reference to the patient's health. However, serious impairment of a woman's health may constitute an ultimate risk to her life, and whether avoiding such a risk actually constitutes preservation of life then becomes a matter of interpretation. (British law states that a woman must not be required to proceed to term if her health will be "wrecked" as a result.) An extremely liberal interpretation by the physician is not always

---

*See also discussions of specific problems in Chapter 12.

upheld by the law; the courts consider inadequately justified abortion a felony. The Roman Catholic Church denounces therapeutic abortion unconditionally as a mortal sin.

If a physician is not prevented from performing a therapeutic abortion by religious doctrine, he must first reconcile in his own mind the ethical theories of utilitarianism (i.e., the philosophy which holds that an act is "good" or "right" if it contributes to the greatest benefit of the greatest number of people) and intentionalism (conscience; an inner sense of moral discrimination, which without reason guides man in his interpersonal decisions); and he must abide by the law.

- A. Neuropsychiatric Disorders: Psychiatrists and obstetricians disagree with each other (and among themselves) on the necessity for abortion in cases of severe or potentially severe emotional illness. It is doubtful, however, if significant benefit is achieved by abortion in any of these cases, and a psychotic woman who submits to abortion may be plagued by severe guilt feelings then or later. Even though the patient expresses suicidal intentions, she rarely takes her life. Institutional psychotherapy without abortion is usually best for the emotionally disturbed pregnant woman.
- B. Renal Disease: Severe bilateral renal insufficiency with azotemia and chronic resistant pyelonephritis with advanced hydronephrosis may be indications for therapeutic abortion. Chronic nephritis is not aggravated by pregnancy in the absence of secondary infection or toxemia of pregnancy.
- C. Heart Disease: (See Classification on p. 284.) Therapeutic abortion is not warranted in patients with class I or class II disability. In class III cases; in patients with atrial fibrillation or coronary occlusion; in those in whom valvulotomy has been tried without success; or in those with a history of cardiac disaster in a previous pregnancy, therapeutic abortion may be considered. If the class IV cardiac patient is too ill for therapeutic abortion, interruption may have to be delayed until improvement has occurred.

    Hypertensive cardiovascular disease rarely jeopardizes the pregnant patient directly, although neglected or inadequately treated eclamptogenic toxemia in certain women who begin pregnancy with a blood pressure greater than 150/90 may cause further permanent vascular damage. Toxemia is often preventable, but must be faced if and when it occurs. Essessential hypertension and cerebrovascular accident or a major ocular hemorrhage during a previous pregnancy are unfavorable prognostic signs. Hypertensive disease alone is almost never an indication for interruption of early pregnancy.
- D. Pulmonary Disease: Marked impairment of pulmonary ventilation with the equivalent of less than one lung in

function (vital capacity less than 1400 ml in the average-sized person) may justify abortion. Pulmonary insufficiency may be the result of thoracic deformity, surgery, infection, or degenerative changes in the lung. Pulmonary tuberculosis is no longer a valid indication for interruption of pregnancy except in rare instances when the disease is unresponsive to chemotherapy.

E. Metabolic Disorders: Diabetes mellitus is not a justification for therapeutic abortion unless progressive loss of vision or progressive Kimmelstiel-Wilson syndrome occur as complications. If the patient is already blind or if the renal lesion is advanced, interruption of pregnancy will not be beneficial.

F. The familial blood dyscrasias, not primarily metabolic in origin, may disturb the metabolism during pregnancy but are not indications for therapeutic abortion.

G. Severe ulcerative colitis may be worsened by pregnancy. When perforations, hemorrhage, or nutritional deficiency become critical, abortion may be necessary.

H. Malignant Disease: Invasive cervical malignancy, stage II breast carcinoma, melanosarcoma, and poorly controlled skin cancer are considered by many to be indications for therapeutic abortion. Leukemia and bowel and thyroid carcinoma are not so considered.

I. Obstetric Complications:
  1. Rubella - The risk of serious damage to the fetus resulting from maternal rubella before the 12th to 14th weeks is now believed to be about 20%. Rubella virus probably causes death of the embryo and abortion in about half of cases during the first month; after the first month, some of the affected embryos survive but are abnormal. Rubella after the 14th week rarely damages the fetus. The severity of the maternal disease has no bearing on the degree of fetal injury by the virus. The diagnosis must be substantiated and age, parity, gravidity, and the religion of the patient must all be considered before the decision to abort or not to abort is made.
  2. Influenza and viral hepatitis occasionally affect the fetus. Predelivery assessment of possible damage is impossible, however, and abortion is not warranted.
  3. A woman's severe sensitization to the Rh factor, her husband's demonstrable Rh-positive status, and the delivery of several erythroblastotic infants, especially of the hydrops fetalis type, indicate a high probability of the disease in all subsequent children. The degree of jeopardy is uncertain, however, and so abortion should not be allowed.

Methods.

A. Dilatation and Curettage: (Illustration on p. 670.) Almost two-thirds of therapeutic abortions are performed transvaginally by dilatation of the cervix, evacuation, and curettage of the uterus. Before the 12th week of pregnancy, the vaginal route is usually chosen for therapeutic abortion unless sterilization is to be performed also, in which case laparotomy and abdominal hysterotomy are required. After the 12th week, abdominal hysterotomy is safer than dilatation of the cervix and evacuation of the uterus from below.

The preoperative preparation is similar to that employed for dilatation and curettage or cesarean section if hysterotomy is chosen. Postoperative management is comparable to postpartal care, although the patient can usually resume full activity in 2-3 weeks.

B. Intra-amniotic Injection of Hypertonic Solutions: Therapeutic abortion after the 14th week and evacuation of the uterus following fetal death can be accomplished medically within 12-14 hours, almost without exception, by aseptic transabdominal aspiration of amniotic fluid and immediate very slow replacement by a similar amount of sterile aqueous 20% sodium chloride or 50% glucose solution. Saline should not be used for patients with eclamptogenic toxemia or other disorders in which sodium restriction is desirable. Labor generally requires only 2-3 hours and appears not to be the result of progestogen block or reduced progestogen production by the placenta.

After voiding (to prevent injury to the bowel or bladder), the patient is placed in the slight Trendelenburg position. A site half-way between the symphysis and umbilicus and slightly lateral to the midline is chosen for amniocentesis. After preparation with antiseptic, the skin is anesthetized with procaine or comparable solution. A No. 14 or 16, 4-6 inch needle with obturator is inserted slowly into the uterine cavity. Ideally, 100-200 ml of fluid are withdrawn. In second trimester pregnancy and missed abortion, only small amounts of amniotic fluid may be available. In such instances, at least 60-90 ml solution should be injected if possible.

The recovered placenta reveals extensive edema and submembranous degeneration. Signs of hypoxia are noted when fetal death follows injection of hypertonic solutions.

C. Irradiation and the use of folic acid antagonists are not recommended for abortion because the results are not reliable and undesirable side effects may occur.

Complications.

Therapeutic abortion is a potentially dangerous operation even in healthy women. Perforation of the uterus, pelvic infection, hemorrhage, and embolism are the most common complications. The primary mortality in elective first trimester abortion is 0.05-0.1% (Scandinavia). A 5% morbidity (fever, pelvic infection) is recorded in the first trimester and over 15-20% in second trimester, state-authorized interruptions of pregnancy.

The mortality is 1-2% in the seriously ill pregnant patient whose physical or emotional disease may justify abortion. This is at least twice the mortality for therapeutic abortion in a healthy woman. The postoperative morbidity is proportionate.

Protracted feelings of guilt and remorse commonly result from interruption of pregnancy, particularly when religious and social conflicts complicate the decision to abort and the patient feels responsible for the loss of the baby.

STERILIZATION

Sterilization is the permanent prevention of pregnancy. Elective or compulsory sterilization is accomplished by surgery or irradiation on women and men who wish to avoid parenthood or are considered unfit to bear or father or rear children because of incapacitating disease, often hereditary. These people often lack the ability or determination to practice contraception, or sterilization may be required because the risks of conception are too great. Individual decision, racial improvement, and relief of poverty are the goals of elective sterilization.

Compulsory sterilization may be recommended by a state board of eugenics in the majority of states in the USA and by similar agencies in numerous other countries, often in response to written application by the patient's family. The board may also initiate the action according to statute subject to appeal in the courts.

Indications.

Most intractable disorders (such as extreme inoperable congenital heart disease), if serious enough to constitute an indication for interruption of pregnancy, are threats to future pregnancies as well. If therapeutic abortion is necessary, sterilization is usually indicated also.

A. Neuropsychiatric: Feeblemindedness, advanced schizophrenia, severe epilepsy.
B. Medical: Familial blood dyscrasias, marked cardiovascular or renal disease.
C. Obstetric: Extreme anti-Rh sensitization in the woman whose husband is Rh positive; uncorrectible uterine abnormality and repeated abortion.
D. Surgical: Stage II carcinoma of the breast; melanosarcoma.

E. Socioeconomic: Frequent pregnancies and inability to rear additional children.

Methods of Sterilization in the Female.

A. Surgical sterilization may be done by bilateral oophorectomy or salpingectomy, hysterectomy, or bilateral tubal closure. Tubal closure is the most commonly used sterilization procedure.

Four main approaches to the tubes are employed: abdominal (over three-fourths of cases), vaginal (occasionally), transuterine (occasionally), and inguinal (rarely).

Tubal closure is accomplished either by ligation or excision. Ligation may be done with segmental resection (Pomeroy) or with crushing (Madlener). Excision may be accomplished by salpingectomy, removal of the infundibular portion of the tube, resection of the isthmic part of the tube (cornual resection), burial of the proximal extremity of the tube beneath the visceral or parietal peritoneum (Uchida), or by cauterization-occlusion of the uterotubal ostia through the uterine cavity.

Surgical reestablishment of the continuity of one or both tubes is successful in about two-thirds of cases following Pomeroy or Madlener sterilization. Pregnancy results in less than half of these patients, however.

B. Irradiation Sterilization:
1. X-ray irradiation is rarely used for sterilization of women. Patients with medical, surgical, or neuropsychiatric conditions which contraindicate surgery or those who refuse surgery may be candidates for roentgen sterilization. A total of 2000 r to the ovaries is generally administered. Biweekly treatments are given to 2 of 4 ports. Therapy is completed in 4 weeks.
2. Radium applied in the cervico-uterine canal is occasionally used for sterilization, usually for women near the menopause who have undergone repeated dilatation and curettage for benign endometrial hemorrhage. The distance from the internal os of the cervix to the ovaries varies widely, even in normal women. A sterilizing dose of 2000 r may be administered in 100 hours, utilizing a tandem of three 1 cm linear sources containing 25 mg of radium filtered by 1 mm of platinum placed in the cervix and uterus (assuming the gonads are 4 cm lateral to the midline at the cervico-uterine juncture).

Sterilization 407

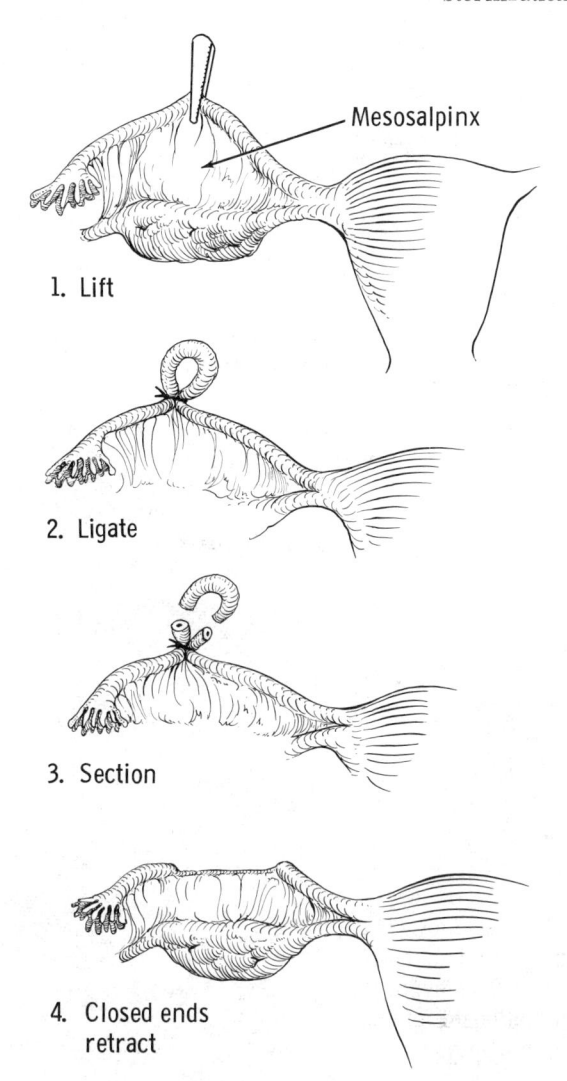

Fig 15-1. Pomeroy method of sterilization.

408 Sterilization

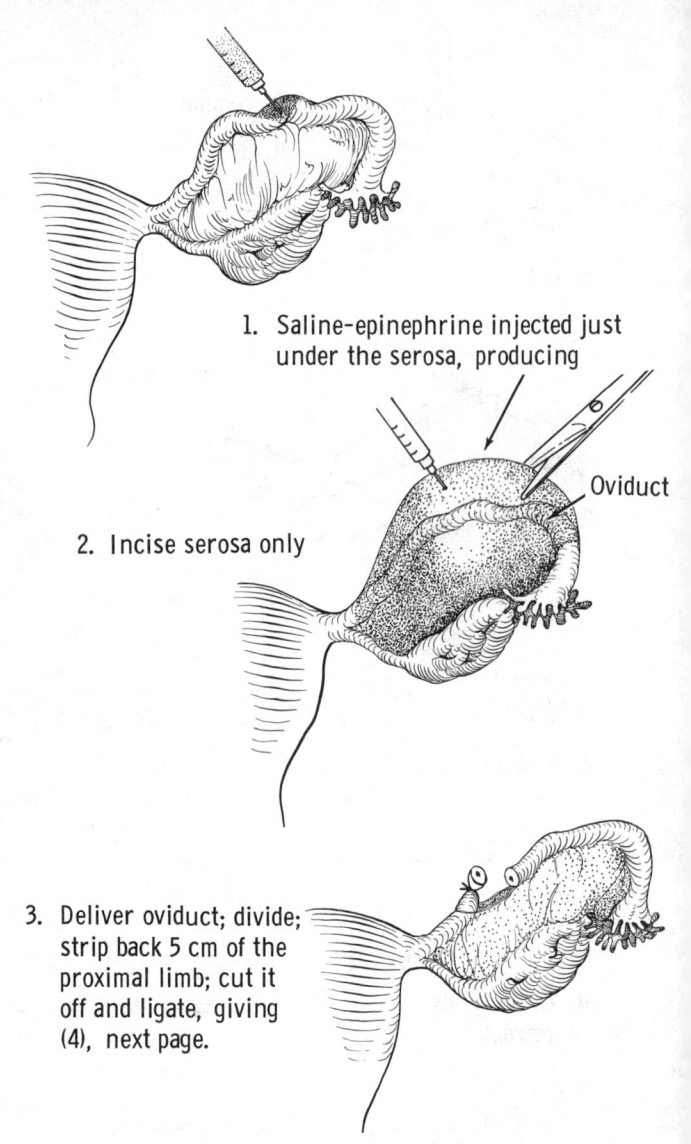

1. Saline-epinephrine injected just under the serosa, producing

Oviduct

2. Incise serosa only

3. Deliver oviduct; divide; strip back 5 cm of the proximal limb; cut it off and ligate, giving (4), next page.

Fig 15-2. Uchida method of sterilization.

Sterilization 409

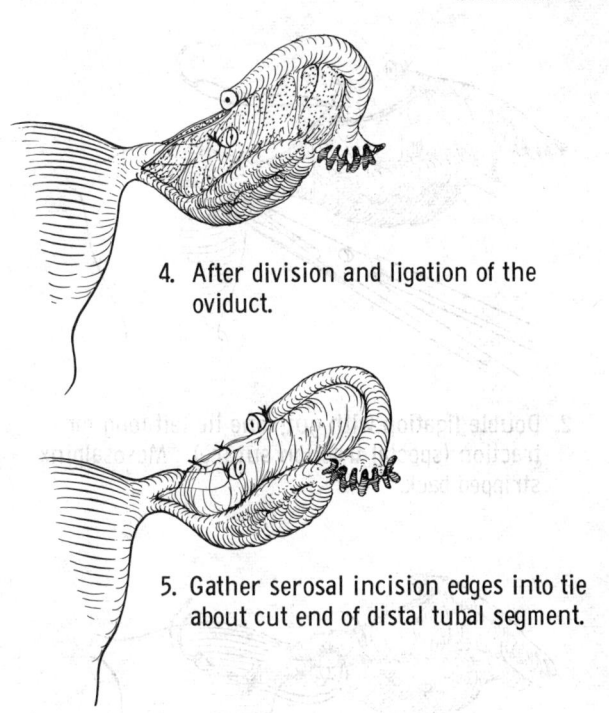

4. After division and ligation of the oviduct.

5. Gather serosal incision edges into tie about cut end of distal tubal segment.

Fig 15-2 (cont'd.). Uchida method of sterilization.

Mesosalpinx

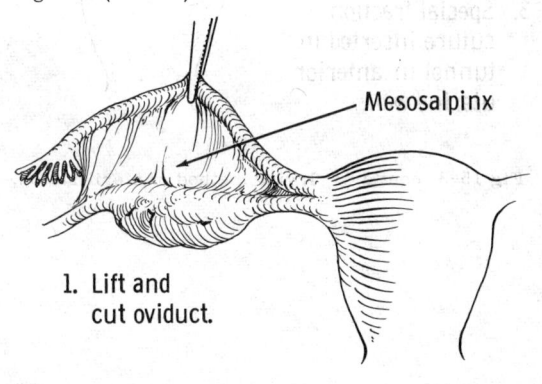

1. Lift and cut oviduct.

Fig 15-3. Irving method of sterilization.

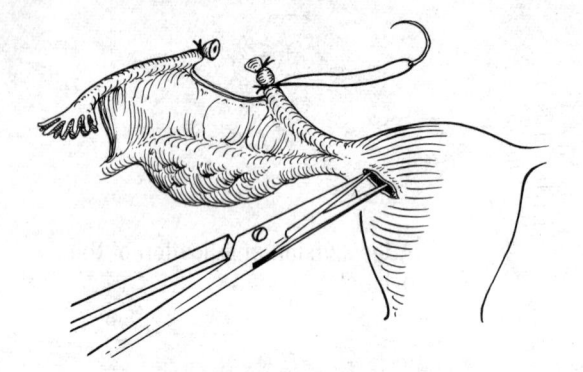

410 Sterilization

2. Double ligation with gut; one tie left long for traction (special traction suture). Mesosalpinx stripped back.

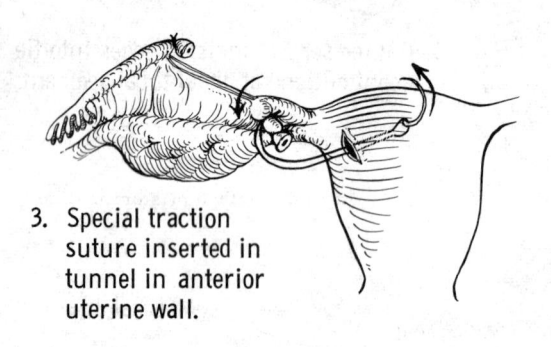

3. Special traction suture inserted in tunnel in anterior uterine wall.

Fig 15-3 (cont'd.). Irving method of sterilization.

Sterilization 411

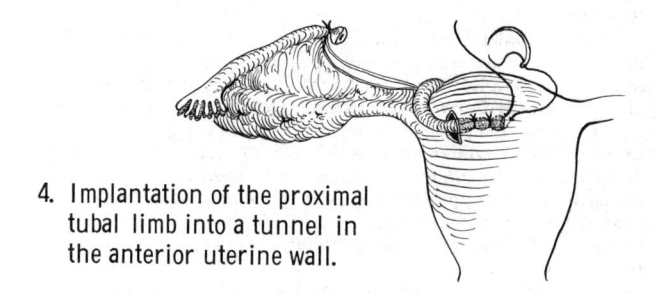

4. Implantation of the proximal tubal limb into a tunnel in the anterior uterine wall.

Figure-8 fixation suture

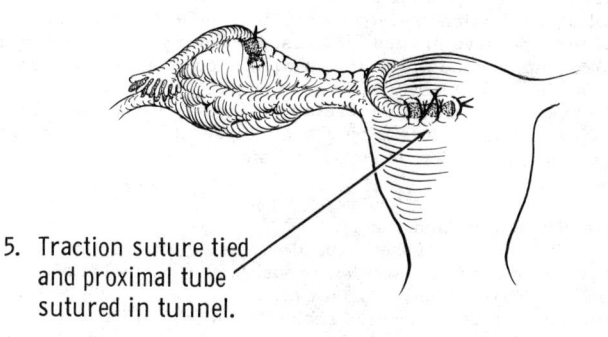

5. Traction suture tied and proximal tube sutured in tunnel.

Fig 15-3 (cont'd.). Irving method of sterilization.

Results.

With tubal interruption alone, no organ is removed; impregnation is the only function denied the patient. The physician must explain that tubal sterilization merely prevents conception. It is not "de-sexing" and will not cause frigidity, vary the menses, or alter the woman's appearance. There is usually no adverse change in sexual function following tubal sterilization; on the contrary, many women who feared pregnancy before the operation report increased satisfaction in sexual intercourse and are pleased with the operative result. However, 5-10% report less frequent orgasm and regret the procedure.

Only bilateral oophorectomy and ovarian damage (x-ray) are considered to be certain methods of sterilization. Abdominal and tubal pregnancies have occurred (though rarely) even after total hysterectomy. Sterilization failures occur in about 1:5000 cases following the Uchida method, 1:2000 cases following ligation, severance, or burying of the proximal end of the tube (Irving), and 1:50 cases following the Pomeroy or Madlener method when sterilization is done at cesarean section (the most difficult circumstance).

Oophorectomy and irradiation sterilization are usually followed within 4 weeks by vasomotor reactions and a gradual diminution in libido or sexual satisfaction during the next 6 months.

Sterilization in Men.

Sterilization of the husband by vas ligation (an office procedure) may be far less dangerous than an operation on the wife if she is for any reason an inappropriate candidate for surgery. This alternative should be offered to the couple who must limit childbearing. Impotence does not result, and re-anastomosis is successful in about 75% of cases.

16...
Emotional Aspects of Pregnancy

Taboos, superstitions, and misinformation regarding menstrual function, sex practices, and childbirth still cause much needless fear and uncertainty among women. Many obstetric and gynecologic illnesses are emotionally induced or are aggravated by emotional factors.

Antepartal care offers an excellent opportunity to study and treat the emotional disorders of women. By fostering greater understanding and encouraging the acceptance of healthy attitudes, the obstetrician can make valuable contributions to the mental health and happiness of his patients and their families. The principal prophylactic measures available are programs of sex information during high school, family life courses in late adolescence, and obstetric advice and counseling during pregnancy. In general, it is felt that more stress should be placed upon the woman's role in rearing children in our complex society than the actual delivery of the baby.

Aims in the Emotional Management of Pregnancy.
A. To assist the patient to accept her pregnancy soon after the last missed menstrual period. Most well-adjusted parents will accept even an unwanted pregnancy. If the patient consciously or unconsciously rejects the pregnancy, mild to severe psychic or somatic complaints soon become manifest.
B. To assist the patient in accepting the child promptly after delivery. The reproductive instinct is often in conflict with personal and social attitudes. Fear and apprehension are commonly associated with the patient's first suspicions that she is pregnant even though she may want the baby. Women having their first baby are suddenly faced with the unknown perils of pregnancy, labor, and delivery. Paradoxic reactions of happiness and resentment are common. Fortunately, by the time the patient sees her doctor, she has usually completely accepted her pregnancy (if the baby is wanted) or has temporarily submerged her fright and resentment in the hope that her symptoms are a "false alarm" (if the baby is unwanted).

The principal adverse psychic factors in pregnancy are as follows: (1) Fear of the unknown, (2) fear of pain during labor and delivery, (3) fear of death, (4) fear of the economic consequences of pregnancy and motherhood, (5) resentment at the imminent loss of personal independence and attractiveness, (6) resentment of the child as a potential competitor for the husband's love and affection, and (7) uncertainty about the role of becoming a parent.

The Emotional Course of Pregnancy.

A. First Trimester: This is the most important phase in the adjustment of the patient, particularly the primigravida. During this interval the patient must either accept or reject her pregnancy. Emotional tensions are manifested as symptoms such as headache, nausea, and easy fatigability. In general, the patient who accepts childbearing as a normal and necessary aspect of womanhood will make a good adjustment. The discomforts of psychosomatic illness are reserved for patients who consider menstruation ("the curse"), sexual intercourse, and pregnancy to be woman's "burden" in life.

The husband is often the "forgotten man" in antepartal care. The physician should welcome him in the office at an early visit, and tell him how pregnancy is progressing and how he can help. Lucid explanations and frank answers to his questions will promote a confident, supportive attitude on his part which will be an important source of satisfaction and assistance to his wife.

B. Second Trimester: When pregnancy progresses on schedule, the patient will feel fetal movements by about the 4th month. This is an exciting and satisfying experience for almost all women.

During the 2nd trimester, relatives and friends often repeat sadistic rumors and recount harrowing experiences to "guide" and sober the patient. The physician must be willing to listen patiently, correct misinformation, and give reassurance as needed.

C. Third Trimester: Tensions mount and anxieties increase as the expected date of confinement (EDC) approaches. Minimize the importance of abnormalities and emphasize the normal features of the pregnancy. The more factual knowledge the patient possesses, the fewer will be her difficulties. Fear of delivery is fear of the unknown; knowledge dispels this fear.

The husband must demonstrate his love for his wife despite her distorted contours. Oversolicitude and too much sympathy have an adverse effect, however.

EMOTIONAL ASPECTS OF LABOR AND DELIVERY

Emotional adjustment to delivery depends upon (1) the patient's emotional stability, (2) the success of the marriage, (3) the couple's desire for a child, and (4) patient-physician rapport. Adequate emotional preparation for labor and delivery will ease the prelabor period, especially for the emotionally immature and apprehensive individual.

Allow the patient to visit the hospital before the onset of labor. Maternity service tours will familiarize the couple with the hospital plan. The patient in labor who enters the hospital in the middle of the night without prior knowledge of hospital procedure may receive a fearsome initiation. Under the worst circumstances, she leaves her husband at the hospital desk and is led down a long, dark corridor by an uncommunicative nurse or attendant—often in cap, mask, and gown. She is undressed, put to bed, shaved, and given a hot enema. Strange individuals do rectal examinations; "shots" may be administered. During all this, painful periodic uterine contractions increase in frequency and severity. The events of the first hours in the hospital increase the patient's inherent fear, and an emotional milieu is created which must be experienced to be appreciated. As tension mounts, pain is intensified.

The dynamics of pain in labor were outlined as follows by Grantly Dick Read:

(1) Gravida + fear = marked tension.

Marked tension + anemia, fatigue, discouragement, panic = severe pain.

(2) Gravida + abnormal pregnancy, poor integration, limited intelligence, previous obstetric disaster = severe pain.

But,

(3) Gravida + normal pregnancy + confidence + relaxation = little pain + good labor.

Pain in childbirth is minimized by patient relaxation. She must utilize her contractions without working against them. A friendly, attentive nurse and an obstetrician who is frequently in attendance can anticipate the patient's concern and estimate her emotional status. The use of relaxing technics and personal attention during labor will reduce her discomfort considerably.

The physician should meet the patient at the hospital or see her shortly after admission, and introduce the resident physician and nurse as a "team" who will assist her during labor and delivery. The physician need not sit for hours with his patient in labor; he may come and go, but must convince the patient that he is actively and successfully supervising her care.

The patient often requests that her husband be permitted to remain with her during labor and delivery. The husband, anxious to be of service, usually agrees and usually is a favorable influence. In general, it is best to limit the husband's participation to occasional brief visits during labor. Thus, he is not excluded and is participating but at the same time is not preventing the patient from relaxing and dozing after analgesia has been administered. The husband usually is excluded from the delivery room because his presence can contribute little to his wife's emotional or physical support. Although there are undoubtedly numerous exceptions, any husband may be a serious potential hazard in the delivery room. He may disconcert the obstetrician or other members of the obstetric team; may require countless explanations; may introduce infection; may feel impelled to object to procedures he does not sufficiently understand; and may interfere with the work at hand by becoming ill or anxious. Most patients do better with professional personnel than with the family in the labor suite.

Many physicians feel that the conscious experience of childbirth is an important factor in maternal acceptance of the baby in the postpartal period, and this seems to be true in animal experiments with drugged births. Heavy analgesia and anesthesia seem to be harmful to the mother and child both physiologically and psychologically. "Natural" childbirth and regional anesthesia reduce these hazards. An exception to this rule might be the unmarried mother whose baby is going to be taken by an adoption agency—in which case it may be desirable to spare her the agony of seeing, hearing, and wanting a child she cannot keep.

EMOTIONAL ASPECTS OF THE POSTPARTAL PERIOD

If the antepartal period has been well managed and there have been no complications, psychic and physiologic adjustments are comparatively easy following delivery. The mother should nurse her baby unless strong aversions or medical problems (e.g., mastitis) interfere. The most important argument in favor of nursing is emotional. A tremendous emotional lift results from being able to nurse the new baby.

Some women do not want to nurse because they believe they will not produce enough milk. The fear that nursing will spoil the beauty of the breasts or will interfere with social activities deters others. Most of these objections can be overcome by explanation of the facts. A "good start" for the child and a "quicker recovery" for the mother are the goals of nursing. If the mother only nurses for several months, this may be sufficient.

When the breasts are full and tender, a temporary emotional depression often occurs ("baby blues"). (See Depressive Reactions, p. 419.) The unfamiliar nursing routine may provoke tears and despondency, and the complete dependency of the infant on the mother entails responsibilities which the mother must accept. This may prove to be difficult until she becomes familiar with the routine of child care and unless she is confident of the assistance of her husband and others. Explanation, demonstration of nursing and child care procedures, and reassurance will help to minimize the dejection of this anticlimax.

A second brief, mild depression may develop about one month after delivery when personal sacrifices and the drudgery of daily duties have taken much of the glamor out of motherhood. Resentment toward the child and the husband is often present. Additional household help, an understanding attitude on the part of the husband and physician, and reassurance usually prevent a serious depression.

The mother may subconsciously consider the child a rival for the husband's affections, and the husband in turn may resent the transfer of his wife's affections to the baby during the first few months after delivery (the "childbirth triangle"). This may lead to jealousy and discontent unless a happy relationship exists between the husband and wife, and the husband should be cautioned to modify his responses in a constructive way for the good of the family.

Aids to Patient-Doctor Communication.

Many of the emotional problems associated with childbearing can be avoided if the patient-doctor relationship is a cordial and confident one. The key to this relationship is communication, and the physician should not hesitate to devote the time necessary to answering his patient's questions and allaying her anxieties. It is good practice, for example, to ask the patient to prepare written questions to be answered at the next visit. Ancillary services as outlined below are valuable supplements to these interviews but should not be relied on exclusively.

A. Publications: Many obstetricians prefer to develop their own materials. The following publications are valuable for both the patient and her husband.

Birch, W.G., and Meilach, D.Z.: A Doctor Discusses Pregnancy. (Budlong Press, 1963.)

Eastman, N.J.: Expectant Motherhood, 4th ed. (Little, Brown, 1963.)

Falls, F. H.: Maternal and Newborn Care. (Donahue, 1959.)

Fielding, W. L., and Benjamin, L.: The Case Against "Natural Childbirth." (Avon, 1962.)

Gruenberg, S. M.: The Wonderful Story of How You Were Born. (For preadolescent children.) (Garden City, 1959.)

Guttmacher, A.: Pregnancy and Birth: A Book for Expectant Parents. (Viking, 1956.)

Hall, R. E.: Nine Months' Reading. (Doubleday, 1960.)

Heardman, E.: A Way to Natural Childbirth. (Williams & Wilkins, 1948.)

Meaker, S. R.: Preparing for Motherhood. (Year Book, 1960.)

Miller, J. S.: Childbirth—A Manual for Pregnancy and Delivery. (Atheneum, 1963.)

Washburn, H.: So You're Going to Have a Baby! (Harcourt, Brace, 1956.)

B. Discussion Groups: Numerous civic and hospital services have organized groups for the presentation and discussion of antenatal and postnatal problems. A doctor or nurse usually acts as moderator. If such meetings are available in the community, the patient and her husband may find them stimulating and informative.

C. Demonstrations of Baby Care, Formula Preparation, Etc: These are generally a part of the hospital nursing service program.

MENTAL ILLNESS ASSOCIATED WITH PREGNANCY

The ability to bear a child does not mean that a woman wishes to have a baby nor that she is psychologically adaptable to the stresses of pregnancy, delivery, and parenthood. Many women have no desire for a child; others have a basic aversion to pregnancy even though they may claim the contrary. In such instances, both the mother and the child may suffer. Depression, anxiety, and feelings of inadequacy are common in such situations.

An emotionally healthy married woman will welcome pregnancy as a step toward maturity. Other conscious motivations are desire to develop a home, to express love, and to gratify her husband.

The fear of pregnancy may be rationalized in many ways, including the following: "It's too soon after marriage" or ". . . after my last baby." "We can't afford it." "My husband is unwilling to accept another obligation." "Our marriage is insecure already." "I'm not well." "I'm absorbed in my career." "I'm afraid of losing my husband's love to the child."

These "reasons" for not wanting a child usually betray an underlying ambivalence toward the feminine role. They may be expressions of unconscious anxiety, conflict, or inadequacy.

On the other hand, there are unhealthy, selfish reasons for wishing to become pregnant, e.g., the desire to stabilize a bad marriage.

The emotional stresses which develop when pregnancy occurs depend largely upon whether the pregnancy was planned and whether one or both parents desires a child. The symptoms of unconscious rejection of the baby are nausea and vomiting, abdominal pain, and diarrhea.

Because even the happiest parents cannot escape some concern regarding pregnancy, positive and negative emotions are almost always present. In some cases the psychic consequences are brief and clinically unimportant; in others, extended and serious. Fortunately, the course of pregnancy is a happy experience for most women.

During the postpartal period even the woman who regarded pregnancy as a joyful time may become tense and disturbed. Nursing is often a problem; some women do not want to nurse, and those who do cannot always produce enough milk. The baby becomes the central figure in the household and the mother its "servant." Responsibilities and obligations are multiplied while personal gratifications and simple conveniences are sacrificed. If the child is in any way abnormal or especially difficult to manage, it may easily seem "too much for one woman to handle." How the mother responds to these challenges is a measure of her emotional stability and maturity.

Psychosis requiring psychiatric intervention occurs in approximately 0.2-0.3% of women during pregnancy and the puerperium. About 15% of psychotic breakdowns occur before delivery, 55% during the fortnight after delivery (most of these during the first 7 days), and the remainder later in the perinatal period.

It is well to bear in mind that pregnancy itself except in rare instances (e.g., toxic psychosis) does not cause psychosis unless the patient is predisposed to psychotic responses to stress. Gestational psychosis and "puerperal insanity" do not exist as entities; and parity is neither significant to the incidence nor the type of emotional illness.

Of the 3 types of psychoses seen postpartum, most are manic-depressive or schizophrenic reactions. Toxic delirium occurs occasionally. Rare types of mental illness are alcoholic psychosis, epilepsy associated with psychosis, and psychosis due to general paresis.

Manic-depressive psychosis: No specific etiologic factor is known, although in many cases there seem to be strong familial predispositions to mental illness. Manic-depressive

420 Mental Illness Associated With Pregnancy

psychosis is usually seen only in adults. In women who develop emotional illness during pregnancy there is often a prior history of a similar disorder.

At least half of psychotic illnesses during or immediately following pregnancy are affective reactions. About 10% of these are major manic or depressive episodes and occur before delivery; the remainder occur during the puerperium. Younger patients are slightly more prone to mania, but in general manic reactions are far less common than depressive ones. Mania or depression (or both) may occur in one pregnancy and not in others; may occur in all pregnancies; or may occur only when the patient is not pregnant.

Jealousy and hatred of the child and rejection of it may reflect (1) the patient's desire to be the "only one" in the husband's affections; (2) aversion toward pregnancy; (3) resentment toward the husband; or (4) a poor sexual adjustment, with guilt feelings regarding contraception, abortion, or religious conflicts.

The patient with manic-depressive psychosis identifies with her mother. The husband is often a mother-substitute, even giving mother-like care. The patient may indulge in fantasies in which another man has fathered the baby or the marriage is denied. Homosexual attitudes are infrequently present.

Manic reactions: These are usually noted 1-2 weeks postpartum and may be preceded by brief periods of depression. Symptoms include agitation, excitement, volubility, inattention, rhyming and punning speech, disorder of dress, and disinterest in food. The patient often becomes dehydrated and exhausted. Manic reactions are brief in duration (1-3 weeks), but the patient can become exhausted early and vigorous initial therapy is most important.

Treat manic reactions by referral to a psychiatrist if possible. Treatment usually consists of electroshock therapy (contraindicated in pelvic infection); phenothiazines or cold packs (or both) if she is debilitated; supportive treatment; and psychotherapy. The prognosis for the child is good if it can be separated from the mother until she has recovered.

Depressive reactions: Periods of despondency are far more frequent than manic states, and are more dangerous for both mother and child. The "baby blues" often deepen and continue into the second week postpartum, and the patient's condition is marked by anxiety, profound fatigue, and anorexia. The amphetamines and antidepressants are of little value. The woman becomes self-accusatory, and expresses inappropriate or bizarre thoughts and feelings. Intense depression often follows during which the patient feels helpless and the future seems hopeless. During this critical interval the disconsolate, despairing mother may kill the child and commit suicide.

The duration of an attack cannot be predicted. Some patients suffer for weeks, others for months. Electroshock therapy usually results in a dramatic improvement, and follow-up psychotherapy is valuable; but recurrences may occur. After repeated attacks the intervals between the depressions are shortened and the ultimate prognosis becomes more grave. The child does well when the problem is recognized and mother and child are separated.

Schizophrenia: This is a psychosis of unknown cause which occurs with greatest frequency in adolescents or young adults. A sudden onset often follows a seemingly contented pregnancy. Abnormal personality reactions before and during pregnancy are almost always present, however.

The split or splintering of the personality results from underlying psychic problems and inability to adjust to adult demands. Abnormally shy, quiet, reserved, sensitive, and suspicious women are more prone to develop schizoid personality reactions during pregnancy. They are exceedingly introspective and easily offended, and are prone to daydreaming.

The baby is invariably rejected. Hostility toward the husband is obvious to the skilled and perceptive physician although frequently not recognized by the patient. The patient often has delusions of immaculate conception or that some other man, perhaps the physician, is the father of the child.

This disorder progresses through avoidance of social contacts and rationalization of failure to complete abandonment of reason for a small, personal world of unreality. Ideas of reference and influence, delusions and hallucinations, complete distortion of emotional responses, excitement, vulgarity, and confusion of thought content are prominent features of the syndrome. Infanticide occurs occasionally, but suicide is rare.

Hospitalization is required. Electroshock therapy followed by psychotherapy is effective in most cases. Exhaustion or pelvic infections are temporary contraindications to shock treatment.

The immediate prognosis for the schizophrenic patient before delivery is fair to good. The prognosis is better if the onset occurs abruptly during the puerperium. Although hereditary tendencies are postulated, the child is not obviously affected by parental schizophrenia.

Toxic deliria: Exogenous or endogenous toxicosis causes behavioral and mental disorders similar to those seen in acute psychosis. The patient is excitable, confused, incoherent, and restless. The sensorium is clouded, and delusions and hallucinations may lead the patient to believe she is fighting for her life. She may try to flee—injuring herself, her baby, and others in the attempt. The causes are as follows: (1) Drugs, occasionally taken with suicidal intent (e. g., alcohol, barbiturates, bromides, opium derivatives, cocaine, marijuana, lead); (2) cardiac or renal failure; (3) metabolic aberrations (hypoglycemia, hypothyroidism); (4) trauma (usually cranial); and (5) acute infections (septicemia, tetanus).

Unless the obstetric patient has eclamptogenic toxemia, a very long labor, is dehydrated, or receives extremely large doses of analgesics, delirium rarely develops.

Delirium clears with removal of the cause and symptomatic, supportive therapy. Discontinue toxic drugs immediately. Restrict the patient's movements as necessary. (Avoid physical restraints.) Force fluids and restore electrolytes. Administer glucose and insulin. Prescribe appropriate antibiotics if infection is likely. Protect the patient and others from harm. Rule out manic-depressive psychosis, schizophrenia, Korsakoff's psychosis, and other types of mental disease.

The prognosis for both mother and child is good when the toxicosis is mild to moderate and exogenous. The prognosis in endogenous toxicosis depends upon the specific medical circumstances (see p. 282).

Emergency Management.

The general physician, obstetrician, or gynecologist should not attempt to treat functional psychoses (schizophrenia, mania, etc) because intensive specialized care and institutional management are almost always required. However, he must be able to treat acute psychiatric emergencies such as antepartal or postpartal psychosis until consultation can be obtained and the patient transferred.

A. Diagnosis: Observe the patient's behavior and movements, looking especially for muscular weakness and paralysis. Listen for speech impairment, disorientation, and delusional or hallucinatory expressions. Perform an adequate physical examination.
B. Allay Fear: Do not promise, agree with, or humor the patient; but calm her with a reassuring, supportive manner, emphasizing illness (not mental problems or "insanity"). Arrange for a favorite relative or friend to remain with or near the patient. Eliminate shadows and noise and exclude nonessential personnel.
C. Avoid force. Restrict but do not restrain the patient.
D. Prevent the patient from harming herself or others. Admit her to a single room on the first floor or to one with barred windows screened on the inside. Remove cords, ties, and sharp or movable heavy objects from the room. Provide special nurses day and night as necessary.
E. Ensure rest. For excitable patients, consider ataractics (promazine, chlorpromazine), sedatives (paraldehyde, barbiturates), warm tubs, and cold packs.
F. Provide adequate simple foods and fluids, observing the patient's preferences insofar as possible. Intravenous or

gavage feedings may be necessary if the patient is completely resistant to eating or drinking.

PSEUDOCYESIS

Pseudocyesis (false pregnancy) is a fantasy reaction noted during the childbearing years in women who have either an intense desire for pregnancy or an extreme fear of it. It occurs once in approximately 1000 general obstetrics cases and is most common in unmarried women or in the infertile married woman. Such patients are severely psychoneurotic or frankly psychotic. Stubborn, illogical insistence that pregnancy exists is characteristic in pseudocyesis.

All of the presumptive symptoms and some of the presumptive signs of pregnancy may be present: amenorrhea (hypothalamic), nausea and vomiting (psychogenic), breast sensitivity (subjective), abdominal protuberance (obesity, subconscious laxity of posture), quickening (misinterpretation), and waddling gait ("playing the role"). There are no probable signs and no positive evidences of pregnancy. On physical examination the physician may be deceived by supposed fetal movements which are usually the result of contractions of the intestines or the muscles of the abdominal wall. However, the small uterus usually can be demonstrated on bimanual examination. In the absence of other disease, the use of certain drugs, or misinterpretation, laboratory tests are negative.

Suicide or a complete psychotic breakdown may occur in patients who are ineptly "convinced against their will" or who are ridiculed. Many patients with pseudocyesis are borderline or actual schizophrenics.

The differential diagnosis of pseudocyesis includes intra- and extrauterine pregnancy, missed abortion, pelvic tumor, and psychopathologic states.

Treatment consists of kindly explanation and psychotherapy, usually by a psychiatrist. Hospitalization may be necessary. Confirmatory vaginal reexamination of all obstetric registrants and early recognition and treatment of significant abnormal emotional attitudes are important preventive measures.

The prognosis depends upon the seriousness of the emotional disorder and the success of psychotherapy.

17...
Delivery in the Home

Selective home delivery is an important phase of maternity care in many parts of the world and is still done in some large cities in the USA and elsewhere. Complicated obstetric cases can now be transported to hospitals—or medical personnel and emergency supplies and equipment brought to the patient and her baby—by improved surface and air transportation. Individualized domiciliary obstetrics will undoubtedly continue to be practiced among the poor, those living in rural areas, when the rapidity of labor prevents transfer to a hospital, and for a large segment of the population during natural catastrophe and war.

In many areas a scarcity of hospital beds and trained medical personnel requires the integration of home and hospital delivery programs. In many of these situations, good antenatal care, delivery of first infants and subsequent abnormal cases in hospitals, and the availability of experienced doctors and nurses have increased the safety of home delivery; maternal and infant mortality and morbidity rates are often below those reported by hospitals in the same region where both uncomplicated and complicated obstetric patients are admitted.

Supervision of midwives is the physician's duty in many countries. All physicians must therefore be familiar with the technics of confinement in the home.

Midwives, general practitioners, and consultant specialists have been incorporated successfully into effective obstetric units. As shown in Fig 17-1, a general practitioner or midwife can call upon or refer patients to numerous services for specialty study and care.

The general practitioner should supervise the midwife in obstetric delivery, and both should be under the direction of a specialist when a patient is to be delivered by a midwife. Obstetricians cannot hope to manage all deliveries personally; their primary function is to manage problem cases.

Selection of Cases for Home Delivery.

Home delivery should be done electively only if the patient has a history of normal pregnancy and a prognosis for probably uncomplicated delivery; in other words, women for whom minimal medical and surgical intervention is anticipated are the best candidates. Individualized judgments must be made

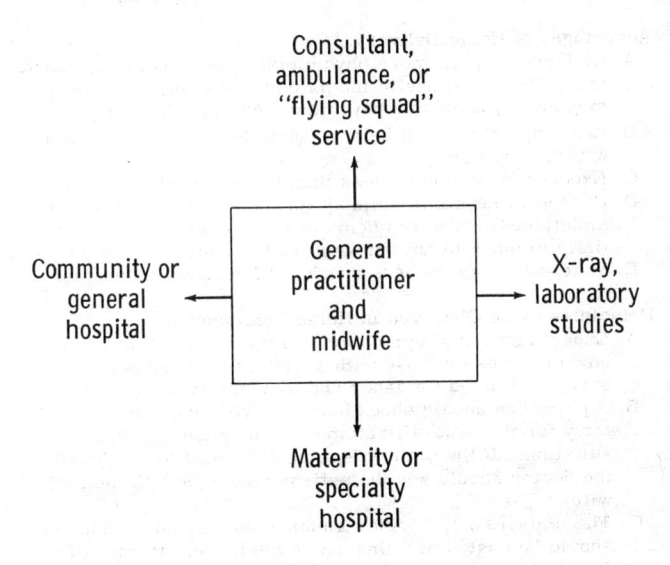

Fig 17-1. Auxiliary services in home delivery obstetrics.

about delivering primigravidas, grande multiparas, patients with the so-called dystocia dystrophy build, etc, in the home.

Contraindications to Home Delivery.

Home delivery is contraindicated for patients requiring forceps rotation, forceps extraction, and general, spinal, or caudal anesthesia. Other contraindications include eclamptogenic toxemia, multiple pregnancy, breech or transverse presentation, antepartal bleeding, elevated anti-Rh titer, a history of premature or post-date deliveries, grand multiparity, and significant medical and surgical complications in previous pregnancies.

Disadvantages of Home Delivery.

A. "Normal" cases chosen for home delivery may become complicated despite the greatest care in selection. It is difficult to predict uterine inertia, prolonged second stage of labor, or postpartal hemorrhage.
B. If emergencies should arise, adequate facilities and personnel are not immediately available.
C. The specialist called to the home to deal with a complicated delivery rarely knows the patient's antepartal course and prior problems.

Advantages of Home Delivery.
  A. Delivery is often more physiologic within known surroundings. The presence of the patient's husband and family may have a favorable psychic effect on some women.
  B. Rooming-in need not be arranged; the baby may remain with the mother.
  C. Expense is frequently less than in a hospital.
  D. Puerperal sepsis is unlikely (provided strict asepsis is maintained). The residents of a home are usually partially immune to any virulent bacteria that may be present.
  E. Maternity hospital beds are freed for complicated cases.

Principles to Be Observed in Home Confinement.
  A. Expert antepartal evaluation is required to eliminate abnormal cases or those with a doubtful prognosis from the group scheduled for labor and delivery at home.
  B. A physician should check home delivery candidates regularly for the best utilization of time, planning, and consultation. If the patient is to be delivered by a midwife, the doctor should see the patient regularly with the midwife.
  C. The midwife's and doctor's names and telephone numbers should be posted prominently in the home. Preparations for confinement should be completed by the 6th month of pregnancy since the patient is likely to be more ambitious before the last trimester and because a sudden premature delivery may occur.
  D. An obstetric specialist should examine pregnant patients vaginally at about the 36th week (with the midwife and generalist present). The pelvic capacity, presentation, size of the infant, etc, can thus be determined.
  E. If a midwife is scheduled to perform the delivery, she should inform the general practitioner when the patient goes into labor. He must then remain on emergency call until the patient is delivered successfully.
  F. Home facilities may be meager or primitive (e.g., poor lighting, few conveniences), and the aseptic field is limited. The precepts of obstetric management are always the same, however, no matter where delivery is accomplished. One can improvise almost everything except water, certain essential instruments and special medications.

REQUIREMENTS FOR HOME DELIVERY

Bedding.
  A supply of linen adequate for the patient's needs during labor, delivery, and the first week after delivery will be required: clean sheets, pillow cases, blankets, and bed pads.

In addition, the patient should obtain a rubber or plastic sheet to protect the mattress; a 4-6 inch stack of unfolded newspapers for padding beneath the patient and for disposal of waste; and light plastic or paper bags and newly ironed ("sterilized") newspapers for storage of sheets and other bedclothing.

Toilet Articles.
A. Soap, towels, wash cloths, sanitary pads.
B. A one-pound roll of absorbent cotton.
C. A bed pan.
D. Three sterile basins: one for the doctor's hands, another for preparing the patient, and one for the placenta.
E. One sterile dipper and 2 kettles: one for sterile hot water, the other for sterile cold water.
F. An ironing board or piece of wood wide enough to be placed under the mattress for elevation of the patient's hips if delivery in bed is likely.

Labor Room.
The mother's own room is usually chosen. It should be clean, light, and attractive. Proximity to a bath and toilet is important. The room should be screened against flies, and measures should be taken to eliminate insect vectors during the lying-in period. Family members with contagious diseases should be excluded.

Delivery Room.
The kitchen is often selected because the light is usually good and a large table is generally available for use as a delivery table. Water, a tub or sink, and a stove for warmth and sterilization are also customarily available.

It is possible to deliver the patient in her own bed if other prerequisites are at hand.

Baby's Room.
The new baby should have his own room if possible. It should be warm, well ventilated, sunny, clean, and quiet. Running water in or near the room is desirable. If the mother wishes to keep the child in her room, simpler facilities than these will be required. Only practical, simple furnishings are necessary: a scrupulously clean baby bed, a newly painted baby basket, or a light bassinet or crib. A shelf, stand, or rack for toilet needs; a closet, bureau, or cabinet for clothing; and a table or bathinette for changing and bathing the baby are desirable but not essential. A low armless chair, clothes racks, and hooks should be provided. A covered diaper pail and paper bags for refuse are necessary. Heavy rugs, coarse hangings, and articles difficult to keep clean should be removed.

The Layette.

Shirts, nightgowns, quilted pads, a plastic or rubber pad, diapers, baby blankets, and flannelet squares should be provided.

Cotton or rayon clothing is preferable to wool because it is easier to launder, cheaper, and does not shrink, and because wool is too harsh for a baby's skin. Allergies are less common with cotton fabrics.

The baby must have his own wash cloths and bath towels. Terry cloth is preferable, and the towel should be at least one yard square so that it can be wrapped around the infant after the bath.

Launder all dry goods, and iron and fold the surfaces together while they are still warm. Store in plastic bags, clean pillow cases, or an ironed newspaper.

The Doctor's and Nurse's Equipment for Home Delivery.

The necessities for the average home delivery can be carried in 2 bags.

A. Doctor's Bag:
  1. Materials -
      Two pairs of rubber gloves, sterile if possible (although gloves can be boiled before use at delivery).
      Two sterile hand brushes.
      One sterile mask, cap, and gown.
      One bar of germicidal soap or detergent.
      One sterile cord tie and dressing.
      One plastic or rubberized apron.
      Labor record and birth certificate.
      One large sterile sheet for draping the patient and one small sheet for instruments.
      Clinistix® and Uristix® for urine glucose and protein.
  2. Medications -
      Meperidine (Demerol®), 1 ml ampules, for analgesia.
      Ergonovine maleate, 0.2 mg tablets, for postpartal bleeding.
      Hydroxyzine (Vistaril®) or other piperazine compound (antihistaminic) in ampules to potentiate analgesia or relieve allergic manifestations.
      Promazine (Sparine®) ampules for use as tranquilizer or to potentiate analgesia.
      Phenobarbital, 0.03 gm ($1/2$ gr) tablets, for sedation.
      Magnesium sulfate solution (10 ml of 25% solution) as antihypertensive, neurosedative medication.
      Calcium carbonate, 1 gm in 10 ml solution (10%) for intravenous use in the event of respiratory depression due to magnesium sulfate.
      Procaine hydrochloride, 1%, 120 ml, for local anesthesia.
      Bichloride of mercury or mercuric cyanide tablets, 475 mg. Two such tablets per quart of water

yield an antiseptic solution of approximately 1:1000 concentration.

Quaternary ammonium chloride solution (12.5%); 30 ml/quart of water (1:1000) will also constitute an effective disinfectant solution.

Silver nitrate, 1% solution in wax plastules, for ocular instillation.

3. Instruments - Boil instruments and then immerse them in an antiseptic solution before use.

One scalpel and one pair of tissue scissors.
One smooth and one toothed tissue forceps.
Three ring (ovum) forceps.
One uterine packing forceps.
Two broad vaginal retractors.
One box of assorted needles: round and cutting.
One needle holder.
Packs of sutures: chromic and plain 00 and 000 size.
Two 10 ml syringes and long needles for local anesthesia.
Four artery forceps.
One sterile tracheal catheter with DeLee mucus trap.
One sterile No. 16 soft rubber catheter.
One pelvimeter.
One sterile measuring tape.
One cord clamp or tie.
One obstetric forceps (Simpson forceps is the most utilitarian).

4. Emergency materials -
   a. Dehydrated plasma and distilled water diluent; tubing and needles for intravenous administration.
   b. Sterile 6 inch gauze roll for vaginal and uterine packing.

The patient's antepartal record, including pelvic measurements, blood pressure readings, serology and Rh titers, x-ray findings, etc, should be available in the home for reference if necessary.

B. Nurse's Bag:

One large sterile sheet for draping the patient and one small sheet for instruments, etc.
Four sterile towels.
One package of sterile 4 × 4 inch gauze sponges.
Two sterile hand brushes and a bar of germicidal soap or detergent.
One oral and one rectal thermometer.
Two pairs of gloves (sterile, if possible).
One stethoscope and sphygmomanometer.
One safety razor and blades.
One rectal tube with funnel.
One flashlight.
Baby scales.

430 Requirements for Home Delivery

> One lifting forceps to remove articles which have been sterilized.
> One sterile 5 ml hypodermic syringe with short and long No. 22 needles.
> Ampules (1 ml each) of oxytocin or ergonovine.
> One plastic or rubberized apron.

Initial Examination at Onset of Labor.
A. Examine the patient (externally and rectally).
B. Administer an enema and shave the perineum.
C. Assist at a shower or give a vigorous bed bath (with special attention to abdomen, legs, and perineum). Use 1:1000 bichloride of mercury solution as a germicide.
D. The patient should wear a clean nightgown or slip.
E. Make her bed with clean sheets (place clean newspapers beneath bed pad).
F. Remove unnecessary furniture, equipment, and litter.
G. Provide a good light and an ample stack of clean newspapers.
H. Sterilize diapers and newspapers by baking if facilities and time are available: dampen "like clothes for ironing," then "bake like bread" for 45-60 minutes in a 375° F oven.
I. Decide whether delivery should be on a table or in bed and make the necessary preparations.

Conduct of Labor and Delivery. (See p. 108.)
Assume that everything but the operative field is contaminated in home delivery. Keep gloved hands, cotton balls, instruments, etc aseptic.

Keep good records on standard hospital forms. As far as possible, simulate a hospital delivery in professional care and consideration for the patient and her family. Moderate analgesia may be administered and episiotomy may be accomplished in the home just as in the hospital.

If an abnormality develops during labor or after delivery which places the patient in jeopardy, call for consultation immediately and arrange for ambulance transfer to a hospital if indicated.

Immediate Postpartal Care of the Mother.
A. Make the patient comfortable, keep her warm, and ensure rest and quiet.
B. Check the fundus every 5 minutes for the first hour; estimate the amount of vaginal bleeding.
C. Elevate the uterus and massage the fundus lightly every 15 minutes for 1-2 hours. (For subsequent management, see p. 128.)

Immediate Care of the Newborn. (See also pp. 127 and 156.)
A premature infant or one which appears to be abnormal should be transferred to a hospital at once.

Handle the baby as little as possible. Wrap him in a clean towel. Cut and tie the cord, using aseptic technic. Oil the infant with liquid petrolatum or baby oil, or apply pHisohex®. Wipe off excess. **Do not bathe the infant.** Insert one drop of 1% aqueous silver nitrate solution into each eye and irrigate with cool boiled water. Dress the infant in a cotton shirt and diaper. Apply a dressing to the cord and wrap a bellyband around his waist. Weigh him and wrap him in a cotton or wool blanket.

Place the baby in a warmed crib, basket, or box away from fire, animals, and vermin. (A box within a box with space around for 5 hot water bottles between the sides is a useful arrangement. **Note:** Do not place hot water bottles at the baby's head.)

Keep the navel and cord stump dry. The cord separates in 5-10 days. If it appears reddened or becomes odorous, touch with 70% alcohol twice daily and dry the navel by exposure to air.

The Placenta.

Inspect the placenta. If it is intact, examine it grossly, count the vessels in the cord and place it in a plastic or paper bag for pathologic study or discard.

18...
Gynecologic History & Examination

OUTLINE OF HISTORY & EXAMINATION

Age, Gravidity, & Parity.

Chief Complaint: List the patient's medical difficulties in her words, in her order of seriousness.

Present Illness: State the character of the patient's health at the onset of her sickness. Narrate the symptomatology in sequence of events. Include facts, dates, and essential details.

Past Medical & Surgical History: Briefly summarize the patient's childhood and later illnesses in chronologic order together with the treatment prescribed for each. Record operations and injuries with dates and outcome.

Obstetric History: Number of previous pregnancies (with dates), duration of pregnancy, character and duration of labor, complications, weight and sex of infant; stillbirths, abortions, neonatal complications.

Family History: Age, health of parents and siblings. Age, cause, date of death of principal relatives. Familial or hereditary abnormalities, diseases, bleeding tendencies. Occurrence of cancer, tuberculosis, diabetes mellitus, syphilis, heart disease, high blood pressure, nervous or mental disorders in the family.

Marital History: Duration of present marriage, age and health of spouse and children, if living, or cause and age at time of death; former marriages; degree of compatibility.

Social History: Occupation, hazards. Church, clubs, reaction to other people. Successes, failures, arrests. Marriages (dates, duration). Health of husbands and children. Success of marriage, coitus, contraception. Sleep, exercise, relaxation, hobbies, intake of alcohol, tobacco, stimulants, sedatives. Medications. Residence abroad or in the tropics.

System Review.

Provide a positive or negative comment for each division in this category but cover the symptoms relative to the patient's chief complaint in the present illness only.

A. General: Describe the patient's health, allergies, skin disorders. Record present weight, average weight,

History & Examination 433

weight prior to the present illness. Include patient's
version of reason for gain or loss.
B. Head and Neck: Pain, tenderness, swelling, restriction
of neck, trauma.
1. Eyes - Vision with and without glasses, double vision,
   irritation, swelling of lids, prominence of eyes.
2. Ears - Hearing, pain, "buzzing," discharge.
3. Nose - Acuity of smell, obstruction to nasal passages,
   bleeding, discharge.
4. Mouth - Condition of teeth, gums, tongue, sensitivity
   of taste, bleeding, chewing difficulties.
5. Throat - Speech, swallowing, condition of tonsils and
   pharynx.
C. Cardiovascular: Skin color (pale, ruddy, dusky), precordial or substernal constriction pain, irregular or labored heartbeat, shortness of breath at rest or exercise.
D. Respiratory: Cough, wheezing, sputum, hemoptysis, chest pain with breathing, chills, fever, night sweats.
E. Gastrointestinal: Appetite, thirst, digestive difficulties (nausea, vomiting, pre- or postprandial pain, hematemesis, food intolerance), jaundice; frequency, character, and color of stools.
F. Genitourinary and Menstrual:
1. Urinary frequency, nocturia, oliguria, dysuria, hematuria, urethral discharge, "sores," swelling, venereal disease.
2. Menarche, last menstrual period (LMP), previous menstrual period (PMP), regularity, duration, amount of bleeding, pain, mucous discharge, intermenstrual or postcoital spotting, menopause (date and symptoms). List pregnancies (including abortions, stillbirths) with dates and complications, obstetric operations.
G. Neuropsychiatric: Skin sensation. Strength, ability to move, walk, work. Ataxia, dizziness, tremor. Headache. "Spells," fits. Acuity of memory. Strange occurrences. Libido.

Physical Examination.
A. General: Appearance of the patient, ambulatory or bed patient. Attitude, color of skin, mucous surfaces. Temperature, pulse, respiration, blood pressure, height, and weight.
B. Head and Neck: Skull size and shape, hair (amount, color, texture), tumors, tenderness, neck swelling, pulsations, deviation of trachea, tracheal tug, mobility.
1. Eyes - Prominence of lids or eyes. Size, shape, pupillary reaction to light, character of conjunctiva and sclera, ocular movements, ophthalmoscopic examination (when indicated).

2. Ears - Hearing, discharge, cerumen, tophi, tenderness, otoscopic examination (when indicated).
3. Nose - Deformity, septal deviation, obstruction, tenderness, discharge, unusual smells, tenderness over sinuses, transillumination of sinuses.
4. Mouth and throat - Lips, gums, tongue, dentition, tonsils, oral pharynx, postnasal discharge, laryngoscopic examination (when indicated).

C. Thorax: Size, shape, symmetry, pulsations, tenderness.
1. Breasts - Size, shape, equality, masses, tenderness, scars, discharge from nipple.
2. Lungs - Inspection of chest: breathing (type, rate, depth), equality of inspiration and expiration.
   a. Palpation - Muscle tone, tenderness, tactile fremitus.
   b. Percussion - Resonance, great vessel and cardiac silhouette, excursions of the diaphragm, gastric tympany.
   c. Auscultation - Quality and intensity of breath sounds, rales (especially post-tussive), whisper and vocal fremitus, friction rub.
3. Heart - Note the point of maximal impulse at apex, abnormal pulsations, retractions or venous distention in neck or other veins.
   a. Palpation - Note the point of maximal intensity. Record in centimeters to the right and left of the midsternal line in centimeters in or near the closest inner space. Palpate the precordial area for shocks and thrills.
   b. Percussion - Outline by direct and indirect methods the borders of the heart and great vessels. Orient the left border of the heart to the midclavicular line.
   c. Auscultation - Character of sounds, intensity of tones, rate and rhythm. Location of murmurs, type and intensity of murmur, transmission of murmur, time of murmur. Compare A_2 and P_2. Friction rubs and post-tussive rales.

D. Abdomen: Note the size, shape, and contour of the abdomen, masses, visible peristaltic waves, prominent veins, herniation.
1. Palpation - Thickness of the abdominal wall (panniculus), tenderness, rigidity, masses, hernias; presence or absence of a fluid wave, palpation of organs, liver, spleen, and kidneys, other masses, costovertebral angle tenderness.
2. Percussion - Dullness in the flanks, fluid shift, position of tumor or organs and bladder.
3. Auscultation - Presence of peristaltic tones, "slush" of shifting fluids.

E. Extremities: Note the size and shape of the hands, color, movements; condition of the fingers and nails; the size and

color of arms; the size and movement of legs and feet.
F. Peripheral Vascular System: Record the blood pressure in both arms, and palpate the arteries for thickness and resilience. Note the type of radial, femoral, distal pedal, posterior tibial, and popliteal pulses. Observe the temperature of the extremities, and note the presence or absence of cyanosis.
G. Nervous System: Cerebral function, cranial nerves, cerebellar function, motor system, sensory system, and reflexes.

GYNECOLOGIC EXAMINATIONS & PROCEDURES

The gynecologic evaluation of each new patient must include blood pressure determination and examination of the heart and lungs. Particular attention must be devoted to the breasts, abdomen, pelvis, and appropriate laboratory studies.

An appraisal of other body systems should be done when indicated by the medical history or unusual findings. Do not dismiss a patient following the initial work-up without detecting a disorder of major consequence if signs or symptoms are present. The gynecologic specialist will frequently refer a patient for consultation, e.g., cardiac or neurologic disease, when indicated. The physician who does not specialize may do whatever evaluation is required for complete diagnosis (although it is unlikely, for example, that this would include a complete ophthalmologic examination). If the patient who is seen for gynecologic complaints is already under the care of another physician, the gynecologic examination should be specific and complete with particular reference to the chief complaint.

Breasts.

Examine the breasts in good direct light with the patient first in a relaxed sitting position. Record abnormalities, using a sketch or diagram for clarity. Note the size, shape, symmetry, and pendulosity of the breasts. Examine for skin and nipple changes and nipple discharge. Smear and fix the discharge for cytologic examination.

Palpate one breast at a time. Hold the fingers flat against the breast and carefully feel with the fingertips, using gentle pressure against the firm chest wall. Evaluate the entire breast systematically from the nipple outward. Distinguish tender regions. Observe breast consistency for thickened or firm zones. Identify the cord-like duct system and any "shotty" or nodular masses, and determine whether masses are fixed to the skin or chest wall. Transilluminate the breast in a darkened room to distinguish solid from cystic tumors. Palpate axillary and supra- and infraclavicular lymph nodes.

Instruct the patient to raise her arms over her head and observe asymmetry or retraction of the nipple or skin. Use oblique light to confirm surface dimpling.

Have the patient bend forward from the erect position to reveal irregularities or dimpling when the breasts fall forward from the chest wall.

Continue the appraisal with the patient supine. Place a small pillow under her shoulder on the side to be examined to "balance" the breast on the chest wall.

Any unphysiologic mass or discharge should be investigated further because of the possibility of cancer.

Abdomen.

Drape the patient in the dorsal recumbent position with her knees slightly flexed to improve abdominal relaxation. Inspect for freedom of respiratory movement, prominence or enlargement of internal organs, asymmetry, scars, and significant skin changes (e.g., rashes, postirradiation telangiectasia).

Palpate the abdomen gently for evidence of muscle guarding, tenderness, rebound phenomenon, herniation, or masses. Palpate firmly for deep masses or sensitivity, especially over the cecum, colon, and bladder. Identify the liver by percussion and palpate its edge; examine the gallbladder and epigastric region. Check for costovertebral angle tenderness and displacement of the kidneys. Consider splenic enlargement.

Pelvis.

A. General Pelvic (Vaginal) Examination: Place the patient in the lithotomy position, appropriately draped. The physician must be seated to visualize the parts adequately. Employ surgically clean gloves and require a female attendant to be present as a chaperone and assistant.
  1. Inspection of external genitalia - Inflamed, hypertrophied, atrophied, ulcerated, and other abnormal areas can be seen almost at a glance. Separate the labia. Look for vaginal discharge at the introitus. Note abnormalities of the clitoris.

     Inspect for skin changes over the perineum, thighs, mons veneris, and perianal region. Note and record the presence of masses and tender areas. Describe discernible external genital lesions.

     Observe the urethral meatus for redness, purulent exudation from Skene's ducts, and other abnormalities.
  2. Vaginal cytology - Before digital examination, obtain vaginal mucus from the posterior vaginal fornix for cytologic examination, using the method recommended by the pathologist who will examine the smear. If a speculum is employed to secure the mucus which will collect in the lower blade, do not use lubricants because they impair the quality of the spread.

3. Speculum examination - Artificial lubrication of the speculum is rarely necessary because vaginal secretions are normally adequate for this purpose when care is used during the speculum insertion. Water may be used if necessary. All cream or jelly lubricants have the disadvantage of interfering with vaginal or cervical cytologic examination, bacterial spreads or cultures, and wet preparations for Trichomonas, Candida, and Hemophilus organisms.

Request the patient to relax and then bear down as with a bowel movement as the speculum is introduced to reduce muscular resistance. Spread the labia with the gloved fingers of one hand, insert the gloved index finger of the same hand into the vagina, and depress the perineum slightly. Do not insert the speculum directly into the vagina but slightly downward and inward to avoid the urethra. Visualize the vaginal canal while inserting and opening the speculum. If a single-blade speculum is used, merely depress it to view the cervix. Progressive observation is necessary to avoid traumatic encounter with a vaginal obstruction, mass, or friable lesion. A good light source is required, preferably daylight or a blue-white spotlight, although some physicians prefer a head lamp or head mirror.

As the blades of the bivalve speculum meet the cervix, open the instrument so that the blades slip into the anterior and posterior fornix to fully expose the cervix. Fix the blades in an open position by tightening the screw lock.

Standard Office Equipment for Pelvic Examination
(See Figs 18-1 to 18-4.)

(1) Standard size Graves speculum for most adult patients.

(2) Large Graves speculum for women with relaxations.

(3) Small Graves speculum for women with a contracted introitus or annular hymen.

(4) Narrow Pederson speculum for women with introital atresia.

(5) A No. 10 Kelly air cystoscope is especially useful for vaginoscopy in children.

(6) A double-ended Sims speculum is employed to demonstrate cystocele, rectocele, or descensus of the cervix, or for lateral vaginal retraction.

438 Examinations & Procedures

Fig 18-1. Kelly air cystoscope for vaginoscopy in children.

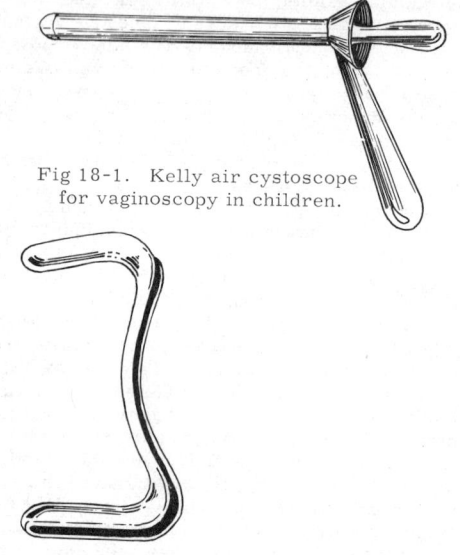

Fig 18-2. Sims vaginal retractor.

Fig 18-3. Graves vaginal speculum.

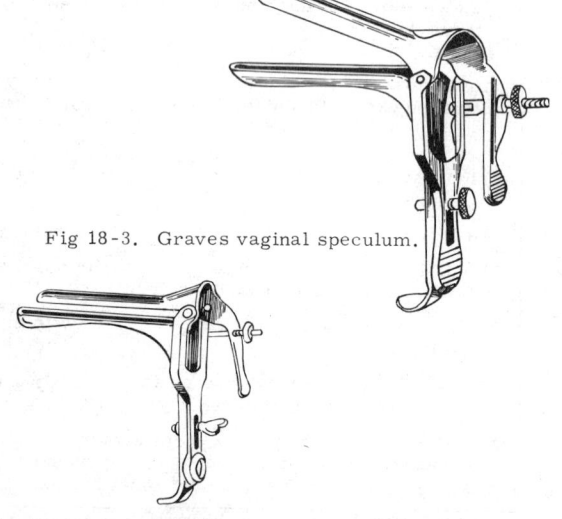

Fig 18-4. Pederson vaginal speculum (narrow blades).

4. Inspection of the cervix - Examine the cervix carefully. Obtain materials for smear and culture from the posterior fornix and cervical os when indicated. Determine the following: (1) Size, contour, and surface characteristics; (2) significant lacerations; (3) displacement; (4) size and configuration of the external os; (5) distortion and ulceration; (6) type and amount of discharge, blood, or fluid originating in the cervical canal; and (7) the character of the cervical canal (in a patulous cervix).

   Touch or gently wipe ulcerations or friable lesions with a cotton-tipped applicator for evidence of contact bleeding. Deliberately move the cervix up and down with moderate force to elicit tenderness on motion. Defer biopsy of suspicious lesions and topical therapy until after bimanual examination to avoid bleeding.

5. Withdrawal of the speculum - Slowly remove the speculum from the vagina while inspecting the vaginal walls. Note the color, the presence or absence of rugae, the apparent thickness of the mucosa, and any abnormalities such as redness, ulceration, or tumors. Be especially alert to observe zones of contact bleeding.

   In cases where cystocele, rectocele, or descensus of the cervix are suspected, open the blades of the speculum widely just within the introitus before complete withdrawal of the instrument and have the patient "bear down." The degree of vaginal relaxation will thus be revealed.

   Firmly "strip" Skene's ducts and the distal urethra immediately after removal of the speculum. Observe, smear, and culture the discharge expressed.

B. Manual Pelvic (Vaginal) Examination: Digital examination is easiest with the patient in the lithotomy position and the examiner standing with his foot on a step or low stool and his elbow on his knee to brace the examining arm and hand. Ideally, use first one hand and then the other in pelvic examination; masses in the right pelvis will be palpated more easily with the right hand, and vice versa.

Insert the gloved, lubricated index finger gently but deliberately into the vagina. Apply slight backward pressure at the fourchet to aid perineal relaxation, to determine the patient's apprehensiveness and resistance, and to note whether the hymen is intact. After a pause to enhance relaxation, slip the middle finger of the examining hand along the forefinger into the vagina.

1. Palpation of the structures of the introitus - Tenderness, masses, and thickening should be noted. With the thumb external and the palm turned downward, feel for enlargement and sensitivity of Bartholin's glands. Investigate the lower vaginal wall for abnormalities. Feel

the urethra for relaxation, local dilatation, masses, and tenderness.

To demonstrate cystocele, rectocele, and descensus of the cervix, turn the hand downward, spread the 2 fingers widely, and ask the patient to strain.

2. Palpation of the cervix - Lightly outline the cervix with the fingers to determine its size, position, contour, consistency, and dilatation. Move the cervix about with moderate vigor to stretch the uterosacral and transverse cervical ligaments. This will usually reveal the degree of freedom of the cervix and unusual pelvic tenderness.
3. Palpation of the bladder base - Feel beneath the bladder to determine sensitivity and unusual structures. Slight tenderness and a suggestion of thickening over the normal ureter at or near its insertion into the bladder are normal.

C. Bimanual Examination: The foregoing procedures require but one unaided hand. The other hand is used on the abdomen to outline the deeper pelvic structures in bimanual examination.

Hold the hand palm down on the abdomen with the fingers together but slightly flexed with the fingers pointed toward the patient's head. Press firmly against the abdominal wall to displace the lower abdominal and pelvic organs toward the fingers in the vagina. The patient should take shallow, rapid breaths with her mouth open to avoid tensing the abdominal wall.

1. Palpation of the uterus - Attempt to depress the fundus of the uterus with one hand while the vaginal fingers are resting against the cervix and lower portion of the corpus. Relaxation of the vaginal walls and fornices may permit examination of all or much of the posterior aspect of the uterus and even the fundus via the cul-de-sac. A normally free uterus can usually be brought well downward and forward by the abdominal hand. This makes possible vaginal palpation of both the anterior wall and the fundus of the uterus.

   Palpate the uterus to determine its position, size, consistency, contour, and mobility, and the patient's discomfort on uterine manipulation. Gently explore the posterior fornix for masses, fullness, fluctuation, and sensitivity. Acute tenderness in this region may temporarily prevent further examination.
2. Palpation of the adnexa - Turn the hand in the vagina so that the palm is upward. Insert the 2 examining fingers slightly posteriorly but high into one of the lateral fornices. Sweep the abdominal examining hand downward over the fingers in the vagina. Attempt to trap the ovary and tube between the 2 hands.

The ovary normally lies just lateral to the uterus near its midportion. If the ovary and tube are not felt initially, check the cul-de-sac, the lateral pelvic wall, or the space anterior to the uterus for a displaced, possibly adherent ovary and tube. If one sweeps the examining hand laterally from the uterine cornu, it may be possible to follow the fallopian tube to the ovary. The ovary is normally slightly tender, which helps to distinguish it from nontender masses, such as fecal material within the bowel. Rectovaginal examination may permit the best delineation of the ovary (see below). Observe the position, size, consistency, contour, and mobility of each ovary. Note any unusual tenderness.

Ordinarily the fallopian tube is not sensitive, but it is so delicate that the normal tube cannot be palpated. Tenderness, swelling, or a cord-like thickening between the ovary and the uterus indicates tubal disease. Inflammation or neoplasia may convert the tube into an enlarged mass which may be mistaken for an ovarian tumor.

Salpingitis, endometriosis, or malignancy may involve one or both adnexa so extensively that these structures and the uterus become a single mass filling the entire true pelvis. The cul-de-sac may be filled or obliterated, and gynecologic landmarks may disappear.

D. Rectovaginal Examination: Rectovaginal examination should be done routinely even though all of the internal genital structures have been palpated satisfactorily on vaginal evaluation. Anal, rectovaginal septal, and even sacral abnormalities may be felt only in this way. The rectovaginal examination is invaluable in children, virgins, and old women, in whom the vaginal introitus is so small that only a single finger can be inserted. Rectovaginal examination is preferred to simple rectal examination because the second finger reaches farther when the first finger is in the vagina.

Rectovaginal examination will permit palpation of the following particularly well: (1) rectocele, (2) an ovary not located by vaginal examination, (3) the posterior uterine wall, (4) cul-de-sac masses, (5) rectovaginal septal masses, (6) sacral nerve trunks, and (7) uterosacral ligaments. Rectovaginal examination may be more informative than two-finger vaginal examination in patients with vaginal stricture, pelvic mass formation, acute pelvic tenderness, and other disorders which interfere with vaginal manipulation.

The patient and the examiner are positioned as for bimanual vaginal examination. Lubricate the second finger of the examining hand liberally and apply the finger to the anus. Have the patient bear down slightly to relax the anal sphincter. Insert the distal half of the finger into the anal canal. Meanwhile, introduce the forefinger into the vagina. The perineal body will then be between the 2 fingers. Encourage the patient to relax by adopting a gentle, slow, deliberate manner. Finally, reach with the tips of both the vaginal and rectal fingers as high as possible in the pelvis. Palpate bimanually, as with the vaginal examination.

To demonstrate rectocele, bring the rectal finger back to the perineal body, removing the vaginal finger. In so doing, the rectal pouch will be entered and its protrusion into the vagina may be evident at the introitus. The patient herself may be able to see a rectocele thus demonstrated if she will hold a mirror at an appropriate angle.

Laboratory Studies.

A. Smears:
1. Bacteria - Obtain smears for bacteria with surgically clean cotton-tipped applicators. Fluid exudate may be obtained from the urethral meatus, Skene's and Bartholin's ducts, from the vaginal walls, the posterior vaginal fornix, and the cervical os. Make a thin spread of the discharge on a clean glass slide and permit it to dry in the air. Methylene blue stain (1% aqueous solution) may suffice for a quick rough appraisal of the type and approximate number of bacteria present. For specific etiologic diagnosis (e.g., pneumococci and gonococci infection), use Gram's stain.
2. Trichomonas vaginalis - Examine separate preparations from the posterior fornix, the cervical os, and the urethral meatus. Moisten a clean cotton-tipped applicator with normal saline. Swab the site of exudation or dip into the discharge with the applicator. Touch a drop of the exudate to a polished slide and apply a fresh cover slip. Examine microscopically immediately (while still warm) for trichomonads. Hollow-ground glass slides are an unnecessary refinement. If a delay of 5-10 minutes is inevitable, the moistened cotton-tipped applicator carrying a small amount of the fluid to be examined may be transferred to 1-2 ml of warmed Ringer's solution and this fluid examined for trichomonads.
3. Candida albicans (monilia) - Employ the same technic as for the demonstration of trichomonads, but use 1-2 drops of potassium hydroxide (10% aqueous solution) on the slide or in the tube to dissolve the epithelial, inflammatory, and red blood cells. The mycelia will be

displayed prominently. It is unnecessary to warm the slide or solution. The material most likely to show mycelia will be the white plaques of "vaginal thrush," which must be rubbed from the mucosa with the cotton applicator.
B. Cultures:
1. Bacteria - Obtain sufficient exudate to saturate a sterile cotton-tipped applicator. Using bacteriologic precautions, place the applicator in a sterile, dry test tube and send it immediately to the bacteriology laboratory for culture and identification. Avoid heating and drying. When gonorrhea is suspected, inoculate a sterile chocolate or blood agar plate at the time of pelvic examination. Place the applicator in a sterile test tube with the customary flame sterilization and send both preparations to the bacteriology laboratory for processing without delay.
2. Trichomonas - Trichomonas vaginalis may be grown on culture media under aerobic conditions, but this is rarely necessary in gynecology. If these organisms are not identified in the "wet smear," careful inspection of the stained exfoliative vaginal cytologic smear (Papanicolaou) will generally reveal their presence.
3. Candida albicans (monilia) - In contrast to Trichomanas, Candida hyphae and spores are frequently missed in the potassium hydroxide wet smear, especially in the absence of curd-like plaques. Therefore, in doubtful cases it is necessary to culture vaginal fluid using Sabouraud's, Nickerson's, or Pagano-Levin medium.
C. Urine: Collect a catheterized urine specimen in a sterile test tube using sterile equipment and technic after thoroughly cleansing the urethral meatus with a mild antiseptic solution.

Other Procedures.

A. Sounding the Uterus: Rule out intrauterine pregnancy before sounding the uterus with a sterile, malleable, calibrated Sims or Simpson uterine sound to determine the patency of the cervical canal, the presence of lesions in the cervix or uterus which will bleed on contact, uterine size, the position of the uterine fundus, and the direction of the uterine canal (before Rubin test or endometrial biopsy).

Carefully wipe the external cervical os with a cotton pledget or gauze sponge saturated with an antiseptic solution. Bend the sound to the estimated curvature of the cervical-uterine axis. The speculum may be surgically clean rather than sterile if one is careful not to touch the blades with the distal 3-4 inches of the sound during its introduction. In the absence of cervical stenosis and extreme flexion of the corpus, gentle sounding of a uterus which is in an approximately normal position causes only very mild, menstrual-like cramps.

Occasionally it may be necessary to draw the cervix toward the introitus to make the os accessible or to straighten the canal. For traction, apply a double-toothed Braun or other suitable tenaculum to the anterior cervical lip in either the frontal or sagittal plane. Warn the patient that she may feel sudden, slight discomfort.

Measure and record the length of the cervical canal and the depth of the uterine cavity. Note points of obstruction, distortion, and bleeding. Be careful to avoid perforation of the uterus.

If sounding of the uterus is impossible with the usual instruments, try a fine, soft wire probe. Hegar dilators (No. 5-10) may be used to dilate the cervix in cervical stenosis and for the diagnosis of an abnormally large (incompetent) internal cervical os.

B. Biopsy:
1. Infiltrate the site of biopsy with procaine (0.5-1% aqueous solution) or its equivalent. If the suspicious lesion is 1 cm or less in diameter, it should be totally excised; if it is larger, only a portion should be taken. Include normal appearing bordering tissue for comparison. One or more fine, nonabsorbable sutures may be required for hemostasis and closure of the defect.

    Excisional biopsy of ulcers, tumors, and other lesions over 1 cm in diameter should be done in an operating room where adequate equipment and assistance for anesthesia and hemostasis are available. Wide margins of normal tissue should be taken.

2. Cervix - Even multiple biopsy of the cervix may be performed in the office with little or no pain or danger, using the Schubert or a similar punch biopsy forceps. Anesthetics are not required because the cervix is relatively insensitive to pain. The Hyams and other similar electrosurgical instruments should not be used because they cause physical changes in the specimen which alter the staining characteristics of the tissue.

    Steady the cervix with a tenaculum; obtain biopsies from the posterior lip first to avoid obscuring other biopsy sites by bleeding. Include samples from the mucosquamous junction. Place tissue fragments in 10% formalin fixative immediately.

    Although the amount of bleeding from biopsy sites is unpredictable, it is generally not excessive and should be controlled without resort to cauterization if possible. Pathologic study of repeat biopsy material or examination of the cervix after surgery for the presence of residual cancer may be complicated by tissue necrosis and inflammation when traumatic or styptic procedures are employed. Control minor ooze with cotton wool or gauze applied with firm pressure. Ligation of individual bleeding points with very fine absorbable catgut should always be done if possible. Interrupted or figure-of-eight hemostasis sutures may be used also. If these measures do not suffice, touch the bleeding areas with negatol (Negatan®), acetone, or 5% silver nitrate solution. Use the electrocautery only as a last resort.

Do a cold knife cone biopsy (and fractional curettage) in surgery. Paracervical or general anesthesia may be required; hemorrhage may necessitate vaginal packing or deeply placed sutures (or both).

3. Endometrium - Sound the uterus (see p. 443) to determine bleeding, contour, points of distortion, and other abnormalities. Utilize a Randall or Weissman tubular barbed curet to obtain strips of endometrium which become threaded into the instrument.

Pass the biopsy curet to the fundus. Stroke it downward against the uterine wall to the cervix in various parts of the uterus to obtain representative bits of endometrium. Finally, secure fragments of the endocervical lining also.

Slight suction from a syringe may be used, but forceful pump or other suction must not be employed or maceration of tissue will result. The tissue obtained can be gently blown into 10% formalin solution by light positive pressure.

If a thorough surgical (therapeutic) curettage is required it should be done in the operating room and not in the examining room.

Contraindications to endometrial biopsy in the office include the following: (1) Possible uterine pregnancy; (2) marked cervicitis; (3) friable, bleeding cervical abnormalities; (4) marked cervical stenosis; (5) profuse bleeding at the initiation of endometrial curettage.

C. Culdoscopy: Culdoscopy is the visualization of the pelvic structures through the vaginal vault and cul-de-sac using an instrument similar to the cystoscope, with a lens system and illumination. It is a hospital procedure and should be attempted only by a physician with adequate experience. Perforation of a viscus, intraperitoneal bleeding, and peritonitis are possible complications.

Culdoscopy may be indicated when the symptomatology is at variance with physical, laboratory, or x-ray findings but laparotomy is not clearly indicated. The procedure is simplest and most successful when minimal abnormal pelvic findings are present. Suspected unruptured ectopic pregnancy, endometriosis, polycystic ovarian disease, atypical pelvic pain, and infertility due to unknown cause may be indications for culdoscopy. The examination makes it possible to avoid laparotomy in many cases, but the patient should be willing to submit to laparotomy if a serious problem is revealed. A fixed cul-de-sac mass, obliteration of the cul-de-sac, or an adherent uterine retroposition are contraindications. Hematoperitoneum prevents visualization. Operative procedures through the culdoscope such as drainage of cysts, biopsy, and fulguration should not be attempted.

In 5-10% of attempts, puncture will be incomplete or visualization unsatisfactory. Diagnostic errors occur in 1-5% of cases.

The procedure is as follows: (See also p. 684.)

1. Administer a hypnotic such as meperidine (Demerol®), 100 mg I. M.
2. With the patient in the knee-chest position and a Sims retractor elevating the perineum, grasp the posterior lip of the cervix with a tenaculum to expose the posterior fornix. Apply an antiseptic solution and then inject 1-2 ml of 1% procaine solution (or equivalent) into the central portion of the fornix. A few minutes later, thrust the sterile culdoscope trocar through the vaginal wall and the peritoneum with one quick movement.
3. Remove the trocar and substitute the sterile culdoscope. Systematically examine the peritoneum, tubes, ovaries, etc.
4. After the examination is completed, remove the culdoscope and expel as much air as possible from the peritoneal cavity through the cannula by exerting pressure on the abdomen.
5. Remove the instrument. It is not necessary to suture the trocar wound; healing will occur within several days.

D. Colposcopy: An expensive microscope (colposcope), high intensity illumination, and special training and experience are required to visualize the vagina and the cervix for the detection of suspicious and early malignant lesions. The colposcope is still considered a research instrument by most gynecologists.

19...
Diseases of the Vulva & Vagina

VAGINAL HERNIAS
(Cystocele, Urethrocele, Rectocele, Enterocele)

Cystocele and rectocele (see Figs 19-1 and 19-2) are herniations of the bladder and rectum, respectively, through faults in the vaginal septa; enterocele (Fig 19-3) is a herniation, usually of intestine, through the cul-de-sac or other pelvic floor defect into the vaginal vault. Cystocele is frequently accompanied by a urethrocele or sagging (not sacculation) of the mid and proximal urethra into the vagina. Most vaginal hernias are multiple and are due to childbirth injuries, but tissue weakness due to any of several causes (postmenopausal estrogen deficiency, obesity, and other causes of increased intra-abdominal pressure, neurologic deficits, operative trauma, congenital defects) is often a contributory factor. Caucasian women develop cystocele and rectocele more often than Negro women.

At least half of all parous women develop some degree of cystocele or rectocele, usually after the menopause, but only about 10% of the lesions become symptomatic. Significant enterocele occurs in all instances of uterine or vaginal vault prolapse.

Vaginal herniations rarely are observed soon after even a traumatic delivery. The defects become evident only months or years later, perhaps following subsequent apparently normal deliveries. The climacteric and the persistent stress of increased intra-abdominal pressure, especially while the woman is in the erect posture, gradually stretches the supports of the damaged bladder, rectum, or pelvic floor. The protrusion may eventually become so large that it presents at the introitus.

Voiding is incomplete with cystocele because some urine always remains in the pouch below the bladder neck. Urinary frequency and urgency incontinence are due to overflow voiding. Residual (stagnant) urine soon becomes contaminated, and urinary tract infection is the result. Urethrocele does not itself interfere with urinary function.

Rectocele enlarges slowly with physical activity and the weight of the abdominal contents. The rectal pouch fills with feces, and constipation becomes a troublesome symptom.

448 Vaginal Hernias

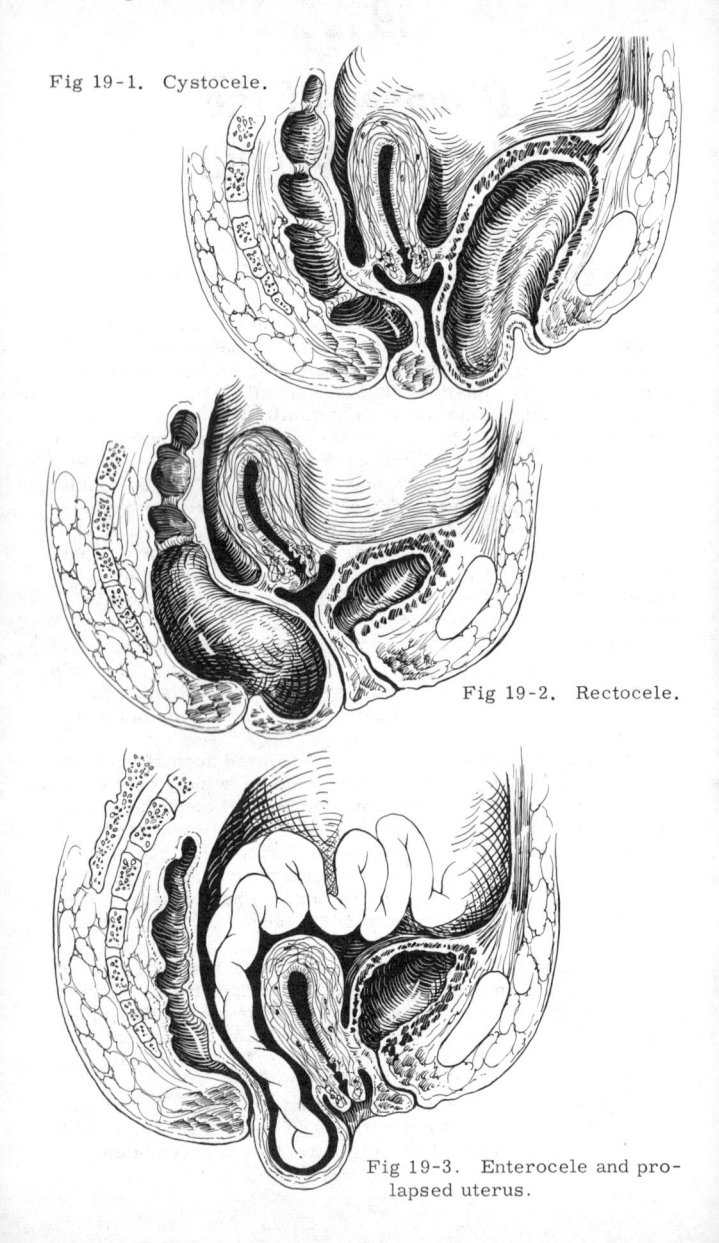

Fig 19-1. Cystocele.

Fig 19-2. Rectocele.

Fig 19-3. Enterocele and prolapsed uterus.

Straining at stool helps to evacuate the rectum, but the force exerted may enlarge the herniation until it distends the introitus.

Clinical Findings.
A. Symptoms and Signs: Cystocele, rectocele, or enterocele of slight to moderate degree is usually asymptomatic, but many women describe a sensation of bladder and vaginal distention and urinary frequency, especially when erect. Stress incontinence of urine develops when injury involves the bladder neck structures. Urethrocele causes no symptoms. Rectocele and enterocele both cause constipation, a "bearing down" sensation, or a feeling of lack of pelvic support and vaginal fullness, particularly when standing.

For evacuation of a large cystocele or rectocele, patients may employ manual reduction of the herniation.

Vaginal hernias can be demonstrated by rectovaginal examination. The rectal finger will enter the rectocele pouch to accentuate the posterior vaginal wall defect. A single-blade vaginal speculum is inserted with the patient in the lithotomy position. Cystocele or rectocele is demonstrated when the patient strains and the instrument is retracted first upward and then downward.

The diagnosis of a small enterocele may be difficult, and some are discovered only at surgery. However, most hernias of this type can be distinguished by slowly withdrawing a bivalve speculum with the patient in the supine position. The bulge of an enterocele may be seen just above that of a rectocele. The diagnosis can be confirmed by performing rectovaginal examination and requiring the patient to cough. An impulse will be felt against the fingertip held against an enterocele (upper bulge) but not a rectocele (lower bulge).
B. X-Ray Findings: Lateral x-rays with contrast medium in the bladder, large bowel, and small bowel may demonstrate a cystocele, rectocele, or enterocele, respectively.
C. Special Examinations: Cystoscopy and proctoscopy will corroborate a diagnosis of cystocele or rectocele. Passage of a firm catheter will demonstrate a urethrocele or cystocele.

Complications.
Urinary tract infection is generally recurrent and often serious.

Damage to the pubococcygeus portion of the levator musculature and the endopelvic fascia, often associated with a large cystocele, weakens the bladder neck and causes incontinence.

Progressive enlargement of a cystocele, usually with uterine prolapse, may result in acute urinary retention.

Most patients with rectocele have hemorrhoids also.

Rectocele may cause obstipation, fecal impaction, and diverticulosis.

Intestinal obstruction occurs rarely in an enterocele containing small amounts of feces.

Differential Diagnosis.

Cysts of vestigial (Wolffian) origin, semi-solid or degenerated tumors of the vaginal septa, and large inclusion cysts may be mistaken for cystocele or rectocele. A large cystocele may overshadow a urethrocele. The fullness of a large, high rectocele, prolapsed and adherent adnexa, markedly retroflexed uterus, soft cervical or uterine myoma, or retained fecal material may be confused with enterocele.

Prevention.

Childbirth injury, obesity, chronic cough, and straining should be avoided. Postmenopausal estrogen therapy is of value. Neurologic disorders should be prevented or treated promptly. Gross enlargement of pelvic and vaginal hernias must not be neglected.

Treatment.

A. Emergency Measures: The lower bowel and bladder must be emptied if acute retention occurs. In enterocele, if incarceration of the intestines is not relieved by placing the patient in the knee-chest position, laparotomy and surgical release will be required.

B. General Measures: The obese female must be encouraged to reduce to her desirable weight. Pelvic tumors must be removed and ascitic fluid drained and reaccumulation prevented. Cough and constipation should be treated appropriately. Cyclic estrogens in small doses are given to postmenopausal women.

C. Specific Measures: Pessaries, especially doughnut, ball, and crescentic (Gehrung) supports, afford temporary symptomatic relief but are never curative. Surgical correction of cystocele, urethrocele, or rectocele by colporrhaphy may be required. Enterocele is repaired surgically by cul-de-sac herniorrhaphy.

D. Treatment of Complications: Bladder drainage and chemotherapy are required for urinary retention and infection. Fecal impaction is relieved by oil instillation, digital evacuation, enemas, and laxatives as required.

Prognosis.

A recurrence rate of 10-15% is reported after vaginal hernia repair.

LEUKORRHEA

Leukorrhea is a usually whitish vaginal discharge which may occur at any age and affects almost all women at some time. It is not a disease but a manifestation of a local or systemic disorder. It is usually due to infection of the lower reproductive tract; other causes include inflammation of other areas, estrogenic or psychic stimulation, tumors, and estrogen depletion. The presence of some vaginal mucus is normal; when soiling of the clothing or distressing local symptoms occur, the discharge must be considered abnormal.

Genital infections, foreign bodies (e. g., pessaries), chemicals (e. g., irritating douches or contraceptives), and irradiation cause leukorrhea. Protozoa, notably Trichomonas vaginalis, cause over one-third of cases; Candida infection is a frequent cause, especially in diabetic patients and during pregnancy; Hemophilus vaginalis infections and gonorrhea and other venereal infections are frequent causes; Mycobacterium tuberculosis is a rare cause; helminths, especially Oxyuris, occasionally cause leukorrhea in children.

Cervical mucus production, principally the result of estrogen stimulation, is the major source of normal vaginal secretion. The vaginal mucosa contains no glands and is not truly secretory. However, estrogen supports a slightly moist, stratified squamous epithelium which produces desquamated cells even in the absence of the cervix and uterus. Progesterone stimulation after estrogen activation increases the glycogen content of exfoliated cells. The maintenance of vaginal acidity is largely dependent upon high levels of estrogen and the presence of lactobacilli (Döderlein's bacilli), which utilize glycogen in their metabolism. Any marked alteration of these relationships predisposes to leukorrhea.

When estrogen and progesterone levels are high, the genital tract resists infection. During childhood and the menopause the titer of these hormones is low or absent, and the thin vulvar and vaginal surfaces are more susceptible to bacterial invasion.

Hyperestrogenism causes the production of cervical mucus in large amounts. Excess mucus production also occurs normally in the newborn, during pregnancy, and as a result of sexual or other emotional stimulation; and pathologically during anovulatory menstrual cycles, with feminizing tumors of the ovary, and after excessive estrogen administration.

Estrogen depletion due to aging, ovariectomy, or pelvic irradiation causes atrophy of the genital tract, a decline of mucus production, and a more alkaline vaginal fluid. This encourages local infection since the lactobacilli are supplanted by a mixed flora or one in which cocci predominate. This alteration also promotes vaginal alkalinity, and the consequent impairment of biologic protective mechanisms encourages the growth of pathogens which may cause leukorrhea.

The most common sites of origin of vaginal discharge (in order of frequency) are the cervix, vagina, vulva, and upper genital tract.

Multiple lacerations of the cervix followed by infection of the glands lead to the production of excessive amounts of alkaline mucus. Leukorrhea increases the vaginal pH, thus promoting the growth of vaginal pathogens.

Vulvitis is often the cause of leukorrhea in children. Vulvitis in the adult may be associated with Trichomonas vaginalis or Candida infections of the vagina, particularly during pregnancy. Leukorrhea due to Trichomonas vaginalis infection usually occurs as a diffuse vaginitis characterized by a thin, yellow-green, occasionally frothy discharge with a fetid odor. Numerous red points ("strawberry patches"), which rarely bleed, are scattered over the vaginal surface and cervical portio.

Trichomonas vaginalis is a venereal infection in most instances. The cervix, urethra, and bladder may be involved secondarily. Because vaginal, oral, and enteric trichomonads are distinctly different morphologically, the gastrointestinal tract can be shown not to be the site of origin of genital trichomoniasis. The vaginal organism can often be traced to the male partner, who harbors the flagellate beneath the prepuce or in the urethra or prostate.

Candida albicans and related yeast pathogens are natural inhabitants of the bowel. They are also found on the skin. Vaginal contamination from these sources is common. The thin vaginal discharge due to Candida infection may have a disagreeable odor. White curd-like collections of exudate are present, and some are lightly attached to the cervical and vaginal mucosa. When these are removed, slight oozing frequently occurs.

Hemophilus organisms are ordinarily found in the respiratory tract. The route of vaginal infection is not clear.

Gonorrheal vulvovaginitis in children is usually due to hand-to-body contact with an infected adult. In adolescents and adults, gonorrhea is sexually transmitted almost without exception.

Metazoal vaginal infestations occur as a result of fecal soiling of the introitus.

Cervicitis may be present even though the appearance of the ectocervix is not remarkable. However, redness and eversion of the cervical os and excessive amounts of mucus may indicate infection. In general, chronic cervicitis is accompanied by a thick, viscid mucopurulent discharge with an acrid (or no) odor.

Table 19-1. Differential diagnosis of causes of leukorrhea.

Color	Consistency	Amount	Odor	Probable Causes
Clear	Mucoid	+ to ++	None	Ovulation, excessive estrogen stimulation, emotional tension.
Milky	Viscid	+ to +++	None to acrid	Cervicitis, Hemophilus vaginalis vaginitis.
White	Thin with curd-like flecks	+ to ++	Fetid	Vaginal mycosis
Pink	Serous	+ to +++	None	Hypoestrogenism, nonspecific infection.
Yellow-green	Frothy	+ to +++	Fetid	Trichomonas vaginalis vaginitis
Brown	Watery	+ to ++	Musty	Vaginitis, cervicitis, cervical stenosis, endometritis, salpingitis; neoplasm of cervix, endometrium, or tube. Post-irradiational.
Gray, blood-streaked	Thin	+ to ++++	Foul	Vaginal ulcer, pyogenic vaginitis-cervicitis (trauma long-retained pessary, forgotten tampon). Vaginal, cervical, endometrial, tubal neoplasm.

Clinical Findings.

A. Symptoms and Signs: Vaginal discharge, with or without itching, may be associated with formication when urine contaminates the inflamed introitus. The patient may complain of pudendal irritation, proctitis, vaginismus, and dyspareunia. The diagnostic features of the discharge are summarized in Table 19-1.

B. Laboratory Findings: Blood findings may suggest low-grade infection. Papanicolaou smears are indicated to rule out malignancy. Specific tests should be performed for the following infections or infestations: trichomoniasis, Hemophilus vaginalis vaginitis, candidiasis, gonorrhea, helminthiasis, syphilis, lymphogranuloma venereum, chancroid, and tuberculosis.

A fresh wet preparation of vaginal fluid should be inspected for motile Trichomonas vaginalis. Hemophilus vaginalis probably will be observed if there is a heavy clouding of the spread, especially the covering of epithelial cells ("clue cells") by myriads of bacteria. Potassium hydroxide (10%) should be added to lake blood cells as an aid in visualization of Candida hyphae and spores. The addition of one drop of Lugol's solution will color the organisms. Intracellular gram-negative diplococci (Neisseria gonorrhoeae) and other predominant bacteria and helminths may be identified by examination of a gram-stained smear. If possible, the vaginal fluid should be cultured anaerobically and aerobically to identify bacterial pathogens. Thioglycollate medium is of assistance in the culture of Hemophilus microorganisms. Candida can be demonstrated by inoculation of Nickerson's, Sabouraud's, Pagano-Levin, or a similar medium. Leukorrhea associated with a positive serology may be due to syphilis; a positive Frei test or complement fixation test suggests lymphogranuloma venereum; a positive dmelcos skin test indicates chancroid. A vaginal smear for acid-fast staining and an inoculum for culture (or guinea pig inoculation) should be secured for suspected Mycobacterium tuberculosis.

Complications.

A. Trichomonas vaginalis vaginitis is often followed by chronic cervicitis, a major factor in infertility. Urinary tract trichomoniasis may cause troublesome symptoms.
B. Candidal vaginal infections may lead to dermatitis of the skin of the thighs and pudendum when the discharge is copious and chafing occurs.
C. Gonococcal vulvar or vaginal infections in infants may be complicated by gonorrheal ophthalmia and blindness. In adults, bartholinitis, skenitis, cervicitis, salpingitis, and peritonitis may occur.
D. Chronic granulomatous ulcerations due to lymphogranuloma venereum may degenerate into malignant lesions, and rectal strictures may develop. Lymphogranuloma venereum causes suppurative inguinal buboes.
E. Tuberculosis of the genital tract, usually secondary to pulmonary or gastrointestinal tuberculosis, may extend to the urinary organs or the peritoneal cavity and its contents.
F. Benign genital tumors may bleed and become infected; malignant tumors may spread locally and metastasize.

Prevention.

The husband should use a condom if infection or reinfection is likely. Sexual promiscuity and borrowing of douche tips, underclothing, or other possibly contaminated articles should be avoided.

Tetracycline therapy over long periods of time should be avoided since it may permit Candida overgrowth.

Treatment.

A. Specific Measures: Treat infection or infestation with the specific drugs listed below. If sensitivity develops, discontinue medication and substitute another drug as soon as practicable. Continue treating the patient during men-

strual flow. Choose a route of administration (e.g., vaginal suppositories, oral tablets) which need not be discontinued because of bleeding.
1. Trichomonas vaginalis vaginitis - It may be necessary to treat the patient during several menstrual periods if necessary; change the medication after 2-3 months in resistant cases. Any of the following may be used:
    a. Metronidazole (Flagyl®), 250 mg orally 3 times daily for 10 days. Treat the husband similarly during the same interval. (**Caution:** This drug may encourage the growth of Candida organisms. Rapid disappearance of leukorrhea due in part to trichomoniasis may mask gonorrhea.) Metronidazole should not be given during pregnancy because of the possibility of fetal complications.
    b. Suppositories of diiodohydroxyquinoline (Diodoquin®); dextrose, lactose, and boric acid (Floraquin®); or carbarsone (Devegan®), one vaginally twice daily for 8 weeks. Additional vaginal insufflation with the same preparation in powder form twice weekly for the first month is also helpful.
    c. Furazolidone-nifuroxime (Tricofuron®) vaginal suppositories, one twice daily for 8 weeks.
2. Candida albicans vaginitis -
    a. Nystatin (Mycostatin®) vaginal suppositories, each containing 100,000 units, one daily for 2 weeks, are most effective.
    b. Propionic acid gel (Propion Gel®), one application vaginally daily for 3 weeks.
    c. Gentian violet, 2% aqueous solution applied topically to the vulva, vagina, and cervical area twice weekly for 3 weeks.
    d. Gentian violet, lactic acid, and acetic acid (Gentia-Jel®), one application vaginally daily for 3 weeks.
    e. Chlordantoin (Sporostacin®) cream, one vaginal application twice daily for 2 weeks.
    f. Candicidin (Candeptin®), one tablet (3 mg) twice daily vaginally and one applicator of candicidin cream daily vaginally for 14 days.
3. Hemophilus vaginalis vaginitis -
    a. Sulfathiazole, sulfacetamide, and benzoylsulfanilamide in cream form (Sultrin®), one application daily for 2 weeks.
    b. Acidified 0.1% hexetidine gel (Sterisil®), one application daily for 2 weeks.
4. Atrophic (senile) vaginitis -
    a. Diethylstilbestrol, 0.5 mg vaginal suppository, one every third day for 3 weeks. Omit medication for one week (to avoid uterine bleeding); then resume cyclic therapy indefinitely unless contraindicated.

456 Leukorrhea

      b. Dienestrol® vaginal cream, one-third applicatorful every third day for 3 weeks. Omit medication for one week, then resume cyclic therapy.
      c. Diethylstilbestrol, 0.2-0.5 mg (or equivalent) orally daily for 3 weeks each month.
   5. Gonorrheal vaginitis - **Caution:** Treatment should not be discontinued until 3 sets of slides or, preferably, cultures of discharge from Skene's ducts and the cervical canal have revealed no gonococci. A STS should be performed before treatment and repeated 2 months later.
      a. Procaine penicillin G, 1-2 million units I.M. every other day for 3 doses.
      b. Sulfisoxazole (Gantrisin®), 1 gm orally 3 times daily for 10 days.
      c. Tetracycline, 500 mg orally initially followed by 250 mg 4 times daily for 5 days. (**Caution:** Do not give tetracyclines to pregnant women unless no other antibiotic will be effective against an infection that must be treated.)
B. General Measures: Use internal menstrual tampons to reduce vulvar soiling, pruritus, and odor. Coitus should be avoided until a cure has been achieved. Trichomonas and Candida infections require treatment of the husband also. Relapses are often reinfections. Re-treat both parties.

    Antipruritic medications are disappointing unless an allergy is present. Specific and local therapy will usually control itching promptly.
C. Local Nonspecific Measures: Occasional acetic acid douches (2 Tbsp of vinegar per liter of water) may be beneficial in the treatment of leukorrhea. (**Caution:** Never use alkaline [soda] douches. They are unphysiologic and often harmful because they inhibit the growth of the normal vaginal flora and raise vaginal pH.)

    Douches are not essential to cleanliness or marital hygiene. Too frequent douches of any kind tend to increase mucus secretion. Irritating medications cause further mucus production.

    In severe, resistant, or recurrent Trichomonas or Candida vaginitis, treat the cervix (even when it is apparently normal) by chemical or light thermal cauterization. Examine the urinary tract and Skene's and Bartholin's ducts and treat these areas if they appear to be reservoirs of reinfection.
D. Surgical Measures: Hospital cauterization, conization of the cervix, incision of Skene's glands, or bartholinectomy may be required. Cervical, uterine, or tubal disease (e.g., tumors or infections) may necessitate laparotomy, irradiation, or other appropriate measures.

Dermatitides of Female Genitalia 457

Prognosis.

Leukorrhea in pregnant, debilitated, or diabetic women is difficult to cure, especially when due to Trichomonas vaginalis, Candida albicans, or Hemophilus vaginalis. Repeated or even continuous treatment for 3-4 months may be required until the patient is delivered or the diabetes is controlled.

The prognosis is good if a specific diagnosis is made promptly and proper intensive therapy given. Treatment of only one of several causes may be the reason for failure of therapy.

DERMATITIDES OF THE FEMALE GENITALIA

Eczema.

"Eczema" is a nonspecific term for a common, pruritic, moist dermatitis characterized by excoriation and crusting, with later lichenification. Eczema is often a contact dermatitis caused by irritants in soap, medications, dyes in clothing, and allergy to wool or silk. Sensitivity tests and exclusion of other dermatitides aid in diagnosis.

Treatment depends upon elimination of the antigen or irritant. Apply Burow's solution twice daily followed by steroid creams.

Psoriasis.

The etiology of this disorder is not known. Pruritic, reddened, slightly elevated, flattened lesions (without the typical silvery scale seen on elbows and knees) are seen in body folds. The elbows and knees are frequently affected by scaly lesions. Psoriasis is a chronic disorder and is often familial. Exacerbations are often noted in the winter.

Treatment includes improved hygiene and soothing medication such as 0.5% hydrocortisone cream applied periodically.

Lichen Rubor Planus.

The cause of this condition is not known. Pruritus accompanies the purplish, raised papules, which have no tendency to ulcerate. Rare vesicles or bullae may develop and, occasionally, atrophy or hyperpigmentation is noted with healing. The disease may follow nervous stress, and the lesions are usually characteristic. The buccal and vulvovaginal surfaces are often involved together with the skin.

No specific treatment is known. Give phenobarbital or tranquilizers as necessary for symptomatic relief. Utilize steroid cream topically.

NONVENEREAL VIRAL INFECTIONS OF THE FEMALE GENITAL TRACT

Herpes Progenitalis.

Herpes simplex virus is the causative agent. The symptoms are local burning and formication. Clusters of small vesicles which are filled with clear fluid develop early. Shallow vulvar ulceration, leukorrhea, and pain develop when the disease becomes chronic or secondary infection occurs. The diagnosis is clinical, but epithelial giant cells with viral inclusions may be seen with Giemsa's stain. The disorder often is recurrent before and during the menses.

The treatment is nonspecific, and the lesions usually heal in 7-14 days. Improve hygiene and prescribe daily acetic acid douches.

Herpes Zoster.

Herpes zoster virus is the causative agent. Severe, persistent burning and aching pain occurs together with small blisters, which are usually unilateral. Zonal vesicular or bullous ulcerative lesions develop along the distribution of one or more sensory nerves. Eventual suppuration and scarring are characteristic.

The treatment is nonspecific. Palliative therapy includes liberal doses of analgesics for pain; rest in bed is helpful. Utilize Burow's compresses. Apply a topical antibiotic ointment such as bacitracin if secondary infection is severe.

One attack generally confers immunity.

Aphthous Ulcers.

A specific virus causes sensitive, small, shallow ulcers in the vulva or vagina. These are covered with a yellowish pseudomembrane. The problem may become recurrent and concomitant with the oral counterpart.

Treatment is palliative. Apply spirit of camphor twice daily to relieve the discomfort.

Molluscum Contagiosum.

An autoinoculable virus with an incubation period of 1-4 weeks is responsible. Asymptomatic pink to gray, discrete, umbilicated, epithelial skin tumors less than 1 cm in diameter develop on the vulva. They have a typical pathologic picture.

Lightly curet away the lesions and apply a topical antibiotic and dressing.

PARASITIC INFECTIONS & INFESTATIONS
OF THE FEMALE GENITAL TRACT

Trichomoniasis.

Trichomonas vaginalis causes a thin, occasionally bubbly, pruritic vaginal discharge. Vulvovaginitis is also described, and numerous reddish points are often seen in the vaginal and cervical mucosa. The diagnosis requires identification of motile trichomonads in wet preparation or culture, or of organisms in a fixed cytologic smear of leukorrheic discharge.

The treatment includes acetic acid douches and specific therapy as outlined on p. 455.

Pediculosis Pubis.

Pediculosis pubis is caused by the Phthirus pubis (crab louse). Intense pruritus accompanies excoriation of the hirsute skin of the pubis, axilla, or scalp. Minute pale-brown insects and their ova may be seen attached to the hair shafts near the skin.

Treat by applying 10% DDT powder or Kwell® cream (1% gamma benzene hexachloride), or apply kerosene to the hairy areas; wash with soap after 30 minutes.

Scabies.

Sarcoptes scabei causes intractable itching and excoriation of the surface in the vicinity of minute skin burrows where the ova have been deposited by the parasites.

Treat by applying Kwell® cream (from the collarbone down) each night for 3 nights. Contacts must be treated also to prevent recurrences.

Enterobiasis (Pinworm, Seatworm).

Oxyuris vermicularis is the usual cause. Nocturnal perineal itching is described by the patient, and perianal excoriation can be observed. This condition is common in children. Apply cellulose tape to the anal region, stick the tape to a glass slide, and examine under the microscope for Oxyuris. Insist that the patient wash her hands and scrub her nails after each defecation. Underclothes must be boiled.

Administer piperazine citrate (Antepar®), 1 gm orally twice daily for 7 days. Repeat after one week. Apply 1% ammoniated mercury ointment to the perianal region twice daily for relief of itching.

MYCOTIC INFECTIONS
OF THE FEMALE GENITAL TRACT

Candidiasis.

Candida albicans, C. krusei, or C. tropica may cause vulvovaginitis. A pruritic irritation of the vulva and vagina

460 Suppurative Infections of Genital Tract

is the patient's complaint; a reddened area with whitish ("scalded") surface is apparent. The process may also involve the skin of the inguinal region and thighs. Vaginitis often accompanies the dermatitis. The disorder is most common in diabetics. A thin, whitish, fetid leukorrheic discharge containing curd-like white flecks of monilial organisms, exfoliated cells, and mucus is present. Diagnosis depends upon demonstration of Candida pseudomycelia in a wet preparation of discharge (especially curds) or in scrapings from the skin. Add one drop of 10% KOH and one drop of Lugol's solution for better visualization of yeast forms. In questionable cases, fluid or scrapings should be cultured in Nickerson's or comparable medium.

Nystatin (Mycostatin®), 0.5 gm as a vaginal suppository twice daily for 10 days, is the accepted treatment. Give vaginal Propion Gel® or Gentia-Jel® 2-4 times at night instead of nystatin, or apply 1-2% aqueous gentian violet vaginally every 2-3 days until improvement is certain.

Fungal Dermatitis.

Microsporum, Epidermophyton, and Trichophyton cause this chronic pruritic skin disorder associated with superficial reddened, dry, scaly, confluent annular dermatitic lesions. Diagnosis depends upon microscopic examination (as for Candida) or culture in Sabouraud's medium.

Apply zincundecate (Desenex®) or 1/4 strength Whitfield's ointment to the skin twice daily for 3 days and then daily for one week.

Deep Cellulitis Caused by Fungi.

Blastomyces, Actinomyces, and Histoplasma are the usual causative organisms. A chronic rectovaginal induration develops, with pain, swelling, tenderness, ulceration, and discharge. Sinus formation is not infrequent. Yellow ray-fungus groupings suggestive of actinomycosis are observed in the discharge.

Treatment is with amphotericin B (Fungizone®), 1 mg/kg in 5% dextrose in water I.V. over a 6-8 hour period to a total dose of 25 mg/kg.

SUPPURATIVE INFECTIONS OF THE FEMALE GENITAL TRACT

Impetigo.

Hemolytic staphylococcus aureus or streptococci are the usual causative organisms. Formication and pruritus are the principal symptoms. Thin-walled vesicles and bullae develop which display reddened edges and crusted surfaces after rupture. Impetigo is common in children, particularly on the face, hands, and vulva.

The patient must be isolated and the blebs incised or crusts removed aseptically. Neomycin or bacitracin cream should be applied twice a day for one week.

Furunculosis.

Furunculosis is due to staphylococcal infection and appears as perifollicular abscesses. Throbbing pain and regional tenderness are described. Pustular areas require incision and drainage. The opened lesions are cultured for organisms.

The patient must be segregated and topical moist heat applied periodically. Systemic antibiotics are prescribed when indicated.

Erysipelas.

Erysipelas is due to beta-hemolytic streptococcal infection and appears as a reddened, slightly raised, and confluent induration. It is a cellulitis of the skin. Fever, vulvar burning and aching, and acute local tenderness are typical manifestations. A rapid onset is usual. The drainage is cultured for beta-hemolytic streptococci.

The patient must be isolated. Continuous hot, wet fomentations should be applied. Intensive treatment with systemic antibiotics such as procaine penicillin G, 1-2 million units I. M. repeated in 12 hours, is indicated.

Hidradenitis. (Infection of the apocrine glands; analogous to cystic acne.)

Staphylococcal infection of the apocrine glands causes soreness and local swelling, with edema, cellulitis, and suppuration, often of the groin. Involvement of apocrine glands establishes the diagnosis.

Treatment consists of hot, wet applications and systemic chemotherapy with antibiotics such as oxacillin or methicillin. Local x-ray therapy may be helpful if the condition is severe or chronic. Excision may be necessary.

Tuberculosis (Usually Vulvovaginal Lupus Vulgaris).

This disorder consists of chronic, minimally painful, exudative "sores" which are tender, reddish, raised, moderately firm, and nodular, with central "apple jelly"-like contents. Ulcerative, undermined, necrotic, discharging lesions develop later. There is some tendency toward healing, with heavy scarring. Induration and sinus formation are common in the scrofulous type. Malignancy and venereal disease must be ruled out and tuberculosis sought elsewhere. Mycobacterium tuberculosis should be identified by acid-fast smear, culture, or guinea pig inoculation.

Wet compresses of Burow's solution are applied. Antituberculosis chemotherapy should be given.

Unusual Ulceration or Granuloma.

Borrelia vincenti or mixed staphylococcal-streptococcal infections and diphtheroids are the usual causative organisms. The symptoms and signs include pain in the vulvovaginal region, discharge, and vaginal bleeding. Early signs are zonal edema and patchy ulceration with grayish pseudomembrane formation. Confluent bleeding, granulomatous lesions develop later. This disorder affects chronically ill females, often children. The organisms must be identified, and malignancy, tuberculosis, and venereal and mycotic infections must be excluded. Biopsy may be required to rule out cancer.

The vulvovaginal area is treated by external dry heat. Vulvovaginal irrigations with 1:5000 potassium permanganate solution twice daily are useful. Systemic broad-spectrum antibiotic therapy is given. Neoarsphenamine, 30% in vegetable oil applied topically twice daily, is beneficial in Vincent's infections.

BARTHOLIN DUCT CYST

A soft swelling within the labia minora at the juncture of its mid and lower thirds usually indicates occlusion of Bartholin's duct. This abnormality is almost invariably the result of pyogenic infection, often with Neisseria gonorrhoeae. Reinfection, usually with streptococci, staphylococci, or Escherichia coli, causes recurrent discomfort and enlargement of the duct. One duct is affected much more commonly than both ducts. Bartholin duct cysts are frequently seen in clinic patients but are not common in private practice.

Bartholin's duct is susceptible to infection because of its narrowness, not because of its transitional cell lining. Infectious organisms become pocketed within the passage, and an abscess forms; inflammation finally resolves, but permanent occlusion of the distal tract causes retention of mucus produced by the gland and a cyst develops. Paradoxically, the gland is almost never as seriously involved as the duct.

Inflammation and obstruction to the discharge of secretions and infectious exudates cause labial swelling. After the infection subsides, distention and occlusion of the duct persists. Reinfection causes recrudescence of signs and symptoms.

Clinical Findings.

A. Symptoms and Signs: The symptoms of Bartholin duct cyst are pain, dyspareunia, and tenderness. The latter depends upon the presence of infection and the degree of distention of the duct. One or both labia are swollen, and the introitus is distorted. A fluctuant swelling (1-4 cm) of the duct and gland can be seen.

B. Laboratory Findings: Leukocytosis with a shift to the left and elevation of the sedimentation rate develop with severe acute infections. Smears and cultures of the ostium of Bartholin's duct, the cervical canal, and the urethral meatus are required for specific bacteriologic diagnosis.

Complications.

Cellulitis of surrounding tissues occasionally is noted.

Differential Diagnosis.

Bartholin duct cyst must be differentiated from inclusion cysts (after vulvar laceration or episiotomy), large sebaceous cysts, hidradenoma, congenital anomalies, primary cancer of Bartholin's gland or duct, and secondary malignancy metastatic to the vulvovaginal area.

Treatment.

Appropriate antibiotics should be employed. Bed rest, local dry or moist heat (or both), and analgesics such as aspirin should be used as indicated. A fluctuant abscess should be incised and drained. Aspiration and injection of antibiotics are of no value. When the lesion is quiescent, the duct should be incised and marsupialized or the diseased duct and gland should be excised.

Cellulitis which does not respond to initial chemotherapy should be treated with broad-spectrum antibiotics.

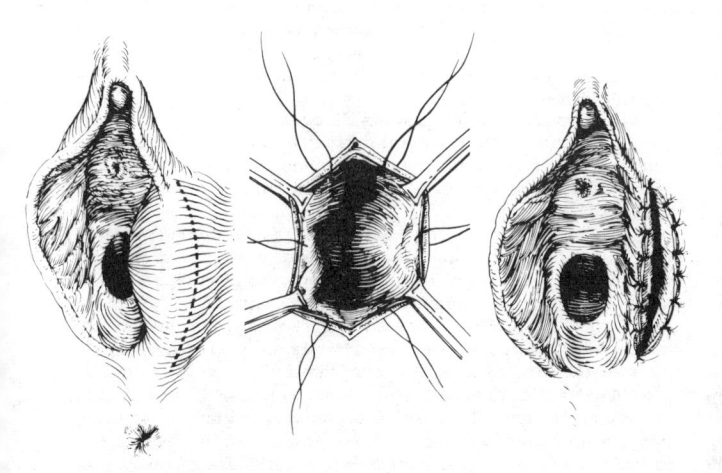

Fig 19-4. Marsupialization of Bartholin's cyst.

Prognosis.

The prognosis is almost invariably good. However, recurrent duct infections, often secondary to coital or obstetric trauma, are the rule.

VULVAR CANCER

Cancer of the vulva is the 4th most common female genital malignancy (following cancer of the cervix, the endometrium, and the ovary). It accounts for 2-3% of female malignancies of all types and about 0.5% of all gynecologic hospital admissions. Epidermoid cancers constitute about 92%; adenocarcinomas, 5%; basal cell carcinomas, 1%; and malignant melanomas, 0.5%.

More than 50% of patients having vulvar cancer are over 50; the average age is about 65 years. However, it may occur at any age and has been reported in infants and children. Dark-skinned races are said to be less susceptible, but vulvar malignancy is diagnosed so commonly among the poor of all races that defective personal hygiene and lack of medical care seem to be more significant than skin color. The coincidence of carcinoma of the vulva and pregnancy is very rare.

The etiology of cancer of the vulva is not known. Many vulvar malignancies develop from or are associated with so-called premalignant conditions. Predisposing and contributing causes include the following:

(1) Leukoplakic vulvitis: This is a chronic inflammatory disorder of the skin and mucous membranes of unknown cause which may occur before the menopause but is usually noted during the climacteric. Since one out of 4 vulvar cancers is accompanied by leukoplakic vulvitis, this condition must be considered precancerous.

(2) Chronic granulomatous disorders: Patients with long-standing condylomata accuminata or venereal disease (especially lymphopathia venereum, lymphogranuloma inguinale, and syphilis) have a much higher incidence of cancer of the vulva than others.

(3) Chronic irritation: Persistent scratching or excoriation of the vulva for months or years as a result of pruritus vulvae may play a part in the development of vulvar malignancy. Friction is considered to be a contributory cause of skin cancer, which is increased by swelling and the development of excrescences such as condylomata. Dryness of the skin surface in old age increases the irritation of contact.

(4) Paget's disease of the skin: Paget's disease is a forerunner of cancer. It arises from apocrine glands, particularly those in supernumerary breast tissue, which may be found in the labia majora. Although Paget's disease of the breast is much more common than its vulvar counterpart, it affects

patients during the same age period (50 years and over) and is morphologically similar in both regions.

(5) Pigmented moles: When stimulated by pregnancy or subjected to prolonged chafing by clothing or perineal pads, these lesions may develop into malignant moles.

(6) Intraepithelial carcinoma: Bowen's disease of the vulvar skin, considered to be in situ cancer by most physicians, may ultimately develop into invasive epidermoid malignancy.

(7) Irradiation: Carcinogenesis resulting from irradiation treatment of nonspecific pruritus vulvae or pelvic cancer has been postulated but never proved.

Carcinoma of the vulva is more closely similar to skin than to genital malignancy because of its origin and external situation. Cancers of the vulva are diagnosed most often (in order of frequency) in the labia majora, the prepuce of the clitoris, the labia minora, Bartholin's gland, and the vestibule of the vagina.

With the exception of most adenocarcinomas, which extend locally and metastasize to remote sites by way of the lymphatics, vulvar cancers begin as intraepithelial surface growths which ulcerate and extend downward and laterally. Only rarely do they grow from a deep site toward the surface. These cancers are slow-growing and, although metastases are unpredictable, the malignant cells probably remain in the regional lymph nodes for a long time before dissemination.

Grossly, cancer of the vulva is classified as ulcerative and nonulcerative, and in each case as everting and inverting. The majority of vulvar cancers are ulcerative everting growths, and almost 60% are in the anterior portion of the vulva. Many are cauliflower-like. The nonulcerative malignancies are firm, smooth, intact tumors, and the overlying skin usually has an "orange peel" appearance. These are rarely pedunculated but may protrude, depending upon their size and situation.

A classical early epidermoid cancer of the vulva is a small, reddened, crusted, slightly exudative, nontender lesion with some peripheral thickening.

Leukoplakic vulvitis is a granulomatous disorder of the genital skin and, to a lesser degree, the mucosal surface of the introitus. It progresses from an early hypertrophic stage through an intermediate leukokraurotic phase to a late kraurotic stage (see Table 19-2).

Patients with chronic variable infections (see p. 467) have fissured or exuberant areas which may include epidermoid cancer. These zones are not typical of carcinoma.

Paget's disease is characterized by a red, moist, granular, nonsensitive area, usually in the labium majus.

Malignant melanomas are usually single, hyperpigmented, raised, ulcerated lesions which bleed easily. No tenderness is described.

Bowen's disease, an in situ carcinoma, may appear as a hyperkeratotic zone in the labial skin. Unless infection or excoriation occurs, the integument is unbroken before invasive cancer develops.

Adenocarcinoma arising in Bartholin's gland is at first indistinguishable from the gland itself. Gross enlargement and induration occur relatively late.

Basal cell carcinoma may be ulcerated, hypertrophic, superficially cicatrizing, or erythematous in type. Either labium (majus or minor) may be affected.

Microscopically, many typical epidermoid carcinomas of the vulva are composed of well differentiated spinal or prickle cells, many of which form keratotic pearls. Occasional mitoses are seen. Malignant cells invade the subepithelial tissues. Leukocytes and lymphocytes infiltrate the stroma and tissues adjacent to the neoplasm. These are grade I cancers. Less well differentiated tumors also occur.

Malignant cells spread to distant sites via the lymphatic drainage channels of the vulva. Cancer cells metastasize to the superficial and deep inguinal and femoral lymph nodes and the external iliac, obturator, and presymphysial lymph nodes. (Cloquet's or Rosenmüller's node, the upper node of the deep group in the femoral canal, just beneath Poupart's ligament, is often invaded by vulvar cancer.)

Because the vulva is a bilateral, joined structure, the lymphatics anastomose and cross, and tumor cells spread from one side to the other by embolic transfer or, more rarely, by permeation of the lymphatic channels. Lymph node metastases are often independent of the size or location of the lesion, the duration of symptoms, and the histologic grade of the malignancy. The more anaplastic the tumor, the more likely it is to metastasize.

The early (hypertrophic) stage of leukoplakic vulvitis (see Table 19-2) is infrequently associated with cancer; the intermediate (leukokraurotic) phase often precedes and accompanies carcinoma; the late kraurotic stage is only occasionally associated with malignancy.

Basal cell carcinoma consists of small rounded, basophilic, neoplastic cells derived from the innermost layers of the epidermis. The cells are arranged irregularly in groupings which often penetrate the underlying connective tissue. Occasional mitoses (but no keratinization) are observed. Basal cell carcinoma differs from the keratinizing epidermoid variety in that it metastasizes late and infrequently. In contrast, malignant melanoma generally spreads early via the venous system. (Both tumors frequently develop local recurrences.)

Table 19-2. Pathologic features of 3 stages of leukoplakic vulvitis.

	Early (Hypertrophic)	Intermediate (Leukokraurotic)	Late (Kraurotic)
Gross	Grayish-white, edematous, thickened.	White with reddened, excoriated, fissured zones.	Pearly-white, thin, parchment-like.
Microscopic Skin or mucous membrane	Surface hyperkeratosis, acanthosis. Separation of midzonal cells. Wide, deep rete pegs. Heavy groupings of basal cells over rete pegs.	Moderate surface hyperkeratinization. Parakeratosis. Blunted rete pegs. Relative hypertrophy of basal, parabasal layers.	Surface hyperkeratosis. All layers greatly thinned. Rete pegs obliterated.
Subepithelial layers	Hyperemia (early). Infiltration with polymorphonuclear neutrophils and lymphocytes.	Moderate hyalinization, homogenization. Obliteration of vessels. Scattered lymphocytes, plasma cells.	Marked hyalinization. Complete loss of elastic fibers. Ischemia. Absent lymphocytes, plasma cells.

Numerous Paget's cells within a disordered epidermis are a diagnostic feature of Paget's disease of the vulva. These large, rounded, vacuolated cells are without prickle projections. The cytoplasm contains mucopolysaccharide. Their prominent, dark nuclei often include several nucleoli. Paget's cells never become keratinized. Malignant change may be noted centrally or peripherally.

Bowen's disease (carcinoma in situ) is characterized by acanthosis, thickening of the rete pegs, loss of stratification of the epithelial layers, disorientation of the cells above the basalis, nuclear hyperchromatism, and numerous mitotic figures. The basement membrane is intact (preinvasive). Other features of Bowen's disease are the increased vascularity of the subepithelial tissues and leukocytic infiltration.

Clinical Findings.

Because of embarrassment or fear of the diagnosis, many women with carcinoma of the vulva do not seek medical care until the disease has reached an advanced stage. Efficient routine physical examinations and a realistic degree of cancer consciousness on the part of the physician will enhance the probabilities of early diagnosis. Nodular ulcerative lesions, especially in postmenopausal women when granulomatous or leukoplakic changes have occurred, are particularly suggestive of vulvar cancer.

A. Symptoms and Signs: Pruritus vulvae is the most common symptom of ulcerative vulvar cancer. Nodulation ("a lump") may be present for months or years before the patient seeks professional advice. Ulceration ("a sore"), an odorous discharge, and bleeding usually occur late, but in postgranulomatous cases are often present early. Lymphadenopathy is always suggestive of carcinomatous metastases. Pain is a late symptom; it depends upon the size and location of the tumor and the presence or absence of ulceration and infection.

There are no generally accepted international criteria for staging cancer of the vulva, but the following modification of Taussig's classification is useful:

Stage (group) I: Tumor less than 3 cm in diameter; no evidence of gland metastases.

Stage II: Tumor 3-7 cm in diameter without subpubic involvement; no positive evidence of gland involvement.

Stage III: Tumor over 7 cm in diameter, or smaller lesions which show deeper infiltration or evidence of gland metastasis.

Stage IV: Any tumor with extension to the vagina, urethra, or subpubic space.

Complications.

A. Without Treatment: Cancer of the vulva, if not treated, inexorably pursues a slow and dreadful course marked by foul odor, bleeding, and soiling; vesicovaginal and rectovaginal fistulas; and breakdown and drainage of inguinal glands containing cancer metastases followed by lymphedema, pain, and thrombophlebitis. The patient usually dies of debility, inanition, or hemorrhage.

B. With Treatment:
   1. Recurrence - Early recurrences may be local or remote; most appear in one year. Incomplete surgery and unrecognized wide dispersion of cancer are the causes. Late recurrences (after 3 years) are almost invariably vulvar and tend to remain localized.

      Wide excision prevents recurrences; lymphadenectomy to the bifurcation of the iliac vessels is required. If cancer reappears after extensive (presumably adequate) surgery, it may be a new growth rather than a recurrence of the original tumor.

   2. Lymphedema of the legs is due to incompetent lymphatic and venous return; it may be caused by postoperative infection and scarring or by recurrence of cancer.

   3. Hernia - Femoral and inguinal hernias result from weakened tissues, severance of Poupart's ligament, and incomplete repair of the musculofascial layers of the abdominal wall after lymphadenectomy.

   4. Vaginal stenosis of marked degree is not common. However, if pregnancy occurs after vulvectomy,

cesarean section may be required because of contracture of the introitus.
5. Prolapse of the cervix and uterus may occur as a consequence of wide, deep excision. To prevent later uterine descensus, an attempt should be made to reconstitute the levator fascia and perineal body, which make up important parts of the pelvic floor for adequate support of the viscera.

Differential Diagnosis.

Basal cell carcinoma of the vulva is identical to the "rodent ulcer" which may occur anywhere on the skin. Adenocarcinoma of the vulva is generally derived from Bartholin's gland, but periurethral and sweat gland cells may also be responsible. Melanocarcinoma may develop from pigmented cells of the lamina basalis of the skin; melanosarcoma may develop from dark-staining cells in connective tissue. Other malignant vulvar tumors are bizarre and exceedingly rare. A few vulvar carcinomas are secondary to breast, kidney, ovarian, bladder, or bowel tumors.

The following manifestations of vulvar cancer may have other causes:
A. Pruritus vulvae may be "nonspecific" (often psychogenic) or secondary to dermatoses (lichen planus, psoriasis), vaginitis (senile vaginitis, Trichomonas or Candida infections), urinary incontinence (relaxed vesical sphincter, neurogenic bladder), and systemic disease (diabetes mellitus, hypothyroidism, allergy).
B. Nodulation may be due to a sebaceous, inclusion, or Bartholin cyst, hidradenoma, or neurofibroma.
C. Ulceration and discharge of the vulva may be caused by venereal or pyogenic infection or by scarring.
D. Lymphadenopathy may represent lymphadenitis.
E. Kraurosis may be due to estrogen depletion (senile vaginitis or vulvitis) or may represent a terminal stage of lichen sclerosis (lichen planus). It is frequently the end stage of leukoplakic vulvitis.
F. Leukoplakia of the vulva may also be caused by leukoderma, syphilis, and scarring.

Prevention.

The early diagnosis and treatment of irritative factors which predispose to vulvar carcinoma will prevent many cases. Precancerous vulvar lesions should be identified and excised promptly. If they are extensive, simple vulvectomy is indicated. Prominent or enlarging pigmented moles of the vulva should be removed before they become malignant.

Treatment.

A. Surgical Measures: Once the diagnosis of vulvar cancer is made, radical surgery should be done unless it is refused or contraindicated. Anemia and metabolic or cardiovascular disease should be treated intensively before surgery. The physician should be encouraging but firm and should make every reasonable effort to convince the patient and her family that the benefits of treatment are worth the substantial risks involved. A patient should not be denied a palliative vulvectomy because she is "a poor operative risk." Expeditious, well planned surgery, perhaps under local anesthesia, is usually well tolerated even by very old women. Relief from the offensive odor, discharge, bleeding, and pain makes surgery worthwhile. With modern surgical technics, anesthesia, and appropriate supportive therapy, at least 80% of patients are operable.

The operation involves (1) wide, deep excision of the entire vulva and (2) extraperitoneal resection of the superficial and deep inguinal, femoral, external iliac, and obturator lymph nodes. Low-grade malignancy does not justify less radical surgery.

An antibiotic such as erythromycin, 250 mg orally 4 times daily, should be administered for 2 days before surgery and for 3-4 days thereafter to reduce the chances of infection following operation. Warm compresses of 1:1000 quaternary ammonium chloride solution 4 times daily for several days are a useful means of debridement of the ulcerated area before surgery.

After the customary abdominoperineal preparation, ulcerative carcinoma should be treated with tincture of iodine and covered with moist gauze. Manipulation during surgery must be avoided. This will minimize operative spread of the tumor and infection.

It is desirable to complete the entire procedure in one operative session if feasible. Gland excision is followed by vulvectomy. If the patient's condition demands a two-stage procedure, vulvectomy should be done first and lymphadenectomy within 3-7 days.

The extent of surgery should not be compromised in order to achieve a primary closure, since in 30-50% of cases closures will partially reopen. Healing by second intention and Tiersch or full-thickness skin grafts are often necessary.

Basal cell carcinoma, quite different in behavior as contrasted with squamous cancer, metastasizes so rarely and so late that most cases can be treated by wide, deep excision without lymphadenectomy. Radical vulvectomy without lymphadenectomy is probably sufficient for cancer which develops in chronic granulomas, because metastases are not likely to occur through lymphatics which have been occluded by infection.

In general, confining the operation to one side is not sufficient, since the multicentricity of malignant and premalignant tissue and the crossing of lymphatic channels favor bilateral involvement.

When glands appear to be involved in the cancer process, a gland biopsy should not be done; the entire gland and all others in that area should be removed.

B. Irradiation: Radiotherapy is not often curative but is of great value in the treatment of recurrent carcinoma, especially the basal cell type. It also is valuable in patients requiring palliation for inoperable cancer and in all instances of known incomplete surgery. Unless metastases are discovered in the lymph glands, supplementary x-ray therapy does not improve the results of surgery sufficiently to justify the skin damage, lymphatic obstruction, and injury to the large vessels, bowel, and urinary tract that it causes.

Prognosis.

With the best available treatment, the five-year arrest rate of cancer of the vulva has risen four-fold in the past 20 years. Over 60% of patients with vulvar cancer who are treated in the large medical centers are alive and well after 5 years if the lymph glands are not involved. When cancer has invaded the nodes, the five-year arrest rate falls to about 15%. Only a rare five-year "cure" is achieved by radical treatment of malignant melanoma.

The operative mortality rate is about 5%. Death may be due to cardiovascular complications, primary or secondary hemorrhage, infection, and venous thrombosis.

CANCER OF THE VAGINA

Primary cancer of the vagina represents about 1% of gynecologic malignancies. It usually develops about 10 years after the menopause, but may occur in children. The upper and lower thirds of the vagina are common sites, but this tumor is multicentric.

At least 90% of primary vaginal cancers are of the squamous cell type; a few are sarcomas, often botryoid in children and old women. Loose connective tissue and a rich vascular and lymphatic circulation favor rapid growth and early dissemination. Tumors of the lower vagina metastasize like vulvar cancers; those in the upper vagina like cervical malignancies.

Painless bleeding is the initial manifestation in about half of cases; leukorrhea in about one-fourth. Less common complaints are a vaginal mass, pruritus, and constipation. Pain, weight loss, and swelling are late manifestations.

There are no typical gross characteristics. Most vaginal tumors are ulcerative and firm. A few are papillary or nodular. Careful physical examination and biopsy are required for diagnosis, although exfoliative cytology may be suggestive.

Clinical Stages of Carcinoma of the Vagina: (**Note**: A carcinoma that has extended to the portio should be classified as carcinoma of the cervix.)

>Stage I: The carcinoma is limited to the vaginal wall.
>
>Stage II: The carcinoma has involved the subvaginal tissues but has not extended onto the pelvic wall.
>
>Stage III: The carcinoma has extended onto the pelvic wall.
>
>Stage IV: The carcinoma has extended beyond the true pelvis or has involved the mucosa of the bladder or of the rectum; however, bullous edema as such does not permit classification as stage IV.

Primary vaginal cancer must be distinguished from extensions of vulvar or cervical malignancies and from metastases of urinary tract, gastrointestinal tract, and ovarian cancer.

Irradiation is the preferred method of treatment in most cases. Radical surgery is usually required for vaginal cancers near the introitus, for sarcomas, and when the bowel, urethra, or bladder is involved with definite localization.

The prognosis depends upon the type, location, and extent of the tumor and the therapy administered. With appropriate treatment, the five-year arrest rate of stage I primary vaginal cancer is about 50%.

20...
Diseases of the Cervix

CERVICITIS

Cervicitis, the most common of all gynecologic disorders, affects over 50% of all women at some time during adult life. It is characterized by eversion due to outward growth of endocervical cells. Chronic cervical infection is the most frequent cause of leukorrhea and is a major etiologic factor in infertility, dyspareunia, and abortion. It may even be a stimulus to the development of cervical carcinoma.

Over 50% of parous women have cervicitis. Cervicitis of variable duration occurs following virtually every delivery because the forcefully dilated cervix inevitably sustains many small lacerations, which become infected. Spontaneous and induced abortion and traumatic instrumentation are likewise often followed by cervicitis.

In nonpregnant women, acute and chronic cervicitis may be caused by gonorrhea which affects the cervix early in the disease. Although specific antibiotics usually destroy the gonococci, secondary invading organisms may persist for months or years as a cause of cervical infection.

Other factors in the pathogenesis of cervicitis are poor hygiene (anal-vaginal contamination), diminished resistance to infection in hypoestrogenism or hypovitaminosis, and irritation caused by pessaries or other foreign bodies.

Cervicitis begins as a surface infection, but the endocervix becomes involved within hours. In 1-2 days, even the remote depths of the cervix are inflamed, and hypertrophy and hyperplasia of the glandular cells follow. Irritation due to infection results in hyperfunction of the glandular epithelium, producing copious leukorrhea. Because the infected glands evacuate poorly, they become dilated, and the fibromuscular supporting framework shields the inflammatory process.

When the columnar endocervical cells and the squamous portio cells are in functional equilibrium, their juncture is just within the external os. If the balance is disturbed by infection or hormonal aberrations, eversion or redness about the external os results. This is an outgrowth of columnar cells from the cervical canal beyond the external os, and new glands develop where glands do not normally exist. With the reestablishment of equilibrium by hormone regulation or elimination of infection, the vaginal and endocervical pH becomes normal and columnar cells regress toward the os. Complete obliteration of evidence of eversion or ectropion may not be possible; however, once columnar cells become established exteriorly, a zone or patch of reddish mucosa persists, and glands in the portio continue to function, a few becoming cystic when their drainage is obstructed. Although the velvety-appearing eversion contrasts with the glistening squamous epithelium of the portio, this does not necessarily mean that it will persist indefinitely as an abnormal area.

"Erosion" is not a proper term for cervical redness except in cases of limited denudation of the mucosquamous junction occurring early in virulent infection or following cauterization. The squamous epithelium is lost for a very brief time in such acute processes and is replaced either by substituted tall columnar cells or squamous elements.

Cervical secretions depend upon hormonal, psychogenic, and irritative stimulation. The production of a thin, clear acellular mucus in average amounts is a major role of the cervix in reproductive physiology. The mucous plug screens out pathogenic bacteria and permits the collection and transport of sperms to the uterine cavity. Reproduction is hindered by contaminated, thick, tenacious mucus or the absence of mucus. Heavy bacterial contamination causes loss of sodium chloride and water from the cervical mucus, and this results in increased viscosity and a decreased pH. Leukocytes and bacteria in the mucus are inimical to sperms and result in a negative Sims-Huhner test (see p. 631).

Clinical Findings.

A. Symptoms and Signs: The most common presenting complaints referable to cervicitis are leukorrhea and infertility.
   1. Leukorrhea - The discharge is white, yellow, occasionally blood-tinged, and thin to mucoid in consistency. It is usually caused by inflammation of the endocervical glandular epithelium. Its characteristics vary with the menstrual cycle. In the absence of infection, the cervical mucus is thin, clear, and acellular at the time of ovulation or after moderate estrogen stimulation. At midcycle the mucus is mucopurulent (even blood-streaked), and may be tenacious and viscid.
   2. Infertility - A thick, viscid, acid, pus-laden cervical mucus is noxious to sperms and prevents fertilization.
   3. Backache - Lymphangitis of the uterosacral structures causes pain which is usually referred to the sacrum.
   4. Lower abdominal pain, dyspareunia, dysmenorrhea - Pelvic congestion and parametritis often cause these symptoms.
   5. Dysuria, frequency, urgency - Urinary distress is

often due to posterior ureteritis and trigonitis secondary to cervicitis.
6. Metrorrhagia - Hyperemia of the infected cervix produces a freely bleeding surface. Such cervical ooze accounts for intermenstrual (often postcoital) spotting.
7. Abortion - Cervicitis is frequently followed by deciduitis and placentitis and leads to abortion early in pregnancy.
8. Cervical dystocia - Fibrosis and stenosis of the cervix may follow a chronic cervical infection. Delayed or incomplete dilatation of the cervix may result.
9. Speculum exposure of the cervix in good light will often reveal a thick mucoid discharge exuding from the canal. Lacerations, eversion, and hypertrophy of the cervix may be apparent, together with occluded superficial cervical glands (nabothian cysts). Patulousness of the deeply lacerated external os exposes the endocervical canal, which may bleed when wiped with a cotton applicator. The portio and the upper vagina usually appear normal in cervicitis.

B. Laboratory Findings: In acute cervicitis, smears and cultures of the cervical discharge reveal a thin purulent spread containing myriads of polymorphonuclear leukocytes. Examination of a smear stained with Gram's stain may disclose intracellular gram-negative diplococci in gonorrhea. Staphylococci, streptococci, and Escherichia coli may also be found. The smear never shows the normal "fern" formation with clinical cervicitis.

In chronic infections the cervical mucus is thick and glutinous and contains clumps of pus cells and cervical debris. Culture usually reveals mixed infection with rods and cocci.

Catheterized urine in patients with cervicitis usually contains only occasional white cells, rare or absent erythrocytes, and no casts. Culture of the urine is generally negative in urethritis and trigonitis secondary to cervicitis.

The white blood count is slightly elevated. The differential count shows a shift to the left.

C. X-Ray Findings: Hysterograms may disclose hypertrophic rugous folds within the endocervical canal and even partial stenosis when a blunt-tipped cannula is used for the injection of radiopaque substance.

Complications.

Leukorrhea, cervical stenosis, and infertility are late sequelae of chronic cervicitis. Chronic infection of the lower and subsequently the upper urinary tract may follow persistent cervicitis. Salpingitis is common with gonorrhea and acute post-abortal cervicitis.

476 Cervicitis

Carcinoma of the cervix usually occurs in parous women. Examination often reveals neglected cervical lacerations and chronic infection. These are now thought to be indirect causes of cervical cancer.

Differential Diagnosis.

Leukorrhea and metrorrhagia are also reported in early carcinoma of the cervix. Vaginal and cervical smears and scrapings and biopsies of the reddened areas are required for a definitive diagnosis. Venereal infections and tuberculous involvement of the cervix must also be considered.

Rectovaginal examination should be done to distinguish the signs and symptoms of pelvic tenderness, induration, and mass formation around and above the cervix when discharge is noted from the cervix.

Prevention.

Prophylactic measures include the following: (1) Avoidance of traumatic delivery and instrumentation. (2) Meticulous postpartal repair of cervical lacerations over 1.5 cm deep. (3) Persistent, methodical treatment of the infected cervix following pregnancy and delivery until healed. (4) Periodic gynecologic examination, vaginal smears and cultures, and prompt therapy of cervical infection. (5) Wider use of total (rather than subtotal) hysterectomy when hysterectomy is indicated.

Treatment.

The selection of the most appropriate treatment depends upon the age of the patient and her desire for pregnancy; the severity of the cervical involvement; the presence of complicating factors (e.g., salpingitis); and previous treatment.

A. Acute Cervicitis: Acute gonococcal and streptococcal cervicitis must be treated promptly and intensively with antibiotics chosen on the basis of sensitivity studies. Procaine penicillin G, 1-2 million units daily for 3 days, is usually specific.

Instrumentation and vigorous topical therapy should be avoided during the acute phase and before the menses, when an upward spread of the infection may occur.

B. Chronic Cervicitis:
1. Medical treatment - Medical treatment should be employed initially for patients during and after the childbearing period. If the patient is unimproved after 2-3 months, minor surgical therapy is indicated.
    a. If the uterus is retroposed, it is restored to normal anteposition if possible and a pessary inserted. This may reduce chronic passive congestion in the cervix and corpus.

b. Chronic cervicitis may be treated with diethylstilbestrol, 1 mg (or equivalent) daily for 15 days beginning with the first day of menstruation, together with sulfisoxazole (Gantrisin®), 1 gm 4 times daily for 3 days and then 0.5 gm daily for the next 7 days. An alternative is to give diethylstilbestrol as above and procaine penicillin G, 600,000 units daily for 3 days beginning on the 10th day of the cycle, when the mucus flow from the cervix is normally free. The criterion of cure is a microscopically clear mucus with the consistency of saliva.
   c. Chemical cauterization of the ecto- and endocervix with 5-10% silver nitrate solution or 2-5% sodium hydroxide solution is effective, especially when done during the midcycle.
   d. Aqueous vaginal creams of low pH are also helpful. Aci-Jel®, one application after an acetic acid douche every night for 3 weeks during the interval, may be used concomitantly with endocrine and antibiotic therapy.
2. Surgical treatment - Before treating cervicitis by surgery, one must consider the results desired; the likelihood of postoperative bleeding, infection, stricture formation and infertility; and the implications for vaginal delivery in future pregnancies. Office dilatation of the cervix and puncture of nabothian cysts may be done at any time during the cycle. Any other type of surgery for cervicitis is contraindicated within 7 days of a menstrual period because of the danger of ascending infection and postoperative infection.
   a. Minor surgical procedures may be employed if the canal is widely exposed by lacerations or for severe chronic cervicitis. These procedures include light electrocauterization with low-frequency current employing a nasal tip or small Post electrode, or mild electrocoagulation with a high-frequency monopolar electrode.

   With electrocoagulation (and electrosurgery), both incision and coagulation are possible, and the penetration of heat and destruction of diseased gland tissue are uniform and controllable. For these reasons, most physicians prefer coagulation to cauterization, although both methods, if used with skill and restraint, will give satisfactory results. Cauterization and coagulation should be done radially. Complications (salpingitis and stenosis of the cervix) are more frequent following cauterization. Only portions of the canal and portio should be treated at any one visit, preferably during the first half of the cycle. In general, undertreatment is best. Several treatments (one week apart) may be required. Anesthesia is usually unnecessary for minor surgical treatment.

Electrotherapy and surgical treatment of chronic cervicitis are applicable during or after the childbearing years. (See Table 20-1.)

Immediately after cauterization, daily acetic acid douches, nitrofurantoin (Furadantin®), sulfonamide cream, or suppositories locally for 3-4 days are prescribed to suppress infection.

   b. If the patient does not respond to minor surgical treatment over a period of 3-4 months, more extensive electrotherapy or major surgery may be required. Wide conization of the cervix (see p. 677) is rarely indicated during the childbearing years because less extreme measures are usually successful. Major surgical procedures for the treatment of cervicitis include Emmet's, Sänger's, or Sturmdorf's trachelorrhaphy, cervical amputation, and total hysterectomy (see p. 678).

C. Treatment of Complications:
1. Cervical hemorrhage - This may follow electrotherapy, trachelorrhaphy, or amputation of the cervix and necessitates suture and ligation of the bleeding vessels. Point coagulation of bleeding areas is often successful. Styptics such as negatol (Negatan®) applied topically with snug vaginal packing are often helpful.
2. Salpingitis - Inflammation of the fallopian tubes usually necessitates the administration of procaine penicillin G, 1.2 million units I.M. daily for 3 days.
3. Leukorrhea - Discharge is usually due to persistent cervicitis caused by pyogenic organisms. In acute cases the endocervix should be cultured and suitable antibiotic treatment given. In chronic cases retreatment of cervicitis is indicated.
4. Cervical stenosis - The gentle passage of graduated sounds through the cervical canal at weekly intervals during the intermenstrual phase following treatment will prevent and correct stenosis.
5. Infertility - Absence of cervical mucus necessary for sperm migration often causes infertility and may be due to too extensive destruction (coagulation, cauterization) or removal (conization, trachelorrhaphy, amputation of the cervix) of the endocervical glandular cells. Diethylstilbestrol (or equivalent), 0.1 mg daily by mouth for 3-4 days prior to and on the day of ovulation, may stimulate the remaining endocervical cells to produce more mucus.
6. Chronic urinary tract infection - The type of antiinfective therapy depends upon the organism and the results of sensitivity tests.

Table 20-1. Pathology and surgical treatment of chronic cervicitis. (After Hyams and Matthews.)

	Grade I (Slight)	Grade II (Moderate)	Grade III (Marked)	Grade IV (Extreme)
Duration	3-12 weeks after infection or delivery	3-12 months after infection or delivery	2-5 years after infection or delivery	18-40 years after infection or delivery
Laceration	Slight	Moderate	Marked	Marked
Eversion	±	Slight	Moderate	Marked
Superficial infection	Slight	Slight	Slight	Moderate
Deep infection	0	Moderate	Moderate	Marked
Nabothian cysts	0	Few	Numerous	Numerous
Hypertrophy	0	0	Slight	Moderate
Treatment	Light cauterization or coagulation	Repeated light cauterization; moderate coagulation; conization.	Repeated moderate cauterization; repeated moderate coagulation; conization; perhaps trachelorrhaphy.	Trachelorrhaphy; amputation of the cervix; perhaps hysterectomy.

7. Carcinoma (see p. 482) - Tissue obtained at conization or amputation of the cervix must be appraised by a pathologist. Later, vaginal and cervical smears, biopsies, or even repeat conization may be required to prove the presence of carcinoma. Treatment depends upon the type and stage of the cancer.

Prognosis.

With a conservative, systematic, and persistent program of therapy, cervicitis can almost always be cured. With neglect or overtreatment, the prognosis is poor. Mild chronic cervicitis usually responds to local therapy in 4-8 weeks; more severe chronic cervicitis may require 2-3 months of treatment.

CERVICAL POLYPS

Polyps are small pedunculated and often sessile or tessellated neoplasms. Those derived from the cervix eventually cause discharge or abnormal bleeding. Most originate from the endocervix; a few from the portio. The etiology of polyp formation is not known, but inflammation is a possible cause. Cervical polyps are common. They may occur at any time after the menarche; the great majority are seen during the functional years, and an occasional one may form after the menopause.

Cervical Polyps

Endocervical polyps are usually red, flame-shaped, fragile growths, rarely over 2 cm in length. They are seen to protrude from the os, are delicate, and bleed easily. A connective tissue framework containing blood vessels centrally and mucus glands peripherally support the neoplasm. The surface is covered by tall, columnar mucus-producing cells typical of those within the endocervical canal.

Ectocervical polyps are pale, flesh-colored, and rounded or elongated, often with a broad pedicle. They arise from the portio and are less likely to bleed than endocervical polyps. Microscopically they are more fibrous than endocervical polyps, having fewer, if any, mucus glands. They are covered by stratified squamous epithelium.

Inflammation, often with necrosis at the tip (or more extensively), is typical of both polyp types. Metaplastic alteration is common, but carcinomatous change occurs rarely. Endometrial cancer may involve the polyp secondarily. Sarcoma rarely develops within a polyp.

Botryoid sarcoma, an embryonal tumor of the cervix (or vaginal wall) resembling small pink or yellow grapes, contains striated muscle and other mesenchymal elements. It is extremely malignant.

Polypoid structures are vascular and often infected, and are subject to displacement or torsion. Discharge commonly results, and bleeding, often metrorrhagia of the postcoital type, follows.

Chronic irritation and bleeding are annoying and cause cervicitis, endometritis, parametritis, and salpingitis if not treated successfully.

Since they are a potential focus of cancer, polyps must be examined routinely on removal for malignant characteristics.

Clinical Findings.

A. Symptoms and Signs: Leukorrhea is the most common sign. Abnormal vaginal bleeding is often reported. Postmenopausal bleeding is frequently described by older women. Infertility may be traceable to cervical polyps and cervicitis.

B. Laboratory Findings: Vaginal cytology will reveal signs of infection and often abnormal cells of Papanicolaou class II-III (see p. 496). Blood and urine studies are not helpful.

C. X-Ray Findings: Hysterosalpingography, using a blunt-tipped cannula, may disclose an occult endocervical polyp in the canal.

D. Special Examinations: Sounding the cervix may reveal a polyp within the canal not yet visible at the os. Surgical dilatation and curettage may be required to outline and remove a polyp high in the canal.

Complications.

All polyps are infected, some by virulent staphylococci, streptococci, or other pathogens. Serious infections occasionally follow instrumentation for the identification or removal of polyps. A broad-spectrum antibiotic should be administered at the first sign or symptom of spreading infection.

Acute salpingitis may be initiated or exacerbated by polypectomy.

It is unwise to remove a large polyp and then do a hysterectomy several days thereafter. Pelvic peritonitis may complicate the latter procedure. A delay of several weeks or a month between polypectomy and hysterectomy is recommended.

Differential Diagnosis.

Masses projecting from the cervix may be polypoid but not polyps. Adenocarcinoma of the endometrium or endometrial sarcoma may present at the external os or even beyond. Discharge and bleeding are present.

Small submucous pedunculated myomas or endometrial polyps arising low in the uterus often result in dilatation of the cervix so that they present just within the os and appear to be cervical polyps.

The products of conception may push through the cervix to be seen as a polypoid tissue mass, but other signs and symptoms of recent pregnancy are notable.

Prevention.

Cervicitis should be treated early and thoroughly. Periodic vaginal examinations may disclose asymptomatic polyps of the cervix.

Treatment.

A. Medical Measures: Culture and sensitivity tests of cervical discharge and appropriate therapy are indicated if infection is present.

B. Specific Measures: Remove the polyp by avulsion, scalpel excision (see p. 669), or high-frequency electrosurgery (all office procedures). All tissue must be sent to a pathologist to be examined for malignancy.

If the cervix is soft, patulous, or definitely dilated and the polyp is large, surgical dilatation and curettage should be done, especially if the pedicle is not readily visible. Exploration of the cervical and uterine cavities with the polyp forceps and curet may disclose multiple polyps or other important lesions.

C. Local Measures: Warm acetic acid douches after polypectomy usually suffice to control an inflammatory reaction. Prophylactic antibiotic therapy is not usually necessary.

Prognosis.

Simple removal is usually curative. All polyps should be examined carefully for evidence of malignancy.

CANCER OF THE CERVIX

Cancer of the cervix is the second most common malignancy in women (breast malignancy is slightly more frequent) and accounts for two-thirds of all malignant disease of the generative tract. Two per cent of women over 40 will develop cancer of the cervix. The average age of patients is 45, but the disease can occur even in the second decade of life and occasionally during pregnancy.

The cause of cervical cancer is not known, but celibacy and nulliparity reduce the statistical risk. Cancer of the cervix is rare among Jewish women, perhaps because of hereditary immunity or because the males are circumcised in infancy.

Squamous cell carcinoma accounts for about 95% of cases and adenocarcinoma for about 5% of malignant epithelial neoplasms of the cervix. An occasional sarcoma is described.

Pathology.
A. Epidermoid Carcinoma: Basal cell hyperplasia and dyskeratosis often precede preinvasive carcinoma, which then becomes invasive cancer in most cases. At least 90% of squamous cell carcinomas of the cervix develop in the intraepithelial layers at or near the squamocolumnar junction. This is initially the preinvasive stage, or carcinoma in situ. Some originate in the epithelium over the portio; others arise from epidermoid, so-called reserve cells found beneath the cylindric epithelium of the glands within the cervical canal, and generally remain occult until extension has occurred.

Epidermoid cancers of the cervix are graded according to the predominant cell type or differentiation of the malignancy. Grade I (Broders) or "spindle cell" (Martzloff) carcinoma is highly differentiated; grade II (Broders) or "transitional cell" carcinoma (Martzloff) is moderately well differentiated; grade III (Broders) is completely undifferentiated.

The histologic criteria for grading squamous cell carcinoma may be expressed more specifically as follows (Warren, Corscaden):

Grade I: Many epithelial pearls, marked keratinization, easily identifiable intercellular bridges, fewer than 2 mitoses per high power field, minimal variation in the size and shape of tumor cells.

Grade III: Infrequent epithelial pearls, moderate keratinization, occasional intercellular bridges, 2-4 mitoses per high power field, moderate variation in size and shape of tumor cells.

Grade III: No epithelial pearls, slight keratinization, no intercellular bridges, more than 4 mitoses per high power field, often marked variation in size and shape of tumor cells; occasional small, elongated, closely packed tumor cells; numerous giant cells.

Malignancy roughly parallels the grade: the undifferentiated variety metastasizes earlier but also responds better initially to irradiation therapy.

B. Adenocarcinoma: Adenocarcinoma of the cervix is derived from the glandular elements of the cervix. It is composed of tall, columnar secretory cells arranged in an adenomatous pattern with scant supporting stroma. A much less common adenocarcinoma is derived from the mesonephric (wolffian) duct remnants within the cervix. In these the cells are small, cuboid, and irregular, and the glandular pattern is less well defined. Adenocarcinoma of the cervix usually is not diagnosed until it is advanced and ulcerative.

During pregnancy, hypertrophy and hyperplasia of the squamous and glandular elements are obvious on biopsy. Intraepithelial as well as invasive carcinoma may also be present, however. Gestational changes should not be permitted to confuse the diagnosis.

Adenocarcinoma is graded as well differentiated, moderately well differentiated, and poorly differentiated. However, precise classification is not possible even after examination of numerous isolated fragments since tissue variability is marked.

C. Invasive Carcinoma: Ulceration always implies necrosis of the superficial epithelium. If extensive necrosis is present, it is imperative that biopsy be done at the margin of the ulcer. A carcinomatous process usually has a firm, somewhat raised edge; the base of the ulcer is indurated, irregular, and granular.

Clinical Findings.

A. Symptoms and Signs: There are no signs or symptoms of noninvasive cancer of the cervix.

Metrorrhagia is the most common sign of malignant and benign cervical ulceration, but hypermenorrhea may be reported, especially in advanced cervical cancer. Leukorrhea, usually sanguineous or purulent, odorous, and nonpruritic, usually is present in invasive cervical cancer. Bladder and rectal dysfunction or fistulas are late symptoms. Pain is present only when obstruction occurs or when local pelvic nerve involvement develops. Anemia, anorexia, and loss of weight are signs of advanced malignant disease.

B. Staging: (Estimating gross spread of cancer of the cervix.) The deeper the malignant cells invade beyond the basement membrane, the wider the extent of primary cancer within the cervix and the more likely that secondary or metastatic cancer has occurred. It is customary to stage cancers of the cervix and lymph node metastases as shown in Table 20-2.

Stage 0+ cervical cancer (microinvasion) is superficial invasion with minimal spread in situ, otherwise morphologically identical with frank epidermoid carcinoma. The diagnosis can be made only by systematic examination of a cone biopsy specimen which has been fixed while held flat on a cutting board. The specimen is then cut into horizontal strips and serial sections of each strip are stained and searched for neoplastic cells. The site of invasion in the cervix is determined by noting the area of the cone from which the pathologic section was obtained.

There are at least 3 types: (1) Invasion characterized by a network of neoplastic cells near the basement membrane which extend slightly beyond the member as a result of progressive proliferation. (2) Infiltration of the stroma by proliferating elements from the base of intraepitheliomatous cell groupings. (3) Invasion of surrounding tissue by isolated neoplastic cells.

Microinvasion must be distinguished from occult cancer in which there are confluent, definite invasive foci of malignancy.

With total hysterectomy and the removal of a wide cuff of vagina, the prognosis approaches that of stage 0. Nevertheless, metastases occur in rare instances.

Table 20-2. Staging and lymph node metastases of cervical cancer.

Stage	Direct Extension	Lymph Node Metastases*
0	None; carcinoma in situ.	None with positive nodes
I	Carcinoma confined to cervix	11% with positive nodes
II	Carcinoma extending beyond the cervix to invade the vagina (except for the lower third) but not spreading to the pelvic wall.	22% with positive nodes
III	Carcinoma extending to the pelvic wall or the lower third of the vagina.	33% with positive nodes
IV	Carcinoma involving the bladder, rectum, or both, or which has extended beyond the limits mentioned above.	77% with positive nodes

*All figures are approximate.

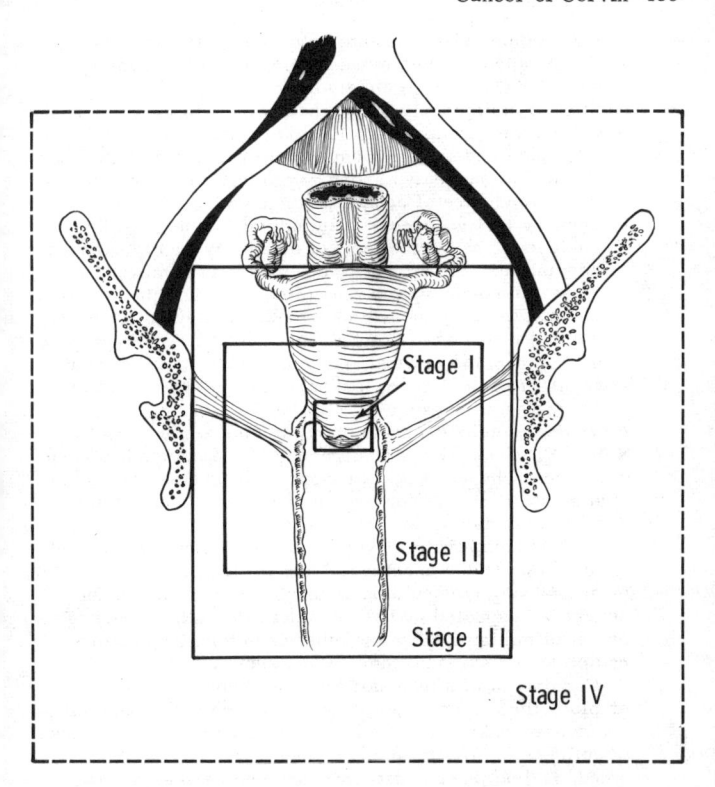

Fig. 20-1. Simple staging of metastases of cervical cancer.

At surgery, the lymph glands most often involved in the spread of carcinoma of the cervix are, in order of frequency, the obturator, hypogastric, common iliac, external iliac, aortic, sacral, and inguinal.

Although the bladder and rectum and the nerves within the pelvis are often invaded in advanced cervical cancer, metastatses to distant organs such as the lungs, liver, brain, and bone tend to be late. They may not be identified clinically but are frequently recognized at autopsy.
C. Laboratory Findings: Blood counts are significant only when anemia has developed as the result of hemorrhage or gross metastases to bone, or following intensive irradiation therapy.

Carcinoma cells exfoliate from the surface of noninvasive neoplasms even more freely than from invasive lesions. Endometrial, tubal, ovarian, or other intraperitoneal malignancies may shed cells which find their way down the genital tract. In an area of cancer, deficient blood supply and infection cause cytolysis. Cytologic study and biopsy of suspected areas have facilitated the early diagnosis and cure of cancer of the cervix.

1. Schiller test - Aqueous solutions of iodine stain the surface of the normal cervix mahogany-brown because normal cervical epithelial cells contain glycogen. Zones of cancer within the epithelium over the cervix do not contain glycogen and remain unstained when painted with Lugol's or Schiller's iodine solutions. Scars, erosion, eversion, cystic mucus glands, and zones of nonmalignant leukoplakia also appear pallid for the same reason.
2. Vaginal smear (Papanicolaou) studies - See p. 495.

D. X-Ray Findings: When malignancy of the cervix has been diagnosed, chest films, intravenous urograms, and other studies should be performed as necessary in an attempt to identify metastases.

E. Special Examinations: Cystoscopy, proctoscopy, vaginal examination under anesthesia, conization, curettage, or even laparotomy should be done when carcinoma of the cervix is suspected or has been definitely diagnosed. The extent of malignant disease must be determined before radiologic or surgical therapy is begun.

Carcinoma in situ is not a visible lesion unless one employs the colposcope. Upon colposcopic examination preinvasive cervical carcinoma usually is seen as an area of dullness or loss of surface sheen. No ulceration is noted, and no irregularity or mass can be seen or felt. Once invasion begins, ulceration and spotting occur. By the time sanguineous vaginal discharge or abnormal bleeding occurs, penetration of the malignancy into the substance of the cervix is certain. Occasionally a small patch of leukoplakia may be found which represents preinvasive carcinoma, or a thickened area in an eversion of the cervix may show these changes. Biopsy or conization of the cervix will be required.

Biopsy should be avoided initially unless a definitely ulcerative and suspicious lesion is noted. Four-quadrant biopsies of the cervix or actual conization of the cervix may be required when repeated, confirmed reports of suspicious or probable exfoliated carcinoma cells is made by the pathologist.

Complications.

A. Metastases to regional lymph nodes occur with increasing frequency from stage I to stage IV.

B. Extension occurs in all directions, the most common being lateral growth of the tumor in the base of the broad ligaments on one or both sides. The ureters are often obstructed lateral to the cervix. Hydroureter and hydronephrosis impair kidney function. Almost two-thirds of patients with carcinoma of the cervix die of uremia when ureteral obstruction is bilateral. Perivascular, perineural, and lymphatic channels facilitate cancer spread.
C. Direct surface extension of cervical carcinoma up the cervical canal may be the path of invasion to the uterus; downward growth of the malignancy often involves the vagina.
D. Posterior extension of malignancy from the cervix along the uterosacral ligaments leads to invasion of the rectum.
E. Anterior extension is followed by invasion of the bladder in stages III and IV.
F. Pain and swelling in the leg, particularly the upper thigh, may indicate lymphatic occlusion and obstruction of the venous return by carcinoma.
G. Pain in the back and in the distribution of the lumbosacral plexus is indicative of neurologic involvement by extending cancer.
H. Pelvic infections may complicate cervical carcinoma, the most common organisms being streptococci and staphylococci. Obstruction of the cervical canal may require drainage of a pyometra and chemotherapy to reduce infection.
I. Death due to hemorrhage occurs in about 10-20% of cases of extensive invasive carcinoma of the cervix. Protracted bleeding will cause anemia.
J. Vaginal fistulas involving the gastrointestinal and urinary tracts are particularly discouraging. Incontinence of urine and feces are major complications, particularly in debilitated individuals.
K. Metastasis to the liver is common, but spread to lung, bone, or brain is rare.

Differential Diagnosis.
A. Eversion and redness around the cervical os caused by infection, irritation, or hormonal imbalance is smooth, soft, and minimally irregular in contrast to carcinoma. It is not exudative and does not bleed easily.
B. The hard chancre of primary syphilis is a shallow ulceration with a glistening surface, oval or circular, with a firm edge and base, which begins as a tiny papule 1-2 mm in diameter and gradually enlarges to 1 cm or more. Minimal serous discharge is noted; bleeding is uncommon. Treponema pallidum may be identified by darkfield examination of the thin exudate. The STS is usually positive.

C. Chancroid (soft chancre) is characterized by an initial vesicle which develops into an irregular, dirty, malodorous ulcer with superficial slough. The edge is frayed and undermined. A double areola, the outer red and the inner yellow, is a characteristic sign. Considerable tenderness is present. Soft, fluctuant, and tender regional lymph nodes (buboes) are present. Giemsa-stained smears from the lesion reveal Hemophilus ducreyi, which may also be cultured from the pus from the buboes.

D. Granuloma inguinale may begin as a vesicle, papule, or nodule. Excoriation of this small elevated lesion results in an eroded, red, freely bleeding base. Other ulcerated areas appear, each with a firm, rolled edge. These coalesce to involve much of the cervix. There is usually no pain and no lymphadenopathy. Wright-stained smears of tissue scrapings reveal characteristic intracellular Donovan bodies.

E. Lymphogranuloma venereum appears first as a small, ovoid, shallow vesicle or firm, elastic nodule. It ulcerates, but the base is clean and does not bleed easily. The lesion has a regular edge with minimal induration, and there is little or no tenderness. A peripheral reddened zone is usually noted. Bilateral soft inguinal buboes appear 1-4 weeks after infection. Lymphogranuloma venereum is caused by a virus which can be identified by the Frei skin test and by complement fixation tests.

F. Cervical tuberculosis is manifested by a submucous nodule, usually 1 cm or less in diameter, which breaks down to reveal a cavity containing yellowish-brown, gelatinous ("apple jelly"-like) contents. The base is granular and covered with a grayish pseudomembrane which bleeds easily. The edge is firm and serpiginous or lupus-like in shape. The lesion is not tender. An inflamed, reddened, somewhat checkered area may be noted peripherally. Mycobacterium tuberculosis may be identified by acid-fast staining technics and by cultures.

G. Abortion of a cervical pregnancy results in a deep, freely bleeding cavity, usually within the cervical canal. Tenderness is absent. Softness and patulousness of the cervix are notable, and hemorrhage is severe. Biopsy of the tissue lining the cavity will usually disclose trophoblastic debris rather than cancer cells.

Prevention.

The causes of cervical cancer are still unknown. Nevertheless, it is known that complete chastity is associated with almost total freedom from this malignancy. Theoretically, then, carcinoma of the cervix (and penis) before middle age may be considered to be a carcinogen induced neoplasm. The

incidence of cervical cancer should therefore be reduced by the following health measures:
- A. Improved Personal Hygiene: Prevention and prompt treatment of vaginitis and cervicitis, male circumcision in infancy, and precoital washing of the penis or habitual use of condoms.
- B. Avoidance of intercourse at an early age; limitation of the number of consorts.
- C. Frequent cancer cytoscreening of all women, especially parous individuals in lower socio-economic brackets and those who are sexually promiscuous.
- D. Prompt removal of suspicious cervical lesions such as epithelial anaplasia, dysplasia, and atypical or equivocal foci.

Treatment.
- A. Emergency Measures: Vaginal hemorrhage originates from gross ulceration and cavitation in the cervix in stage II-IV carcinoma. Ligation of bleeding points and suturing are impractical. Styptics such as negatol (Negatan®), 10% silver nitrate solution, or acetone are effective, although later slough may result in further bleeding. Vaginal packing is helpful. Ligation of the uterine or hypogastric arteries has been lifesaving when other measures have failed.
- B. General Measures: The patient should be admitted to the hospital for thorough study and rest before therapy is begun. Vaginal, urinary, and pelvic infections should be eradicated before surgery or irradiation. Anemia must be corrected and nutrition improved. The debilitated patient should be kept in the hospital for supportive therapy during x-ray and radium treatment; if exposures are poorly tolerated, discharged patients should be readmitted.

    Pain may be controlled with analgesics such as aspirin compound with codeine, 8 or 15 mg ($1/8$ or $1/4$ gr), 1 tablet 4 times daily as necessary. Give camphorated opium tincture, 4-8 ml 4 times daily as necessary for diarrhea. For urinary frequency and dysuria, give bladder sedative mixture, 4 ml every 4 hours as necessary.
- C. Local Measures: Plain warm water douches are permitted when necessary during x-ray therapy and after radium treatments for comfort and hygiene.
- D. Irradiation Therapy: Irradiation is generally considered to be the best treatment for invasive carcinoma of the cervix. Irradiation with x-ray, Co^{60}, radium, the cyclotron, the linear accelerator, etc, is employed. All stages of cancer may be treated by this method, and the medical contraindications to irradiation are fewer than to radical surgery. Optimal results have been achieved with ex-

ternally applied roentgen therapy combined with intracavitary and paracervical vaginal radium therapy.

The objectives of irradiation treatment for cervical cancer are (1) the destruction of primary and secondary carcinoma within the pelvis and (2) the preservation of tissues not involved in malignancy. The amount of irradiation required to destroy cancer varies from patient to patient. A cancerocidal dose for cervical carcinoma is about 8000 r administered over a period of 4-5 weeks.

It is impossible to administer homogeneous cancerocidal irradiation throughout the pelvis without damaging vital structures such as bowel, bladder, ureters, and blood vessels. The cervix can be treated intensively, however, because it has a high tolerance to radiation. The structures immediately lateral and posterior to it are damaged more easily, and so must be protected from exposure to high doses. The cervix can tolerate 24,000 r, but the bladder and ureter will be destroyed by doses higher than 10,000 r and the bowel by doses higher than 7000-9000 r. Major blood vessels will survive approximately the same exposure as the intestine. Therefore, dosage is dictated both by the radiosensitivity of cancer cells and the vulnerability of unaffected tissues. In practice, the experienced gynecologist or radiologist applies as much irradiation as possible to the cancer within a reasonable time, with particular concern for the neighboring organs.

The skilled management of cervical cancer depends more upon an understanding of the accepted principles of therapy than upon detailed familiarity with radium applicators, the many types of roentgen equipment, and other technics employed. Radium therapy is used to destroy cancer in the cervix; x-ray therapy is used to destroy cancer which may have progressed beyond the primary site. Both methods are employed concurrently over a period of about 5-6 weeks, although some physicians choose to start with one and some with the other. Physicians who prefer to begin therapy with x-ray do so because they feel that the spread of cancer beyond the cervix is what generally kills the patient and that containment and destruction of cancer within the lymphatics beyond the primary lesion are the primary objectives of therapy. X-ray therapy will usually (1) eradicate cervical infection, (2) control hemorrhage, and (3) reduce the size of the tumor. A further advantage is that roentgen exposures are far less uncomfortable for the patient early in therapy than surgery for the insertion of a radium source.

Physicians who prefer to begin therapy with radium do so in the conviction that the cancer should be treated within the cervix as soon as possible to prevent metastases. Statistical evidence for the superiority of one method over the other is equivocal.

When vaginal contractures, a cervical stump, or the patient's condition preclude radium therapy, x-ray may be used alone. Radium alone is often employed when the cancer is small and medical or surgical problems contraindicate protracted x-ray therapy.

Numerous methods have been developed for the application of radium in the treatment of cervical cancer. The objective of all methods is to deliver 8000 r to point A (see below) with radium alone, utilizing 1-2 administrations over a period of 1-2 weeks.

1. Manchester technic - One of the most logical and popular methods is the Manchester technic (Tod and Meredith). In this approach 2 points in the pelvis are selected as landmarks for calculation of irradiation dosage: Point A is 2 cm lateral to the cervical canal and 2 cm above the lateral vaginal fornix (at the level of the internal os); i.e., point A is the point at which the ureter is crossed by the uterine vessels, or the zone of first concentration of lymphatics beyond and lateral to the cervix. Point B is 3 cm lateral to point A at the same level. Point B is almost to the pelvic wall and represents a lymph gland focus adjacent to the iliac vessels. This is a pelvic site for metastatic cancer from the cervix.

   Intracavitary and paracervical radium in standard loadings of "units" is used to deliver a constant dose rate to points A and B irrespective of the combination of Manchester applicators used. The ratio of radium in the uterus and in the vagina with the Manchester technic is slightly over 1.5:1. The unit is 2.5 mg radium in a 1 cm linear source (needle). Filtration (of single tube loadings) is achieved by 1 mm of platinum to reduce alpha and beta irradiation, thereby minimizing unfavorable local reactions. An intrauterine tandem with 2 (or, at the most, 3) linear sources is employed. One unit is left within the cervix and the equivalent of 2 units for each linear source is positioned within the uterine cavity.

   The number of units placed in the uterus depends upon the depth of the cavity; the number of units in the ovoids (rounded rubber forniceal applicators) or the size of these applicators is determined by the capacity of the vagina and particularly the fornices. The ovoid with the smallest diameter carries 3 units of radium; the largest contains 5 units. Gauze packing of the vagina is necessary to retain the radium applicators.

   The contribution of the paracervical radium-containing rubber ovoids depends upon their effective radium content, the thickness of the 3 graduated ovoids, and rubber spacers, all of which are used to vary the distance of the radium from points A and B. The dosage depends upon the amount of radium inserted and the distribution employed.

Rubber applicators for carrying radium tubes in tandem are available in 3 lengths for the deep, average, and shallow uterus. By employing paracervical radium applicators, a cross-fire is established. This is far more effective than a radium tandem placed in the cervix alone or radium placed only in the vagina.

The optimal predetermined dosage from radium alone to point A is 8000 r in 144 hours. The 8000 r is delivered in 2 sessions of 2-3 days each, the first preceding x-ray therapy and the second following it. (For patients over 65 years of age, the dosage usually is reduced to 6500 r.)

The addition of external x-ray therapy augments this technic. An x-ray dose of 3000 r is given through 2 anterior and 2 posterior ports to the parametrium (point B) within 4 weeks.

2. The Curie (Paris) technic utilizes radium sources placed in an intrauterine tandem. A radium applicator is placed in each fornix; these are held by a bent spring to distend the fornices. An applicator is pressed against the cervix at the external os. Vaginal packing is employed to retain the radium. Low intensity of the sources and protracted treatment are the principal features of this method of treatment.

3. The Stockholm technic employs (1) an intrauterine tandem containing linear radium sources (no radium is left in the cervical canal), (2) metal boxes containing radium needles placed in each fornix, and (3) a box-applicator applied to the cervix. Snug vaginal packing is required. This method delivers high doses over a relatively short period of time.

4. During pregnancy, cervical cancer is treated as outlined below:

    a. First trimester - Deliver 6000 r of x-ray radiation of the pelvis through each of 4 ports. Concurrently, give 2 courses of intra- and paracervical radium, and await spontaneous abortion.

    b. Second trimester - Deliver intra- and contracervical radium. In 7-10 days, perform an abdominal (classical) hysterotomy. Two weeks after surgery, begin 6000 r of x-ray radiation, and then give a further course of intra- and contracervical radiation during the last week of x-ray therapy.

    c. Third trimester - Perform classical cesarean section at viability. In 7-10 days, begin 6000 r of external x-ray radiation, and then give 2 courses of intra- and paracervical radium one week apart, the first during the last 7-10 days of x-ray therapy.

E. Surgical Measures: Total hysterectomy with the removal of a wide vaginal cuff is the surgical treatment of choice for the woman over 40 years of age with in situ carcinoma of the cervix. In the younger woman who wishes to have another baby, deep conization of the cervix may be acceptable. This is a calculated risk even though the woman understands the necessity for vaginal smears every 6 months for an indefinite time.

Radical total hysterectomy (Wertheim) together with pelvic lymphadenectomy is utilized in the treatment of stage I and stage II carcinoma by surgeons skilled in the technic required for this extensive procedure. The five-year arrest rate of cervical cancer by this operation is as good as with irradiation in selected cases. Obesity, advanced age, and serious medical problems which are likely to complicate surgery or convalescence greatly reduce the number of candidates for elective cancer surgery. All patients and surgeons considered, the hazards of the operation exceed those of irradiation therapy, the most common serious complication being urinary tract fistula formation.

Nevertheless, the Wertheim operation and pelvic lymphadenectomy are often employed as the definitive treatment of cancer of the cervix if (1) the patient is pregnant, (2) large uterine or adnexal tumors are present, (3) the patient has chronic salpingitis, (4) the small or large bowel adheres to the uterus, (5) the patient is under 35 years of age and demands ovarian tissue conservation, and (6) the patient refuses or abandons irradiation but is a good surgical risk.

In a small proportion of patients with cancer of the cervix treated initially with radium and x-ray, recurrence or persistence of the malignancy will be noted within the cervix or vaginal vault. A Wertheim hysterectomy and lymph node resection may be indicated for good risk patients in this group because of the serious hazards of repeated irradiation.

Where recurrence or extension of cervical cancer involves the bladder or bowel, eventration operations are occasionally justified. This type of surgery should be attempted only when metastases to the pelvic glands have not occurred and when the patient is fully aware of the problems of colostomy and urinary diversion.

Prognosis.

The earlier the stage at which cancer is found, the better the prognosis. Preinvasive cancer commonly is diagnosed in women 30-40 years of age, but most patients with invasive carcinoma are 40-50 years old. Hence, 5-10 years are required for carcinoma to penetrate the basement membrane

494 Cancer of Cervix

and invade. After invasion, death usually occurs in 3-5 years in the untreated patient.

Reported survival figures according to the stage at which the cancer is discovered vary widely. In 5 recent studies, the percentage of five-year survivors has fallen into the following ranges:

> Stage 0:   100%
> Stage I: 70-85%
> Stage II: 50-55%
> Stage III: 20-35%
> Stage IV: 0-20%

The over-all cure rates in the 5 studies varied from 35% to 50%.

. . .

EXFOLIATIVE CYTOLOGIC STUDY; PAPANICOLAOU SMEAR*

Examination for characteristic neoplastic cells in the exfoliated cells from the secretions, exudates, transudates, or scrapings of various internal organs and tissues may permit a diagnosis of early malignancy which cannot be established by other technics. Exfoliative cytology has been so valuable in the detection of early cancer of the uterus and uterine cervix that it is usually performed as a routine part of the annual examination for all women.

Exfoliated cells may also be obtained from the oral mucosa, trachea and bronchi, stomach, rectum and colon, urinary tract, serous sac fluids, cyst fluids, synovial fluids, cerebrospinal fluid, glandular excretions, and exudates. Methods for obtaining, collecting, and preserving such materials may vary slightly according to the pathologist's preference. Staining and interpretation of the smears should be done only by properly trained and experienced pathologists or cytologists.

Vaginal Aspiration and Cervical Scrapings.†

A. Vaginal Smears: Material from the vagina can be obtained by aspiration or with a spatula or cut tongue depressor as shown on p. 497.

B. Cervical Scrapings: After vaginal fluid is obtained, a vaginal speculum (moistened in warm water) is inserted and the cervix is visualized. No lubricant should be used. The second specimen is taken from the region of the squamocolumnar junction by scraping with a cut tongue depressor or plastic spatula. Because this is the focus from which most cancers of the cervix develop, these scrapings provide the most reliable specimen for finding carcinoma in situ. (Specimens should always be taken from any area of the cervix which is clinically abnormal.)

While the scrapings taken directly from the cervix provide material for highly accurate interpretation, the vaginal smear gives reliable results as well, ranging from 70 to 98%. The advantage of the vaginal smear is that it may reveal malignant cells not only from the cervix but also from the endometrium, the ovaries, and even the parametrium and other peritoneal surfaces.

---

*Reproduced, with permission, from Krupp, Sweet, Jawetz, and Biglieri, Physician's Handbook, 14th Ed. Lange, 1966.
†The combined smear technic shown and described on pp. 497-9 is that recommended by the Cytopathology Laboratory, Johns Hopkins University School of Medicine. Modified, redrawn, and reproduced, with permission, from John K. Frost and Betty Jane McClellan, Clinical Cytopathology Techniques for Specimen Preparation, 2nd Ed., 1962.

Mailing the Specimens.

Smears to be mailed to a laboratory for staining and interpretation should remain in the alcohol fixative for at least one hour. Place a second, clean glass slide on each for protection, and fit the slides into the mailing container. Wrap the history form around the container and secure with a rubber band for further protection of the slides against breakage in mailing.

Laboratory Reports.

The cytologic report from the pathology laboratory usually describes the cell specimens as (1) normal, repeat in one year; (2) suspicious, repeat immediately; or (3) positive, take biopsy. Any additional information of value is, of course, added.

Vaginal cytology for cancer is reported as follows:

American Cancer Society	Papanicolau	
Normal	I	Negative for malignant cells
Suspicious	II	Negative for malignant cells but containing atypical benign elements (including those with radiation changes)
	III	Markedly atypical cells suspicious of malignancy
Positive	IV	Probably malignant cells
	V	Cells cytologically conclusive of malignancy*

*Note: Vaginal cytology **never** justifies an unequivocal diagnosis of cancer; tissue (biopsy, curettings, etc) is required for confirmation before definitive therapy.

Perhaps the most important caution relates to the "suspicious" smear. Repeat smears should be taken at once to pinpoint the source of danger since Trichomonas infection, atrophic changes, or other clinical conditions unrelated to cancer may be the reason for the abnormal or atypical cells.

Note: In no case, including that of the positive smear, is treatment justified until definitive diagnosis has been established through biopsy studies.

Exfoliative Cytologic Study 497

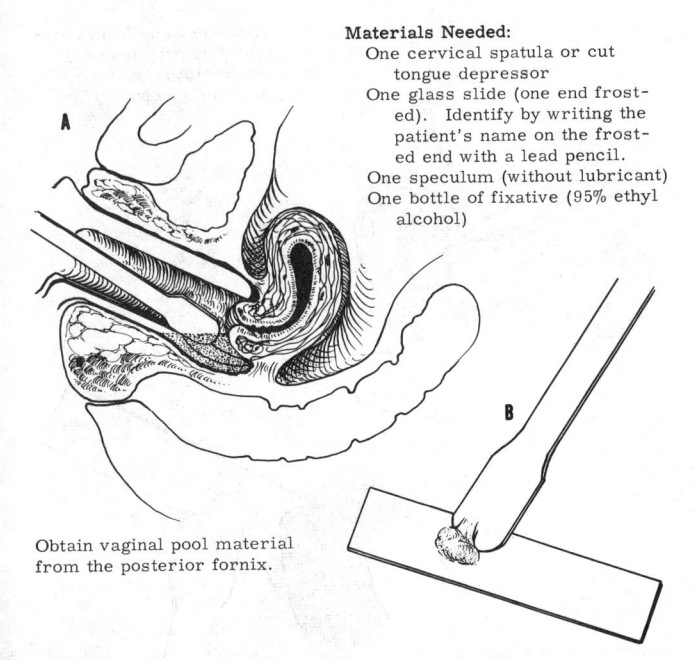

Materials Needed:
One cervical spatula or cut tongue depressor
One glass slide (one end frosted). Identify by writing the patient's name on the frosted end with a lead pencil.
One speculum (without lubricant)
One bottle of fixative (95% ethyl alcohol)

Obtain vaginal pool material from the posterior fornix.

Place adequate drop 1 inch from the end. **Do not smear.** Continue as in C, next page.

General Rules in Obtaining Specimens.
(1) Use a separate bottle of fixative for each patient.
(2) The bottle of fixative should be open and readily accessible before the specimen is obtained. Cells dry rapidly once they are spread out on the glass slide, so that the slide must immediately be dropped into the fixative when the smear has been made.
(3) Alcohols other than ethyl alcohol will not fix the smear properly and lead to difficulty in interpretation. Even a small amount of methyl or isopropyl alcohol may contaminate a large bottle of ethyl alcohol and lead to poor results. When in doubt, all old fixative should be discarded and fresh fixative should be obtained from the cytopathology laboratory.
(4) Talcum powder or starch should be wiped from the gloved finger before the smear is made so that it will not obscure the cells.

[Cont'd. on next page.]

498   Exfoliative Cytologic Study

Obtain cervical scraping from complete squamocolumnar junction by rotating spatula 360° around external os, high up the endocervical canal.

Quickly remove and mix with lower part of vaginal pool drop. Smear and fix as shown on next page.

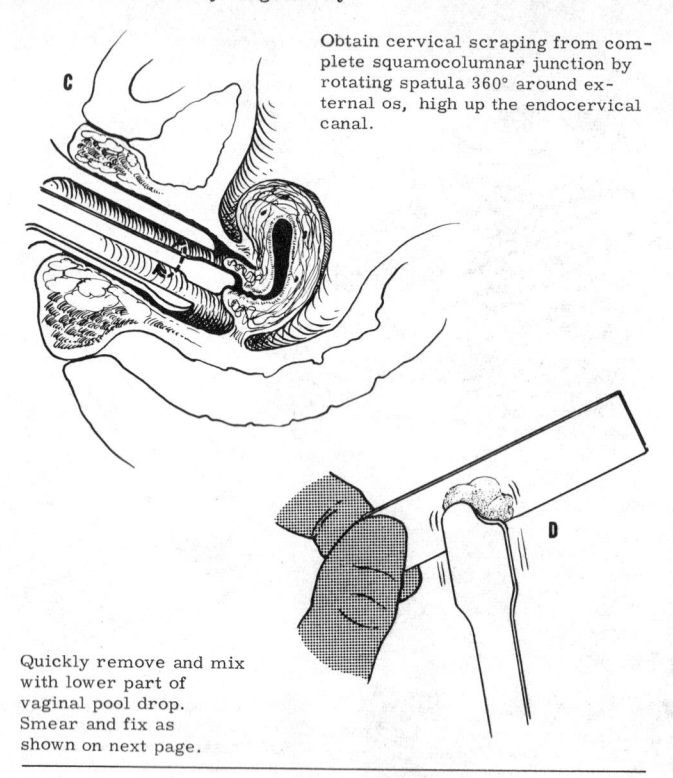

(5) Cotton swabs, if used, must not be contaminated by epithelium from the manufacturer's, examiner's, or patient's skin. They should be prepared just before use by picking up a small amount of nonabsorbent cotton with the tip of an applicator stick and rolling against the coat sleeve or clean towel.

(6) The speculum must be introduced with no lubricant. If necessary, normal saline or vaginal fluid may be used to moisten the speculum and assist introduction.

(7) Bleeding and douching within the previous 24 hours are not contraindications to specimen collection. Specimens should be obtained when the first opportunity arises. These conditions do yield a higher percentage of unsatisfactory specimens, however, and the patient should be advised that it may be necessary to repeat the study in order to ward off anxiety if repeat study should become necessary.

Exfoliative Cytologic Study 499

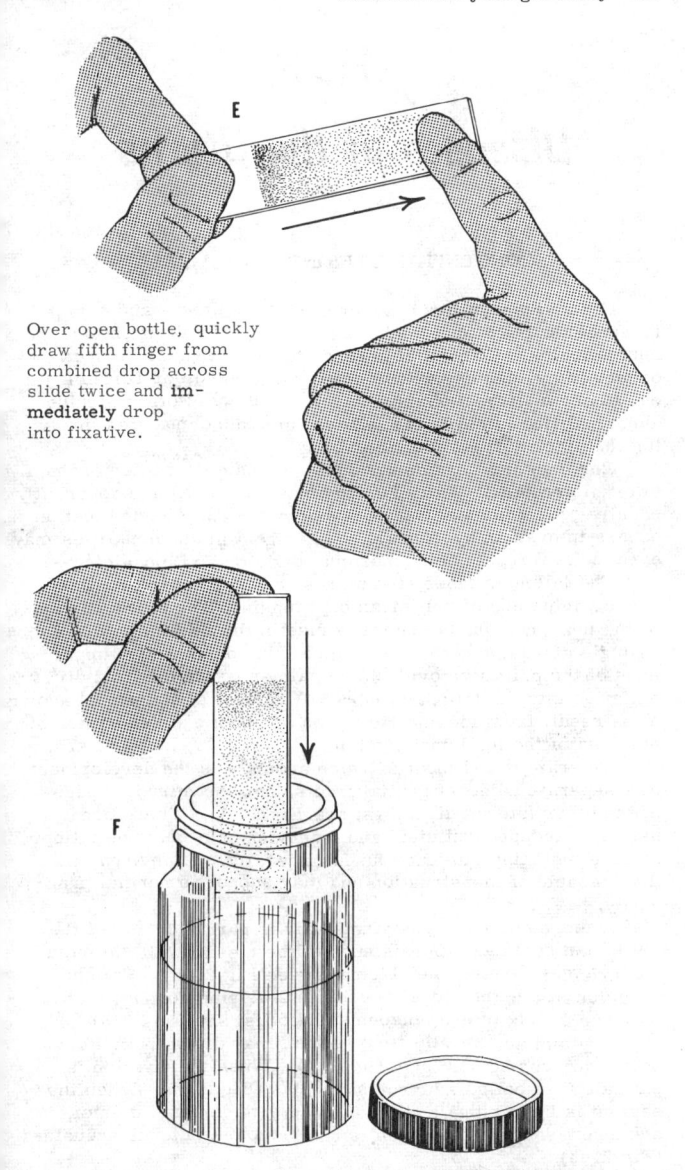

E

Over open bottle, quickly draw fifth finger from combined drop across slide twice and **immediately** drop into fixative.

F

21...
Diseases of the Uterus

CONGENITAL UTERINE ANOMALIES

Clinically significant anomalies of the uterus and cervix (absence, duplication, or distortion) occur in about one in 1000 females. Congenital absence of the uterus and cervix occurs in ovarian dysgenesis (ovarian agenesis of Turner) due to chromosomal aberration; the etiology of other uterine abnormalities is not known. Associated abnormalities involving the urinary tract are common.

Chromosomal sex determines the basic character of the internal genitalia. Paired X chromosomes (XX) are apparently required for a normal uterus and cervix. An XO combination occurs in ovarian dysgenesis. Other genital abnormalities may occur with irregular chromosomal division and mosaicism.

The fallopian tubes, the uterus, and the upper two-thirds of the vagina are of müllerian duct origin. The lower portions of the müllerian ducts generally fuse in the midline to develop a single uterus, cervix, and vagina. In contrast, the upper ends of the primitive oviducts remain separate for final differentiation into the fallopian tubes. A variety of congenital anomalies result from incomplete fusion or abnormal resorption of portions of the müllerian system.

The rarest and most extreme anomaly is the development of 2 separate adjacent genital tracts, one the mirror-image of the other (uterus didelphys; see Fig 21-1). There are usually 2 independent uteri and 2 cervices but only one fallopian tube inserting into each fundus laterally. Each organ is then capable of menstruation and may support a normal pregnancy.

A more common type of anomaly is partial fusion of the müllerian ducts with persistence of the mesial walls to include 2 cervices (uterus duplex bicornis; see Fig 21-2). Failure of fusion at a higher level results in 2 uterine corpora with only one cervix (uterus bicornis unicollis; see Fig 21-3).

A complete, usually firm septum may divide both uterine bodies (uterus septus; see Fig 21-4). When the division is partial, it is called a uterus subseptus (Fig 21-5). When the septum is but a ridge and the uterine exterior and interior are heart-shaped, the organ is referred to as uterus arcuatus (Fig 21-6).

Rarely, one müllerian duct may fail to develop (uterus unicornis). If it is not too small it usually functions normally.

Gross developmental deficiencies are of special obstetric and gynecologic concern, but microscopic variations rarely are of clinical importance. Whether normal function is possible or not depends upon the degree of deviation and the ultimate size of the uterus.

Clinical Findings.
A. Symptoms and Signs:
 1. Nonpregnant women - Amenorrhea occurs with absence of the uterus, occlusions of the cervix, and imperforate hymen; oligomenorrhea with uterine hypoplasia; and dysmenorrhea with uterine maldevelopment.
 2. Pregnant women - Abortion, premature labor, and delivery will occur if the fetus overdistends the maldeveloped uterus. Malpresentation and lack of engagement may occur if the contour of the uterine cavity is abnormal. Dystocia may be caused by inadequate, poorly coordinated forces of contraction or soft tissue obstruction (as with congenital cervical stenosis or in a uterus bicornis bicollis). Postpartal hemorrhage may be due to uterine atony or lacerations of the uterus or birth canal.
B. X-Ray Findings: Hysterosalpingography, often augmented by pneumoperitoneum, is the most effective diagnostic procedure for detection and delineation of uterine anomalies in nonpregnant women.
C. Special Examinations: Laparotomy is rarely justified for the diagnosis of müllerian dysplasia, but the uterus and adnexa should be examined for abnormal development whenever laparotomy is done for other reasons. Peritoneoscopy, culdoscopy, and culdotomy may be employed when developmental uterotubal abnormalities are strongly suspected.

Complications.
Hematometra or infection may occur in an obstructed horn of a double uterus. Perforation of a congenitally deformed uterus during instrumentation and uterine rupture during pregnancy or labor are serious complications.

Differential Diagnosis.
Neoplasms of the uterus and adnexa may suggest a bicornuate uterus. Malposition of the corpus with adherence of the tubes and ovaries may be mistaken for an abnormally formed uterus. Unilateral tubal occlusion (due to many causes) must be considered when a presumptive diagnosis of uterus unicornis is made.

502 Congenital Uterine Anomalies

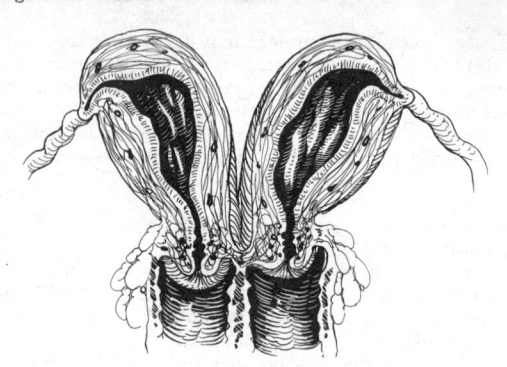

Fig 21-1. Uterus didelphys.

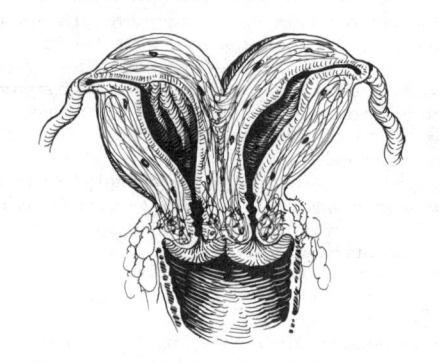

Fig 21-2. Uterus duplex bicornis.

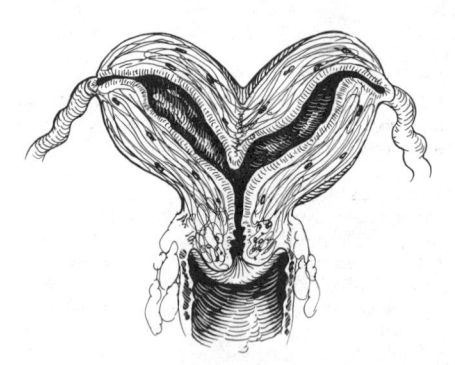

Fig 21-3. Uterus bicornis unicollis.

Congenital Uterine Anomalies 503

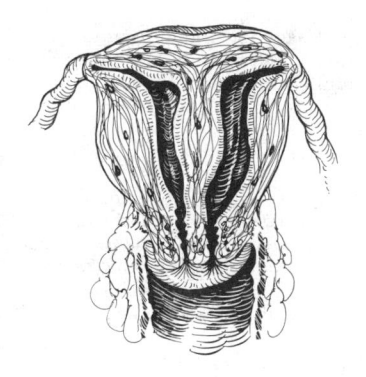

Fig 21-4. Uterus septus.

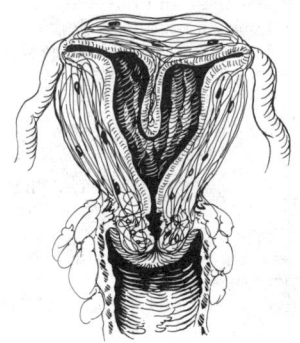

Fig 21-5. Uterus subseptus.

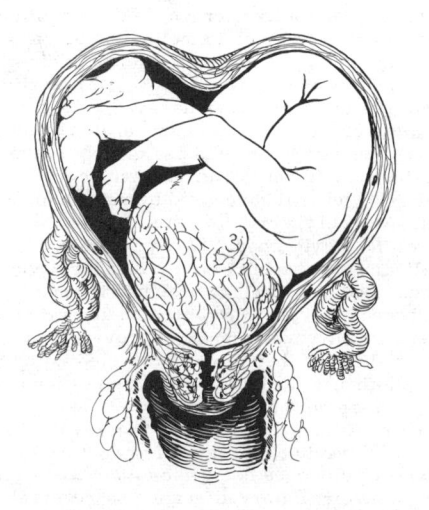

Fig 21-6. Gravid uterus arcuatus.

Treatment.

Consider operation for septal excision and unification of the uterus after repeated abortion which is related to a uterocervical anomaly. Remove a diminutive horn of a double uterus when abnormal bleeding, tumor formation, or obstruction develops on the deformed side.

Prognosis.

The prognosis depends upon the extent of the abnormality. Pregnancy and the delivery of a normal infant are not usually prevented by minor degrees of anomalous development. Fetal salvage is reasonably good after unification operations, even with vaginal delivery.

Familial repetition of anomalies of the female generative tract is rare.

MALPOSITIONS OF THE UTERUS
("Tipped Uterus")

Significant displacement of the uterus may cause signs or symptoms such as pelvic pain, backache, menstrual aberrations, and infertility. Displacement may be lateral, anterior, or posterior. Virtually all women with symptoms which may be due to displacements are premenopausal. Almost all postpartal patients have a temporarily "tipped uterus."

The uterus is not a fixed organ, and the position may vary transiently as a result of pelvic inclination or prolonged sitting, standing, or lying. The body of the uterus is directed forward in 80% of women; in the remaining 20%, retroposition will be noted. Fewer than 5% of these, however, will have a bona fide complaint referable to posterior version of the uterus. Normally, the cervix is directed posteriorly in the vaginal vault in nulliparas. After parturition, the cervix is often in the vaginal axis, an attitude caused by retrodisplacement of the corpus. The cervix and uterus often are aligned following relaxation of the pelvic floor. Laxity of the transverse cervical and round ligaments accounts for a posterior deviation in uterine position. Moderate uterine prolapse is usually associated with a retroposed uterus. Retroversion and retroflexion are more or less synonymous terms. Retroversion implies that the axis of the body of the uterus is directed to the hollow of the sacrum, although the cervix remains in its normal axis. If angulation of the corpus on the cervix is extreme, retroflexion is recognized. Retrocession implies that both cervix and uterus have gravitated backward toward the sacrum. Acute anteversion probably does not cause either obstruction to uterine discharge or circulatory alteration—a reversal of opinion of a generation or more ago. Free dextroversion or levoversion is of little clinical importance unless tumors, shortened supports, or other disorders are present. Adherent lateral deviation of the uterus indicates primary pelvic disease, e.g., salpingitis. Enlargement of the uterus, whether by pregnancy or tumor, may alter the relative position of that organ. Pelvic infections or endometriosis may obliterate the cul-de-sac; a pyo- or hydrosalpinx may drag the corpus backward and downward by its weight, whereupon adhesions add restriction to cause immobility. (See Figs 21-7 to 21-10.)

The patient's complaints uncommonly arise solely as the result of free retroposition. Nevertheless, dysmenorrhea and menometrorrhagia may be due to utero-ovarian congestion; backache is frequently caused by similar turgescence or taut uterosacral ligaments. Prolapse of the ovaries accounts for dyspareunia in uterine retroposition. Infertility occasionally results from anterior displacement of the cervix because the ejaculate in the seminal pool in the posterior fornix does not bathe the cervix.

Constipation due to displacement of the bowel or pressure by the uterine fundus on the rectum is possible but unlikely. Bladder dysfunction secondary to malposition of the uterus rarely occurs.

During early pregnancy, a retroposed uterus may become incarcerated, often because of adhesions, thus causing acute urinary retention. In addition, because adherence prevents normal uterofetal growth and development, abortion may result.

Clinical Findings.
A. Symptoms and Signs: Pelvic pain, backache, abnormal menstrual bleeding, and infertility are commonly but uncritically related to malposition of the uterus. A combined abdomino-retrovaginal examination should be done to determine uterine position, and the degree of misalignment of the uterus and cervix as well as adherence and tumefaction should be estimated.
B. X-Ray Findings: Hysterography will reveal malposition of the uterus especially when both AP and lateral films are obtained. Pneumoperitoneum or contrast media placed within the rectum and bladder will enhance hysterography, especially when malposition is related to pelvic tumors.
C. Special Examinations: In the nonpregnant patient, gently insert a sterile curved uterine sound into the uterine cavity after applying a topical antiseptic to the external cervical os and distal canal. The direction of the instrument will indicate the position of the corpus.

506 Malpositions of Uterus

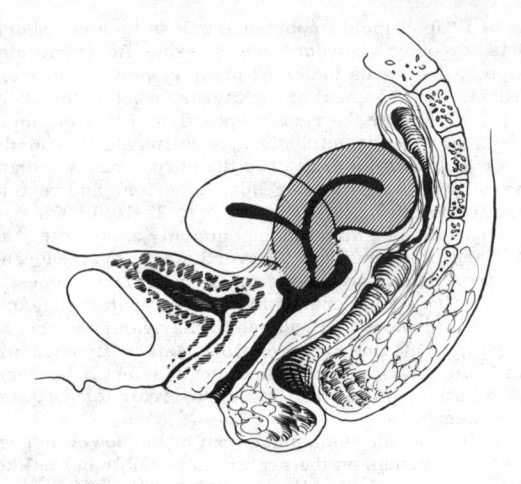

Fig 21-7. Retroflexion of uterus.

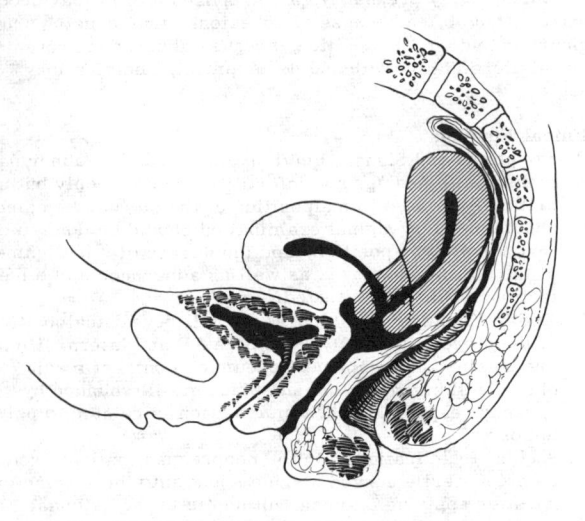

Fig 21-8. Retrocession of uterus.

Malpositions of Uterus 507

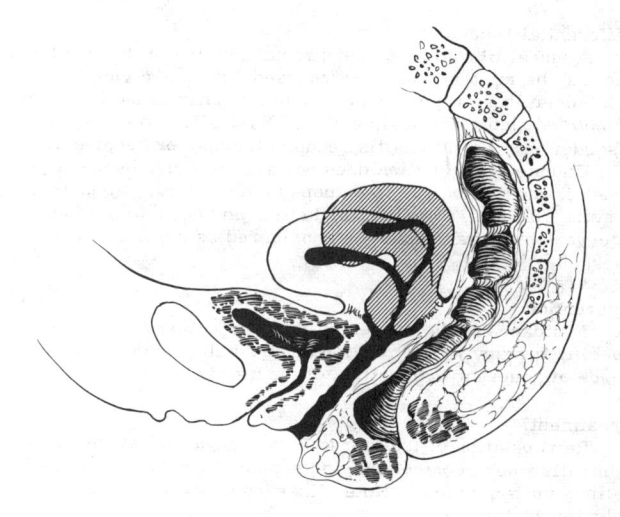

Fig 21-9. Anteflexion of uterus.

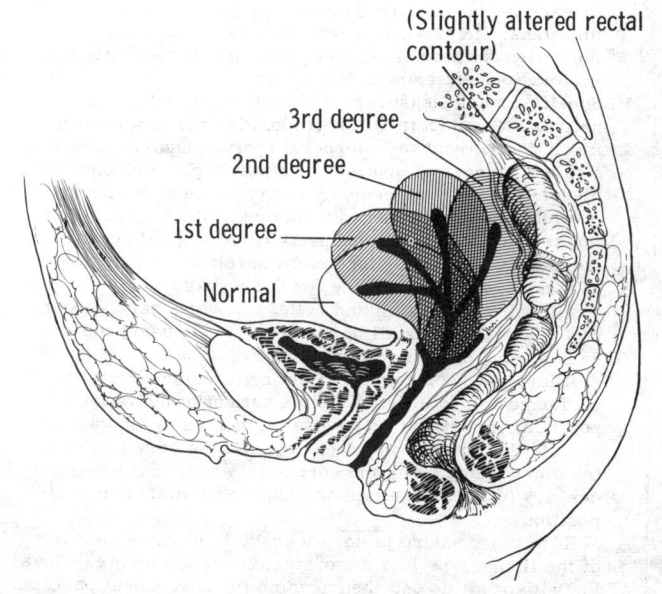

Fig 21-10. Degrees of retroversion of uterus.

Malpositions of Uterus

Differential Diagnosis.

A fundal fibroid or ovarian tumor resting in the cul-de-sac may be mistaken for a retroposed fundus and vice versa.

Adherent retroposition of the uterus may cause the same symptoms as uterine malposition. Basically, however, the disorder may be salpingitis, endometriosis, or neoplasia.

Uterine retroposition does not usually cause backache, which is most often due to orthopedic disorders. Abnormal posture, fatigue, myositis, arthritis, and herniation of an intervertebral disk should be considered as possible causes of backache.

Prevention.

Avoidance of the causes of pelvic infection and early, specific therapy when infection occurs will reduce the incidence of adherent malposition of the uterus.

Treatment.

Retroposition of the uterus is now regarded as important clinically when replacement and support by a vaginal pessary relieve the symptoms. **Note**: Knee-chest exercises are of questionable value.

A. Emergency Measures: Elevate an incarcerated, nonadherent uterus, especially when the patient develops acute urinary retention during pregnancy or when abortion threatens. Rectovaginal manipulation of the corpus with the patient in the knee-chest position may facilitate the restoration of uterine anteposition.

B. Specific Local Measures: In the nonpregnant patient neither an asymptomatic retroposition nor a normally involuting retroposed puerperal uterus requires treatment. For the gynecologic patient with pelvic pain or abnormal bleeding and for the recently delivered woman with subinvolution and persistent lochia or bleeding, reposition the uterus and insert a properly fitted vaginal pessary (see below). Unless discomfort develops, permit the pessary to remain in place for 6-8 weeks and record the result. If anteversion and relief follow pessary support, no further therapy will be necessary. Reinsert the pessary after 2 months if symptoms recur.

Bimanual replacement of the retrodisplaced uterus is performed as follows: With the patient in the lithotomy position, insert one or 2 gloved fingers into the vagina, elevate the fundus, and press against the cervix. With the other hand, bring the corpus forward. Fit a vaginal pessary of the Hodge type to support the uterus in anteposition.

If this procedure is not successful, insert a pessary of the Hodge type into the posterior vaginal fornix. Have the patient sit up and then assume the knee-chest position.

Malpositions of Uterus 509

Uterus elevated

Uterine anteversion encouraged

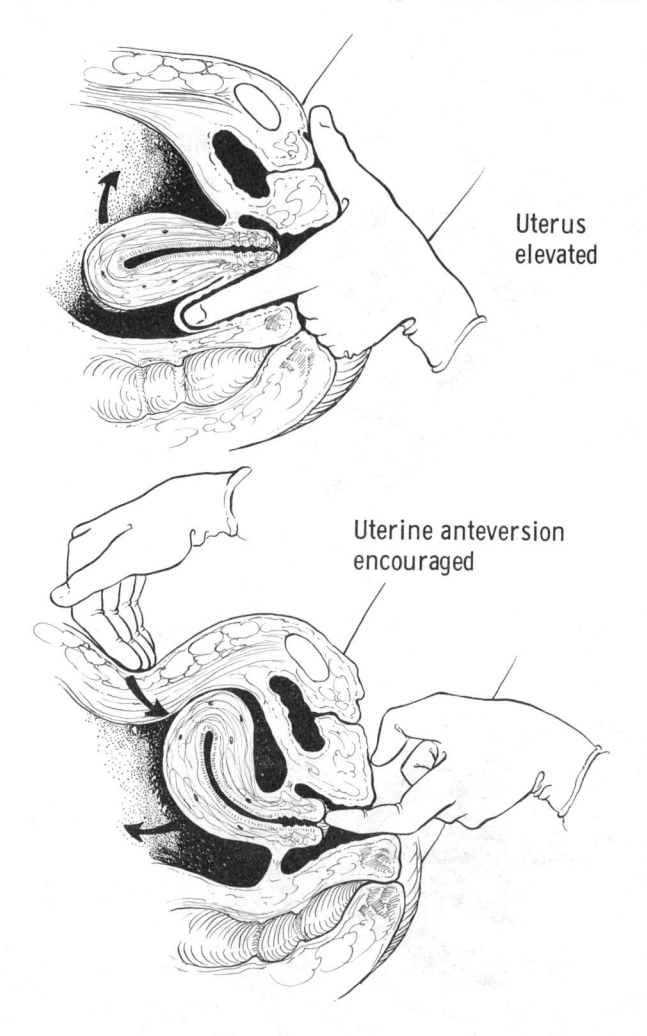

Fig 21-11. Bimanual replacement of uterus.

510 Malpositions of Uterus

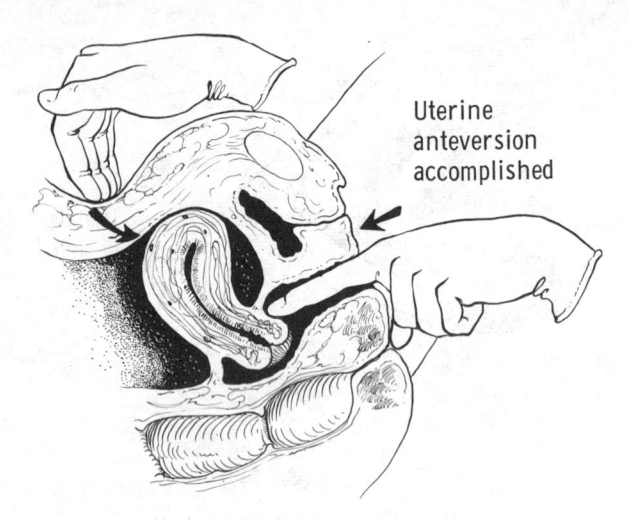

Fig 21-11 (cont'd.). Bimanual replacement of uterus.

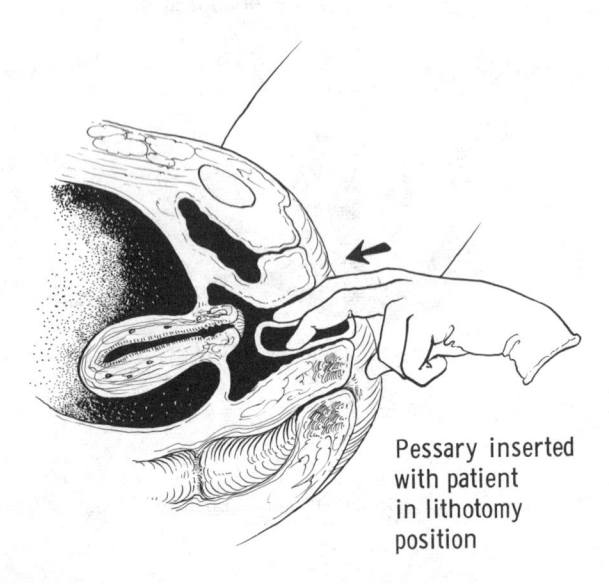

Fig 21-12. Insertion of Hodge pessary if bimanual replacement of uterus is not successful.

Malpositions of Uterus 511

Patient in knee-chest position. Uterus anteverted and pessary seated.

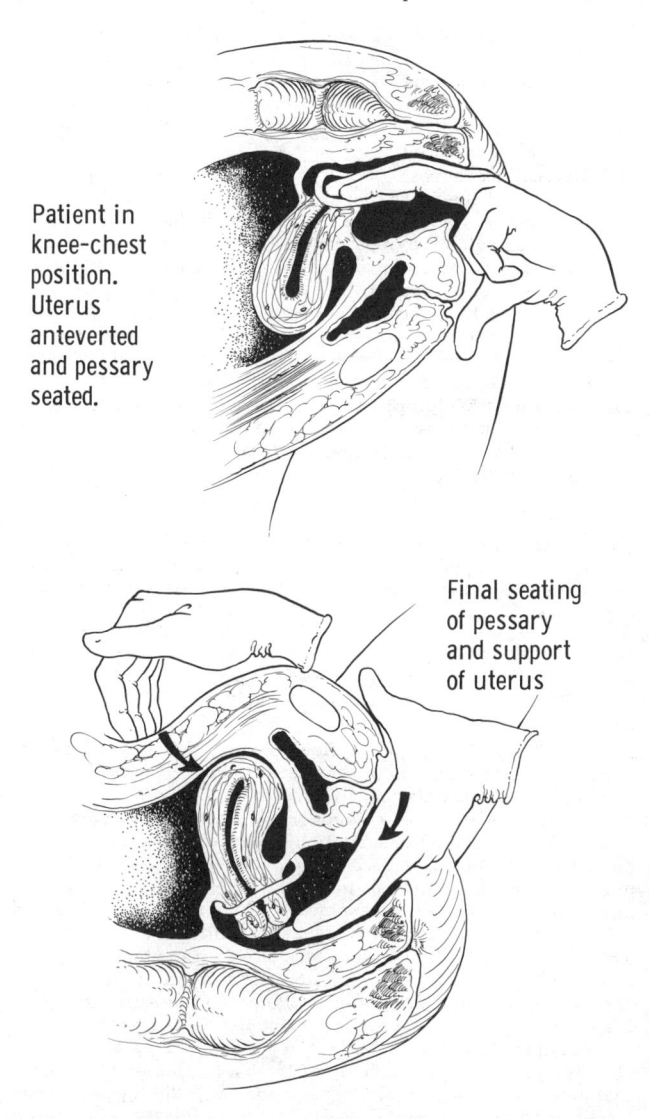

Final seating of pessary and support of uterus

Fig 21-12 (cont'd.). Insertion of Hodge pessary if bimanual replacement of uterus is not successful.

Apply pressure on the lateral bars of the pessary and displace the cervix backward while the patient coughs; the nonadherent uterus will usually fall forward. Require the patient to slip slowly into the prone and then into the lithotomy position. Seat the pessary to maintain the uterus in forward position.
C. Surgical Measures:
1. Suspend the uterus as a primary procedure when repeated replacement of the corpus by the use of a pessary has alleviated symptoms and signs or when adherence of the uterus and prolapse of the adnexa are probable causes of disability.
2. Suspend the uterus as a secondary procedure as a concluding step in surgery done to eliminate specific pelvic disease such as chronic recurrent salpingitis or progressive pelvic endometriosis.
D. Treatment of Complications: Occasional warm acetic acid douches may relieve irritation and prevent discharge caused by a vaginal pessary. (Even a well-fitted one may cause irritation.)

Prognosis.

If correction of the uterine malposition follows an accurate diagnosis of symptomatic displacement, the prognosis is good; it is poor if uterine suspension is done without a convincing indication.

UTERINE PROLAPSE
(Descensus Uteri)

Uterine prolapse (pelvic floor hernia, pudendal hernia) is the abnormal protrusion of the uterus through the pelvic floor aperture or genital hiatus. It occurs most commonly in postmenopausal, multiparous Caucasian women as a gradually progressive, delayed result of childbirth trauma; congenital anomaly; musculofascial weakness, which may account for uncommon prolapse in nulliparous women; pelvic tumor; or sacral nerve disorders, especially injury to S1-4 (as in spina bifida), diabetic neuropathy, caudal anesthesia accidents, and sacral tumors. It is usually associated with enterocele, cystocele, and rectocele. Ascites and internal genital tumors accelerate the development of prolapse. Corrective surgery for uterine prolapse accounts for about 15% of major gynecologic operations.

The principal components of the basin-like pelvic floor are the pelvic bones (including the coccyx), the levator musculature, and the endopelvic fascia. Normally, the pelvic floor supports and contains the pelvic viscera and withstands increased intra-abdominal pressure during straining, lifting, or

Uterine Prolapse 513

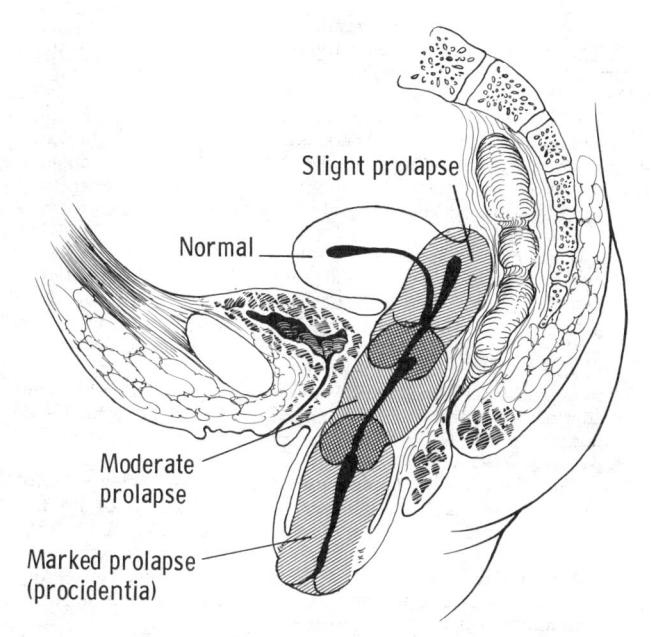

Fig 21-13. Prolapse of the uterus.

coughing when the individual is erect. A potential weak zone of the pelvic floor is the central anterior portion where the slot-like pelvic aperture permits the urethra, vagina, and rectum to penetrate the pelvic floor. The puborectalis and pubococcygeus muscles and iliococcygeus portions of the levator muscle group lateral to the pelvic aperture act as a sphincter mechanism for the conduits. Injury to the levator musculature, the endopelvic fascia, or cardinal and uterosacral ligaments may occur during delivery of a very large baby, with a long or tumultous labor, as a result of a badly executed forceps delivery or breech extraction.

Both retroposition and prolapse of the uterus develop as a result of relaxation of uterine supports. When the corpus is in the vaginal axis, the uterus exerts a piston-like action with each episode of increased intra-abdominal pressure.

The degree of uterine prolapse parallels the extent of separation or attenuation of its supporting structures. In slight intravaginal or incomplete prolapse, the uterus descends only part way down the vagina; in moderate prolapse, it descends to the introitus and the cervix protrudes slightly beyond; in marked or complete prolapse (procidentia), the entire cervix and uterus protrude beyond the introitus and the vagina is inverted.

Anterior and posterior vaginal relaxation as well as incompetency of the perineum often accompany prolapse of the uterus. Cystocele is more common than rectocele in prolapse because the bladder is easily carried downward.

For unknown reasons the cervix often becomes elongated in prolapse. Prior to the menopause, the prolapsed uterus hypertrophies and is engorged and flabby. After the menopause, the uterus atrophies. In procidentia, the vaginal mucosa thickens and cornifies to resemble skin.

Clinical Findings.

A. Symptoms and Signs: Most patients with uterine prolapse have a history of at least one traumatic or operative delivery. Nevertheless, the symptoms are often minor even with considerable degree of prolapse. A sense of heaviness or "dragging" in the low back, pelvis, or inguinal regions, often ascribed to enteroptosis, is related to traction on the uterine and cervical ligaments by the inadequately supported uterus. A firm, mobile mass is palpable in the lower vagina.

In premenopausal women with prolapse, leukorrhea or menometrorrhagia frequently develops because of uterine engorgement. Infertility is often related to excessive discharge. Once well established, however, pregnancy usually continues to term. After the menopause, excessive vaginal mucus and bleeding may be due to trophic ulceration and infection of the prolapse.

Compression, distortion, or herniation of the bladder by the displaced uterus and cervix may be responsible for accumulation of residual urine, which leads to urinary tract infection, frequency and urgency, and overflow voiding. Incontinence is rare. Constipation and painful defecation occur with prolapse because of pressure and rectocele. Ease and completeness of voiding and defecation may follow manual reduction of the prolapse by the patient. Cramping and obstipation may follow intestinal constriction within a large enterocele.

Pelvic examination in the supine or standing position, first with the patient at rest and then straining, will demonstrate downward displacement of a prolapsing uterus. Traction on a tenaculum applied to the cervix, particularly when the patient is standing, will disclose the maximal degree of descensus.

Herniation of the bladder, rectum, or cul-de-sac is also diagnosed by vaginal examination. A prolapsed uterus is invariably accompanied by an enterocele, the dimensions of the enterocele sac being dependent upon the size of the pelvic floor defect and degree of uterine descent. The tubes and ovaries are drawn downward by the prolapsing uterus. Uterine or adnexal neoplasms and ascites which may be associated with uterine prolapse should be noted.

Rectovaginal examination may reveal a rectocele; an enterocele may be behind and perhaps below the cervix, but above a rectocele. A metal sound or firm catheter within the bladder may be used to determine the extent of concomitant cystocele.

Complications.

Leukorrhea, abnormal uterine bleeding, and abortion may result from infection or disordered uterine or ovarian circulation in prolapse. Chronic decubitus ulceration may develop in procidentia; but whether the ulcers predispose to cancer is uncertain. Urinary tract infection is common with prolapse because of cystocele, and partial ureteral obstruction with hydronephrosis may occur in procidentia. Hemorrhoids result from straining to overcome constipation. Small bowel obstruction may occur within a deep enterocele.

Differential Diagnosis.

Prolapse of the uterus must be distinguished from hypertrophic cervical elongations or tumors of the cervix or uterus, cystocele, rectocele, uterine inversion, fecal impaction, or a large bladder stone. Myomas or polyps may coexist with prolapse of the uterus to cause unusual symptomatology.

Despite the variety of possibilities, the history and physical findings in uterine prolapse are so characteristic that the proper diagnosis is usually not a problem.

Prevention.

Avoidance of obstetric trauma, and postpartal exercises (Kegel) to strengthen the levator musculature, will prevent or minimize prolapse. Prolonged cyclic estrogen therapy for postmenopausal women will often conserve the strength and tone of the pelvic floor constituents.

Treatment.

A. General Measures: Palliative therapy with bed rest and a well fitted pessary (e.g., soft or firm doughnut-type, Gellhorn, or Menge pessary) may give relief if surgery is refused or is contraindicated. Prescribe acetic acid douches, medicated tampons, or chemotherapy for ulceration. Give estrogens in suppository or vaginal cream form to elderly patients. Treat urinary tract infection, diabetes mellitus, or cardiovascular complications appropriately. Prescribe laxatives or enemas for constipation. Ulcerated areas should be biopsied; surgical dilatation and curettage are indicated to investigate bleeding and rule out cancer.
B. Specific Measures: Selection of the surgical approach depends upon the patient's age and desire for menstruation,

pregnancy, and coitus and upon the extent of prolapse. Uterine suspension or ventrofixation is not effective in the treatment of prolapse since attachments give way and the cervix continues to elongate.

In young women, restore the pelvic floor. The Manchester-Fothergill operation is preferred if conservation of the uterus is important. Otherwise, vaginal hysterectomy with correction of hernia defects may be elected.

In postmenopausal women who are sexually active, vaginal hysterectomy and repair are preferable to interposition procedures. In elderly patients, colpocleisis or colpectomy is often chosen.

C. Treatment of Complications: Infection of the operative area or of the urinary tract may require antibiotic therapy. Prescribe a pessary or reoperate for recurrence.

Prognosis.

Prolapse of the uterus may remain unchanged for months or years, but it will never regress and will ultimately progress unless corrected surgically. The age of the patient is less important than her medical status in the surgical prognosis. Nevertheless, the likelihood of cure of prolapse after proper preparation and well chosen, properly performed surgery is excellent.

. . .

PESSARIES

The pessary is a prosthesis of ancient lineage, now made of rubber or plastic material, often with a metal band or spring frame. A great many types have been devised, but fewer than a dozen are basically unique and specifically helpful.

Pessaries are principally employed to support the uterus, cervical stump, or pelvic floor hernias. They are effective because they reduce vaginal relaxation and increase the tautness of the pelvic floor structures. Little or no leverage is involved. The retrodisplaced uterus remains forward after it is repositioned and a pessary inserted because the tension produced on the uterosacral ligaments draws the cervix backward. In most cases, adequate support anteriorly and a reasonably good perineal body are required; otherwise, the pessary may slip from behind the symphysis and extrude from the vagina.

Indications and Uses.
A. Obstetric: (1) Threatened abortion presumed to be due to marked uterine retroposition and chronic passive conges-

tion. (2) To promote healing of trophic cervical ulceration associated with prolapse during pregnancy. (3) Relief of acute urinary retention due to retroposition of the uterus in midpregnancy. (4) Prevention or relief of postpartal subinvolution or retroversion.
B. Gynecologic: (1) Poor risk patients or those who refuse surgery for uterine prolapse or other genitourinary hernias. (2) As a preoperative aid in healing of cervical stasis ulcerations associated with uterine prolapse. (3) Reduction of cystocele or rectocele. (4) Alleviation of hypermenorrhea, dysmenorrhea, or dyspareunia related to free uterine retroposition and adnexal prolapse. (5) To determine whether hysteropexy will relieve backache due to retroversion. (6) Correction of urinary stress incontinence by exerting pressure beneath the urethra or improving the posterior urethrovesical angle. (7) As an aid to conception in the management of infertility, since the cervix may be displaced anteriorly, away from the posterior fornix seminal pool, or there may be angulation of tubes or chronic passive congestion secondary to retroposition. (8) To facilitate hysteropexy by holding the uterus in position for surgery.

Contraindications.

Pessaries are contraindicated in acute genital tract infections and in adherent retroposition of the uterus.

Types of Pessaries. (See Figs 14 and 15.)

A. The Hodge pessary (Smith-Hodge, or Smith and other variations) is an elongated curved ovoid. One end is placed behind the symphysis and the other in the posterior vaginal fornix. The anterior bow is curved to avoid the urethra; the cervix rests within the larger posterior bow. This type of pessary is used to hold the uterus in place after it has been repositioned.
B. The Gellhorn and Menge pessaries, both of which resemble a collar button, provide a ring-like platform for the cervix. The pessary is stabilized by a stem which rests upon the perineum. These pessaries are used for the correction of marked prolapse when the perineal body is reasonably adequate.
C. The Gehrung pessary resembles 2 firm letter U's attached by crossbars. It rests in the vagina with the cervix cradled between the long arms, thus arching the anterior vaginal wall to reduce a cystocele.
D. A ring pessary, either of hard vulcanite or plastic composition or the soft "doughnut" type, distends the vagina and elevates the cervix. Cystocele and rectocele are reduced considerably by a ring pessary.
E. A hollow plastic ball or sponge rubber (bee cell) pessary functions much like a ring pessary and is used for simi-

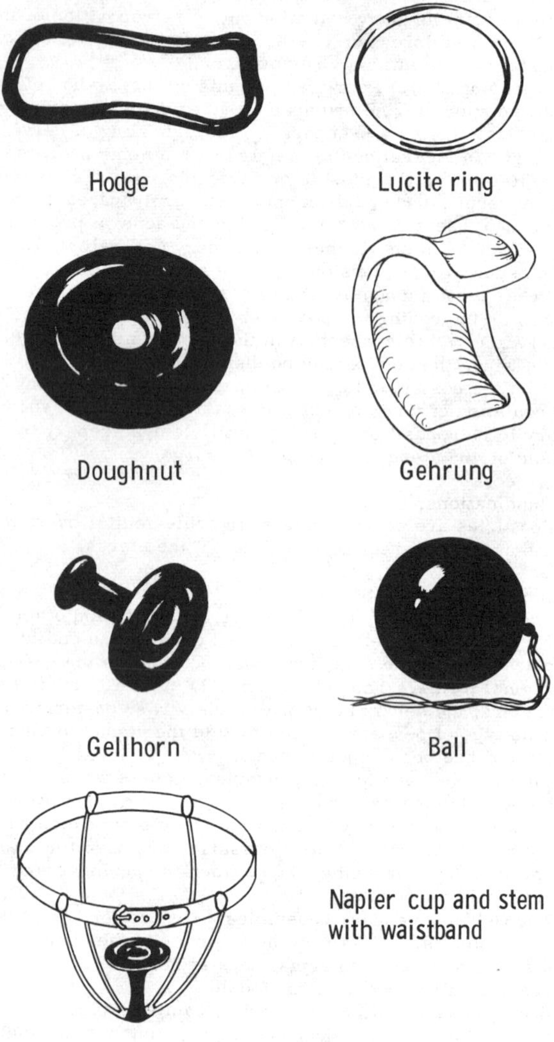

518 Pessaries

Hodge

Lucite ring

Doughnut

Gehrung

Gellhorn

Ball

Napier cup and stem with waistband

Fig 21-14. Types of pessaries.

Pessaries 519

Hexagonal bee cell pessary

Bee cell pessary compressed for insertion

Bee cell pessary in place

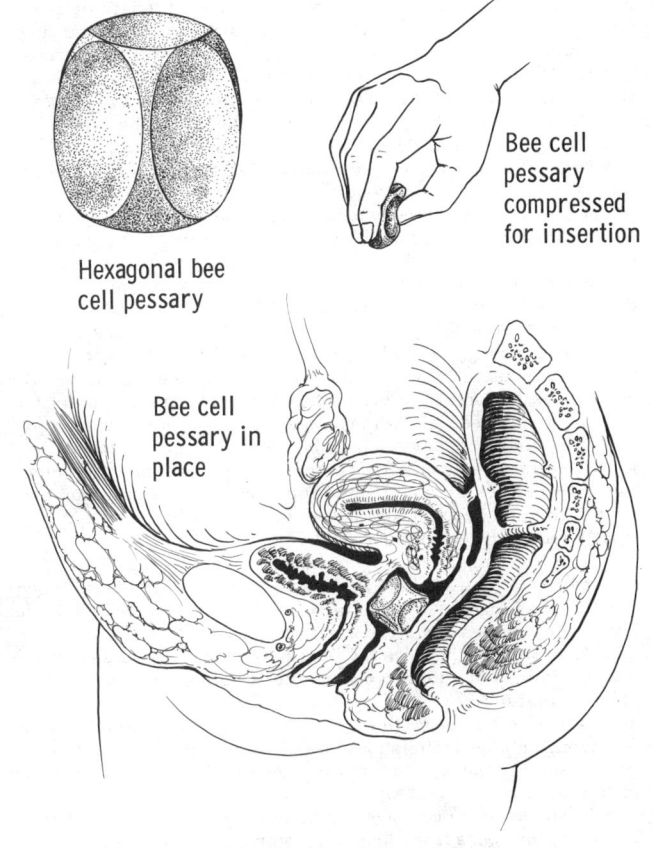

Fig 21-15. Bee cell pessary.

lar purposes. A moderately intact perineum is necessary for retention.

F. A uterine supporter (Napier pessary) is a cup-stem arrangement supported by a belt. This device elevates and holds the cervix and uterus in place. It is used in cases of marked prolapse when the perineum is incompetent, especially in a patient who cannot sustain surgery.

Fitting of Pessaries.

Pessaries which are too large will cause irritation and ulceration. Those which are too small may fail to remain in place and protrude. To determine the proper length of a pessary, pass a pair of uterine dressing forceps, using the finger as a guide, into the vagina to the top of the posterior vaginal vault. Mark the shank of the forceps at the introitus with a finger or piece of tape. Withdraw the forceps and measure the distance from the marked point to the tip of the blades. This dimension minus 1 cm is the appropriate length of the pessary. To obtain the width (assuming that an ovoid rather than a round pessary is required), introduce the forceps to about the level of the cervix and separate the handles until the blades touch the walls of the vagina. Note the distance between the handles, and then close the instrument and withdraw it. Separate the handles to the distance noted and measure the distance between the tips of the blades. This measurement represents the greatest diameter of the pessary.

The pessary should be lubricated and inserted with its widest dimension in the oblique diameter of the vagina to avoid painful distention at the introitus. With a finger of the opposite hand, depress the perineum to widen the introitus.

The Hodge pessary should be rotated slightly after it is in the vagina; using the forefinger of one hand, the posterior bar may then be slipped behind the cervix. The anterior bar should then be brought upward so that the pessary will be wholly within the vagina (i.e., no portion of it visible).

The forefinger should pass easily between the sides of the frame and the vaginal wall at any point; otherwise the pessary is too large. A solid vulcanite pessary can be molded in hot water and reshaped for a better "fit."

After fitting the pessary, the patient should be asked to stand, walk, and squat to determine if pain occurs and if the uterus remains in proper position. The patient should be shown how to withdraw the pessary if it becomes displaced or is uncomfortable. She should be cautioned that a contraceptive vaginal diaphragm cannot be used while a vaginal pessary is in place.

Frequent low pressure acetic acid douches are helpful while vaginal pessaries are being worn. Pessaries should be removed and cleaned once every 4-6 weeks, or a pessary of slightly different size and shape can be substituted. During pregnancy—and as a preoperative trial in gynecologic patients—a pessary should be worn for approximately 3 months. In many cases during pregnancy, if uterine retroposition is corrected with a pessary, the uterus will remain forward after it is removed.

Pessaries rarely are curative, but they may be used for months or years for palliation with proper supervision.

A neglected pessary may cause fistulas or favor genital infections, but it is doubtful that cancer ever occurs as a result of wearing a pessary.

. . .

MYOMA
(Fibroid, Fibroid Tumor, Fibromyoma)

Myoma—the most common neoplasm of the female genital tract—is a discrete, rounded, firm, pale pink, benign uterine tumor composed of smooth muscle and connective tissue. It causes at least 10% of gynecologic problems and is slightly more common in women who have not borne children and among women of dark racial groups. In the USA, myomas are found in 10% of Caucasian and 30% of Negro women at age 30; by age 50, the incidence increases to 30% and 50%, respectively. In some African tribes myomas are uncommon, however.

The cause of myoma formation is not known. Myomas develop from immature smooth muscle cells sheathing myometrial arterioles; they include but are not derived from connective tissue. Because they resemble fibromas, myomas are also called fibroids, fibroid tumors, and fibromyomas.

Uterine myomas have been produced experimentally by administration of estrogens in massive doses, but production of myomas in humans by hormonal or other means has not been authenticated. In the newborn, minute myomas may be present but they do not develop until after puberty. After the menopause, their growth is stimulated by greater than physiologic doses of estrogens. The dependence of myomas on hormonal stimulation and vascular nutrition is well demonstrated in pregnancy; these tumors generally increase in size after the first trimester and subside promptly after delivery.

The uterus may contain many myomas in various stages of development and degeneration. As many as several hundred have been found; only 2% are solitary. Some grow to massive size; the largest recorded weighed over 100 lb.

Each tumor is limited by a pseudocapsule—a potential cleavage plane for surgical enucleation. Vascular channels enter at the periphery and arborize within the tumor.

On cut section a typical developing myoma reveals a pattern of whorls of smooth muscle and fibrous connective tissue in varying proportions. The myelocytes are remarkably uniform in size, and the nuclear cytoplasm gives a characteristic benign appearance. Young myomas are well vascularized; older ones are not. Telangiectasia or lymphectasia is occasionally seen.

Uterine myomas originate in the myometrium and are classified by anatomic location (see Fig 21-16). Intramural myomas cause the uterus to contract so that the tumor is urged toward the cavity (submucous) or to the peritoneal surface (subserous). A myoma becomes intraligamentous when it extrudes retroperitoneally between the leaves of the broad ligament. Adherence to the bowel or other intra-abdom-

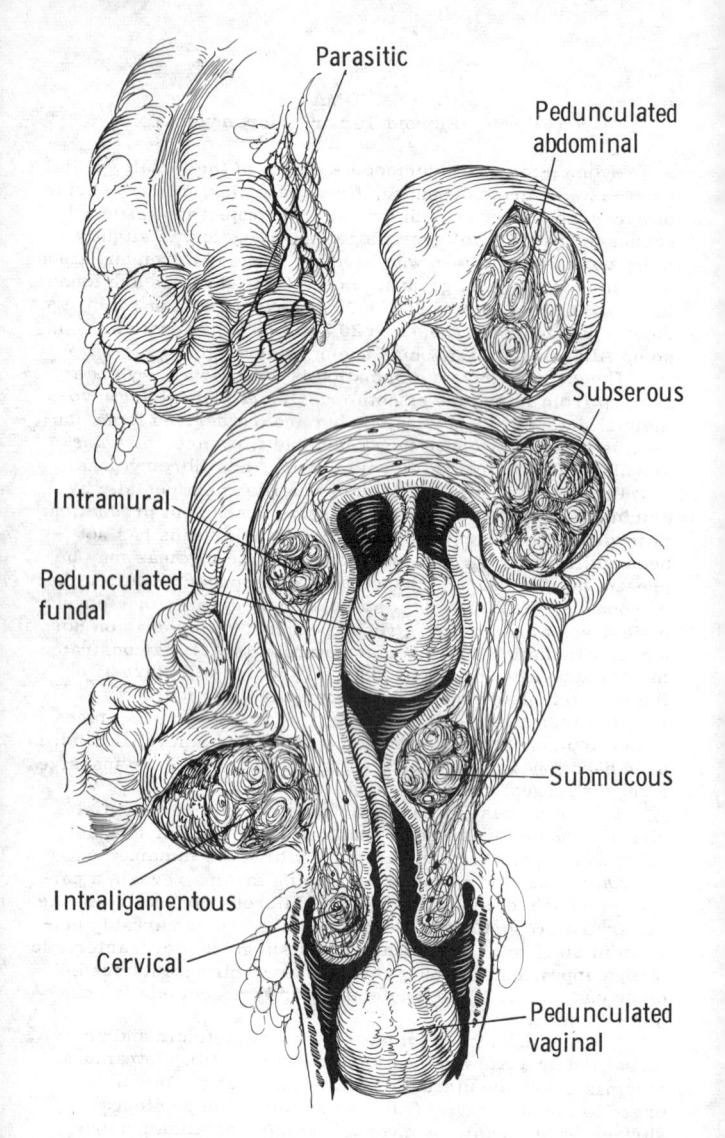

Fig 21-16. Myomas of the uterus.

inal structures is rare. A myoma eventually becomes parasitic when its blood supply is derived from the new attachment. It then separates from the uterus or retains only a few adhesive bands to the parent organ.

Two to 3% of uterine myomas are cervical in origin.

Differential Diagnosis.

Uterine enlargement or irregularity may be due to any of the following in addition to myoma: pregnancy, adenomyosis, benign hypertrophy, subinvolution, congenital anomaly; adherent adnexa, omentum, or bowel; and sarcoma or carcinoma. Even when the diagnosis of myoma has been made, other neoplastic diseases, cervicitis, cervical stenosis, and other gynecologic disorders must be considered.

Complications.

The complications of myoma are benign degeneration and malignant change.

A. Benign degeneration is of the following types:
1. Atrophic - Signs and symptoms regress or disappear as the tumor size decreases at the menopause or after pregnancy.
2. Hyaline - Mature or "old" myomas are white but contain yellow, soft, and often gelatinous areas of hyaline change; these tumors are usually asymptomatic.
3. Cystic - Liquefaction follows extreme hyalinization; physical stress may cause sudden evacuation of fluid contents into the uterus, peritoneal cavity, or retroperitoneally.
4. Calcific (calcareous) - Subserous myomas are most commonly affected by circulatory obstruction causing precipitation of calcium carbonate and phosphate within the tumor; torsion causes pain.
5. Septic - Circulatory inadequacy may cause necrosis of the central portion of the tumor, followed by infection. Acute pain, tenderness, and fever result.
6. Carneous or red - Thrombosis, venous congestion, and interstitial hemorrhage are responsible for bright coloring. During pregnancy, when carneous degeneration is most common, edema and hypertrophy of the myometrium occur. The change in the myoma is not the same as in the myometrium; there is a resultant anatomic discrepancy affecting the blood supply with infarction, aseptic degeneration, autolysis, and extreme pain.
7. Myxomatous or fatty - This uncommon and asymptomatic type follows hyaline and cystic degeneration.

B. Malignant change is generative, not degenerative. Leiomyosarcoma develops in about 0.1-0.5% of patients with myoma. (The incidence is uncertain because not all myomas are studied microscopically.)

Clinical Findings.

A. Symptoms and Signs: Symptomatology depends upon the situation, size, and state of preservation of the tumor and whether or not the patient is pregnant.
   1. Site - Intramural, subserous, or intraligamentous tumors may distort or obstruct other organs, causing pain or bleeding. Submucous tumors remain asymptomatic until they become large enough to displace neighboring viscera. They may cause dysmenorrhea, leukorrhea, hypermenorrhea, or metrorrhagia (especially if pedunculated and protruding through the cervix). Torsion of a sessile submucous tumor may cause acute recurrent pain. Cervical tumors cause vaginal discharge, vaginal bleeding, dyspareunia, and infertility. Large cervical tumors may fill the true pelvis, displacing other pelvic structures and thereby occluding the cervical canal and impeding labor. Parasitic tumors cause intestinal obstruction if they are large or involve the omentum or bowel.
   2. Condition of patient - In nonpregnant women myomas may or may not cause problems. About 25%, however, cause abnormal uterine bleeding. Some patients complain of pelvic fullness or heaviness. Backache and neurologic complaints are rarely reported.

      Before or after pregnancy, myomas may cause pelvic pressure and distention (due to excessive size and weight); urinary frequency (due to displacement of neighboring organs); menometrorrhagia (due to erosion of the endometrium); constipation (due to pressure on contiguous structures); dysmenorrhea (due to increased uterine contractility); retention cysts (due to reduced ovarian circulation); and infertility (due to obstruction of the genital tract).

      In pregnant women, myomas may cause the following additional hazards: Abortion (due to atrophic endometrial changes); malpresentation or abortion (due to distortion of the uterine cavity); failure of engagement (due to displacement of the uterus); premature labor (due to increased uterine irritability); pain (due to torsion or to degeneration of the tumor); dystocia (due to obstruction of the birth canal); and desultory labor and postpartal hemorrhage (due to reduction of uterine contractility).

B. Laboratory Findings: Anemia may be present as a result of abnormal uterine bleeding and infection. Leukocytosis is present with myoma and endometritis or carneous, septic degeneration. The white count is elevated to 20,000/cu mm. The sedimentation rate may be increased.

C. X-Ray Findings: A plain film of the pelvis may show phlyctenular opacities if calcific degeneration has occurred.

Hysterography (contraindicated during pregnancy) may reveal a cervical or submucous tumor.
D. Special Examinations: In the nonpregnant woman, vaginal examination under anesthesia and surgical dilatation and curettage may be necessary to delineate myomas. The tumor may be outlined by the curet as a protrusion from the uterine wall.

Prevention.

Estrogens in large doses should not be given to postmenopausal women with uterine fibroids.

Treatment.

Selection of the most appropriate method of treatment depends upon symptomatology, the size and location of the tumors, their state of preservation, the patient's age and parity, her present pregnancy status, her desire for future pregnancies, and her general health.
A. Emergency Measures: Blood transfusions may be necessary to correct anemia. Surgery is indicated for acute torsion of a pedunculated myoma or intestinal obstruction caused by a pedunculated or parasitic fibroid. Myomectomy is contraindicated during pregnancy, however, except for a torsive fibroid, since it causes abortion which cannot be prevented by administration of hormones.
B. Specific Measures:
  1. Nonpregnant women - Asymptomatic, small myomas require only periodic observation and reassurance. Several years after the menopause, myomas are rarely palpable even though they were at one time as large as a 14-week pregnancy. Intramural and subserous myomas do not require surgery unless they are larger than a 14-week pregnancy, multiple, or distorting. Cervical myomas larger than 3-4 cm in diameter should be removed surgically.
  2. Pregnant women - Uterine surgery will jeopardize the fetus. If a myomatous uterus is no larger than a six-month pregnancy by the 4th month of gestation, an uncomplicated course is probable. If a fibroid mass—especially a cervical myoma—is the size of a five- or six-month pregnancy by the second month, abortion will probably occur. (However, a few patients have delivered viable infants at term.) Defer surgery until 6 months after delivery, when involution of the uterus and regression of the tumor will be complete.
C. Supportive Measures: Give preoperative counsel to the patient and her husband before hysterectomy or oophorectomy regarding the effects of the operation on menstruation, menopause, and libido.
D. Surgical Measures: Preserve the uterus during the childbearing years, if possible.

1. Myomectomy (contraindicated during pregnancy) permits excision of multiple myomas and restoration of normal uterine contours and function. It is the treatment of choice during the childbearing years. Place a rubber tourniquet snugly around the uterus beneath the round ligaments and tubes to control bleeding. Employ transcervical drainage after entry into the uterine cavity.
2. Total hysterectomy is necessary when myomectomy is so extensive as to leave the uterus grossly distorted and incompetent. Abdominal hysterectomy is indicated for removal of large tumors (especially intraligamentous fibroids), exploration of the abdomen, and coincidental appendectomy and treatment of endometriosis or chronic salpingitis. Subtotal abdominal hysterectomy is required when salpingitis or endometriosis make removal of the cervix extremely difficult. If the ovaries are diseased or if their blood supply has been destroyed, oophorectomy is necessary; otherwise, the ovaries should be preserved. Vaginal hysterectomy may be employed if the corpus is no larger than a 14-week pregnancy and if the uterus is mobile and descends appreciably. Associated cystocele, rectocele, and enterocele may then also be corrected. Subtotal vaginal hysterectomy has been virtually abandoned in favor of total vaginal hysterectomy because of its technical difficulty and because there is no advantage to leaving the cervix intact.

E. Other Measures: X-ray irradiation is employed when major surgery is contraindicated in the nonpregnant woman. Dilatation and curettage (perhaps under local anesthesia) must be done first to rule out cancer. Irradiation castration—not the direct effect on the tumor—causes myomas to regress and become asymptomatic within 6 months. **Caution:** Radium should not be used for submucous tumors, since slough and infection will follow.

Prognosis.

Surgical therapy is curative. Pregnancy is possible after multiple myomectomy. Cesarean section may be necessary if the uterine cavity has been entered widely or if the uterine wall has been weakened. Menopause will not occur prematurely following a well executed hysterectomy if normal ovaries are left intact.

CARCINOMA OF THE ENDOMETRIUM
(Corpus or Fundal Cancer)

Adenocarcinoma of the endometrium is the second most common female genital malignancy, exceeded only by cervical cancer, and accounts for more than 90% of endometrial neoplasms. Almost 3% of women between 20-50 will develop the disease if their life span continues into old age; about 10% of women with hypermenorrhea just prior to the menopause have it. It is most prevalent in women between 60-70 years of age; only occasionally is it diagnosed in patients under 35 years of age. Large-boned, heavy, mesomorphic, or endomorphic women seem more susceptible. The incidence is 3 times as high in nulliparous as in parous women. The ratio of cancer of the cervix to cancer of the endometrium varies from about 8:1 in women 35-40 years of age to 1.5:1 in women 65-70 years of age.

There are 2 theories of the development of carcinoma of the the endometrium: (1) that susceptibility to cancer is a hereditary tendency (10-20% in certain families) which is intensified by estrogen stimulation; and (2) the focal development theory, which postulates that cancer occurs as a result of mitotic mutation within one or more areas of the endometrial lining, spreads to involve all strata of the endometrium, and eventually invades the myometrium and metastasizes. Inasmuch as cancer is rarely influenced by variations in the endometrial cycle or its functions, the original mutation is assumed to be an independent growth.

A hormonal aberration has long been suspected in the development of endometrial cancer for the following reasons: (1) Large unphysiologic doses of estrogen administered over a prolonged period have been thought capable of stimulating the endometrium to the point of cancer development. (2) Estrogen-producing ovarian tumors are occasionally associated with adenocarcinoma of the endometrium. (3) Benign endometrial hyperplasia in postmenopausal women who have not received endocrine products is often followed by cancer. (4) Delayed menopause permits continued estrogen stimulation of the endometrium. However, traditional "Swiss cheese hyperplasia" of the endometrium and adenocarcinoma are not often seen, and adenocarcinoma often develops in women who have been surgically castrated and in patients who have undergone irradiation treatment for nonmalignant uterine disease. It therefore seems more likely that estrogens may hasten the development of endometrial carcinoma in patients with a familial predisposition to cancer.

Obesity, diabetes mellitus, and hypertension often are said to be commonly associated with endometrial cancer, but no theories of specific metabolic deficiencies have been substantiated. Endometrial polyps and uterine myomas do not cause adenocarcinoma of the endometrium, nor does radium in the dosage employed in the treatment of abnormal uterine bleeding (artificial menopause). The underlying causes of bleeding and the age of the patient probably explain the cancer without the need to implicate radium.

Primary cancers of the endometrium are almost invariably of the following types:

(1) Adenocarcinoma: Obviously derived from the endometrial elements.

(2) Squamous cell carcinoma: Arising from squamous rests, perhaps the isthmic portion of the uterus near the endocervical canal. This is a rare lesion which usually extends by surface spread initially.

(3) Adeno-acanthoma: A variant of adenocarcinoma including squamous cells derived presumably by metaplasia. Not surprising are the malignant characteristics displayed by many of these epidermoid cells. Metastases often disclose both cell varieties; hence, they may simply be variations of the parent cell type, and both are regarded as malignant.

(4) Carcinosarcoma: A double cancer displaying malignant adenocarcinomatous elements and sarcomatous changes. It is a rare lesion which may arise from embryonal rests.

(5) Endometrial sarcoma: Originating from the endometrial stroma; chondrosarcoma, myxosarcoma, etc.

Early malignant lesions originating in the endometrium are generally minute, in situ changes confined to the functionalis layer, but the cancer finally involves most, if not all, of the endometrial surface. Fortunately, invasion of the myometrium and metastasis occur relatively late. When invasion of the uterine wall does occur, the lymphatics are involved first and the venous and arterial channels later. On rare occasions adenomyosis of the uterus becomes the primary focus for the development of endometrial malignancy, either adenocarcinoma or sarcoma.

Primary carcinomas of the endometrium may be staged as follows:

Stage 0: In situ and noninvasive carcinoma of endometrium.

Stage I: Carcinoma confined to the corpus.

Stage II: Carcinoma involving the corpus and cervix.

Stage III: Carcinoma which has extended outside the uterus but not outside the true pelvis.

Stage IV: Carcinoma which has extended outside the true pelvis or has obviously involved the mucosa of the bladder or rectum.

(**Note:** On occasion it may be difficult to decide whether the cancer involves the endocervix only or both the corpus and the endocervix. If a clear differentiation is not possible upon examination of a specimen obtained by fractional curettage, adenocarcinoma should be classified as carcinoma of the corpus and epidermoid carcinoma as carcinoma of the cervix.)

The over-all impression or stage seems to bear a general relationship to the patient's survival, although staging of an adenocarcinoma of the uterus is not generally satisfactory because of variations in the appearance of specimens from different portions of the lining of the cavity. A well differentiated adenocarcinoma, formerly called an "adenoma malignum," is merely a grade 1 lesion. Others show intermediate degrees of differentiation, and extremely bizarre, unclassifiable types are also seen. Two-thirds of all adenocarcinomas are graded as 1 or 2 on a scale of 1-4.

Endometrial carcinoma may spread in any of the following ways: (1) Within the endometrium as a surface growth into the cervical canal. (2) Into the myometrium to the peritoneum and parametrium. (3) Through the tube to the ovaries. (4) To the uterine and cervical lymphatics. (5) To the uterine arteries and veins.

As the malignancy progresses, the uterus usually becomes larger, more globular, and irregularly softened. The cervix may soften and the os may appear slightly patulous. Many cases of adenocarcinoma in postmenopausal women are not diagnosed because the cervix is stenotic and closed while the malignancy continues to develop within the fundus. Extension of the cancer to the cervix may occur, and pyometra or hematometra is commonly associated with this type of carcinoma. When endometrial cancer involves the endocervix, the iliac, obturator, and sacral lymph nodes are seeded (just as with primary cervical carcinoma).

Obstruction of the cervix and the damming of blood and mucus-containing malignant cells within the uterine cavity permits a reflux of fluid-containing cancer cells into the fallopian tubes; neoplastic cells finally escape from the fimbriated ends of the tubes to be implanted lateral and posterior to the uterus, just as with retrograde menstruation and the development of the endometriosis. However, lymphatic spread is more common than transtubal progression.

Vaginal metastases occur in 10-15% of patients following hysterectomy; most of these are in the vaginal vault or along the urethra 1-2 cm from the urethral meatus. Vaginal metastases may be blood-borne, disseminated through the lymphatics, or implanted at operation. Hematogenous metastases in the liver, lungs, and bones are not common.

Endometrial carcinoma causes hypermenorrhea or metrorrhagia during the functional years and postmenopausal bleeding in older women. This bleeding is apparently related to cancer, although functional aberration of the endometrium may also be involved.

A thin vaginal discharge, often yellow or brown, may occasionally be described instead of, or in addition to, the spotting. When obstruction of a senile cervix prevents drainage of discharge, a slow, progressive, painless enlargement of the uterus occurs followed by muco- or hematometra. The uterine wall becomes extraordinarily thin, and if drainage is not established, rupture of the uterus will follow.

Clinical Findings.

A. Symptoms and Signs: The possibility of endometrial carcinoma must be considered in all patients with abnormal uterine bleeding. Cancer of the corpus is the cause of about two-thirds of cases of menopausal menometrorrhagia and postmenopausal bleeding. Abnormal uterine bleeding is the initial symptom in about 80% of cases of adenocarcinoma of the endometrium. A watery, serous or sanguineous, malodorous vaginal discharge is occasionally described. Pain occurs late in the disease or when intrauterine infection occurs.

Menometrorrhagia is noted in about 50% of women who develop fundal cancer at the menopause, and 30% of these are found to have had abnormal menstrual bleeding for more than 10 years. Postmenopausal patients with endometrial carcinoma often report delayed menopause or abnormal bleeding although it is difficult to distinguish spotting which is the result of cancer from benign menometrorrhagia. Only pressure and general fullness within the pelvis are described by most patients with muco- or hematometra.

The contour and consistency of the uterus cannot be relied upon in the diagnosis of malignant endometrial change. Although the uterus is often softened, smooth and globular, occasionally with invasion of the myometrium by cancer, the fundus may become firm and irregular, suggesting myoma. In stage III cases, the cancer will have spread beyond the confines of the uterus so that an adnexal mass, masses within the cul-de-sac, or distant metastases are to be expected.

B. Laboratory Findings: The sedimentation rate may be elevated in advanced cancer and when pyometra is present. Cytologic examination of vaginal smears may show endometrial carcinoma cells whether or not symptoms are present. Aspirated material from the upper endocervical canal should also be examined. Study of all slides will increase the accuracy of diagnosis. In about 20% of cases exfoliated carcinoma cells either do not reach the vaginal pool (because of cervical occlusion) or they are lysed by enzymatic action. Endometrial carcinoma cells often appear in groups and clusters and are smaller than endocervical cells. Unfortunately, the accuracy of diagnosis of endometrial cancer by vaginal cytology is only about 80-85%, whereas in cervical cancer cytodiagnosis is about 95% accurate.

C. X-Ray Findings: Hysterosalpingography is helpful in the diagnosis of cancer of the endometrium. Hypertrophic folds of the endometrium, an irregular bulky tumor tending to fill the cavity, or gross papillary excrescences within the uterine cavity suggest adenocarcinoma, partic-

ularly when there is a history of abnormal uterine bleeding (pregnancy excluded). The contrast media should be injected with minimal pressure—sufficient to fill the uterus without distending the tubes—to avoid transtubal spread of the malignancy.
D. Special Examinations:
1. Surgical dilatation and curettage is by far the best procedure for the diagnosis of endometrial cancer. Fractional curettage, taking samples of the endocervical canal as well as the fundus, enables the pathologist to identify the site of origin and the extent of spread of cancer.
2. The Clark test consists of gently passing a blunt, curved uterine sound through the endocervical os into the uterine cavity. Further manipulation is avoided and the sound is removed. Bleeding constitutes a positive test. Unfortunately, although this may be indicative of malignancy, benign polyps, submucous myomas, and even an early pregnancy may also cause bleeding. Tissue is required to make the diagnosis of cancer.
3. Examination under anesthesia provides valuable information, particularly in obese and tense women or when the degree of restriction of the adnexa and uterus is difficult to determine on initial examination.
4. Aspiration biopsy of the endometrium, utilizing the suction curet, is a simple and fairly effective means of diagnosis. An adequate amount of tissue can often be obtained in this manner without anesthesia. Water suction is not necessary; a Luer-Lok® syringe provides sufficient negative pressure.

Differential Diagnosis.

Although cystic glandular hyperplasia of the endometrium is never a precursor of cancer, adenomatous (atypical) hyperplasia may be, particularly when it is of long standing or when premenopausal ovulatory failure and abnormal uterine bleeding have recurred. Repeat curettage in 4-6 months usually is indicated to prove the persistence of the disorder.

The differentiation of papillary adenocarcinoma of the endometrium and adenomatous or atypical hyperplasia may be extremely difficult. Successive biopsies after several months or repeat surgical curettage may be necessary to determine the presence of actual malignant change. Special stains are not required to make the diagnosis. The following comparison may be helpful.

Adenocarcinoma may involve the uterine cavity secondarily. It may extend to the endometrium from the tubes or the cervix. Ovarian, bladder, bowel, and breast cancers also spread to the endometrium.

Table 21-1. Differentiation of adenocarcinoma and atypical hyperplasia of the endometrium.

Atypical Hyperplasia	Adenocarcinoma
1. Premenopausal. Menometrorrhagia common.	1. Postmenopausal
2. Unusual degree of proliferative epithelial activity; pseudostratification of nuclei or actual stratification of cells, frequently in the smaller glands.	2. Glandular epithelium stratified. Anaplastic changes in the closely packed polyhedral cells with darkly staining nuclei containing many mitoses. Gland atypia is slight. Glands closely packed or moderately atypical with epithelium appearing normal in some places.
3. Metaplasia of glandular epithelium on occasion, suggesting tubal syncytial or squamous epithelium.	3. Undifferentiated cells in glands resembling solid epidermoid cancer.
4. Glands often markedly increased in number with almost no tissue. Atypical glandular convolutions and intraglandular involutions.	4. Glands increased in number with many irregular and bizarre convolutions. Invasion of the stroma common in highly malignant types; necrosis common. Papillary pattern characteristic. Reactive inflammatory infiltration almost always in stroma.
5. Presence or absence of mitoses of little value. Mitoses common to both.	5. Presence of atypical or bizarre mitoses.
6. May become cancer.	6. Is cancer.

Adenocarcinoma of the cervix is composed of taller, larger cells which have a greater tendency toward the formation of large acinar patterns (in contrast with endometrial cancer elements). Sections containing adenocarcinomatous tissue from the cervix usually also contain more stroma than tissue derived from endometrial cancer.

Adenocarcinoma cells arising in wolffian duct remnants in the lateral aspect of the uterus or cervix are less well differentiated and contain curious frayed or irregular elements.

Carcinosarcoma is diagnosed by the recognition of sarcomatous and adenocarcinomatous elements. Sarcoma of the endometrium is usually of the stromal or spindle cell variety. Polypoid intracavitary growths are typical.

Complications.

Mucometra, hematometra, and pyometra may be followed by salpingitis before the menopause, and this may be followed by peritonitis. Rupture of the uterus or transtubal spread of the fluid to the peritoneal cavity may occur. Perforation of the uterus may complicate curettage, particularly when the fundus is soft and ill-defined. Bleeding through such a perforation into the abdominal cavity or parauterine spaces is uncommon but may lead to infection at the site of penetration. Metastatic spread to the vaginal vault or lower vagina, the ovary, tubes, and peritoneal cavity, as well as the distant organs, are grave complications.

Prevention.

Routine screening of all women by periodic vaginal smears will disclose many incipient as well as clinical cases of endometrial cancer. Dilatation and curettage should be done promptly on patients who report abnormal menstrual bleeding or postmenopausal uterine bleeding. In women who have recently received estrogens and are bleeding, discontinue the hormone and obtain vaginal smears as soon as bleeding ceases. Repeat smears and secure endometrial biopsy 3 months later, even if the first cytologic or tissue preparations are not suggestive of cancer.

Pelvic examination of postmenopausal women every 9-12 months is necessary for the recognition and correction of cervical stenosis and other gynecologic problems.

Treatment.

A. Emergency Measures: Drainage of an infected, fluid-distended uterus must be done without delay to avoid progression of infection. Perforation of the stenotic, occluded cervix usually requires an anesthetic and a small cruciate incision with a bistoury-type blade. Culture the discharge and obtain bacteriologic sensitivity tests and cytologic evaluation. Insert a small mushroom catheter or rubber drain; suture it fast within the cervix, and allow it to remain for 2-5 days.

When a pyometra is drained, instrumentation should be avoided or extension of the infection and cancer may occur. Surgical curettage or aspiration biopsy should be done when infection has subsided, about one week after drainage of the uterus.

B. Supportive Measures: The patient with endometrial cancer is often in an age group in which other diseases are prevalent. She is apt to be weak, anemic, diabetic, or hypertensive. Such complications must be treated medically and the patient restored to reasonable health before specific therapy.

C. Local Measures: Daily acetic acid vaginal douches should be employed to reduce the amount of vaginal pathogens during preparation of the patient for definitive therapy.

D. General Measures: Examination under anesthesia and surgical dilatation and curettage should precede virtually every hysterectomy. Gross and microscopic evaluation of the endometrium is recommended before major surgery involving the uterus. Even a delay of several days between the 2 stages of the operation is justified to permit close pathologic study of the curettings. If cancer is discovered, more extensive surgery will be required.

Cystoscopy, proctoscopy, chest x-ray, and intravenous urography should also be done in a search for extension of cancer.

E. Specific Measures: Treatment of carcinoma of the endometrium depends upon the age and general condition of the patient; the type, grade, and stage of the malignancy; and the availability of adequate surgical or irradiation therapy. If the patient is a good surgical risk, preliminary intracavity radium therapy is generally employed unless the uterine cavity is distorted by large myomas or is excessively deep or infected. Multiple small sources of radium are preferred. Platinum radium containers holding approximately 2-5 mg each are inserted to fill the uterine cavity for homogeneous irradiation of the uterus. (This is far more appropriate than a radium tandem or even an intrauterine Y-shaped radium applicator.) The dosage depends upon the size of the uterus, the stage of the tumor, and whether surgery is likely to follow irradiation.

Even with well planned, well executed radium therapy, which causes uterine shrinkage, destroys much and often all recognizable carcinoma, and permits resolution of infection, 30-50% of patients will be found to have residual cancer in the operative specimen 4-6 weeks following the irradiation. Often this is because adenocarcinoma is resistant to irradiation and it is difficult to irradiate an irregularly shaped uterine cavity.

The central feature in the treatment of adenocarcinoma of the endometrium is total hysterectomy and bilateral salpingo-oophorectomy. For the patient without extension of cancer, infection, or debility, surgery alone is extremely successful. The use of radium will not reduce the incidence of peritoneal or lymphatic metastases, but it will probably reduce the incidence of vaginal metastases or recurrence within the vagina. When the tumor involves the endocervix or the portio vaginalis, vaginal and intrauterine irradiation with radium, administered as for the treatment of primary cervical cancer, is often prescribed.

When the uterus is considerably enlarged or when extension has occurred, deep x-ray therapy together with intrauterine or intravaginal radium (or both) may be utilized. This is often only palliative therapy, however, especially when the peritoneum is involved and the tumor has extended beyond the pelvis.

Extrafascial total abdominal hysterectomy, sacrificing both tubes and ovaries, is usually done 4-6 weeks following completion of irradiation in stage I and II cases. Stage III problems may require exenteration. Stage IV patients are inoperable.

A wide vaginal cuff should also be removed. Preliminary packing of the cervix with gauze saturated with tincture of iodine may be helpful in preventing spill and implantation of carcinoma.

Radical hysterectomy of the Wertheim type together with pelvic lymphadenectomy is not commonly utilized because of the advanced age and poor condition of many patients. Extended surgery for the uncomplicated patient will improve the five-year arrest rate in cases where the cervix is involved but there is no other apparent extension.

F. Treatment of Complications: Cervical stenosis, causing retention of mucoid, purulent, or sanguineous material within the uterus of a patient with endometrial carcinoma, requires gentle dilatation of the cervix. Avoid vigorous curettage, or dissemination of cancer and infection may follow. A rubber catheter drain should be sutured in place and left for 2-5 days. Employ broad-spectrum antibiotics if infection is present.

Spontaneous perforation of the uterus by cancer and spillage of infected contents into the peritoneal cavity requires drainage of the uterus via the cervix and of the peritoneal cavity via the posterior cul-de-sac.

Retrograde spread of endometrial cancer through the tubes may involve the adnexa, pelvic peritoneum, and bowel. This must be prevented by giving the best available surgical and irradiation therapy for destruction of fundal cancer in and near the uterus.

The administration of intracavitary radium is occasionally followed by peritonitis. The radium must be removed promptly when infection is clinically apparent. Prescribe a broad-spectrum antibiotic and order blood transfusions if the patient is anemic.

Adenocarcinoma originating in the endometrium discovered within the cervical stump or vaginal wall requires radium or roentgen administration, or both (preferably supervoltage therapy). X-ray therapy is also used when residual or recurrent carcinoma involves the peritoneum or the adnexal regions.

Prognosis.

A compilation of worldwide experience in the treatment of adenocarcinoma of the endometrium through the League of Nations (1959) reveals the salvage in stages I and II, operable group, at 5 years to be 72%; in the inoperable group, the arrest rate was 46%. Patients with stage III lesions had a five-year survival of only 22%. The employment of irradiation only (usually radium plus x-ray) yields a five-year survival of 20-40% depending upon the stage of the disease and the adequacy of irradiation.

Treatment by surgery alone, without irradiation pre- or postoperatively, of stage I patients will result in a lower salvage than when surgery and irradiation are combined.

In recurrent cases, the five-year cure rate following retreatment (usually irradiation) is 15-25% in most modern clinics.

SARCOMA

Sarcomas are heterogeneous, highly malignant tumors of mesodermal origin constituting 2% of all uterine malignancies. The corpus of the uterus is affected more frequently than the cervix.

The etiology is not known; parity or gravidity has no etiologic significance. The condition occurs most frequently in postmenopausal women, but even infants may be afflicted.

About 25% originate in myomas. Anatomically, about 55% are derived from smooth muscle (leiomyosarcoma) by heteroplasia; 40% are mixed mesenchymal or mesodermal tumors probably derived from endometrial stroma cells; less than 5% are carcinosarcoma. The remaining 5% develop from such structures as blood vessels (angiosarcoma) or from connective tissue (reticulum cell sarcoma).

Histologic examination of immature, undifferentiated forms of the tumor will not determine malignancy. Great variation in cell size, hyperchromatism, and more than 5 mitoses per high power field indicate high-grade malignancy. The classical division of sarcomas into histologic types is as follows: (1) Spindle cell (usually leiomyosarcoma). (2) Mixed cell (most often mixed mesenchymal tumors). (3) Round cell (generally endometrial sarcoma). Sarcoma may be classified as primary (originating in the musculature of the uterine wall or stroma of the endometrium) or secondary (discovered in a preexisting myoma or area of adenomyosis). Primary sarcomas are further classified as follows:

(1) Leiomyosarcomas are homogeneous, pink or grayish, soft, and "meaty" with minimal fibrous structure; there is no capsule or limiting membrane. The tumor invades the myometrium with spread of tumor tissue within tissue spaces

and along blood vessels; sarcoma soon penetrates these channels and metastasizes rapidly to lungs and liver.

(2) "Recurrent fibroids" (low-grade leiomyosarcomas) are pathologically benign. They are, however, clinically malignant tumors because they invade other spaces. They are often found in the cervix after subtotal hysterectomy.

(3) Mixed mesenchymal tumors contain embryonic striated muscle, osteoid elements, fat, and edematous polymorphous tissue. They develop in the wall of the uterus, but may be found in the cervix and resemble pale grapes as they protrude through the os (sarcoma botryoides). Elderly women are affected almost as often as children.

(4) Endometrial stromal cell sarcomas display pale, smooth, firm, polypoid "cockscomb"-like extensions which protrude into the uterine cavity and invade the myometrium.

(5) Carcinosarcoma resembles endometrial stromal cell sarcoma grossly and contains epithelial cells in an adenomatous pattern combined with round cell sarcoma.

(6) Angiosarcomas are delicate and highly vascular, invading the myometrium without restriction; they arise from blood vessels.

(7) Reticulum cell sarcoma is a loose, poorly organized and vascularized connective tissue tumor.

(8) Secondary sarcomas may be leiomyosarcomas (occurring in about 0.1-0.5% of myomas) or, rarely, endometrial stromal cell sarcomas (occurring in areas of adenomyosis within the uterine wall).

Sarcomas begin as localized silent tumors, but they become diffuse and symptomatic upon extension into the myometrium. Development is gradual; pain, obstruction, and inflammation do not occur until the tumor is moderately advanced. Erosion into the uterine cavity or formation of polypoid growths causes leukorrhea and abnormal bleeding. Metastases occur early via the blood stream, although sarcomas also grow by extension.

Clinical Findings.
A. Symptoms and Signs: A rapidly enlarging uterus or myoma may suggest sarcoma in a young girl or postmenopausal woman. Protrusion of polyps through the cervix is ominous. Common complaints are abnormal uterine bleeding, abdominal enlargement, leukorrhea, urinary frequency, and pelvic discomfort. Late manifestations are loss of weight, pain, orthopnea, jaundice, and edema of the legs.
B. Laboratory Findings: Anemia, increased sedimentation rate, and eosinophilia are reported in well established sarcoma.
C. X-Ray Findings: Radiopaque coin-shaped densities in the lung fields indicate pulmonary metastases.

D. Special Examinations.
1. Vaginal cytology may disclose malignant cells of endometrial sarcoma and mixed mesenchymal tumors, but rarely leiomyosarcoma.
2. Biopsy of polyps and dilatation and curettage confirm the diagnosis.

Complications.

Relentless local extension and distant metastases occur despite therapy in most cases.

Differential Diagnosis.

Rapidly growing myomas (particularly submucous fibroids) are usually benign during the period of menstrual activity; postmenopausally they may be stimulated to resume growth by large doses of estrogen.

Neoplastic carcinoma should be considered in the differential diagnosis. Epithelial cells are present only in the uncommon carcinosarcoma.

Diagnosis of sarcoma depends upon thorough pathologic study, including numerous sections and special stains. The presence of "giant cells" and hyperchromatism may indicate degeneration rather than malignancy.

Treatment.

Treatment consists of Wertheim-type hysterectomy, and bilateral salpingo-oophorectomy. Irradiation therapy may retard tumor growth but does not significantly increase life expectancy.

Prognosis.

Without treatment, sarcoma of the uterus is fatal within 18 months in 75% of patients. After therapy, approximately 18% survive 5 years.

ADENOMYOSIS

Adenomyosis is a proliferative process wherein benign endometrium, including glands and stroma, has passed into the wall of the uterus beyond the basalis; it usually involves the posterior but sometimes involves the anterior or cornual regions.

The condition has also been called "adenomyoma," which implies an isolated, distinct regional abnormality. However, a scattered, diffuse type also occurs. Neither type has a sharp limitation or pseudocapsule. "Endometriosis interna" is erroneously used as a synonym; the symptomatology of the 2 is different.

The etiology of adenomyosis is not known. It is unlikely that it could develop primarily from wolffian rests within the uterine wall. The condition is infrequent in nulliparas; multiparas are affected 4 times as frequently as primiparas. Rapid reduction in size of a markedly distended uterus may "fold" the endometrium into the uterine wall at delivery; however, this does not explain adenomyosis when it occurs in nulliparas. It is found in 20% of hysterectomy specimens. It causes difficulty in approximately 70% of proved cases; about 30% of cases are asymptomatic and discovered by accident. Adenomyosis is generally symptomatic between the ages of 45-50; it is rare after the menopause.

The uterus is enlarged (often symmetrically), irregularly firm, and vascular. Incision reveals a coarse, stippled, or granular trabeculation with small yellow or brown cystic spaces containing fluid or blood. Cut surfaces appear convex and bulging, exuding serum. The endometrial-myometrial juncture is often irregular, with the endometrium dipping down into the myometrium. The abnormal zone contains and is surrounded by coarse and whorled strands of muscular tissue.

Adenomyosis is confirmed when both of the following are present: (1) penetration of the endometrium into the myometrium of more than 2 low power (50 ×) fields; and (2) associated muscle hypertrophy and hyperplasia.

A grossly yellow specimen suggests stromal adenomyosis (stromatosis). This is a low-grade stromal cell sarcoma. The stroma exceeds the glandular elements, plugs of which are found within tissue spaces and in vessels.

Pain and abnormal uterine bleeding may be caused by (1) increased vascularity of the uterus pre- and comenstrually, or (2) poor vascular control secondary to weakening of myometrial contractility by ectopic endometrium. Intramyometrial bleeding probably does not occur during menstruation, but blood or hemosiderin deep in the myometrium is occasionally seen later in the cycle. Ectopic glands usually resemble those in the basalis; they respond to progesterone in only 20% of patients.

Extension of adenomyosis from the uterine cornu into the tube occurs in 15-20% of patients (salpingitis isthmica nodosa). It rarely causes infertility because both tubes are not usually blocked.

Clinical Findings.
A. Symptoms and Signs: Adenomyosis is diagnosed and later confirmed at surgery in 65% of patients in the 40-50 year age group with complaints of abnormal uterine bleeding, increasingly severe dysmenorrhea, and an enlarging, firm, tender uterus.
B. X-Ray Findings: Contrast hysterography may be diagnostic, but the medium must penetrate the glands.
C. Special Examinations: Pelvic examination should be done just prior to or during the early phase of menstruation.

Areas of adenomyosis are softened and tender as a result of the blood vessel dilating effect of estrogen (Halban's sign).

Complications.
There are no acute phenomena. Chronic, severe anemia may result from persistent hypermenorrhea. Stromal adenomyosis is rare, originating as an indolent sarcoma in an area of adenomyosis. Equally rare is the development of adenocarcinoma in an area of ectopic endometrium.

Differential Diagnosis.
A. Submucous Myoma: Myomas are present in 50-60% of cases of adenomyosis, but the 2 disorders have different symptomatology. Myomas may cause excessive and progressive metrorrhagia and pain. The uterus is firm and nontender. Discomfort occurs if the myoma is pedunculated and in the process of extrusion. Dilatation and curettage are diagnostic.
B. Endometrial Cancer: Also diagnosed by dilatation and curettage.
C. Idiopathic Hypertrophy of the Uterus: This diagnosis must be considered if hypermenorrhea occurs without dysmenorrhea or uterine tenderness.
D. Pelvic Congestion Syndrome (Taylor): Chronic complaints, often continuous pelvic pain and menometrorrhagia, in emotional or hysterical patients should be considered. The uterus is enlarged, symmetric, and minimally softened; the cervix is cyanotic and somewhat patulous.
E. Pelvic Endometriosis: Pre- and comenstrual dysmenorrhea, adherent adnexal masses, and "shotty" cul-de-sac nodulations are typical. This disorder is associated with adenomyosis in about 15% of patients.

Treatment.
Maximal benefit is obtained by surgery: Hysterectomy is best because en bloc excision is required in the absence of a capsule or distinct margin. The ovaries should not be sacrificed unless diseased, even at age 40-50 years. Other accompanying abnormalities such as vaginal relaxation should be corrected.

X-ray and radium therapy will eliminate ovarian function, arrest progress of adenomyosis, and stop pain and bleeding. While therapeutically effective, irradiation should be used rarely in women under 40 because it induces menopause.

Estrogen and androgen therapy are not effective.

Prognosis.
After corrective surgery the prognosis is good.

ENDOMETRIOSIS

Endometriosis is extrauterine occurrence of endometrium; it most often involves the visceral peritoneal surfaces and may cause pelvic pain, infertility, and abnormal uterine bleeding. Seventy-five per cent of patients with endometriosis are 30-40 years of age. The disorder is more common in women who marry late and in nulliparas. In gynecologic in-patients the ratio of white to Negro patients is 2:1. Endometriosis is discovered in 5% of obstetric and gynecologic patients.

Endometriosis may originate in any of the following ways: (1) as a result of temporary occlusion of the cervix so that menstrual flow passes through the tubes into the abdominal cavity, where it may implant; (2) by peritoneal (celomic) metaplasia; (3) by vascular and lymphatic dissemination; (4) from embryonic rests; or (5) by surgical implantation.

Aberrant endometrium is found in many different situations: in the ovaries, tubes, and over the posterior surface of the uterus; over the anterior surface of the rectum; and even in the appendix.

The sigmoid colon and rectum are often involved in a firm, crescentic or annular, constricting tumefaction. Endometriosis may also distort and obstruct the ureters or invade the bladder. Endometriosis is also reported in the cervix, vulva, umbilicus, pelvic lymph nodes, and operative abdominal and vaginal scars following uterine surgery.

Minute (never large), rounded, raised, cystic "blueberry spots" of endometriosis are scattered over the pelvic structures. Discolored "powder-burn" points and minute stellar scars are characteristic. Dense fibrinoplastic distorting adhesions restrict the organs involved. The uterus is immobilized in retroversion; the cul-de-sac is obliterated. The tarry endometriotic cysts in the ovary may be microscopic or large (up to 20 cm in diameter). They contain chocolate colored, thick, grumous material, the residue of old hemorrhage (chocolate cysts of the ovary).

The endometrial implants are identical to uterine endometrium: tubular or simple branched epithelial glands or lymphoid-like stroma (or both). The histologic characteristics of ectopic endometrium depend upon the type and amount of circulating ovarian hormone and the response of the ectopic endometrium to these endocrine products. During pregnancy, endometriotic foci react by developing typical decidua.

Malignant change, e.g., adenocarcinoma or stromal cell sarcoma (stromal endometriosis or stromatosis), is rare in endometriosis.

Ectopic endometrium, like uterine endometrium, responds to steroid sex hormones. The response is conditioned by the presence of either adenomatous or stromal tissue, or both; the site and viability of the ectopic endometrium; the phase of the endometrium in endometriosis at the time of examination; and the extent of endometrial involvement and the degree of reaction by underlying tissue.

Endometriosis is unresponsive when pressure within the cyst reduces the function of the endometrial cells; when menstrual bleeding grossly disrupts the cystic epithelial lining; or when scarring or thrombosis diminishes the circulation to the lesion.

Most extrauterine foci may be considered miniature uteri because they bleed at menstruation. The greatest response is to estrogen and progesterone in ovulatory cycles. Egress of blood, especially from buried lesions, is not always possible, however. Blood distends and infiltrates the surrounding tissues. Slow, partial absorption and phagocytosis of blood products follow. Chemical irritation causes the bowel and omentum to seal off many endometriotic bleeding points. Gradual enlargement of the lesions, adherence, and scarring occur.

Comenstrual pain, swelling, tenderness, and mass formation are typical of endometriosis during the functional years. During pregnancy, the discomfort of endometriosis generally ceases, and in the majority of cases remissions occur following delivery of a fetus carried to viability. Necrosis of decidua, dissolution of the endometriosis, and healing occur in these instances. The menopause terminates the activity and progress of endometriosis unless large, repeated doses of estrogen are administered.

Clinical Findings.
A. Symptoms and Signs: Pre- and comenstrual pelvic pain is practically constant, beginning a few days to a week before the menses and increasing in severity until the flow has virtually ceased. Dysmenorrhea is generally most marked where the endometriosis is advanced. Pain, due to local engorgement and regional bleeding, is often of a "grinding" type and may be referred to the inguinal regions, hips, or toward the rectum or coccyx depending upon the situation of the endometriosis. One-third of patients have no pain despite typical pelvic findings. A definite diagnosis is not possible until after laparotomy and tissue appraisal; symptomatology alone, in the absence of pelvic findings, is not sufficient to establish the diagnosis.

Painful defecation occurs if the lesions are on the bowel or in a rectovaginal septum. Dyspareunia of the acquired, deep-thrust type occurs in ovarian and cul-de-sac involvement. Infertility may result from peritubal and ovarian endometriosis. Hypermenorrhea and shortening of the menstrual interval (more rarely metrorrhagia) occurs when the ovary is the site of ectopic endometrium. Bleeding occurs from the rectum or bladder at the time of the menses when these organs are invaded.

B. X-Ray Findings: Endometriosis must often be differentiated from inflammatory or malignant disease. The colon is involved in 50% of extensive cases of endometriosis, and may be shown by barium enema x-rays to be fixed and constricted in one area; thickened regionally by a plaque or concentric stenosing lesion with sharp demarcations; restricted in motion with rounded, intraluminal projections (rare).
C. Special Examinations: Pelvic examination in the absence of a history of salpingitis will reveal an adherent, retroverted uterus; shotty nodulation in the cul-de-sac, adnexal induration and ovarian cyst formation; and increased pelvic tenderness just prior to and during menses. Sigmoidoscopy and cystoscopy may reveal bleeding only at the time of menstruation.

Complications.

Tubal, bowel, and ureteral obstruction have been reported in endometriosis. Destruction of the ovary may complicate ovarian endometriosis. Rupture of large endometriotic cysts—particularly during pregnancy, when the enlarging uterus disrupts adhesions—may lead to intra-abdominal bleeding and a low grade chemical peritonitis.

Differential Diagnosis.

Endometriosis must be distinguished from infection and neoplasia:
A. Postabortal or Postgonococcal Salpingitis: Salpingitis is initiated by an acute illness; endometriosis is gradual in development. Fever and elevation of the white count and sedimentation rate are unlikely in endometriosis; they are common in salpingitis.
B. Pelvic Tuberculosis With Involvement of the Ovaries, Tubes, Cul-de-Sac, and Bowel: Pain, particularly the crescendo-type dysmenorrhea and dyspareunia, varying with the menstrual cycle; painful defecation; and bleeding from the bowel and bladder are not typical of pelvic tuberculosis. Debilitation and anemia occur with tuberculosis.
C. Ovarian Cancer With Pelvic Implants: Pre- and comenstrual pain, dyspareunia, infertility, and abnormal menses do not occur. Ascites often accompanies pelvic carcinoma.
D. Bowel Malignancy: This is an intrinsically silent tumor which rapidly invades the intestinal wall from within; secondarily, it causes adherence and tumor formation. Bloody stools accompany cancer of the colon. Minimal periodic bleeding from the bowel occurs even in severe endometriosis involving the colon.

Prevention.

Annual examination of all women during the childbearing years is recommended.

Treatment.

Women with suspected mild endometriosis should be examined every 6 months until the menopause or until the diagnosis is confirmed or ruled out.

A. Medical Treatment: Relieve pain by giving analgesics such as codeine, 0.03 gm ($^{1}/2$ gr), and aspirin, 0.6 gm (10 gr), orally every 4-6 hours when necessary during the immediate premenstrual interval. Married women desirous of children should be urged to become pregnant without delay. Infertility studies, including Rubin tests and hysterosalpingography, may release peritubal adhesions and obliterate kinks and distortions of the oviducts caused by endometriosis.

B. Endocrine Therapy: Pregnancy or pseudopregnancy will halt the spread of endometriosis in many cases, although amenorrhea must continue for at least 4 months to be beneficial.

   1. Estrogens - Diethylstilbestrol, 1 mg orally beginning on the first day of the period and increased to a total of 7 mg, may be given for the first week; double the daily dose the second week, and then give 25 mg daily, the dosage being increased by 25 mg weekly until a total daily dosage of 100 mg is reached. This is continued for 4 months. To avoid hypermenorrhea, the dose is then decreased by 25 mg weekly to 5 mg daily over the next 2 months, whereupon 1 mg is given each day for one month and then stopped. Remission of symptoms is usually complete during this treatment, but about 30% of patients have recurrences.

   2. Androgens - Methyltestosterone, 5-10 mg sublingually daily, generally relieves pain and retards the growth of endometriosis. With the smaller dose, ovulation usually continues and pregnancy often occurs. The patient must be observed for signs of virilization and the drug discontinued if they appear.

   3. Progestogens - Norethynodrel with mestranol (Enovid®), 10 mg orally daily for 2 weeks beginning on the 5th day of the menstrual period and increased by 10 mg every 2 weeks until 40 mg daily are being given, induces pseudopregnancy. The drug should be given for 6-9 months for optimal effect. Sodium restriction should be stressed to avoid undue fluid retention. Diuretics such as hydrochlorothiazide (Hydro-Diuril®), 50 mg orally every third day, will temporarily reduce edema secondary to steroid therapy.

C. Surgical Treatment:
   1. Incidental endometriosis - Small foci should be excised or cauterized during surgery for other indications.
   2. Moderately extensive endometriosis -
      a. Under 35 years - Resect the lesions, free adhesions, and suspend the uterus but avoid sacrificing repro-

ductive ability. About 20% of such patients become pregnant, although 50% must undergo surgery again later when the disease progresses.
  b. Over 35 years - If both ovaries are involved, both ovaries and tubes and the uterus may have to be sacrificed. If only one ovary is affected, its removal may be sufficient.
 3. Very extensive endometriosis - Excision of both ovaries, tubes, and the uterus is almost always required regardless of the woman's age. Induced pseudopregnancy may improve the patient's status so that an easier and less radical operation will be feasible.
D. X-Ray Treatment: If surgery is contraindicated or hazardous, castration doses of x-ray irradiation will relieve the symptoms and cause almost complete regression of the lesions. Nevertheless, one must obtain a definite diagnosis of extensive endometriosis, either by biopsy at exploratory laparotomy or from a previous operation, before this is justified.
E. Treatment of Complications: Bowel obstruction or ureteral occlusion due to endometriosis will require laparotomy for confirmation and decision regarding definitive therapy. Resection and reanastomosis may be required. If removal of the ovaries or roentgen castration is accomplished, the stenotic areas usually resolve spontaneously. Signs of intraperitoneal bleeding or peritonitis will require exploratory surgery, even during pregnancy.

Prognosis.

When infertility is not an insurmountable problem or when conservative therapy preserves reproduction, the prognosis is favorable in early and even moderately advanced endometriosis. In advanced endometriosis when castration is not permitted, the prognosis is unfavorable. With appropriate treatment, reproductive capacity is usually regained if endometriosis is minimal; in moderately extensive endometriosis, fertility can be restored in about 20% of women; few women with extensive endometriosis can ever conceive even with the most intensive treatment.

22...
Diseases of the Fallopian Tubes

ANOMALIES OF THE FALLOPIAN TUBES

Congenital absence or distortion of the fallopian tubes is frequently associated with anomalies of the uterus or ovaries. It may occur as a result of aplasia or dysplasia of the müllerian ducts or regional injury to the tubes during fetal life.

Any variation—absence, atresia, shortening, or lengthening—may be evident and is usually unilateral.

The resultant clinical problem, of course, is infertility.

SALPINGITIS
(Pelvic Inflammatory Disease [PID])

Inflammation of the fallopian tubes may be acute or chronic and unilateral or bilateral. It accounts for 15-20% of gynecologic admissions to large hospitals serving indigent populations. It is more common in urban areas, especially where gonorrhea is prevalent, obstetric care is poor, and tuberculosis is not well controlled.

Almost all cases are due to bacterial infection, usually with gonococci, streptococci, staphylococci, tubercle bacilli, or mixed flora. Rare types include Actinomyces infection and Schistosoma and Oxyuris infestations. A mild, transient, supposedly sterile or "physiologic" salpingitis has been reported to occur during the intermenstrual period. A "menotoxin" or other irritant derived from decomposed blood and endometrial debris has been postulated as the cause.

Gonorrheal infections are responsible for 65-75% of cases. The gonococcus spreads across the mucosal surface of the cervix and endometrium to the endosalpinx. Streptococcal salpingitis, especially that caused by anaerobic strains of enterococci, is still a common sequel of obstetric mishaps. Ascending bacterial infections, notably gonorrhea and postabortal or postpartal infections, almost always involve one or both fallopian tubes within 1-3 days after the initial infection. Childbirth and postabortal infections cause about 10% of cases. Infection caused by staphylococci or streptococci reaches the tubes by the lymphatic and vascular pathways in the parametrium and mesosalpinx.

Tuberculous infection now accounts for fewer than 5% of cases of salpingitis in the USA. It occurs via descending hematogenous spread from a pulmonary, intestinal, or urinary tract focus. Tuberculous salpingitis is usually not diagnosed until many months or years after recognition of the primary tuberculous lesion. Mixed infections with staphylococci, streptococci, pneumococci, Pseudomonas organisms, and others are often responsible for recurrences or treatment failures.

Factors which predispose to salpingitis include the following: Transvaginal instrumentation of the cervix and uterus (especially before and during menstruation), operative delivery, cervical contraceptive pessaries, peritonitis of bowel origin, degenerative cervical or uterine tumors, and hysterosalpingography performed with excess of oily medium.

Women in the childbearing age group are most commonly affected, though the condition is rare during pregnancy. Prepuberal girls and postmenopausal women may also develop salpingitis (usually tuberculous).

Chronic salpingitis (often inappropriately called pelvic inflammatory disease) is one of the principal causes of female infertility, menstrual disorders, and gynecologic disability.

Pathology.

The process of tubal inflammation may pass through various stages. Acute pyogenic infection may become chronic, and chronic pyogenic salpingitis may develop into chronic hydrosalpinx or tubo-ovarian abscess, either of which may result in fixed retroversion with bilateral tubo-ovarian masses. Specifically, the pathologic findings are as follows:

A. Acute Stage:
  1. Gonococcal - Both tubes are generally dependent, injected, and edematous. The tube contains a purulent exudate which may drain from the swollen, fimbriated extremity. Peritonitis frequently accompanies fulminant salpingitis, and fibrinous adhesions soon wall off the uterus, tubes, ovaries, and perhaps loops of bowel and omentum. Occlusion of the distal extremities of the tubes is the rule. Occasionally the tube and ovary are so closely involved that a tubo-ovarian abscess is created (Fig 22-1). Early microscopic examination of stained sections shows severe inflammation of the mucosa; deeper structures soon become involved. Plical swelling, turgescence of all layers, and gross exudation into the lumen of the tube are typical.

  In spite of the initial virulence of Neisseria gonorrhoeae, it is usually impossible to identify this organism in the fallopian tube after 1-2 weeks even when

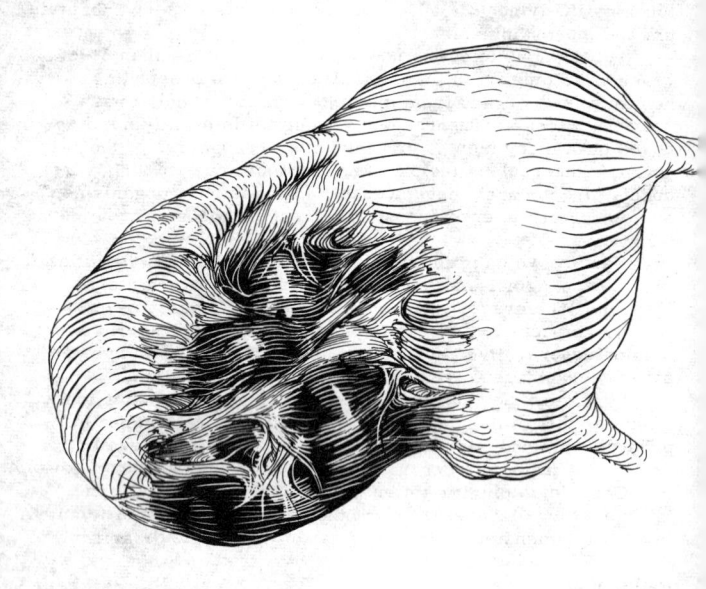

Fig 22-1. Tubo-ovarian abscess.

untreated gonorrheal infection of other tissues is obviously present. Secondary invaders, usually a mixed group of cocci, replace the gonococcus. Reinfection of the tubes by gonococcal organisms does not commonly occur.
2. Due to other pyogenic infections - One or both tubes will resemble those seen in acute gonococcal salpingitis, but the swelling and induration are usually more marked in postabortal or puerperal salpingitis. Parametritis often is present, but adherence of the tube to the ovary with resultant tubo-ovarian abscess is less likely to occur with staphylococcal or streptococcal infections. Microscopic examination shows infiltration of interstitial tissues with polymorphonuclear cells. The muscular layer of the tube is swollen and red, and cloudy swelling of the cells is prominent. Mucosal inflammation and exudation into the tubal lumen often are relatively slight.
3. Tuberculous - A sero-exudative reaction in the tube with the development of tubercles often occurs, especially in the deeper layers of the endosalpinx and the inner muscular layers.

B. Chronic Stage:
1. Gonococcal - The tubes become fluid-filled and "retort-shaped"; curved, bulbous, thickened in certain areas and thinned in others. Both ends are usually closed. The tubes are frequently adherent to the ovary, uterus, or other neighboring structures. Subdiaphragmatic or subhepatic adhesions, also involving the bowel and omentum, may indicate prior upper abdominal peritonitis due to salpingitis. As the infection resolves, the exudate in the tube is reabsorbed; however, up to 180 ml of thin, tawny, serous fluid may remain in the occluded tube (hydrosalpinx). Adhesions usually persist, although they may disappear completely for unknown reasons. If considerable distention of the tube occurs, the plicae become flattened and the microscopic pattern on cross-section is referred to as hydrosalpinx simplex. Agglutination of numerous rugous folds, with minimal distention of the tube by fluid, results in hydrosalpinx follicularis. Patchy loss of the endosalpingeal mucosa, scar tissue formation, and the persistence of lymphocytes and plasma cells in the mucosa of the tubes are to be expected. Repeated acute infections in the absence of pyosalpinx formation result in a firm tubal enlargement, the consequence of thickening of the wall of the tube (chronic interstitial salpingitis). Partial or complete closure of the bulbous ends of the tubes, with inversion and agglutination of the fimbriated processes, are notable findings. The tubes usually are tightly adherent to the ovary or the posterior aspect of the broad ligament. Reabsorption of a tubo-ovarian abscess leaves a tubo-ovarian cyst. With repeated episodes of salpingitis, the heavy infected tubes drag the uterus backward into the cul-de-sac where it becomes densely fixed in retroposition.
2. Due to other pyogenic infections - The tube may remain thickened, densely adherent, and inflamed for weeks or months after the initial infection. Microscopic findings consist of abscess formation, destruction of the integrity of the tube, and lymphocyte and plasma cell accumulations.
3. Tuberculous - The tubes are thickened, rigid, rather straight, and occasionally adherent. Small raised, pale, firm tubercles may be seen beneath the serosal surface. The fimbriated extremities may be everted, and seropurulent fluid may drop from the ostium. Caseation and multiple minute cold abscesses within the tube can be observed on stained sections. Granulomatous infiltration, necrosis, and tubercle formation are usually present. Giant cells may be difficult to find in certain areas.

Clinical Findings.

A. Symptoms and Signs: The symptoms and signs depend upon the infectious agent and the type, extent, and stage of infection.

In the acute phase, lower quadrant pain, the most common complaint, is unilateral or bilateral depending upon whether one or both tubes are involved. In acute salpingitis the pain is severe, aching, often cramp-like but not wholly remitting, and nonradiating. Pain is often described as dyspareunia or dysmenorrhea of the comenstrual and postmenstrual type. Severe sacral backache (referred pain) may be present.

In about 10% of cases of nontuberculous salpingitis, a piercing right upper quadrant pain with radiation toward the back occurs. The pain may localize below the right costal margin. It is the result of accumulation of purulent exudate below the diaphragm.

Shaking chills and a high, intermittent fever up to 104° F (40° C) are often present. Menstruation almost always exacerbates salpingitis because of the pelvic engorgement with which it is associated. Menstrual disturbances occur. Other findings include profuse, seropurulent leukorrhea; thin, purulent discharge from Skene's and Bartholin's ducts (in gonococcal infections); slight enlargement and tenderness of the uterus (in postabortal salpingitis); and marked bilateral adnexal tenderness without mass formation. Adynamic ileus is usually present in acute salpingitis.

The onset and course of tuberculous salpingitis are insidious; an explosive, dramatic onset is rare.

In the chronic phase of salpingitis, the character of the pain depends upon the extent of the disease. Symptoms and signs include purulent discharge from Skene's ducts, Bartholin's duct cysts, mucopurulent leukorrhea, menometrorrhagia or hypermenorrhea, a tender unilateral or bilateral pelvic mass, severe sacral backache (referred pain), abdominal tenderness and adnexal restriction without abdominal rigidity, dyspareunia, low-grade fever, and, occasionally, sudden passage of several ounces of thin clear or straw-colored fluid (hydrops tubae profluens). Hydrosalpinx may in rare instances discharge via the uterine cornu.

B. Laboratory Findings: Cervical and urethral smears, suitably fixed and stained, may reveal Neisseria gonorrhoeae. Cervical smears may reveal Clostridium welchii in certain instances of criminal abortion. Cervical and urethral cultures should be obtained if smears are not diagnostic of gonorrhea in suspect cases. Chocolate agar plates and tubes of nutrient broth containing just enough of the media to moisten the swab should be

Salpingitis 551

inoculated and incubated at 37°C under anaerobic conditions. In 36 hours they should be smeared, stained, and examined for N. gonorrhoeae. Cervical or uterine cultures inoculated on both blood agar and nutrient broth and maintained aerobically and anaerobically will usually aid in the identification of the pathogen and help to establish its sensitivity to antibiotics in postabortal and puerperal infections.

In acute salpingitis, the white count may be as high as 20-30 thousand/cu mm and a marked shift to the left is always present; the red cell count is normal. In tuberculous salpingitis the white and red counts are often within normal limits; increased numbers of monocytes and a relative lymphopenia may be described.

C. X-Ray Findings (in Tuberculous Salpingitis):
1. Hysterography often reveals evidence of tuberculosis. The uterus fills slowly with the contrast media; the corpus is trumpet-shaped, with a fuzzy or shaggy convex inner outline and the fundic and lateral shadows bulge.
2. Salpingography may not be possible because of occlusion of the tubes after suppurative salpingitis. In other cases, contrast media may fill the tubes to reveal tuberculous changes. A flat film before injection of radiopaque fluid may reveal calcific tubo-ovarian densities. The tubes fill, if at all, by slow, jerky progress of the media. Uneven, blurred beading, segmentation, or sacculation—even fistula formation—are revealed. These changes are more likely to be seen in the isthmic and ampullar portions of the tubes. The tubes are relatively straight, rigid, and drooping, often with diverticula near the fimbriated extremities. They are usually narrowly patent, and both are usually affected. Contrast filling of the blood and lymph vessels occurs occasionally.

D. Special Examinations (in Tuberculous Salpingitis):
1. Culture of menstrual discharge for Mycobacterium tuberculosis - Collect sanguineous fluid in a contraceptive diaphragm or in a test tube worn vaginally (or aspirate blood from the posterior vaginal fornix) on the first or second day of the period. Inoculate into Petragnani's or Sabouraud's medium; incubate at 37°C for 4 weeks. Smear, fix, and stain for acid-fast organisms. (Nonpathogenic acid-fast bacteria are smaller and more readily stained than Myco. tuberculosis.)
2. Guinea pig inoculation - Collect menstrual blood on the first or second day of flow, as above; inject 2-3 ml intraperitoneally into 2 guinea pigs; sacrifice the animals in 4-6 weeks and examine for evidence of tuberculosis.

3. The Mantoux intradermal test or the skin patch test - If strongly positive, suspect an active tuberculous focus, possibly tubal.
4. Endometrial biopsy may give evidence of endometrial tuberculosis.

Complications.

Salpingitis rarely remains confined to the tube; the peritoneum, ovary, and the distal intestinal and urinary tracts soon become involved.

Complications of gonococcal, streptococcal, or staphylococcal salpingitis include the following:

(1) Torsion of the swollen, deformed adnexa.

(2) Rupture of tubo-ovarian or other abscesses into a neighboring adherent viscus: The initial step in abscess formation may have been due to ovulation resulting in infection of a corpus luteum. Sometimes tubo-ovarian abscesses may drain spontaneously into the bladder or may point laterally above the pelvic brim, in which case incision and drainage may be feasible. Rupture into these areas may be considered fortunate, since rupture into the peritoneal cavity may have lethal consequences. Pyosalpinx or pelvic abscess may become localized in the posterior cul-de-sac. Unless surgical drainage is instituted through the vagina, spontaneous rupture into the rectum may occur.

(3) Diffuse generalized peritonitis which may extend beyond the pelvis to the upper abdomen (especially on the right side): This is far more devastating than the acute tubal disease itself. Gonococcal septicemia and endocarditis occur rarely. Metastatic gonococcal abscess formation, especially in the bones and joints, has been reported. Broad ligament cellulitis, pelvic thrombophlebitis, periphlebitis, lymphangitis, and pulmonary septic embolism are critical complications of streptococcal or staphylococcal salpingitis.

(4) Intestinal obstruction.

(5) Infertility: About 50% of patients with tuberculous salpingitis seek medical assistance with no other complaint than infertility. It is common even after mild, short-lived gonococcal, streptococcal, or staphylococcal salpingitis.

Differential Diagnosis.

A history of previous salpingitis is helpful in identification of the residuals of pelvic infection.

Salpingitis must be differentiated from appendicitis and ectopic pregnancy so that appropriate therapy can be given.

To differentiate between appendicitis and acute right-sided salpingitis, palpate the patient's abdomen while she lies in different positions. If the point of maximal tenderness, originally felt over the region of the right ovary and tube in the horizontal position, disappears or diminishes markedly while the patient is in the Trendelenburg position, appendicitis is the more likely diagnosis.

The tetrad of symptomatology—menstrual abnormality followed by uterine bleeding, pelvic pain, and pelvic mass—is indicative of ectopic pregnancy in the majority of women during the functional years.

Salpingitis isthmica nodosa is characterized by areas of nodular thickening of the isthmus of the fallopian tube. On section, glandular spaces are observed to be interspersed with an irregularly hypertrophied myosalpinx. Cells suggestive of chronic inflammation may be present. This disorder is bilateral in about one-third of cases, and less than one-half of cases are due to infection. Few cases are diagnosed preoperatively. The outstanding clinical problem is infertility due to tubal occlusion. Treatment consists of salpingectomy and wedge resection of the cornu.

Prevention.

Many cases of salpingitis can be prevented by early diagnosis and treatment of cervical and uterine neoplasms (which may become infected); by avoidance of obstetric and instrumental trauma; by discarding cervical and uterine contraceptive pessaries; and by hygienic and anti-infective measures to prevent and control infection.

Treatment.

A. Specific Measures:
  1. Gonococcal, streptococcal, and staphylococcal salpingitis - Penicillin is effective against gonococci, most strains of streptococci, and many types of staphylococci. An initial dose of 1.2 million units of penicillin G, I. M., followed by 600,000 units/day I. M. for 5-7 days, will cure most uncomplicated cases. Larger doses, often combined with other antibiotics or given intravenously at regular intervals (or both), may be required in virulent or persistent infections.

      Streptomycin, usually given with penicillin, broadens the chemotherapeutic attack, especially in mixed pyogenic infections. Give 1 gm I. M. followed by 0.5 gm I. M. 4 times daily.

      Chloramphenicol (Chloromycetin®) and the tetracyclines are also effective in the treatment of non-tuberculous salpingitis. Give 500 mg orally and then 250 mg every 6 hours for one week. The intravenous dosage is about half the oral dose.

      Sulfonamide therapy is less effective but may be warranted in penicillin-resistant infections. Sulfisoxazole (Gantrisin®), 2 gm orally followed by 1 gm orally every 4 hours for one week, is usually sufficient.

2. Tuberculous salpingitis - Streptomycin, 1 gm I. M. twice weekly; isoniazid, 150-300 mg orally daily; and aminosalicylic acid, 12-20 gm orally daily (depending upon tolerance) must be continued for at least 6 months.
B. General Measures: Complete bed rest in Fowler's position during the acute stage aids in localization of the infection. A hot water bottle or hot pad to the hypogastrium relieves lower abdominal pain. Pelvic pain can be relieved with heat applied deep in the pelvis by diathermy (or equivalent), especially when an abdominal and vaginal electrode is used, or with warm water or warm air circulation in the vagina using the Elliott or a similar apparatus or warm (gallon) vaginal douches. Aspirin, 0.3-0.6 gm (5-10 gr), and codeine, 30-60 mg ($1/2$-1 gr), orally every 4 hours as necessary, are usually sufficient to relieve pain, although morphine may be necessary at first in severe acute infections.
C. Surgical Measures:
1. Acute salpingitis - Abdominal surgery is contraindicated. If the peritoneum is opened in error, the tubal inflammatory process should not be disturbed and the abdomen should be closed immediately without drainage. Colpotomy or extraperitoneal drainage of large pelvic abscesses may be required.
2. Chronic salpingitis - Every effort must be made to treat the patient medically to conserve organs and function. Surgery is indicated, however, when conservative management fails, repeated exacerbations occur, and disability develops. Pelvic abscesses should be drained through the vagina or extraperitoneally. Large pelvic masses are less common with antibiotic and other methods of medical treatment.

In general, it is a good rule to be conservative. When this has failed, a vigorous, definitive surgical approach to the problem should be adopted. If tubo-ovarian masses are not present and the patient is young, simple bilateral cornual resection and preservation of both tubes and ovaries may be curative without sacrificing ovarian function. If both tubes and ovaries are extensively diseased despite prolonged medical therapy, bilateral salpingo-oophorectomy and hysterectomy, total if possible, are indicated even in a young woman. Assuming that the diseased tube can be removed by careful dissection, the ovary should not be removed if it appears to be reasonably normal. If a bilateral salpingectomy is required, the uterus and cervix should be removed. The vena cava and the infundibulopelvic vessels should be ligated after repeated pulmonary septic embolization.

Salpingostomy after acute salpingitis has seldom proved satisfactory, even with the most modern technics.

Prognosis.
The earlier and more adequate the treatment, the better the prognosis. While inflammation usually resolves rapidly, tubal obstruction occurs in many cases. Recurrent salpingitis with subsequent infertility usually occur if an abscess develops within or near the tube.

CARCINOMA OF THE FALLOPIAN TUBES

Primary cancer of the fallopian tube (characteristically unilateral) is almost always an adenocarcinoma. It is the least common malignancy of the müllerian system; only about 600 cases have been described in the literature. Metastatic carcinoma, usually from the endometrium or ovary, is more common.

Most cases occur in nulliparous postmenopausal women. Salpingitis is probably not an etiologic factor because of the disparity of incidence between tubal cancer and tubal infection.

Carcinoma of the fallopian tube usually occurs in the ampullary or fimbriated portion; the right tube is more frequently involved than the left. The tube in the area of carcinoma is rounded at first but later becomes fusiform or even sausage-shaped. The surface is glistening and red or purple; the tube is firm but not hard or nodular.

The tube contains yellow-brown grumous necrotic cancer tissue and dark-brown or straw-colored fluid of sanguineous origin. Minute hemorrhagic points are commonly present. The fimbriated extremity is usually closed. Perforation occurs when the malignancy extrudes or grows through the fimbriated end, and the tube, ovary, and uterus are ultimately bound together in an irregularly-shaped fixed mass.

Carcinoma of the fallopian tube may be (1) papillomatous, (2) adenomatous, or (3) medullary or solid. Microscopically it is characterized by anaplastic and pleomorphic cuboidal cells on a sparse framework of connective tissue. These cells remain within the lumen at first and then spread or penetrate through the wall. Metastases occur first through the lymphatics and then via the blood stream.

Clinical Findings.
  A. Symptoms and Signs: Unfortunately, growth and spread of carcinoma of the fallopian tube often are rapid, and manifestations do not usually occur until the malignancy is well established. Pain or bleeding is the most frequent complaint when symptoms do occur. Hemorrhage

into the tube, torsion, or pressure on the tubal mass may
cause symptoms varying from lower quadrant aching to
constant pain and sacral backache. Distention of the tube
with blood and invasion of the uterine cornu by the cancer (or other tubal disease) may result in sudden passage
of a thin serous or sanguineous fluid associated with relief of discomfort. Abdominal enlargement or intestinal
obstruction is usually a late manifestation. Ascites is
not often present.

On pelvic examination, a small, rounded or elongated,
slightly tender pelvic mass, at first separate from the
uterus and ovary and later indistinguishable from them,
may be felt. A primary tubal cancer rarely exceeds 10
cm in diameter. An adnexal mass in a postmenopausal
woman always suggests tubal (or ovarian) cancer.

When the tumor is primary and small, associated pelvic disease such as a large myoma may interfere with
palpation of the somewhat distended tube. Routine transection of the tubes should therefore be done in the course
of surgery for other pelvic masses.

B. Laboratory Findings: Vaginal smears have been reported
to be positive for malignant cells in a number of cases of
tubal carcinoma, but the site of origin cannot be identified in this way.

C. X-Ray Findings: Hysterosalpingography may be of value.

D. Special Examinations: Culdoscopy or culdotomy may be
diagnostically helpful. Dilatation and curettage will only
disclose tubal cancer which has extended to the endometrium.

Differential Diagnosis.

In the premenopausal woman, exclude the following in
differential diagnosis: Salpingitis, tubal pregnancy, ovarian
enlargement and carcinoma, endometrial disease, hydrosalpinx, and a soft pedunculated myoma. Tubal tuberculosis
often produces a highly adenomatous picture which can be
mistaken for tubal cancer, particularly the papillomatous type.

Treatment.

Total hysterectomy and bilateral salpingo-oophorectomy,
followed by x-ray therapy in the dosages usually given for the
treatment of ovarian cancer, are required for both primary
and secondary tubal carcinoma.

Prognosis.

Even with the best diagnosis and treatment, the five-year
survival rate is less than 15%.

23...
Diseases of the Ovaries

FIBROMAS AND SARCOMAS OF THE OVARY

Fibromas of the ovary are unilateral, firm, nonfunctional benign tumors of mesenchymal origin composed principally of fibrous connective tissue. They usually occur in postmenopausal women and represent about 5% of ovarian tumors.

Most fibromas are small; a few will weigh as much as 5 pounds. In appearance they are smooth, round, and lobulated. Their weight may cause pedunculation of the gonad, leading to torsion and degeneration. Fibromas are poorly encapsulated and rarely adherent. Sectioning discloses dense grayish or white tissue. Gritty inclusions sometimes are found. Zones of degeneration with gelatinous or small cystic spaces often are seen within the soft portions. Microscopic examination shows a monotonous pattern of elongated fibrocytes which appear as trabeculations within a parenchyma of variable density.

Adenofibroma, a variation of fibroma, appears rough, fissured, and coarsely lobulated, and is covered by a single layer or pseudostratum of darkly-staining cuboid cells. Strands and clumps of cells suggestive of smooth muscle are occasionally interspersed between the fibrocytes.

Fibromyomas differ from fibromas only microscopically in the inclusion of smooth muscle.

Sarcoma of the ovary, one of the rarest of gonadal tumors, also develops in fibromas. These cancers are usually of the spindle cell type, although chondrosarcomas, osteosarcomas, and myxosarcomas also have been reported. Many ovarian sarcomas are probably of teratogenous origin.

Fibromatous tumors are associated with **Meigs's (Demons-Meigs) syndrome**, characterized by a solid benign tumor of the ovary, with transudative hydrothorax and ascites. Cure follows removal of the tumor.

These tumors are predominantly of connective tissue origin or content (fibroma, thecoma, granulosa cell tumor, Brenner tumor). However, all ovarian growths can produce ascites and hydrothorax. Ascites accompanies approximately 20% of fibromas, but Meigs's syndrome is far less common (about 100 authentic cases reported). Ascites (with or without hydrothorax) can occur in the absence of a pelvic mass with cardiac, renal, and hepatic disorders. Carcinoma, particularly of the tail of the pancreas, also may cause ascites.

The abdomen enlarges and the patient complains of orthopnea, tachycardia, and a feeling of oppression in the chest. Torsion often occurs, causing agonizing pain in the affected lower quadrant and nausea and vomiting. Larger tumors cause a sense of pelvic heaviness. The tumor is usually palpable on pelvic examination.

Shifting dullness of the abdomen and hydrothorax are apparent upon palpation and percussion. The tumor may not be palpable until after abdominal paracentesis.

Peritoneal and thoracic fluid in Meigs's syndrome is a clear, pale yellow transudate. Epithelial cells are few, and leukocytes are rare. Chest x-ray may demonstrate fluid in one or both thoracic cavities. Pneumoperitoneum after paracentesis may clearly delineate the fibroma.

Meigs's syndrome should be considered in every woman over 40 years of age in whom a relapsing unexplained pleural or peritoneal transudate is discovered. Meigs's syndrome must be distinguished from primary pulmonary, cardiac, and abdominal disease causing hydrothorax and ascites.

The fibroma must be differentiated from granulosa and theca cell tumors.

An exploratory laparotomy is advised. Upon removal of the fibroma, abdominal and chest fluid will usually disappear spontaneously within a week.

Recovery is to be anticipated following the removal of a fibromatous ovarian tumor. If sarcomatous change has occurred, the prognosis is grave.

CYSTADENOMA & CYSTADENOCARCINOMA
(Pseudomucinous & Serous Cystadenomas)

Cystadenomas are the most common of ovarian neoplasms, representing 70% of all ovarian tumors. These tumors produce no hormone and are most common in women between the ages of 45 and 65. The relative frequency of serous to pseudomucinous cystadenoma is about 1:1.

Pseudomucinous cystadenoma grows more sluggishly and becomes larger than the serous type; some have been reported to weigh over 45.5 kg (100 lb). These tumors may be derived from the ovarian surface epithelium, or they may be of teratogenous origin. They are usually multilocular; contain a thick, viscid, brownish liquid; are lined by tall columnar epithelial and goblet cells; and are sheathed by a tough membranous capsule. About 5% are found to be malignant at surgery.

Serous cystadenomas do not become as large as pseudomucinous cystadenomas; most weigh 4.5-9 kg (10-20 lb).

Originally, they are unilocular, filled with a thin yellowish fluid, are lined by cuboidal or short columnar cells, and then tend to develop multilocular spaces and papillary excrescences on both their inner and outer surfaces. Serous cystadenomas, like the pseudomucinous type, are also contained in a parchment-like capsule. Small sand-like, sharp, calcareous concretions (psammoma bodies) are often present within the tumor. Serous cystadenomas are believed to arise from invagination of the germinal epithelium of the surface of the ovary.

A great variety and complexity of these tumors is possible. Some contain only a few folds or broad-based papillary processes. These may be fibrotic, partially hyalinized, and covered by a single layer of cells which are quite innocent in appearance. At the other extreme is an almost solid carcinoma with pleomorphism and only a few remaining identifiable glandular areas.

Malignant change in cystadenoma is characterized by the following: (1) Excessive proliferation and extensive stratification of cells. (2) Intricate pattern with increased glandular elements. (3) Sparse stroma in proportion to epithelial cells. (4) Anaplasia: immature cells, variation in size and shape of cells and nuclei, numerous nucleoli, many undifferentiated cells, and numerous mitotic figures. (5) Invasion of the stroma or the capsule by glandular elements with intralocular cyst formation.

Cystadenomas are silent tumors because they do not produce hormones. Symptoms are produced only when the tumor becomes large enough to cause increased abdominal girth and weight gain, pelvic heaviness, constipation, and urinary frequency.

Abdominal examination generally discloses an insensitive, rounded pelvic-abdominal mass which may fill the entire true pelvis. The upper margin should then be measured in centimeters above or below the umbilicus. A fluid wave should be sought. Hydrothorax may also be noted. This cannot be classed as Meigs's syndrome because malignant cells are often found in the tumor and in the abdominal fluid.

Laboratory findings are not diagnostic. The sedimentation rate may be elevated, and eosinophilia may be present.

Abdominal x-rays reveal a rounded area of increased density. Psammoma bodies (small calcific conglomerates) within the acini of the tumor can occasionally be seen.

While pseudomucinous cystadenomas may develop a well defined pedicle, the serous type does not usually do so. Unless perforation, infection, or rupture ensues, the tough membranous capsule is rarely adherent.

Complications may occur as a result of malignant change. These are due to extension or rupture. Intestinal obstruction may develop.

The differential diagnosis must include dermoid cyst,

semi-solid tumor (especially dysgerminoma), secondary involvement by malignancy from the gastrointestinal tract or breast, and thyroid and retroperitoneal tumors.

Yearly pelvic examination of all women will reduce the incidence of this tragic disorder. All ovarian cysts over 7 cm in diameter and which persist for over 90 days should be removed.

Unless the tumor ruptures or torsion occurs, emergency measures are not necessary. In any case, surgery is required. It should be preceded by preoperative bowel preparation. Preoperative x-ray examination should include chest x-ray and intravenous urography to determine kidney function and the course and patency of the ureters.

A large incision must be made and peritoneal fluid aspirated before the pelvis and abdomen are palpated. The fluid is then sent to the laboratory for the preparation of a sediment "button" and a pathology report of the presence or absence of malignant cells. Trocar aspirations of the cyst should be avoided unless the tumor is too huge to remove through the incision because spill is undesirable.

If the tumor is benign, oophorocystectomy should be performed. The tumor must be considered malignant if any of the following are present: gross papillar formation or a solid mass within the tumor, or moderate papillar formation outside the tumor. Total hysterectomy and bilateral salpingo-oophorectomy is then indicated. It may be necessary to resect the bowel or do a colostomy if resectable tumor involves the gastrointestinal tract. Even if the case is considered inoperable, one should remove everything carcinomatous if feasible. Radiation or intraperitoneal injection of chlorambucil (Leukeran®) or similar nitrogen mustard drug may be elected if peritoneal or visceral metastases are found.

Approximately 50% of serous cystadenomas will become clinically malignant and will at least involve the opposite ovary. Only about 5% of pseudomucinous cystadenomas become definitely cancerous with involvement of the opposite gonad and other structures.

Barely 25% of patients with cystadenocarcinoma can be operated upon with the expectancy of cure. Three-fourths of women with this tumor are found to have a far-advanced, incurable cystadenocarcinoma, generally of the serous variety.

VIRILIZING LIPOID CELL TUMORS OF THE OVARY

Under this category are included a number of rare unilateral, yellowish, glassy, semisolid, relatively small neoplasms which usually cause masculinization and occur most commonly in women over 50 years of age. This category includes luteomas, luteinomas, luteoblastomas, functional hypernephroid tumors, gynandroblastomas, masculinovoblastomas, corticoadrenal tumors, hormonally active adrenal carcinomas, and virilizing hilus cell tumors of the ovary.

There are at least 3 possible theories of origin. These tumors may arise (1) as adrenal rest tumors of the ovary; (2) as abnormally luteinized, atypical granulosa cell tumors or arrhenoblastomas; or (3) as pseudo—Leydig cell tumors, perhaps of hilus cell origin.

These poorly encapsulated tumors are rarely adherent unless they are malignant. Areas of degeneration and internal hemorrhage are common. Clusters and sheets of at least 2 cell types are seen microscopically: (1) moderately large polyhedral cells with small basophilic nuclei and a generous eosinophilic cytoplasm containing lipoid inclusions, similar to cells in the reticular zone of the adrenal cortex; and (2) large, rounded cells with moderately deeply-staining basophilic nuclei containing prominent nucleoli and a clear cytoplasm. (This latter type is reminiscent of Leydig cells of the testis.) A light supporting framework of connective tissue is usually present.

Virilization occurs and amenorrhea or oligomenorrhea is present. Hirsutism with a masculine hair distribution and balding, odorous perspiration, acne, and clitoral hypertrophy are notable. The patient is often obese. Hypertension, polycythemia, and diabetes mellitus have occasionally been described. Many of these tumors are small and nonpalpable, so that an adnexal enlargement may not be recorded.

17-Hydroxycorticosteroid or 17-ketosteroid excretion is elevated. A high pregnanetriol level may be reported.

About 20% are malignant. Distant metastasis is a late complication.

These tumors must be differentiated from other ovarian tumors (especially arrhenoblastoma), primary adrenal cortical tumors, and adrenal cortical hyperplasia.

Removal of the adnexa on the affected side is necessary. If the site of origin is the adrenal gland or a mesoblastic tumor which has metastasized to the ovary, more radical surgery will be required. Palliation by x-ray therapy has been disappointing because many of these tumors are radio-resistant.

Refeminization occurs after the complete excision of a virilizing lipoid cell tumor. Lowered voice quality and bristly hair are not reversible.

MESONEPHROMA

Mesonephromas are a small group of nonfunctional ovarian tumors, clinically indistinguishable from papillary serous cystadenoma. They occur before puberty, but are

562 Arrhenoblastoma

usually discovered after age 35. They are probably of teratogenous origin. About 200 cases have been described, but many are unreported. They are important because malignant change occurs in about 30%.

The tumor is grayish brown, smooth, free, semi-soft or cystic, and fairly well encapsulated. It is occasionally adherent. Friable tissue and thin serous fluid fill the locules and tissue spaces and there are areas of cystic degeneration and even hemorrhagic extravasation. Most tumors are 10-20 cm in diameter when first discovered.

Microscopically, loose connective tissue supports a gross acinar or papillary pattern of cuboidal cells having clear cytoplasm and small, dark, elongated nuclei. Many of these cells are widely spaced, bulge outward, are "hobnail" or peg-like in appearance, and have their nuclei parallel to the lumen. Tuft-like invaginations occasionally protrude into smaller cysts. These produce a glomerulus-like configuration, but no central tuft of vessels is present. Some tubules or cystic spaces contain acidophilic granular material. Solid nests or clumps of cells with distinct outlines containing pleomorphic nuclei and almost water-clear cytoplasm can often be found in mesonephromas.

The symptomatology is identical to that of papillary serous cystadenoma (see p. 558). When malignant, both ovaries and the neighboring structures will be involved and moderate ascites will occur.

Mesonephromas must be distinguished from the cystadenomas and cystadenocarcinomas, clear-cell kidney carcinomas metastatic to the ovary, and undifferentiated carcinomas of uncertain type. Periodic acid—Shiff reagents stain mesonephroma clear cells and pseudomucinous cystadenoma tissue red. This contrasts with a negative reaction in serous cystadenoma.

Excision of the adnexa is required. If malignant change or spread is noted, bilateral salpingo-oophorectomy and panhysterectomy are indicated. Roentgen therapy is only palliative because these tumors are only slightly radiosensitive.

The prognosis is good if the tumor is benign. Many mesonephromas are histologically benign and clinically malignant, however; when malignant, the outlook is unfavorable.

ARRHENOBLASTOMA

Arrhenoblastoma is a rare ovarian tumor (fewer than 175 cases have been reported) which occurs most frequently during the reproductive years and is assumed to arise from sexually ambivalent cells noted in the ovary of the 6-7 week embryo or to be of teratoid origin. The tumor is unilateral (more often on the right side), and may be minute or may fill the entire pelvis. Twenty-five per cent become malignant, but metastases are usually late.

Grossly, most arrhenoblastomas are grayish to yellow-brown, firm, and poorly encapsulated. They may become soft because of internal hemorrhage, degeneration, and cyst formation secondary to necrosis.

Microscopically, tubules or columns of cells and, frequently, interstitial type cells are seen in a heavy, often partially hyalinized connective tissue stroma. The architecture of the majority of these tumors suggests the structure of the immature testis. The degree of functional activity of an arrhenoblastoma usually depends upon the presence of numerous actively secreting interstitial cells and not upon its degree of maturity or whether it is histologically benign or malignant. In general, no definite conclusion about malignant potential can be drawn from the histologic appearance of the tumor. Metastatic foci are often less well differentiated than the original tumor, and their ability to produce hormone may be lost.

Arrhenoblastomas are usually hormonally active, producing androgenic substances which cause both defeminization and virilization, manifested by varying degrees of amenorrhea, acne, hirsutism, recession of the hair-line at the forehead, slight alopecia, loss of feminine contours, breast and genital atrophy (but clitoral hypertrophy), and deepening of the voice. Arrhenoblastomas of the nonfunctional type cause the signs and symptoms of a solid ovarian neoplasm. Androgen hormone secreted by a masculinizing neoplasm probably does not exert an effective inhibitory action on the anterior pituitary because the follicle-stimulating hormone (FSH) is not appreciably depressed. Hence, involution of the contralateral ovary is unlikely.

Blood tests may reveal polycythemia. Thyroid function tests may be low. Urinary 17-ketosteroids are slightly or moderately increased; etiocholanolone may represent 75% of the 17-ketosteroid fraction. The dehydroepiandrosterone level is strikingly high. The estrogen, hydroxysteroid, and FSH levels are normal or minimally reduced.

Arrhenoblastoma must be distinguished from adrenocortical disorders, a much more frequent cause of masculinization, which usually cause less virilization and a much more pronounced elevation of the urinary 17-ketosteroids.

Early investigation of defeminization may reveal an early masculinizing disorder of the ovary or adrenal gland which can be removed before malignant spread or virilization occurs.

Superfluous hair should be removed and acne treated. Arrhenoblastoma should be removed surgically together with other pelvic reproductive organs unless the patient desires children and the tumor is clinically and histologically benign, in which case unilateral oophorectomy and salpingectomy generally are sufficient. Hormonal evaluation should be repeated after several months to determine recurrence.

Irradiation therapy of malignant residue or recurrence is discouraging, although an occasional arrhenoblastoma is radiosensitive.

Estrogen therapy does not reverse androgenic hormone effects.

After the removal of an arrhenoblastoma, feminization recurs within several months in the otherwise normal premenopausal woman who has adequate function in the remaining ovary. Masculinization is slow to regress; coarse hair, deep voice, and clitoral hypertrophy may persist unchanged or in considerable degree.

Many arrhenoblastomas eventually undergo malignant change. Pregnancy may be permitted after 8 months if a recurrence of the neoplasm is not observed.

SECONDARY OVARIAN NEOPLASMS

In 10% of cases of fatal malignant disease in women, the ovary is found to be secondarily involved by metastasis or extension of malignancy, usually from the uterus or the ovary (although one-third represent metastasis from stomach cancer). The gastrointestinal tract, breast, thyroid, kidney, or adrenals may also be the primary foci.

The **Krukenberg tumor** is the most interesting carcinoma metastatic to the ovaries. It usually originates in the stomach, intestine, or gallbladder or, on very rare occasions, in the breast and thyroid. Grossly, it is large, buff-colored, firm, solid, moderately large, lobulated, often kidney-shaped, nonadherent, and bilateral. A heavy but easily stripped capsule covers the parenchyma which is composed of firm and softer, often minutely cystic, tissue.

Two microscopic features are diagnostic: (1) coarse, abundant, occasionally edematous stroma, and (2) islands of moderately large epithelial cells with mucin-laden or vacuolated cytoplasm and eccentrically placed, hyperchromatic nuclei. Such cells resemble signet rings. If the tumor does not display these classic details, it is not termed a Krukenberg tumor but simply a secondary ovarian cancer.

Other cancers metastatic to the ovary usually are similar in morphology, but not in function, to their primary tumor.

There are no specific signs or symptoms. These neoplasms are generally insidious until the process is extensive. Most secondary ovarian cancers do not produce hormones. The Krukenberg tumor is often outlined first in the abdomen by external or pelvic examination. Amenorrhea, dyspepsia, postprandial epigastric discomfort, slight weight loss, and mild anemia may then be noted. Ascites is rarely present.

Gastric washings occasionally recover cancer cells. Achlorhydria and a positive guaiac test may be recorded. The x-ray appearance of the lesion in the stomach is not striking considering the size of the ovarian tumors.

The importance of these secondary ovarian cancers is that they must be distinguished from primary ovarian tumors. Secondary involvement of the contralateral ovary is common in primary ovarian cancer. Only an occasional colon cancer involves both ovaries. A similar prospect is likely for most cervical, breast, or urinary tract carcinomas, and for melanosarcomas.

Palliation is all that can be offered. Radiation therapy and radical gynecologic or other definitive surgery are futile because the cancer is widely disseminated by the time it reaches the ovary.

Certain tumors, such as carcinoma of the thyroid, may grow slowly, so that individual, more distant metastases may be excised with some hope for limited prolongation of life and health. However, cancers which are primary in the gastrointestinal tract are widely dispersed and beyond more than palliative treatment by the time the ovary is involved.

OVARIAN CYSTS

A cyst is a sac which contains fluid or semi-solid material. Ovarian cysts may develop at any time but are most common from puberty to the menopause. Most are small and clinically unimportant, and only a few require removal. Ovarian cysts range in size from microscopic to a large pelvic mass, and may cause difficulty by enlargement, pulsion, traction, torsion, or rupture.

Most cystic enlargements disappear within a few months. Cysts which do not disappear in that time are often inflammatory or endometrial or may have malignant potentialities.

The following factors must be considered in any ovarian enlargement: size, persistence, bilaterality, adherence, hormone production, surface nodulation, papillar formations or neighboring irregularities, and ascites. Surgery is generally required if a tense ovarian enlargement progresses to more than 6 cm in diameter within 4 months.

Abdominal pain, bleeding, or a palpable pelvic mass may require exploratory laparotomy. Treatment is based upon an estimate of whether the growth is benign or malignant, the consequences of their development, and the risk of their removal or destruction.

Classification of Ovarian Cysts.
(1) Functional cysts (follicle, granulosa lutein, theca lutein).
(2) Inflammatory cysts (tubo-ovarian).
(3) Endometrial cysts (endometriomas).
(4) Inclusion cysts.

Functional Cysts.

Follicle and corpus luteum cysts are normal transient physiologic structures.

A. Follicle (Retention) Cysts: Follicle cysts are common, frequently bilateral and multiple cysts which appear at the surface of the ovaries as pale blebs filled with a clear fluid. They vary in size from microscopic to 4 cm in diameter (rarely larger). These cysts represent the failure of an incompletely developed follicle to reabsorb. They are commonly found in prolapsed adherent ovaries or when a thickened, previously inflamed ovarian capsule prevents extrusion of the ovum. Symptoms are usually not present unless torsion or rupture with hemorrhage occurs, in which case the symptoms and signs of an acute abdomen are often present. Large or numerous cysts may cause aching pelvic pain, dyspareunia, and occasionally abnormal uterine bleeding. The ovary may be slightly enlarged and tender to palpation, and the vaginal smear will often show a high estrogen level and a lack of progesterone stimulation.

Salpingitis, endometriosis, lutein cysts, and neoplastic cysts must be considered in the differential diagnosis.

Most follicle cysts disappear spontaneously within 60 days without any treatment; when symptoms are disturbing, warm douches, pelvic diathermy, and reestablishment of ovulation may be helpful. Ovulation may be simulated following 5 days of therapy with a single injection of progesterone in oil, 5 mg I.M.; or hydroxyprogesterone caproate (Delalutin®), 1.25-2.5 mg I.M. Ovulation may be induced with clomiphene citrate (Clomid®), 50 mg orally daily for 5 days.

Pain as the result of a prolapsed adherent ovary may require laparotomy. Ovariectomy is justified in disabling and chronic or recurring salpingitis. Malignant change does not occur.

Any cyst which becomes larger than 5 cm in diameter or which persists longer than 60 days probably is not a follicle cyst.

B. Lutein Cysts: Two types are recognized: (1) granulosa lutein cysts, found within a corpus luteum; and (2) theca lutein cysts, associated with a proliferative hydatidiform mole, chorio-epithelioma, or chorionic gonadotropin therapy.

1. Granulosa lutein cysts - Corpus luteum cysts are functional, nonneoplastic enlargements of the ovary caused by the unexplained increase in secretion of fluid by the corpus luteum which occurs after ovulation or during early pregnancy. They are 4-6 cm in diameter, raised, and brown; and are filled with brown serous

fluid. A contracted blood clot is often found within the cavity.

Corpus luteum cysts may cause local pain and tenderness, and either amenorrhea or delayed menstruation followed by brisk bleeding after resolution of the cyst. They are usually readily palpable. Corpus luteum cyst may encourage torsion of the ovary, causing severe pain; or it may rupture and bleed, in which case laparotomy is usually required to control hemorrhage into the peritoneal cavity. Unless these acute complications develop, symptomatic therapy is all that is required. The cyst will disappear within 2 months in nonpregnant women, and will gradually become smaller during the last trimester in pregnant women.

It is necessary to distinguish between a cystic corpus luteum and a corpus luteum cyst. The former is much smaller and is a normal variation of no clinical importance.

2. Theca lutein cysts - Theca lutein cysts range in size from minute to 4 cm in diameter. They are usually bilateral, are filled with clear straw-colored and occasionally bloody serous fluid, and are found only in association with hydatidiform mole, chorio-epithelioma, or gonadotropin therapy.

Abdominal symptoms are often minimal. A sense of pelvic weight or ache is described at times. Rupture of the cyst may result in intraperitoneal bleeding. Continued signs and symptoms of pregnancy, especially hyperemesis and breast paresthesias, are also described.

Laboratory studies disclose startlingly high titers of chorionic gonadotropin. Curettage should be done if there is any question of ectopic pregnancy, retained products of conception, a proliferative mole, or chorio-epithelioma. The remote possibility of bilateral papillary cystadenoma should be considered in the differential diagnosis.

Ovarian surgery is not required inasmuch as the cysts disappear spontaneously following elimination of the molar pregnancy, destruction of the chorio-epithelioma, or discontinuation of chorionic gonadotropin.

Inflammatory Cysts (Tubo-Ovarian Cysts).

Distortion and adherence of the tube and ovary as the result of salpingitis following acute gonorrhea, an infected abortion, or appendicitis cause an inflammatory adnexal mass up to 15 cm in diameter with cyst formation.

Severe and persistent pelvic pain is typical. Metrorrhagia or hypermenorrhea occurs concomitantly. If the pain

568 Ovarian Cysts

is unilateral, acute appendicitis, intrapelvic bleeding, and endometriosis must be ruled out.

The white blood count and sedimentation rate are markedly elevated. Pregnancy tests will be negative.

Antibiotics, analgesics, and local heat will give relief. Surgery is not indicated if appendicitis and ectopic pregnancy can be ruled out unless symptoms do not subside in 2-3 weeks, in which case salpingo-oophorectomy is performed.

Endometrial Cysts (Endometrioma).

Functional ectopic endometrium which implants on the ovary* retains its ability to bleed periodically with the proper hormonal stimulus. Alternate oozing and healing with each period results in cyst formation.

These cysts vary from microscopic in size ("powder burns") up to 10-12 cm in diameter. Dense adhesions to neighboring viscera are common.

The interior of the cyst is filled with thick, chocolate-colored old blood. The cyst wall is found to contain active endometrial glands. Local bleeding occurs from the stroma at the time of the period. Hemosiderin, pseudoxanthoma cells, and chronic inflammatory elements with fibrosis are recognized.

Symptomatology includes infertility, hypermenorrhea, dyspareunia, and secondary or acquired dysmenorrhea. The dysmenorrhea is generally premenstrual or occurs during menstruation, and is of an aching, crescendo, or curious "grinding" type, with referral of the pain toward the sacrum and rectum.

Laboratory tests are not diagnostic.

Not all "chocolate-like cysts" are endometrial in origin. Bleeding into any cystic cavity will later yield decomposed blood. The wall of a corpus luteum will show a yellowish lining zone. Papillary processes or thickened areas of actual neoplasia will be seen in cystadenomas.

See p. 544 for treatment of endometriosis.

The treatment of large ovarian endometriomas is surgical resection of the cyst to leave as much functioning ovarian tissue as possible. Smaller points of endometriosis can be destroyed by the electrocautery.

Inclusion Cysts.

These are small cysts (generally of microscopic proportions) seen just beneath the surface of the ovary in post-inflammatory states or after the menopause. A minute amount of serous fluid fills the single locule.

The germinal epithelium becomes turned-in or buried in one small area, perhaps within a fissure.

No discomfort or disability results from these cysts,

---

*See Endometriosis, p. 541.

which are usually found by the pathologist. It is postulated that cystadenomas may originate from inclusion cysts because of unknown growth stimuli.

No treatment is required for inclusion cysts. Cystadenomas are easily recognized and should be resected.

HYPERNEPHROMA
(Hypernephroid Ovarian Tumor)

Hypernephroma of the ovary is a rare rounded, grayish, fairly well-encapsulated, semi-solid, aggressive adenocarcinoma probably mesonephric in origin. The tumor is occasionally virilizing. It is usually discovered in postmenopausal women who have progressive painless abdominal enlargement and a unilateral ovarian tumor.

Hypernephromas are composed of moderately large, round or cuboid cells with a clear, often vacuolated cytoplasm and small hyperchromatic nuclei. The epithelial cells are supported by a light stromal framework. Hypernephromas are not highly vascularized. Secondary cystic or hemorrhagic areas may develop in the parenchyma. This neoplasm resembles the so-called clear-cell carcinoma of the kidney (Grawitz tumor). Nevertheless, a confusing variation of pattern is common. At times the tumor suggests solid serous cystadenocarcinoma, adrenal cortical neoplasm, and mesonephroma.

Treatment is similar to that employed for ovarian cystadenocarcinoma (see p. 558). The prognosis depends largely upon the stage of the tumor.

THECA CELL TUMOR
(Thecoma)

Theca cell tumors are uncommon functional, feminizing ovarian neoplasms derived from ovarian stromal anlagen. They occur most frequently in young girls and postmenopausal women, and vary in size from minute nodules to masses 30 cm in diameter. The tumor is almost invariably unilateral.

Granulosa cells and theca cells are almost always found together. The ratio of incidence of theca cell to granulosa cell tumors is often 1:8. A few thecal elements will be found even in well differentiated granulosa cell tumor. The tumor is designated as a "granulosa-theca cell" or a "theca-granulosa cell" depending upon which cell variety is predominant.

These tumors are rounded, smooth, yellowish, and rarely adherent. A definite capsule is lacking. On section the tumor is densely fibrous with much stromal connective tissue; vascularization is often deficient. It is firm unless liquified by hyalinization or other degenerative change. A pattern of whorls may resemble a fibroma, especially in older thecomas, but fat stains reveal intracellular lipids in thecomas.

Stained sections of the tumor will show connective tissue elements with interspersed islands and strands of theca cells. Silver stains will reveal reticular fibrils. Sudan-type stains reveal the presence of lipids. Lipid material intracellularly, which is doubly refractile with polarization, indicates luteinization; extracellularly, it indicates degeneration. In a poorly preserved tumor, hyalin frequently replaces both theca and granulosa cells; and fibroblastic elements, which may also display collagenous degeneration, become prominent. Numerous luteinized theca and granulosa cells indicate that the tumor has recently produced considerable steroid sex hormone. Distinctly pleomorphic nuclei with numerous mitoses showing a tendency to invade cell groups are indicative of malignant changes.

There are 3 theca cell types in thecomas: (1) Slender spindle-shaped cells with elongated nuclei and a scant cytoplasm containing fat droplets similar to theca interna cells of the mature and regressive graafian follicle. (2) Ovoid or plump cells with rounded or oval nuclei and an abundant lipid-laden cytoplasm resembling theca interna cells immediately prior to rupture of the graafian follicle. (3) Polyhedral cells (theca lutein cells) having heavy fibrillary projections with an affinity for silver stains. They have moderately large nuclei and ample cytoplasms full of lipoid substance and are similar to enlarging theca interna cells after rupture of the graafian follicle.

Clinical and laboratory findings are identical with those of granulosa cell tumors. As is true of granulosa cell tumors also, theca cell tumor may virilize rather than feminize in rare instances.

As the cause of abnormal uterine bleeding, theca cell tumors must be differentiated from idiopathic precocious puberty, granulosa cell tumors, and uterine neoplasms. Meigs's syndrome (ascites and hydrothorax) may result, just as with ovarian fibroma. Partially degenerated theca-granulosa cell tumors are often mistaken for fibromas of the ovary. A sure diagnosis may require numerous sections and special stains.

Unilateral oophorectomy will usually cure a patient with a benign theca cell tumor. Malignant tumors require total hysterectomy and bilateral salpingo-oophorectomy.

Experience with x-ray therapy for treatment of the very rare malignancies of the theca cell type is inadequate for evaluation.

Because of the low incidence of malignancy (1%) in theca cell tumors, the prognosis is excellent after surgery.

DYSGERMINOMA
(Ovarian Seminoma)

Dysgerminoma is a nonfunctioning, potentially malignant ovarian tumor. (About 4% of all primary malignant ovarian tumors are dysgerminomas, and approximately one-third of dysgerminomas are cancerous.) Dysgerminoma is bilateral in one-third of cases, and is most common in females 10-30 years of age. It is thought to be of teratogenous origin. Although usually small when found (4-7 cm in diameter), dysgerminomas may grow rapidly to fill the entire pelvis. The tumor is often discovered in patients with underdeveloped secondary sex characteristics, e.g., female pseudohermaphrodites. (The same tumor found in a male is called a seminoma.) It is grayish-brown, smooth, rounded, thinly encapsulated, non-adherent, semi-solid, and "rubbery." On section the surface is edematous in appearance and soft, almost brain-like, in consistency. There are no septa—only a tenuous connective tissue framework.

Microscopically, 2 cell types are always seen: (1) Unusually large, rounded cells with vesicular, coarsely granular cytoplasm, and (2) many scattered small lymphocytes. The elements are loosely arranged with no typical pattern. The lymphocytes invariably infiltrate the tumor. Hemorrhagic extravasation and cystic degeneration are common. Anaplasia and pleomorphism may be noted, but grading is impossible.

Symptoms are usually due to abdominal enlargement caused by rapid tumor growth and ascites. Acute pain may result if the thin capsule ruptures. Weakly false-positive pregnancy tests have been reported in some cases. Malignancy must be suspected when a neoplasm grows rapidly, is firmly adherent or bilateral, or is accompanied by ascites.

Other nonfunctioning ovarian tumors (e.g., teratoma, cystadenoma) must be considered in the differential diagnosis.

Ovariectomy is required. If malignancy is suspected, both ovaries, the uterus, and the tubes should be removed. If the tumor is small and unilateral, and if the patient desires to maintain reproductive function, oophorocystectomy may be feasible.

Although dysgerminomas are quite radiosensitive, only temporary remission follows irradiation therapy. Nitrogen mustards may be used to control recurrent cases.

Prognosis is generally guarded because it is usually impossible to distinguish the benign from the malignant form by microscopic study. It is particularly serious in young patients, and very poor when extension or metastasis occurs.

Underdevelopment of secondary sex characteristics is not affected by removal of the tumor.

BRENNER TUMOR OF THE OVARY

This is a yellowish-brown, solid, nonadherent, fibroepitheliomatous mesenchymal neoplasm which usually affects postmenopausal women. Brenner tumors are almost always unilateral and very rarely secrete a hormone. Brenner tumors represent about 1% of primary ovarian tumors, approximately 400 having been studied and described in the medical literature. They are believed to arise from Walthard cell rests, but are occasionally found in the wall of a pseudomucinous cystadenoma. Malignant change is very rare.

This nonencapsulated tumor is composed of epithelial-like cells surrounded by trabeculations of very dense connective tissue. The epithelioid cells have a clear cytoplasm and accept a pale basophilic stain. They are similar to transitional cells of the urinary tract. The dark nuclei have a longitudinal groove which makes them resemble coffee beans. The epithelioid cells and the fluid within the tissue spaces stain positively for mucopolysaccharides in the same way as pseudomucinous cystadenoma cells. The basophilic connective tissue is unusually dense. Occasional areas of eosinophilic hyalinization are seen. Small degenerative cysts develop, but large, necrotic, or hemorrhagic zones are rarely observed. Degeneration destroys the epithelioid cells in the occasional Brenner tumor. Such a neoplasm might be described as a "fibroma with holes."

Unilateral pelvic discomfort and a sense of fullness and heaviness in the lower abdomen are described. Torsion results in severe pain. Ascites or Meigs's syndrome occasionally coexist with the larger Brenner tumors, which grow to about 30 cm in diameter. Most tumors, however, are less than 2-3 cm in diameter, are asymptomatic, and are discovered incidentally at surgery for other reasons.

On gross observation Brenner tumors are occasionally mistaken for nonfunctional granulosa or theca cell tumors because of their yellow color. Fibromas must also be considered; they also are firm but are usually pearl-gray, not yellow.

Treatment consists of surgical removal, preserving the uninvolved portion of the ovary. If a pseudomucinous component is also present, oophorectomy is recommended.

TERATOID TUMORS OF THE OVARY
(Dermoid Cysts & Teratomas)

Teratoid tumors may represent imperfect parthogenesis. They are composed of one, 2, or 3 germinal layers which may grow into any possible combination of imperfectly formed structures. If one type of tissue predominates, the appearance will be that of a single-tissue tumor; such is the case in struma ovarii, the thyroid (iodine-containing) tumor of the ovary. Teratoid tumors occur primarily in women 18-40 years of age. Dermoids account for 10% and solid teratomas for 0.1% of all ovarian tumors. About 15% are bilateral. Dermoid cysts, the most common type of teratoid tumor, contain ectodermal (and often mesodermal) tissue in the form of macerated skin, hair, bone, and teeth; the cyst is filled with a heavy, greasy sebaceous material and other structures as mentioned. A long pedicle is often present. Dermoid cysts may be minute; most weigh less than a pound.

Embryoma is the term applied to the solid teratoma containing poorly developed organs.

Microscopically, the dermoid is lined by stratified squamous epithelium typical of epidermis. Sudoriparous and sebaceous glands and hair follicles are numerous. Vestiges of many organs may be identified in teratoids, depending upon their organization and development.

Epidermoid carcinoma occurs uncommonly in dermoids. Sarcomatous change occurs much more rarely but is occasionally found in infancy and childhood.

Since the contents of dermoids are light, they "float" upward in the abdomen, elongating the ovarian pedicle. The symptomatology usually relates to this freely-shifting lower abdominal tumor. Constipation, reduced bladder capacity, and a sense of pelvic pressure occur in patients with teratoid tumors over 10 cm in diameter. Sudden, excruciating, continuous unilateral pelvic pain develops with torsion. Gangrene or trauma may rupture a teratoid, and severe chemical peritonitis results. Ascites is rare with benign teratoids.

During pregnancy, a dermoid may become wedged in the true pelvis to obstruct the birth canal.

About 5% of struma ovarii produce thyroxin, which causes signs and symptoms of hypermetabolism.

Urinalysis and blood studies will not identify most teratoid tumors. However, a rare malignant teratoma, the chorio-epithelioma, produces chorionic gonadotropin, which is excreted in the urine. A positive pregnancy test may be reported.

I^{131} uptake studies of a woman with an adnexal tumor and hypermetabolism but no goiter may disclose localization of radioactivity in the pelvis (struma ovarii) and not over the thyroid.

X-ray films disclose bone and teeth in dermoids and contrast in density between the cyst and nearby structures.

All adnexal tumors and pedunculated myomas must be considered. Most dermoids are found anterior and superior to the uterus (Küstner's sign).

Even large dermoid cysts which have not undergone torsion or rupture often can be resected to preserve functional ovarian tissue. A twisted cyst must not be untwisted for fear of discharging emboli. An oophorocystectomy should be performed. The opposite ovary should be incised or aspirated (with a large needle) to determine if the tumor is bilateral.

Bilateral salpingo-oophorectomy and total hysterectomy are required if the teratoma is malignant. X-ray and radium therapy are of no value.

The gravida with a dermoid blocking the pelvic inlet should be placed in the knee-chest position. Displacement of the tumor out of the pelvis is then often possible by vaginal manipulation. If this cannot be done, the cyst should be removed immediately. Care should be taken not to spill the contents into the pelvic cavity. Teratomas should never be needled through the cul-de-sac for therapeutic or diagnostic reasons because leakage into the abdomen causes serious complications (chemical peritonitis, adhesion formation, and obstruction).

The prognosis is usually excellent. Malignant change, though uncommon, implies a poor prognosis.

GRANULOSA CELL TUMOR
(Folliculoma)

Granulosa cell tumors, the most common ovarian neoplasms of sex gland derivation, represent 3-4% of all ovarian tumors. They are solid tumors which vary in size from microscopic to 9 kg (20 lb), and often produce estrogens. A rare tumor may be virilizing, however. Granulosa cell tumors are most often seen in women 50-70 years of age. Ten per cent are bilateral. Both granulosa and theca cells are invariably found together in these tumors. About 15-20% are malignant, but metastasis is almost always confined to neighboring genital organs.

The tumors are rounded or ovoid and somewhat lobulated. They are composed principally of granulosa cells arranged in pseudo-follicles or rosettes which resemble primordial follicles. On section the cell contents are soft and vascular with a poor supporting framework. In the more solid portions the tumor is almost invariably yellowish-brown in color. Some division or trabeculation is occasionally seen. These tumors are retained by a fragile, thin capsule, which in large tumors is easily damaged during examination or at surgery.

Granulosa cells themselves are small, with a scant cytoplasm. The cells contain dark, granular, or vesicular nuclei which take a deep basophilic stain; they tend to occur in rather closely packed clusters. Circular or star-shaped groups of granulosa cells around a degenerating central cell or space (Call-Exner bodies) presumably represent attempted duplication of a graafian follicle. The difference, of course, is that there is no ovum in the center but only a few nondescript, degenerated connective tissue elements. This causes a punched-out or empty appearance of these pseudo-follicles. The better differentiated granulosa cell tumors contain many of these folliculoid arrangements.

Call-Exner bodies seem to break up cords or strands of granulosa cells which vary in maturity and differentiation. The supporting matrix is fragile, and vascular channels are numerous. When the tumor is quite anaplastic, large areas of packed granulosa cells avoid any pattern, but here and there the follicle groupings distinguish the tumor. Where considerable pleomorphism is noted, the cells show many of the characteristics of carcinoma. Nevertheless, there are no histologic criteria for determining the degree of malignancy in granulosa cell tumors.

Tumors which seem to be well differentiated resist degenerative changes. The reverse is certainly true, particularly where gross areas of pseudocyst formation or hemorrhage into the tumor have occurred.

The stroma of granulosa and theca cell tumors is quite characteristic, and a close relationship between the ovarian stroma, the theca cells, and granulosa cells has been demonstrated. The stroma consists in large measure of elongated connective tissue cells which develop long, dendritic reticular fibrils. Insinuated between these, less well differentiated cells are commonly seen. Certain of these latter appear to have epithelioid characteristics, and many are actually theca cells. Each such cell is found to be surrounded by a proliferation of reticulum fibrils, as shown by the Foot silver stain. In contrast, aggregations of well-differentiated granulosa cells form clusters which are surrounded as a group by whorls of reticular fibers.

In general, the higher the grade of differentiation or maturity of the granulosa cells, the greater the likelihood of hormone production, as is evidenced by luteinization or by the collection of lipoid granules within the cytoplasm of the cells. Considerable luteinization is usually seen in active, older tumors.

Granulosa cell tumors, including granulosa cell carcinomas, are divided into 4 principal microscopic patterns: (1) Folliculoid arrangement, with large or small acini surrounded by a rim of granulosa cells suggesting the graafian follicle. The theca interna may be scant or absent. The central cavity contains fluid, often bloody. (2) The cylindromatous pattern, with dense columns of cells separated by fibrous septa of connective tissue. These are less well differentiated than the folliculoid type. Partial luteinization occurs. These tumors may suggest Brenner tumors at first glance, though Brenner cell tumors contain no lipoid material and connective tissue is far more extensive. (3) The diffuse form, without pattern, in which granulosa cells are seen between planes of connective tissue. (4) A system of tubules may be noted in another type in which cells arrange themselves in a single row around a central acinus as though it were a duct. Such an arrangement suggests Pick's adenoma, although the latter does not contain lipoid bodies.

A trabeculated form, a gyrate form, and one suggesting moiré silk have also been described. These are purely descriptive terms and are not very useful. The folliculoid pattern contains the Call-Exner bodies to a greater degree than in most other types.

The effect of the production of large amounts of estrogen depends upon the age of the individual and her functional status. In children, this causes early development of pubic hair, hypertrophy of the breasts, and enlargement of the labia, cervix, and uterus. Advanced bone age and early epiphysial closure (dwarfism) will occur if hormonal stimulation is continued for a long time. Pelvic examination in such cases generally discloses an adnexal mass. In the functional years, menometrorrhagia is usually the only finding.

In pregnancy the principal problem is rupture of the tumor and hemorrhage.

In postmenopausal women refeminization and reinstitution of uterine bleeding occur. Generally speaking, however, this is not true menstruation but abnormal bleeding of an irregular type, and the flow is often more profuse and prolonged than with normal menses.

Granulosa cell tumors may cause pain because of torsion or pulsion of the mass. Abdominal distention usually occurs only with very large tumors or, in the case of malignant tumors, with regional spread or ascites. Masculinization is characterized by development of male hair distribution, coarsening of the features, amenorrhea, deepening of the voice, and hypertrophy of the clitoris. Rare androgenicity in a group of otherwise feminizing neoplasms is not adequately explained.

On pelvic examination, the smallest granulosa cell tumor may not be palpable; those that are palpable may be almost any size. They generally are mobile, rarely adherent, and often soft or semi-cystic. If the woman is slender, firmer areas also may be felt. Ascites and Meigs's syndrome may occur. Hemorrhagic ascites and fixation of the tumor suggest malignancy.

Laboratory findings consist of elevated urinary estrogens and a high degree of cornification as demonstrated in the vaginal smear.

Granulosa cell tumors have a very thin capsule which is easily ruptured either by stressful movements or too vigorous pelvic examination. About 20 such cases have been recorded in the past 10 years. With rupture of the tumor, gross intra-abdominal hemorrhage occurs, and patients should be hospitalized as abdominal emergencies. Metastases of the tumor to the opposite ovary, endometrium, and vagina are frequent, but distant spread is uncommon and almost never extensive.

The differential diagnosis includes the following: (1) multiple follicle cysts of the ovary; (2) other functional ovarian neoplasms, such as theca cell tumors with cystic degeneration; (3) ovarian adrenal rest or lipoid cell tumor of the ovary; and (4) other causes of postmenopausal bleeding or abnormal menstruation. There are times when the tumor is so poorly differentiated and so obviously malignant that it may be considered an anaplastic carcinoma, particularly because this type of granulosa cell carcinoma does not usually produce steroid sex hormones.

The probability of a granulosa cell tumor being present is about 1:100 in patients with postmenopausal bleeding; if postmenopausal bleeding is associated with an ovarian tumor, the chances are 1:5.

Treatment consists of surgical removal. In patients in the functional or prepuberal years, benign tumors are removed by ovariectomy; in postmenopausal women, total hysterectomy and bilateral salpingo-oophorectomy are indicated. If the patient is young or if the question of malignancy has not been settled, it may be best to remove the tumor and await the pathologist's complete report. Reentry for more radical surgery may be performed if the presence of a definite cancer or its extension is established.

Roentgen therapy has not proved to be of great value. Even mega-voltage x-ray is ineffectual in controlling most recurrences although the hormone-secreting function of the tumor is usually destroyed by x-ray. This gives the impression that the tumor is highly radiosensitive because the symptoms regress after x-ray therapy. Adequate surgery, however, is still the best therapeutic weapon.

The histologic findings are not reliable for prognostic purposes, nor can malignancy be judged by the degree of endocrine activity. The clinical course and stage of the tumor are the most helpful prognostic guides. Many five- or even ten-year arrests have been credited to surgery. Late recurrences (one after 33 years) have been recorded, however.

STEIN-LEVENTHAL SYNDROME
(Polycystic Ovarian Disease)

The Stein-Leventhal syndrome is an uncommon disorder characterized by bilaterally enlarged polycystic ovaries, secondary amenorrhea or oligomenorrhea, and infertility. About 50% of patients are hirsute, and at least 10% are obese. The syndrome affects females between the ages of approximately 15-30 years. About 2-3% of cases of female infertility—those secondary to failure of ovulation—are due to polycystic ovarian disease. The disorder is presumably of endocrine origin.

The slightly enlarged, sclerocystic ovaries with smooth, pearl-white, shiny surfaces but without surface scarring or indentations have been called "oyster ovaries." Many small, fluid-filled follicle cysts lie beneath the thick fibrous capsule. The ovarian stroma is often edematous but rarely luteinized. Hyperplasia and luteinization of the theca interna generally is observed.

A presumptive diagnosis of Stein-Leventhal syndrome often can be made from the history and initial physical examination. A normal puberty and early adolescence with reasonably regular menses is followed by episodes of amenorrhea which become progressively longer. The enlarged ovaries are identifiable on pelvic examination in about 50% of patients.

Urinary 17-ketosteroids are minimally elevated but estrogen and FSH excretion is normal. Some patients have an increased Δ-4-androstenedione and 17-α-hydroxyprogesterone output; others excrete considerable amounts of dehydroepiandrosterone. Adrenocorticosteroid hormone titers are normal. Basal body temperature records and endometrial biopsies confirm anovulation.

Pelvic pneumoroentgenography, culdoscopy, culdotomy, or laparotomy will reveal the ovarian abnormality.

Adrenocortical hyperplasia or tumor is ruled out since signs of defeminization and masculinization are absent and adrenal function is normal. A virilizing ovarian tumor is an unlikely diagnosis because the ovarian enlargement is bilateral.

Give cortisone, 50 mg orally b.i.d. for 2-3 months. Clomiphene citrate (Clomid®), 50 mg orally daily for 1-2 months, may be helpful. If ovulatory cycles do not resume, wedge resection of one-third to one-half of each ovary should be considered. The majority of patients will respond to the above regimen, and infertility is often overcome. Hirsutism and obesity are not affected by cortisone or surgery.

OVARIAN CORTICAL STROMAL HYPERPLASIA

Focal or diffuse proliferation of partially luteinized stromal cells in the ovarian cortex is observed occasionally in menopausal and, particularly, postmenopausal women. Progressive stromal hyperplasia occurs in affected middle-aged patients, whereas the disorder usually resolves in older women. The cause is not known, although a strikingly high frequency of association has been observed with slightly increased estrogen production, endometrial hyperplasia, or cancer of the endometrium or breast. Whether hyperfunction of the ovary is primary or secondary is still debated.

Minimal enlargement and rounding of surface contours of

the ovaries coincide with the accumulation of plump, ovoid, variably luteinized stromal cells in the cortex. No cysts develop. Multinodular, partially confluent stromal hyperplasia is the most common pattern. Small cortical granulomas composed of peripheral stromal cells and central epithelioid elements, chronic inflammatory cells, and lipid-containing debris are encountered by the pathologist.

Cortical stromal hyperplasia may be suspected when slight, persistently increased estrogen production continues after the menopause. Hyperestrogenism is best diagnosed by the vaginal smear. Postmenopausal uterine bleeding may also be reported.

Exogenous estrogen and feminizing ovarian tumors cause similar signs and symptoms.

The patient should be re-examined at frequent intervals. Laparotomy and resection of the ovaries are not justified on a presumptive diagnosis. If genital or breast cancer can be ruled out, spontaneous regression of the ovarian stromal hyperplasia is likely after age 60-70.

OVARIAN HYPERTHECOSIS

Hyperthecosis is a rare ovarian abnormality which occurs in premenopausal women and is characterized by amenorrhea, obesity, defeminization, and even mild virilization. Both ovaries contain numerous follicle cysts, hyperplasia, and hyperactivity of theca cells, with marked luteinization of theca and cortical stromal cells. The cause is not known; abnormal ovarian or adrenocortical function may be responsible.

Hyperthecosis ovarii may be an extreme degree of the polycystic ovary syndrome. Urinary 17-ketosteroid, estrogen, and corticoid excretion is normal. The glucose tolerance test often is slightly elevated for unknown reasons.

Definite hyperadrenocorticism can be ruled out by cortisone suppression and ACTH stimulation tests.

Cortisone therapy, as used in the Stein-Leventhal syndrome, has been ineffectual. Bilateral wedge resection of the ovaries most often corrects amenorrhea, and masculinization is arrested.

ARGENTAFFIN (CARCINOID) TUMORS

Argentaffin (carcinoid) tumors are not rare. Most originate in the appendix, but ovarian argentaffinoma may occur. An ovarian mass, vasomotor symptoms, and a positive urinary 5-hydroxyindoleacetic acid test suggest the diagnosis. Surgical removal is usually curative.

OOPHORITIS

Isolated infection of the ovary is very rare. However, oophoritis may accompany puerperal infection, mumps, tuberculosis, mycosis, severe regional infections (e.g., tubal sepsis and appendicitis), and nematode infestations. Women in the reproductive years are most often affected.

Infective organisms reach the ovary in the following ways: (1) Via the lymphatics (following dilatation and curettage, attempted criminal abortion, puerperal sepsis, salpingography). (2) Via the fallopian tubes (gonorrhea, schistosomiasis). (3) Via the blood stream (mumps, distant abscesses, wound infections, pulmonary tuberculosis). (4) Via the peritoneal fluid and contiguous intra-abdominal infections (pelvic tuberculosis and actinomycosis). The microorganisms most often responsible for oophoritis are the streptococci (usually hemolytic or anaerobic types), colon bacilli, staphylococci, gonococci, and tubercle bacilli (in that order).

The ovary is generally resistant to infection. Nevertheless, the point of rupture of the follicle or the forming corpus luteum itself may provide an entrance for bacteria. Little tendency toward healing is noted once deep cortical or medullary infection is established.

Ovarian infection usually starts as a peri-oophoritis. Inflammation and adherence of the ovary, tube, bowel, and omentum follow, progressing to an ovarian or tubo-ovarian abscess.

With a gonococcal or post-abortal ovarian abscess, the ovary is a tender, rounded, discrete, fluctuant mass up to 15 cm in diameter, and it may be adherent to a swollen, distorted tube.

In tuberculous and mycotic oophoritis, the lesion consists of an adherent, firm callus, riddled by numerous cavities filled with grumous material. Invasion of the neighboring structures causes purulent effusion and secondary fistula formation.

The symptomatology of the suppurative form of oophoritis is similar to that of gonococcal or pyogenic salpingitis. In the nonsuppurative variety, pain, fever, and menstrual abnormalities appear in the advanced stage of the disease, together with ovarian (and other) adherent pelvic masses. Intestinal obstruction or fistula may develop.

The white count is elevated with a shift to the left, and the sedimentation rate is accelerated. In nonsuppurative oophoritis, anemia is present.

Films of the lung fields, gastrointestinal barium meal, and intravenous urography may be helpful in identifying the primary site of tuberculosis or mycosis. Bacterial staining, culture, and guinea pig inoculation of aspirate or drainage material may reveal the primary organism. Tubal occlusion may also be demonstrable.

Chronic suppurative oophoritis must be distinguished from salpingitis and endometriosis. Chronic nonsuppurative oophoritis may resemble regional ileitis, ulcerative colitis, carcinoma, syphilis, and lymphogranuloma venereum of the bowel.

Prompt definitive, adequate treatment of pelvic infections will usually prevent oophoritis.

Give procaine penicillin G, 1-2 million units, and streptomycin, 1 gm stat. For the next 3-5 days give 600,000 units of procaine penicillin G and 0.5 gm of streptomycin twice daily. Dilatation and curettage should be performed following an incomplete or criminal abortion. Treat tuberculosis or mycotic infection with appropriate chemotherapeutic agents.

The patient should be hospitalized if fever persists or if pain is severe. Give blood transfusions as required for anemia, and intravenous fluids for dehydration. Give codeine, 0.06 gm (1 gr), and aspirin, 0.6 gm (10 gr), every 4-6 hours as necessary for pain.

Drain large abscesses extraperitoneally or through the cul-de-sac when fluctuant and superficially pointing. Remove suppurative adnexa in chronic oophoritis. Avoid surgery in tuberculous or mycotic oophoritis until after 6-9 months of chemotherapy. Large residual masses or fistulas may then be treated surgically.

Treat complications as for infected abortion. (See p. 249.)

When early oophoritis yields to medical management, the prognosis is good for fertility and normal ovarian function. It is poor when severe acute or chronic oophoritis requires prolonged medical or surgical therapy.

24...
Urologic & Bowel Complications in Obstetrics & Gynecology

URINARY STRESS INCONTINENCE

Urinary stress incontinence is the involuntary leakage of urine through an intact urethra and bladder under the stimulus of increased intra-abdominal pressure. Unexpected loss of urine may occur while coughing, laughing, sneezing, or lifting heavy objects. Slight degrees of urinary stress incontinence are noted in 50-60% of females in all age groups; most cases occur in women who have suffered childbirth injuries or who have developed weakness of the pelvic floor structures following menopause. About 20% of major elective gynecologic surgical procedures are partially or wholly for the purpose of correcting this annoying disorder.

Urinary stress incontinence is the result of congenital defects or acquired disorders of the urinary tract, pelvic organs, pelvic musculature, or nervous system. Developmental anomalies include congenital urethrovesical widening, anomalous urethra, spina bifida, and deficient tissue tone. The most important single cause of the acquired type of urinary stress incontinence is trauma to the bladder control mechanism. Injury most frequently results from prolonged or difficult labor or instrumental delivery, especially forceps rotations and midforceps extractions. Nonoperative trauma, including penetrating injuries to the perineal area, is also causative. Cystourethrocele, uterine descensus, pelvic floor relaxation, compression of the bladder by the pregnant uterus, ascites, pelvic tumors, and reduced pelvic circulation are etiologic factors. Loss of muscle tone as a result of aging and, particularly, estrogen deficiency may cause minor anatomic or neurologic deficiencies to become clinically evident. In many cases neurologic disease or injury (e.g., conduction anesthesia complications) will cause urinary stress incontinence even though the anatomic structures are relatively normal. For reasons difficult to explain, psychogenic difficulties also may lead to poor control of urinary function.

Patients who undergo operation for the correction of uterine prolapse or cystocele occasionally develop urinary stress incontinence not present before surgery in spite of a seemingly good anatomic result. The surgeon's failure to restore normal anatomic relationships (allowing free movement of the bladder and urethra) and to tighten all essential fascial planes often explains the functional difficulty.

Clinical Findings.

A. Symptoms and Signs: The clinical evaluation of the incontinent patient requires a complete review of the onset and any diseases or traumatic events which may be pertinent. Any type of pelvic surgery, obstetric procedures, and labors should be analyzed. A search should be made for associated urinary symptoms, especially those suggesting infection.

The complete physical examination should emphasize developmental and neurologic disorders; abdominal masses, zones of tenderness and herniation or fullness; cystourethrocele and rectocele; uterine size, shape, position, and descensus; and adnexal abnormalities. The urethra should be sounded for strictures and to determine the caliber and direction of the urethra. Local fullness may indicate a urethral diverticulum. The tone of the rectal sphincter and the pubococcygeus muscle should be evaluated by requiring the patient to contract these muscles over the examining fingers.

Many patients experience transitory episodes of incontinence with severe emotional or physical stress, but as a rule only the more seriously affected seek medical care. The vast majority of cases are reported in multiparous women over 45, many of whom have undergone pelvic surgery, in some instances for the treatment of urinary stress incontinence.

Most patients have urinary stress incontinence only when erect, with respiratory effort, or upon sudden straining or change of position, e.g., rising from a chair. Voluntary control of the bladder is reduced temporarily by distraction or increased intra-abdominal pressure, or both, which in turn raises the intravesical pressure to a point beyond which urine can no longer be retained. Urinary incontinence with stress is more likely to occur when the bladder is full. The amount of urine lost varies widely.

Most women with true urinary stress incontinence report dysuria or urgency, but frequency of urination may occur with residual urine and associated cystocele, descensus of the uterus, or reduction of bladder capacity by pelvic tumors or bladder fixation. The presence of residual urine usually implies urinary infection, though it may not be symptomatic.

B. Laboratory Findings: Stained sediment from a centrifuged specimen of urine should be examined for bacterial infection, which may cause urgency incontinence. A serologic test should be performed to rule out the possibility of central nervous system syphilis. Diabetes mellitus and multiple sclerosis should also be considered.

C. X-Ray Findings: In incontinent parous women, AP and lateral cystourethrograms usually reveal sagging of the bladder, which is greatly increased by cystocele; altered silhouette and normal relationships of the bladder and urethra, depending upon the direction and degree of displacement in prolapse of the uterus, uterine suspension, pregnancy, and pelvic tumors; and funneling of the proximal urethra. In the lateral views only, one may note the formation of an obtuse angle, rather than a straight line, at the posterior urethrovesical junction; a reduction in the angle made by the anterior aspect of the bladder and urethra; and descent and posterior rotation of the bladder with straining while the urethra remains more or less fixed beneath the symphysis. The following anatomic changes should be sought in cystourethrograms: (1) patulousness of the posterior urethra; (2) descent of the bladder neck below the median inferior point of the symphysis; and (3) marked reduction of the posterior urethrovesical angle. Weakness of the pubococcygeal muscle, abnormal advancement of the bladder on the uterus, pelvic tumors, and zones of induration or tenderness may be significant. Pertinent abnormalities include loss of sensation in the distribution of the sacral nerves, e.g., atrophy of the pelvic muscles and weakness of the rectal sphincter, and deficiencies in locomotion.

Cinefluorography discloses a voluntary relaxation of the female pelvic floor during voiding which causes a wide funneling of the posterior urethra. As intra-abdominal pressure increases, flattening (almost to the point of obliteration) of the posterior urethrovesical angle occurs, and urine passes. The act of voiding in the female is different from that in the male because women have no individual detrusor muscle which contracts to open the internal sphincter at the urethrovesical neck. Ectopy of the urethra or bladder, causing these structures to be out of natural alignment behind the symphysis, reduces the patient's ability to relax the base of the bladder and posterior urethra. This prevents the increase in the urethrovesical angle which is required to empty the bladder.

D. Special Examinations:
  1. "Trigone test" - Procaine, 2 ml of 0.5% solution (or equivalent), is injected just beneath the mucosa of the urethra at the urethrovesical junction. After anesthe-

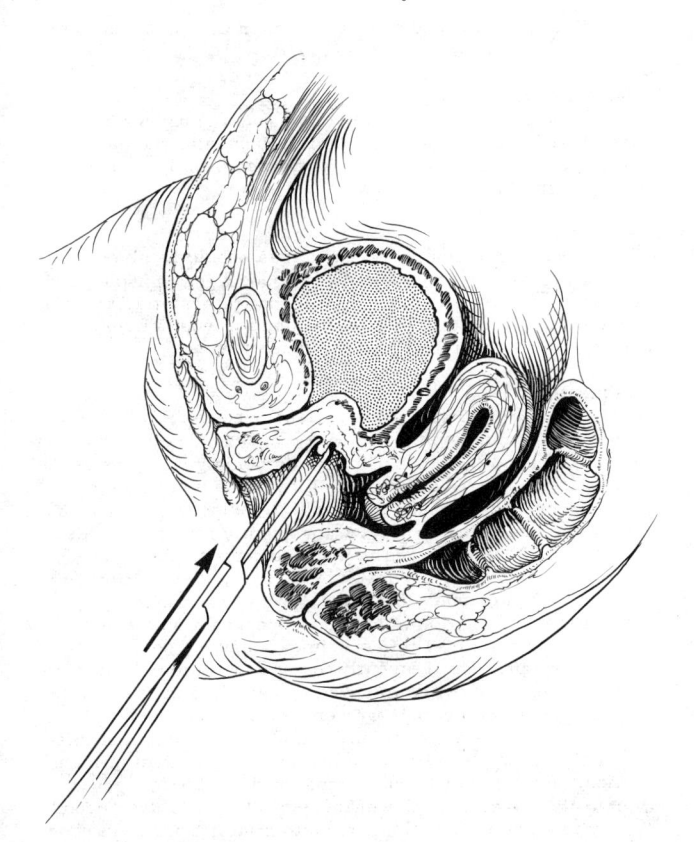

Fig 24-1. Trigone test.

sia has become effective, 200 ml of water are injected into the empty bladder. Allis clamps are placed on the vaginal mucosa beneath the bladder neck. The exact site of the bulge is noted when the patient strains with the bladder moderately full. Patients with a relaxed vesical neck and reduced urethrovesical angle will lose urine when they strain or when the clamps are depressed, but incontinence can be checked by elevating the clamps. Thus, elevation of the bladder neck and improvement in the acuteness of the anterior urethrovesical angle with surgery may be expected to benefit the patient postoperatively.

2. Urethroscopy and cystoscopy often are required to reveal developmental irregularities.

Differential Diagnosis.

Paradoxic incontinence (overflow voiding) usually is caused by residual urine due to a developmental anomaly or neurologic disease. Urgency incontinence usually is due to urethritis or bladder infection.

Prevention.

Antepartal and postpartal exercises should be given as described below to strengthen the pubococcygeal muscles and other pelvic floor structures. Avoidance of obstetric trauma, especially difficult or ineptly performed forceps delivery, will do much to prevent urinary stress incontinence.

Treatment.
A. Medical Treatment: If the patient is cooperative, medical treatment should be tried for at least 3-4 months before surgery is considered. Myasthenia gravis, extreme obesity, asthma, diabetes mellitus, and other medical disorders which cause or aggravate urinary stress incontinence should be controlled by specific measures. Estrogens should be given in cyclic dosage to postmenopausal estrogen deficient women, e.g., diethylstilbestrol, 0.25 mg orally daily for 3 weeks each month.

Firm contraction of the pubococcygeal muscle and sphincter ani 20-30 times 3 times a day for several months, and less frequently for an indefinite period thereafter, usually will be followed by complete cure or at least satisfactory improvement (Kegel exercises). The patient often is unaware of the important function of this portion of the levator musculature in the control of urination. Lack of conscious control of the pubococcygeal muscle, together with weakness of this structure secondary to aging, laceration, or birth injury, results in poor supportive closure of the posterior urethra.
B. Surgical Measures: Patients who do not respond to exercises may be candidates for surgery, particularly when cystocele or prolapse of the bladder and uterus is present. Numerous operations have been devised for the correction of urinary stress incontinence; all seem to achieve their effects by tightening fascial planes. A combined abdominal-vaginal approach gives a better chance of success than a strictly abdominal approach. There are 4 principal types:
1. Sling formation for the urethra for repair of cystocele or urethrocele.
2. Plication of the urethra - The Kelly operation consists of plication of the so-called pubovesical fascia to narrow and support the urethra.

3. Lengthening of the urethra, e.g., Brunkow urethral advancement, Lapides' operation.
4. Replacement of the urethra and bladder in its normal position behind the symphysis, e.g., Marshall-Marchetti-Krantz operation, anterior vaginal suspension.

C. General Measures: Prevention of postoperative overdistention of the bladder generally requires the use of an inlying catheter for 4-5 days or until the patient is able to void without retaining more than 100 ml of residual urine.

Anti-infective therapy, e.g., sulfisoxazole (Gantrisin®), 1-2 gm 4 times a day, often is given postoperatively to prevent and treat urinary tract infections.

In the postmenopausal woman, oral or parenteral estrogen therapy should be given in cyclic dosage for at least one month before surgery and indefinitely thereafter.

Prognosis.

Cooperative patients who do not have severe lesions or anomalies (particularly those with weak pubococcygeus muscles) can achieve satisfactory continence on medical therapy alone in at least 50% of cases. The over-all surgical cure rate with the first operation is about 85%, and half of the remainder can be cured by a second operation. The success rate is over 90% if the vaginal-abdominal approach is used. When the abdominal approach is used, the cure rate is slightly lower because cystoceles often cannot be repaired adequately and perineorrhaphy cannot be done.

Patients with serious developmental abnormalities and those with severe tissue damage due to trauma are not cured easily. Where urologic disease is congenital or acquired, medical and surgical treatment often fail. Patients who have sustained more than 2 operations for correction of urinary stress incontinence have a poor prognosis if for no other reason than that the formation of dense scar tissue prevents normal urethral and bladder function.

URETHRAL CARUNCLE

A small reddened, sensitive fleshy excrescence at the urethral meatus is called a caruncle. Most caruncles represent eversion (ectropion) of the urethra or infections at the urinary meatus (or both), but vascular anomalies or benign or malignant neoplasm may also cause caruncle formation. The vast majority of caruncles are benign; persistent and progressive lesions may be cancerous. Caruncles may occur at any age, but postmenopausal women are most commonly affected.

Caruncles are categorized according to type as follows (combined types also occur): (1) Papillary caruncles are flame-shaped and delicately tesselated, have a rich vascular supply, and are covered with stratified transitional or squamous cells. Gross infection may or may not be present. (2) Granulomatous caruncles are inflammatory processes usually due to bacterial infection, although they may also be caused by lymphogranuloma venereum and syphilis. (3) Vascular caruncles usually have an angiomatous pattern and are frequently infected.

Clinical Findings.
A. Symptoms and Signs: A caruncle appears as a small, vividly red, sessile or flattened mass protruding from the urethral meatus. It usually bleeds, exudes, or causes pain, depending upon its cause, size, and integrity. Dysuria, frequency, and urgency are common urinary symptoms. Bleeding and leukorrhea are usually not severe except when malignant change has occurred. Dyspareunia or other types of local discomfort are frequently described, particularly during the climacteric. Malignant caruncles are firm, on a wide base, have a distinct margin, and are friable and hemorrhagic. Local ulceration, urethritis, and vulvitis may develop.
B. Laboratory Findings: Specimens for cytologic examination, bacterial smears, cultures, and biopsies should be obtained. If syphilis is suspected, dark-field examination is required; if lymphgranuloma venereum is a possibility, a Frei test or complement fixation test is indicated.

Prevention.
Estrogen therapy for postmenopausal women and avoidance of local irritation will probably prevent caruncle formation.

Treatment.
A. Specific Measures: Venereal disease is treated with appropriate measures. If the patient is postmenopausal and has not been receiving steroid sex hormone therapy, estrogens are applied topically (diethylstilbestrol vaginal suppositories, 0.5 mg every other night for 3 weeks) before specific therapy.

If tests are negative for malignancy and the lesion is not large or severely infected, light fulguration under local anesthesia or excision may be performed with care not to cause stricture. Repeated light fulguration is preferable to extensive coagulation initially. Fulguration may be repeated if benign caruncle recurs. Topical anti-infective therapy (e.g., nitrofurazone [Furacin®]) is indicated before and after cauterization or excision.

Urethral Diverticulum   589

   If malignant change has occurred, radical resection or irradiation therapy is required.
B. General Measures: A bladder sedative compound may be given to relieve urinary distress.
C. Treatment of Complications: The urethral meatus must be dilated after therapy if stenosis develops.

Prognosis.

The prognosis is excellent in benign cases but guarded when malignant change has occurred.

URETHRAL DIVERTICULUM

Urethral diverticulum is a sacculation caused by: (1) congenital cystic dilatation of paraurethral (wolffian) remnants; (2) infection of the paraurethral gland with rupture or trauma to the urethra; or (3) urinary, obstetric, or gynecologic injury. Most patients are 40-50 years old and multiparas.

The mid or distal third of the urethra is the usual site. With congenital malformation, the cystic structure, usually 1-4 cm in diameter, may be a single or multiloculated cavity. One or more minute ostia connect the diverticulum with the urethra. Symptoms are due to the sacculation and local inflammation. Complaints may be acute or chronic and constant or intermittent, but chronic infection with periodic acute exacerbations is the most common clinical picture. Calculi are present in 10-20% of patients.

Clinical Findings.
A. Symptoms and Signs:
   1. Urinary distress - Pain with voiding, urgency, dysuria, frequency, and nocturia are due to infection or urethral distortion. The complaints are similar to those of cystitis, and there is often a feeling of inability to empty the bladder.
   2. Dribbling after urination (pseudoincontinence) - The postvoiding leakage may be urine or purulent or bloody fluid, the result of evacuation of the diverticulum.
   3. Discharge - A urinous or bloody purulent discharge at the meatus following stripping of the urethra represents diverticulum contents.
   4. Vaginal pain - This is usually more severe before and after the menses. Dyspareunia, urethral tenderness, and pelvic discomfort are caused by inflammation or distention of the diverticulum.
   5. Indefinite anterior vaginal fullness or soft mass on digital examination - This is periodically painful and best felt over a catheter or cystoscope.
   6. Malaise, chills, fever - Manifestations of acute infection.

B. **X-ray Findings:** Radiopaque contrast fluid studies generally will outline the diverticulum.
C. **Special Examinations:** A small urethral sound may demonstrate a slight stricture of the urethra and the diverticulum just beyond.

Panendoscopy with a large caliber instrument to dilate the ostium will reveal the diverticular opening in most cases although the opening may be small and obscured by mucosal folds or granulation tissue.

Complications.

Urethrovaginal fistula may follow unsuccessful diverticulectomy or spontaneous rupture (often during labor), erosion by stone, incisional drainage, or fulguration of the cystic abnormality. Transitional cell carcinoma or adenocarcinoma may develop in urethral diverticula. Stricture of the urethra may be a consequence of extensive or complicated surgery.

Differential Diagnosis.

Urethritis, venereal or nonspecific, is a diffuse process; urethral abscess is a phase of diverticulum development. Urethrocele is not a swelling or herniation but a disengagement of the urethra from the symphysis. Gartner's duct cysts and inclusion cysts do not communicate with the urethra. Tumors near or involving the urethra may be primary or secondary. They are firm, semifixed, and nontender.

Treatment.

Broad-spectrum antibiotic therapy and warm vaginal douches generally will resolve the acute inflammatory phase in 3-5 days, but chronic infection almost always persists.

Transvaginal diverticulectomy usually is necessary for permanent relief in all but very small or persistently asymptomatic (large ostium) sacculations. An indwelling urethral catheter should be left in place for 10 days.

URINARY TRACT INJURIES FOLLOWING OBSTETRIC & GYNECOLOGIC SURGERY

Urinary fistulas and obstructions are occasional serious postoperative complications of obstetric and gynecologic surgery. Fistulas may occur in any part of the urinary tract and result from direct or indirect injury; occlusions usually involve the ureter and occur as a result of angulation or obstruction by a suture, scarring after injury or infection, or as a complication of the treatment of pelvic malignancy. The incidence of urinary tract injury in large medical centers in the USA is about 0.8% following major gynecologic surgery and 0.08% in operative obstetrics.

Postpartal fistulas of the bladder and urethra are generally caused by extreme pressure of the presenting part or by instrumentation. A history of prolonged labor and operative delivery is usually present. Many fistulas are the result of technical surgical errors (poor exposure, operative ineptitude, or distortion of anatomy); hematoma formation (incomplete hemostasis, failure to institute drainage when indicated); and infection (neglected hematoma or contaminated urinary extravasation). Deep sutures, mass ligatures, and overdistention of the bladder also cause bladder injuries and fistula formation.

The ureter is often involved in fistula formation or stenosis, but the kidney is rarely damaged directly during gynecologic surgery. Many types of fistulas (singly or in combination) may be diagnosed after operation or delivery: ureterovaginal, ureterovesical, ureteroperitoneal, ureteroenteric, vesicovaginal, vesicouterine, vesicocervical, and urethrovaginal. Some fistulas are minute; others represent loss of a major segment of the urinary tract. Strictures are confined to narrow structures, e.g., the ureter and urethra. Partial or complete closure of one or both ureters is not uncommon, but stricture of the female urethra rarely occurs postoperatively.

Clinical Findings.

A. Symptoms and Signs: The symptomatology depends upon the site of the injury (unilateral or bilateral), the degree of damage (partial or complete), and the direction of urine drainage (external, intraperitoneal, or retroperitoneal).

Unilateral ureteral injury usually causes flank pain, tenderness, and fever but does not alter the urinary volume. It may indicate constriction of the ureter, fistula, and infection. Escape of urine from the abdominal or vaginal incision indicates probable ureteral or bladder fistulas (or both). Ileus often follows urinary obstruction, extravasation, and infection. Urinary infection, especially with partial obstruction of the ureter, results in chills, fever, renal pain, and costovertebral and loin tenderness. Fever develops when a ureter to an infected kidney is ligated. In the absence of preexisting bacteriuria, complete obstruction of one ureter usually is asymptomatic. If leakage of urine is into the peritoneal cavity, there will be signs of free peritoneal fluid and peritoneal irritation. Progressive degeneration and necrosis of a damaged area in the urinary system or temporary pocketing of extravasated urine may account for delayed leakage (up to 3-4 weeks postoperatively).

Uremia ordinarily does not follow unilateral ureteral injury and intraperitoneal leakage because much of the extravasated urine is reabsorbed and excreted by the opposite kidney. Signs of perirenal or psoas abscess follow retroperitoneal extravasation of urine.

Anuria and uremia follow complete bilateral ureteral occlusion. Oliguria follows partial obstruction of both ureters, a large vesicoperitoneal fistula, or occlusion of the urethra. Dehydration, shock, lower nephron nephrosis, and congestive heart failure should be ruled out.

B. Laboratory Findings: The PSP test indicates the degree of renal tubular function by excretion of a foreign dye. About one-half hour before the test is started, 400 ml of water are given to the patient to drink. Half an hour later 1 ml (6 mg) of dye is injected I.V. Urines are collected at the end of one-half and one hour and water added to dilute the urine specimen to 1000 ml. A sample of the diluted mixture is compared in a colorimeter with a standard. Normally, 60-70% of the dye is excreted in 2 hours; excretion of less than 50% is an indication of renal insufficiency. Passage of the dye verifies the patency of at least one ureter in cases of postoperative oliguria provided adequate hydration and a normal blood pressure have been maintained.

C. X-Ray Findings:
1. Ureteral obstruction, fistula, or extravasation -
   a. Excretory urography - The freshly occluded kidney will not excrete the contrast agent well, thus assisting in diagnosis. The urogram is an excellent screening test, but the presence of excessive intestinal gas reduces the clarity of the roentgenogram.
   b. Retrograde urography - A ureteral catheter may be blocked by an occlusion or it may be inserted easily. (A radiopaque catheter should be used so that the level of the obstruction can be observed on the film.) Injection of a contrast medium into a Braasch-bulb catheter may reveal a fistula above the bulb fixed in the most distal portion of the ureter.
   c. Plain film (AP) of the abdomen - This may suggest retroperitoneal extravasation of urine or psoas abscess by revealing a mass, obliteration of the psoas muscle contours, or displacement of intestinal gas shadows.
2. Bladder fistula and extravasation - An AP scout film of the pelvis should be obtained. The bladder is filled with 50 ml of radiopaque medium such as iodopyracet (Diodrast®) or acetrizoate (Urokon®) in 200 ml of water and a second film taken. The bladder is then drained and a third film obtained at once. Slight extravasation not visible in the second film may be clearly seen in the third.
3. Urethral occlusion or fistula - This may be visualized by taking lateral x-ray films promptly after the in-

jection of 5 ml of I.V. urography medium mixed with an equal quantity of water into the urethral meatus.
D. Special Examinations:
1. Passage of a urethral catheter may reveal an obstruction.
2. Urethroscopy often will expose an obstruction, perforating suture, or fistula.
3. Cystoscopy may disclose a large vesical fistula, but direct visualization is disappointing in the identification of small fistulas. Distention of the bladder with water for water cystoscopy may complicate the problem further by causing gross extravasation of fluid through the defect.
4. To differentiate a ureterovaginal from a vesicovaginal fistula -
   a. The bladder is distended with a solution of 5 ml of indigo carmine in 200 ml of water. In the absence of ureteral reflux (rare), a fistula will be revealed by the presence of blue fluid. Severe chronic cystitis may cause vesicoureteral reflux. When this is likely, 50 ml of an aqueous x-ray contrast medium are added to the indigo carmine solution, the bladder filled, and an AP film of the pelvis obtained to demonstrate backflow as well as the extravasation.
   b. A vaginal pack or snug menstrual tampon which has been moistened with an aqueous solution of sodium carbonate or bicarbonate is inserted. The bladder is injected with 200 ml of water containing 10 ml of methylene blue. The catheter is removed, avoiding any spill which might discolor the pack, and a 1 ml ampule containing 6 mg of PSP is administered I.V. The vaginal pack is removed in 30 minutes. If the pack is stained blue, the presumptive diagnosis is vesicovaginal fistula; if the pack is red, the defect is probably a ureterovaginal fistula; if the pack is multicolored, a ureterovesicovaginal fistula may be present.
5. Retrograde study of the urinary system - If ureteral catheters pass readily to both renal pelves and recover clear urine, ureteral injury, except perhaps a crushing injury or a small perforation, is excluded. If one of these complications seems likely, the catheter is secured in the ureter for splinting and drainage for the 10-14 days necessary for healing.

Complications.

Peritonitis is the most serious complication and may end in death. Anuria or oliguria may be associated with uremia and may also lead to death. Other complications are psoas or perirenal abscess, thrombophlebitis, incontinence of urine, and diarrhea. Urinary tract infection may follow obstruction, as might hydroureter, hydronephrosis, nephrolithiasis, ureterolithiasis, and marked bladder distention.

Differential Diagnosis.

Some fistulas follow irradiation, particularly radium therapy, for cancer of the cervix or the body of the uterus; some may be associated with the treatment of granulomas following pressure by a pessary, tuberculosis, lymphogranuloma venereum, and schistosomiasis. Clear, yellowish, odorless drainage from the abdominal wound may represent ascites or exudative peritoneal fluid, an antecedent of wound dehiscence. Thin, brownish discharge from an abdominal or vaginal suture line may be serum from a seroma or hematoma. In ureteral obstruction oliguria or anuria may be due to shock, dehydration, or lower nephron nephrosis; abdominal distention may indicate dynamic ileus caused by intestinal obstruction or adynamic ileus due to peritonitis; fever may be due to an infected wound, peritonitis, or thrombophlebitis; and kidney pain and costovertebral or flank tenderness may be due to nephrolithiasis, ureterolithiasis, or pyelonephritis.

Prevention.

Adequate preliminary studies of the urinary tract and full knowledge of the anatomy and pathology involved are essential before surgery. The ureters should be catheterized and identified initially in all difficult cases and the wire stylet left in a ureteral catheter for identification to keep the ureter from being cut or clamped. All structures must be identified before clamping, incision, and ligation and care taken so that there is no undue traction and needless denudation of the ureter and the base of the bladder. Only fine absorbable sutures in or around the urinary tract should be used. Pressure is applied, rather than multiple ligatures, for hemorrhage, and a single bleeding point secured. The course of the ureters is traced at the completion of each abdominal operation. The ureter is splinted with an inlying catheter, the bladder drained with another catheter, and the area drained extraperitoneally in suspected or actual urinary tract injury.

Sufficient doses of appropriate antibiotics are utilized for treatment of infection. The surgeon himself should remove ureteral catheters after surgery if it is decided not to leave them in place. A "hang" may indicate ureteral constriction. No oily solutions should be injected into a lacerated portion of the urinary system or a sinus tract, since granuloma may develop.

Treatment.
A. Emergency Measures: Shock, blood loss, and dehydration are treated as indicated and the bladder catheterized.

If oliguria or anuria is present, a PSP test is ordered. Specific gravity should be checked and the patient weighed.
B. Specific Surgical Measures:
1. Bilateral ureteral stricture - If both ureters are obstructed and the patient is a poor surgical risk, nephrostomy or unilateral tube ureterostomy is performed using the largest child's urethral catheter that will enter the ureter. The other kidney should not be left obstructed for more than a few days. As soon as the patient becomes a satisfactory operative risk, the second blocked kidney is relieved by nephrostomy or tube ureterostomy. Deligation alone is not satisfactory unless the suture is obvious and deligation can be performed easily. If deligation is done, a splinting catheter is inserted through a longitudinal incision several cm above the point of obstruction, passed to the kidney and bladder, brought out through the urethra, and fixed to a Foley retention catheter for 10-14 days, at which time both may be removed. The retroperitoneal area is drained through a separate lower quadrant or flank stab wound.

    A gallbladder T tube can be used in lieu of a catheter as follows: (1) The cross-arm of the T is notched at the vertical segment. (2) The ureter is incised longitudinally several cm above the defect. (3) The tube is inserted so that the lower arm splints the point of injury. (4) The upper arm is fixed in the proximal ureter and the long arm carried out retroperitoneally through a stab wound in the flank. (5) A drain is placed in the retroperitoneal space underlying the T tube and allowed to remain until drainage ceases (about one week after the removal of the tube).

2. Vesicoperitoneal fistula - Laparotomy should be performed as soon as the diagnosis is established. The edges are freshened and the fistula closed without tension in 2 layers: one continuous or both interrupted, using 000 chromic catgut. The mucosa should be avoided in suturing. The bladder is drained by cystostomy or with a Foley retention catheter, and suction drainage employed for 10-14 days.

3. Vesicovaginal fistula - Local infection is treated by removing old sutures and concretions and by giving systemic antibiotics. Repair is indicated as outlined for vesicoperitoneal fistula. In general, one should wait 4 months or more after injury before attempting closure. If there are no other contraindications, one may take a calculated risk in selected cases and perform earlier repair after preparation with prednisone, 10 mg 4 times daily, and massive doses of broad-spectrum antibiotics for 7 days. All but large inac-

cessible, immobile vesicovaginal fistulas (85-90% of total) should be closed transvaginally.
4. Ureterovesicovaginal fistulas - These should be closed abdominally. The procedure at operation is to freshen the edges, excise scar tissue, free restrictions, and close without tension. Relatively few fine, removable nylon monofilament or silver wire interrupted mattress sutures should be employed, avoiding the mucosa. Monofilament sutures should never be buried, nor should purse-string sutures of any sort be employed.

Reimplantation of the severely damaged or severed ureter into the bladder (ureteroneocystostomy) is preferred to ureteroureterostomy on the same side. Ureteroneocystostomy should be attempted only when the proximal ureter is long enough to permit anastomosis without tension. A splinting catheter is inserted into the ureter, brought out through the urethra, and fixed to a Foley retention catheter for 10-14 days, at which time both may be removed. The bladder is drained by cystostomy or with a Foley retention catheter, and suction drainage employed for 10-14 days.

Ligation of the damaged ureter and sacrifice of the kidney on that side is almost always contraindicated. A renal abscess may develop, necessitating a much more serious operation (nephrectomy) than restoration of the continuity of the urinary system. Moreover, the opposite kidney may be, or may become, grossly deficient.

Prognosis.

Many ureterovaginal fistulas will heal if a ureteral catheter splint and an extraperitoneal drain are inserted promptly after the fistula is diagnosed. However, because serious, symptomatic ureteral stenosis and severe chronic urinary tract infection develop in the majority of cases, a reanastomosis procedure such as a ureteroneocystostomy, which ordinarily heals and functions well, is preferred.

Very small vesicovaginal fistulas often close spontaneously if the bladder can be kept collapsed and infection prevented.

Urethral fistulas are notoriously resistant to spontaneous closure if a urethral catheter is employed. Many heal well, however, if simply repaired and if cystostomy is used instead of a urethral catheter.

Only minor strictures of the urethra and ureter can be widened with bougie dilatation. Extensive scarring will require a plastic or reanastomosis operation.

INTESTINAL INJURIES IN OBSTETRIC & GYNECOLOGIC SURGERY

Surgical accidents such as laceration, incision, crushing, or puncture of the intestine may be discovered at operation or soon thereafter. Such injury is usually associated with distortion, unusual displacement of the abdominal contents, poor exposure, lack of surgical knowledge, or haste. Most operative damage occurs with pelvic tumor, chronic inflammation, or after previous surgery. About 5% of gynecologic operations involve primary or secondary bowel surgery.

Adherence of the intestine to the abdominal wall, dense organized adhesions, a large neoplasm, extensive infection, and endometriosis increase the hazard of injury to the gut. Sharp or blunt separation may be causal, but poor differentiation of margins of adherent organs always complicates dissection. Postoperative bleeding and infection follow extensive, initially unrecognized intestinal trauma. Even if a defect is closed at surgery, it may bleed or leak later. Peritonitis, pelvic abscess, fecal fistula, evisceration, septic embolization, and death are the sequelae.

Fever, severe anorexia, nausea and vomiting, abdominal pain, distention, tenderness, and guarding develop a few days after the complicated operation. A vague abdominal mass may be outlined. Spreading sepsis, purulent or fecal drainage from the incision, or dehiscence often follow 7-10 days after surgery. Laboratory tests indicate an acute infectious process; anemia may be evident. X-ray studies are rarely diagnostic. Moreover, the introduction of a contrast medium may enlarge the intestinal defect.

The differential diagnosis includes incisional, urinary, or respiratory infection and intestinal obstruction.

In serious surgical intestinal injury cases, especially those involving the colon, complete bed rest in Fowler's position must be instituted. Other measures include initiation of gastric suction, establishment of fluid and electrolyte balance by parenteral means, replacement of blood loss, and administration of antibiotics such as penicillin and streptomycin. Enemas are contraindicated. Analgesics should be provided until bowel function is reestablished (in about 10 days).

The bowel should be inspected at surgery, bleeding controlled, and defects repaired. The suture line must be transverse, never longitudinal, or circular constriction will result. Interrupted intestinal nonabsorbable sutures are preferred.

In wounds of the serosa and the muscularis, a single row of sutures will suffice. One or 2 mattress sutures will generally close puncture wounds satisfactorily.

When the mucosa of the bowel has been opened, contamination of the peritoneal cavity should be assumed and spill limited by suction, laparotomy packs, and elevation of the edges of the defect. Two layers of sutures should be employed: the first in the muscularis, and the second in the superficial muscularis and serosa. A Penrose-type drain is inserted through a stab incision to the site of repair.

When widespread bowel damage or its invasion by tumor is noted, segmental resection, "aseptic anastomosis," and drainage should be considered, if feasible. Repair of the bowel, proximal tube enterostomy, peritoneal drainage, and later definitive surgery may be necessary for poor-risk patients.

If intestinal obstruction or dehiscence develops, the problem is corrected by re-operation. A "pointing" pelvic abscess is drained transvaginally or extraperitoneally. Critical sepsis is much more likely from an injury to the large bowel rather than the small bowel.

When spreading peritonitis or large pelvic abscess develops, the prognosis becomes grave.

25...
Abnormalities of Menstruation

ABNORMAL UTERINE BLEEDING

Abnormal uterine bleeding refers to both menstrual and nonmenstrual disturbances. The former include uterine bleeding in excess of the normal period or prolonged beyond 7 days at the expected time of the menses (hypermenorrhea, menorrhagia), and uterine bleeding more often than at intervals of 24 days (polymenorrhea). The latter include irregular flow at times other than the menstrual period (metrorrhagia).

Abnormal uterine bleeding is a matter of concern to almost all women at some time from the menarche to the menopause. The bleeding is always annoying, often debilitating, and occasionally critical. Accurate diagnosis and prompt therapy are mandatory for the maintenance of good health.

Abnormal uterine bleeding may result from local or systemic disorders and from psychogenic causes. It often is presumed to be caused by an enlarged, irregular uterus or an adnexal tumor. Additional studies or curettage often disclose an entirely different but serious abnormality as the cause. The amount and periodicity of blood loss are important measures of menstrual function. Regular menstrual periods of average flow are generally ovulatory; abnormal uterine bleeding should not be ascribed to ovulation or anovulation without knowledge of the patient's history, physical examination, and laboratory studies.

Hypermenorrhea (menorrhagia) may be caused by myoma, endometrial polyposis, irregular shedding of the endometrium, functional hypertrophy of the uterus, blood dyscrasias, and psychic problems. Polymenorrhea may be due to a short cycle (proliferative phase less than 10 days or secretory phase less than 14 days) or to premature interruption of the bleeding cycle due to physical or emotional stress. Metrorrhagia may be due to hormonal imbalance or miscellaneous pelvic abnormalities. Hormonal causes include endometrial hyperplasia, ovulation bleeding ("mittelschmerz"), excessive estrogen administration, anovulatory bleeding, and hypo- or hyperthyroidism. Pelvic disorders which cause metrorrhagia include disturbed pregnancy (abortion, hydatidiform mole, chorio-epithelioma); cervical and endometrial polyposis; submucous myoma; carcinoma or sarcoma of the cervix, corpus uteri, or fallopian tubes; and endometritis (postabortal or due to tuberculosis or cervical stenosis).

Clinical Findings.

A. Symptoms and Signs: The symptoms are best revealed by the history, which includes the type, amount, and duration of flow, character of related pain, last menstrual period (LMP), and previous menstrual period (PMP). The patient's general health, previous illnesses, surgery, and accidents are described. Congenital development and metabolic abnormalities and bleeding tendencies in relatives are recorded. The menstrual record is reviewed: menarche; usual interval; average duration; amount of flow; discomfort before, during, and after menstruation; previous leukorrhea, pruritus, and intermenstrual bleeding. All medications taken, including those for the control of abnormal uterine bleeding, must be identified: estrogens may increase bleeding; androgens may suppress the flow. The ovary produces measurable steroid sex hormones until about age 65. Ovarian function should not be eliminated or reduced simply to control uterine bleeding. Continued ovarian function protects against coronary sclerosis, vulvovaginitis, urinary tract infections, and osteoporosis.

Significant signs include the following: edema and increased vascular patterns of the abdomen and lower extremities due to venous obstruction; fullness of the abdomen due to enlarged organs, tumors, or fluid; tenderness and guarding of the abdominal wall due to inflammation, pulsion, traction, torsion, and obstruction; dullness due to inflammatory or neoplastic process; shifting dullness due to ascites; herniation, often due to tumor or fluid; distinctive cutaneous lesions due to obscure vulvovaginal abnormalities; adenopathy due to infection or neoplasia; swelling, tenderness, or discharge from Skene's or Bartholin's glands due to infection or tumor; and deformity and altered reflexes due to the cause of abdominal and back discomfort.

Rectovaginal examination may reveal tenderness, induration, nodulation, mass formation, and the presence of peritoneal fluid. A separate rectal examination may confirm, modify, or reject previous impressions.

B. Laboratory Findings: Vaginal smears should be obtained before digital examination for cytologic and bacteriologic study. Vaginal smears taken during active bleeding and fixed in alcohol-ether can be laked of red cells after fixation by applying 1% hydrochloric acid. The epithelial detritus which remains may reveal tumor cells or trophoblastic squamae from a uterine abortion.

Table* 25-1. Diagnosis of hematologic causes of abnormal uterine bleeding.

	Thrombasthenia, Pseudohemophilia	Idiopathic Thrombocytopenic Purpuras	Secondary or Symptomatic Purpura
Coagulation time	Normal	Normal	Normal
Clot retraction	Decreased	Slow, poor	Slow, poor
Platelet count	Normal	Very low	Decreased
Bleeding time	Increased	Increased	Increased
Capillary fragility	Increased	Increased	Increased

*Adapted from Krupp & others, Physician's Handbook, 14th ed. Lange Medical Publications, 1966.

Scrapings or biopsies of ulcerated or hyperplastic areas in the vaginal canal and cervix are secured. Application of Schiller's or Lugol's iodine solution will identify abnormal zones. Other tests should include Hct, urinalysis, and STS. Systemic diseases, some of which are revealed as bleeding diatheses, may be disclosed by the bleeding time, clotting time, clot retraction time, leukocyte and platelet counts, and tourniquet test for capillary resistance. (See Table 25-1.) Infection and leukemia also may be determined by a white count with differential and sedimentation rate.

Leukorrheal discharges should be investigated for trichomonads, Candida organisms, Neisseria gonorrhoeae, and Hemophilus vaginalis. Abnormal thyroid function should be appraised.

C. X-Ray Findings: A flat film of the abdomen, hysterosalpingography, cystography, and barium enema studies of the abdomen may reveal tumors, fluid levels, and distortions. Roentgenograms are ordered only when abnormalities are suspected.

D. Special Examinations: An examination under anesthesia, biopsy, and surgical curettage will usually be necessary to establish the diagnosis, e.g., occult neoplasm, polyps, or submucous fibroids. Cancer of the cervix or endometrium may be revealed by a cone or four-quadrant biopsy of the cervix and differential curettage of the cervix and uterus.

Complications.

Continued or excessive blood loss leads to anemia which, in turn, often is followed by local as well as systemic infec-

602 Abnormal Uterine Bleeding

tion. Neoplasms cause bleeding, discharge, pain, and infertility. Cancer developing in the cervix, uterus, and tubes may be lethal when delay in diagnosis and treatment is permitted.

Prevention.

Periodic medical and gynecologic evaluation and early treatment of diseases capable of causing uterine hemorrhage will prevent many cases of abnormal uterine bleeding.

Treatment.

A. Emergency Measures: For acute blood loss the patient is placed in the Trendelenburg position and sedation, intravenous fluids, and blood transfusions are given. Hemostasis is achieved by surgical dilatation and curettage. This procedure is both diagnostic and therapeutic.

Excessive uterine bleeding due to almost any cause may be checked temporarily (1-2 days) with hormonal preparations. The choice of medication is determined by the condition of the endometrium, the severity of bleeding, and the availability of drugs.

The steroid sex hormones check bleeding by suppressing pituitary production of gonadotropins and reducing endometrial vascular dilatation and permeability. Large doses will modify the morphology of the endometrium strikingly after 1-2 days.

Progesterone lack during a late menstrual cycle allows irregular, profuse, or prolonged bleeding in cases of unopposed estrogen stimulation. Thus, anovulatory bleeding is controlled by progesterone. Estrogens may be administered for several weeks prior to and during progesterone therapy to prevent early break-through bleeding.

Androgen therapy is not advised for adolescent or young adult women. Acne, irreversible hirsutism, and permanent voice change often result even when the dosage of methyltestosterone (or its equivalent) is kept below 200-300 mg/month. This medication should be used only in later life, if at all.

Pitressin exerts an oxytocic effect in the nonpregnant patient but does not alter the character of the endometrium. This hormone is valuable when bleeding must be checked for 1-2 days prior to curettage.

The following hormonal preparations will control hemorrhage in selected cases:
1. Diethylstilbestrol, 25 mg orally every 15 minutes for 8 doses or 100 mg I.M. twice a day for 2 days.
2. Norethynodrel with mestranol (Enovid®), 15 mg orally daily for 2 days.
3. Norethindrone (Norlutin®), 15 mg orally daily for 2 days.
4. Medroxyprogesterone acetate (Provera®), 7.5 mg orally daily for 2 days.
5. Conjugated estrogens (equine) (Premarin®), 20 mg I.V.

Abnormal Uterine Bleeding 603

     6. Testosterone enanthate (Delatestryl®), 200 mg I. M.
     7. Deladumone® (testosterone enanthate, 90 mg, and estradiol valerate, 4 mg), 1 ml I. M.
     8. Estradiol diproprionate (Ovocylin®), 2.5 mg I. M.
     9. Estradiol benzoate (Progynon®), 1.6 mg I. M., and estradiol valerate (Delestrogen®), 20 mg I. M.
    10. Pitressin tannate in oil, 10 pressor units (2 ml) I. M. (Shake well to suspend active principle.)

B. Specific Measures: After biopsy and curettage the following routines may be employed for several months for the control of further bleeding:

1. Estrogens and progestogens - To control hypermenorrhea (not metrorrhagia) the following may be used: Progesterone aqueous suspension, 35 mg I. M. on the 24th day after the onset of the last period; hydroxyprogesterone caproate (Delalutin®), 125 mg I. M. on the 21st day; norethindrone (Norlutin®), 10 mg orally daily for 7 days beginning on the 21st day; norethynodrel with mestranol (Enovid®), 10 mg orally daily for 7 days, beginning on the 21st day; and medroxyprogesterone acetate (Provera®), 5 mg orally daily for 4 days beginning on the 21st day.

2. Androgens - After age 45, androgenic substances may be administered following biopsy and curettage to check abnormal bleeding, increase libido, and enhance anabolism. Side effects may appear, and one should be aware of their development. The following routine may be used: Testosterone enanthate (Delatestryl®), 200 mg I. M.; after 10 days, methyltestosterone, 10 mg sublingually daily for 2 weeks; medication is discontinued for 7 days; then methyltestosterone, 10 mg sublingually every other day for 3 weeks of each month for 2 months.

3. Thyroid hormone - Hypermenorrhea and metrorrhagia often are noted in hypothyroidism. Oligomenorrhea or amenorrhea accompanies hyperthyroidism if the periods are altered. Thyroid hormone will improve menstrual function if a deficiency in thyroid hormone production is the only problem. It should not be used for all patients with abnormal menstrual periods. Euthyroid individuals may be harmed by this medication. Endogenous thyroxin production is suppressed during and for several weeks after thyroid therapy.

4. Chorionic gonadotropin - A short postovulatory phase can be extended by the administration of chorionic gonadotropic hormone, 1000-2000 units I. M. daily for 12 days following ovulation. This may increase fertility by extending the luteal phase.

5. Adrenal cortical hormones - The Stein-Leventhal syndrome may be treated with prednisone, 5 mg (or equivalent) orally daily for 2-3 months. The corticosteroids

are not indicated in patients who have excessive or
intermenstrual bleeding.
6. Irradiation - X-ray and radium therapy should be
reserved for poor risk or menopausal patients. In
complicated cases, this can be done under local anesthesia. Limited irradiation in the amount required
for biologic sterilization varies directly with ovarian
functional capacity and age. In women under 35 years
of age, approximately 1250 r to the ovaries will be
required; over age 35, 800 r will usually suffice.
C. Surgical Measures: Surgical curettage may reveal polyps,
submucous myomas, and abnormal endometrium. Intractable abnormal uterine bleeding, particularly after age
40, may require hysterectomy, but conservation of normal appearing ovaries is preferred.

Prognosis.

In the absence of cancer, large tumors, or salpingitis,
about 50% of patients with hypermenorrhea and almost 60% of
patients with metrorrhagia will resume normal menstrual
periods after curettage alone. The addition of thyroid hormone or progesterone, when indicated, will increase the recoveries by an additional 10-15%.

POSTMENOPAUSAL VAGINAL BLEEDING

Postmenopausal vaginal bleeding is abnormal sanguineous
flow from the generative tract 6 months or more following
cessation of menstrual function. The type, amount, and duration of bleeding are unrelated to the cause. Local pelvic disorders of systemic diseases are etiologic, and bleeding may be
derived from malignant lesions anywhere in the generative
tract.

Pelvic cancer is the most serious etiologic factor. Cancer
of the cervix or endometrium accounts for 35-50% of cases.
Other causes, in approximate order of frequency, include excessive or prolonged estrogen administration, atrophic vaginitis, physical injury, cervical or endometrial polyposis, hypertensive cardiovascular disease, submucous myomas, trophic
ulcers of the cervix associated with prolapse of the uterus,
blood dyscrasias, and endogenous estrogen produced by feminizing ovarian tumor.

Postmenopausal women, like premenopausal women, may
bleed from any type of endometrium. One can divide endometrium obtained from postmenopausal women into 3 basic types:
(1) functioning (implying hormone stimulation), (2) nonfunctioning (inactive, atrophic), and (3) malignant (cancerous).
Many endometrial specimens obtained from postmenopausal
patients will be actively proliferative. The most exaggerated
variety is cystic glandular hyperplasia displaying unequal

glandular development, edema of the stroma, and augmented vascularity. The relative number of benign mitotic figures in the endometrium is a good index of estrogen stimulation.

Adenomatous or atypical hyperplasia of the endometrium is diagnosed occasionally. Disparity in the size and shape of the glands with invaginations and pseudostratification of the glandular epithelium and slight to moderate activity of the stroma are characteristic. No positive evidence of malignant change is present in this type of specimen. Whether this endometrial pattern represents a neoplastic trend, a "premalignancy," or overactivity is still being debated. Nevertheless, atypical hyperplasia and actual adenocarcinoma are occasionally discovered together. Whether this is coincidence or progression to cancer is not known. Inactive endometrium is atrophic or senile. Some dilatation of the glands occurs, but a decadent epithelium and a sparse, shrunken stroma is the rule.

Bleeding from a proliferative or hyperplastic endometrium probably occurs as the result of a sudden, marked fall in the blood estrogen level. Hormone fluctuations are due to metabolic alterations of production or to degradation. Exclusive of therapeutic estrogen hormone withdrawal, these variations in hormone titer are unpredictable.

There is ample proof of postmenopausal endocrine activity (vaginal cytology, endometrial histology, and blood and urinary sex steroid assay). The production of estrogen probably continues in the ovary for 10-15 years after cessation of the menses. In addition, even small granulosa or theca cell tumors may produce large amounts of estrogen during the climacteric. The adrenal cortex also develops gonadal-type steroids. Exogenous or endogenous estrogens may account for postmenopausal endometrial activity and subsequent bleeding.

Accessory causes of bleeding from any type of endometrium include (1) infection, (2) vascular fragility, and (3) varices or congenital vascular anomalies.

Bleeding from an atrophic endometrium is often due to a senile thinning of the functionalis layers to virtually expose capillary loops which may rupture during episodes of increased intravascular pressure, especially with hypertensive cardiovascular disease.

A benign polyp bleeds from its surface or pedicle as the result of mechanical trauma, circulatory disturbances, and infection. Torsion and infection explain bleeding from submucous myomas.

Adenocarcinoma may be focal or extensive. With the exception of early, "in-situ" cancers, the midzonal and basilar layers are usually involved in adenocarcinoma. Anaplasia and pleomorphism will be present. Carcinomatous invasion of vascular channels and sterile as well as bacterial necrosis may account for bleeding in cancer patients. Carcinogenesis by therapeutic doses of steroids is unlikely, but estrogen may create a favorable environment for the development of cancer induced by other (unknown) agents. There is no evidence that either parity or nulliparity predisposes to postmenopausal vaginal bleeding.

Clinical Findings.
A. Symptoms and Signs: Postmenopausal vaginal bleeding may be painless or painful. Discomfort depends upon the patency of the cervix, the amount and rapidity of blood loss, the presence of infection, or torsion of a tumor. Bleeding varies from a bright ooze or brownish discharge to frank hemorrhage. Patients may report a single episode of spotting or profuse bleeding for days to months.
B. Laboratory Findings: Vaginal cytology may disclose the presence of exfoliated neoplastic cells, infectious organisms (e.g., trichomonads, Candida, bacteria) diagnostic of specific forms of vaginitis, or free basal cells and white cells (but no cornified epithelial cells). This indicates probable vaginal atrophy or infection.
C. Special Examinations: Passage of a sound through the cervix into the uterus will demonstrate cervical stenosis and hematocolpos; will cause an intracervical or endometrial cancer to bleed (Clark's test); or may outline a cervical or uterine tumor. An aspiration biopsy or suction curettage often provides adequate endometrial tissue to diagnose cancer, endometrial hyperplasia, or endometritis.

Complications.
Although it is not known whether atypical endometrial hyperplasia can or will progress to adenocarcinoma, persistence or recurrence of atypical hyperplasia after thorough curettage may presage cancer. Failure to diagnose a pelvic carcinoma or to adequately treat a malignancy may be a fatal mistake. Unsuccessful therapy of a genital or urinary tract infection may lead to abscess formation or septicemia. Neglect of a functional granulosa cell tumor of the ovary may permit its growth and the development of malignant characteristics.

Differential Diagnosis.
Blood may originate from a disease process in the lower genital tract. Bleeding from the urethra (caruncle, carcinoma of the urethra or bladder) or from the anus (hemorrhoids, fissure in ano, cancer) may be erroneously reported as vaginal hemorrhage.

When a postmenopausal patient is receiving unspecified medication for "nervousness," flushes, or arthritis, exogenous estrogen therapy must be considered and the drug identified. Estrogens may cause break-through bleeding when prescribed in uninterrupted dosage.

A functional ovarian tumor or carcinoma of the fallopian tube may cause bleeding but may not be palpable.

Prevention.

Periodic (6-12 months) vaginal smears and gynecologic examinations should be arranged and indiscriminate, continuous, or excessive estrogen treatment avoided. Examination under anesthesia and surgical curettage are important when repeated vaginal smears are reported class III or IV. Intracavitary radium should not be used for "benign" causes when bleeding is uncontrolled by dilatation and curettage. Inadequate, improperly applied irradiation therapy may palliate, but not eliminate, an occult cancer missed at previous surgery. Another dilatation and curettage is required.

Treatment.

Treatment depends upon the etiology of bleeding. Surgical dilatation and curettage, together with polypectomy when indicated, is sufficient operative treatment for almost two-thirds of patients with the complaint of postmenopausal vaginal bleeding.

A. Emergency Measures: The patient should be hospitalized at once for hemorrhage and all possible causes of bleeding investigated. A dilatation and curettage is performed if bleeding is coming from above the external cervical os. The site of bleeding is biopsied and sutured if it is ulcerative or tumorous.
B. Specific and Surgical Measures:
  1. All steroid sex hormone therapy must be discontinued until bleeding has been explained and checked for at least 3 months.
  2. A complete gynecologic evaluation and urinary, gastrointestinal, and hematologic examinations are necessary to determine the cause of bleeding.
  3. Vaginal cytology and biopsies of vaginal or other lesions which may be cancer also are necessary.
  4. The cervix is coned and a differential curettage performed if bleeding is from the upper genital tract. If cancer is not found but endometrial hyperplasia is diagnosed, vaginal smears are obtained each month and curettage repeated in 3 months without hormone therapy.
  5. Laparotomy must be considered if an adnexal tumor is palpated in association with persistent endometrial hyperplasia (assuming no estrogen therapy).
  6. Cancer from any source requires definitive treatment.
  7. Total hysterectomy and bilateral salpingo-oophorectomy may be indicated for recurrent postmenopausal

bleeding after the second curettage (in the absence of estrogen therapy).
   8. If atrophic vaginitis alone is determined to be the cause of the bleeding, cyclic estrogen therapy is instituted.
C. Supportive Measures: Explanation, reassurance, and mild sedatives are important supportive measures for the anxious patient. Antibiotics, hematinics, and dietary supplements are ordered respectively for infection, anemia, and nutritional deficiency. Daily acetic acid vaginal douches are prescribed for clinical vaginitis.
D. Treatment of Complications: If uterine perforation occurs during curettage, bleeding into the peritoneal cavity, bladder, or rectum may occur, in which case a total abdominal hysterectomy may be required and other damage repaired. Infection is treated with antibiotics.

Prognosis.

Dilatation and curettage and estrogen therapy will generally correct postmenopausal vaginal bleeding in the absence of cancer or a feminizing ovarian tumor. The prognosis in women whose bleeding is due to severe neoplastic disease depends upon the extent of invasion and the success of antitumor therapy.

AMENORRHEA

Amenorrhea (failure to menstruate) is a symptom rather than a disease. Pregnancy is the most common cause. The regularity of the menses is a delicate index of physical and mental health and may be the first indication of a physiologic disorder. When menstrual periods have not begun by the 18th year, an abnormality may be assumed.

Amenorrhea is a common complaint. It may be categorized as "primary," when menarche has never occurred; or "secondary," when a previously established menstruation ceases. It may also be classified as physiologic or pathologic. Physiologic amenorrhea exists prior to puberty, during pregnancy and the puerperium, and after the menopause. The average age at menopause is 49; only about 5% of women cease to menstruate normally before age 40. Pathologic amenorrhea may follow malnutrition; tumors or metabolic disorders involving the pituitary, thyroid, adrenal, or ovary; and abnormal growth and development of the uterus, cervix, or vagina.

Menstruation is the end-point in a complex intraglandular coordination. Disorders involving one area of function will often be reflected in other areas with resultant amenorrhea. These are determined by a review of systems or levels of function as follows:

(1) Cortex and hypothalamus: Malnutrition, anorexia nervosa, depressive psychoses, stress, travel, schizophrenia, pseudocyesis.
(2) Pituitary: Chromophobe adenoma, Sheehan's disease, Simmonds' disease, eosinophilic adenoma, basophilic adenoma.
(3) Thyroid: Myxedema, Graves' disease.
(4) Adrenal: Addison's disease, Cushing's syndrome.
(5) Ovarian: Gonadal dysgenesis (Turner's syndrome), ovarian insufficiency (after surgery, infection, or irradiation), arrhenoblastoma, hilus cell tumor, Stein-Leventhal syndrome, granulosa-theca cell tumor.
(6) Uterine, cervical, vaginal: Congenital absence or obstruction (imperforate hymen), endometrial destruction (tuberculosis).

Clinical Findings.
A. Symptoms and Signs: Difficulties associated with amenorrhea can be elicited by a careful history, physical examination, and laboratory studies. Physical findings will be consonant with those referable to a particular disease or syndrome. The patient's age and her social, physical, and emotional status must be considered together with the physiologic and pathologic disorders which may result in amenorrhea. Both pregnancy and physiologic failure of ovarian function (menopause) must be considered before extensive diagnostic studies are begun.
B. Laboratory Findings: Diagnostic aids used in the study of amenorrhea are as follows: (1) electroencephalography for tumors or intracranial disorders; (2) follicle-stimulating hormone (FSH) determinations, which are low in pituitary deficiency and high in ovarian failure; (3) butanol-extractable iodine (BEI) or protein-bound iodine (PBI) studies to reveal thyroid dysfunction; (4) urinary 17-ketosteroid and pregnanediol levels to indicate adrenal or ovarian disease; (5) vaginal cytology to estimate the degree of estrogen stimulation (if a series is obtained, cyclic variations may be noted); (6) Aschheim-Zondek test to diagnose pregnancy, hydatidiform mole, or chorioepithelioma; (7) endometrial biopsy for determination of endometrial responsiveness to hormonal stimulation; (8) BBT determination for abnormalities in the menstrual cycle; (9) pregnanediol studies to elucidate hormonal function; (10) culdoscopy for determination of anatomic ovarian abnormalities; and (11) chromosomal studies, e.g., buccal or vaginal smear to clarify ovarian dysgenesis.
C. X-Ray Findings: Films of the sella turcica often reveal compression-atrophy of the clinoid process in pituitary tumor formation. Adrenal neoplasms frequently are visualized by intravenous urography or retroperitoneal

pneumography studies. Ovarian enlargement has been outlined by roentgenography after pneumoperitoneum. X-rays of other areas (e.g., chest) are ordered as indicated. Hysterosalpingography may be of value in outlining uterine abnormalities, but this test should be omitted if pregnancy is suspected.

D. Special Examinations: Visual fields should be plotted to note a constriction indicative of pituitary tumor.

The presence of adequate estrogen and a functional endometrium may be established by injecting progesterone (Delalutin®), 3 ml I. M., or equivalent. Uterine bleeding after 5-7 days constitutes a positive test. If bleeding does not occur, priming the endometrium with estrogens (diethylstilbestrol, 1 mg daily for 3 weeks) should cause withdrawal bleeding if the patient is hypoestrogenic and the endometrium is functional.

Treatment.

The objective of therapy is initiation of spontaneous ovulatory cycles and their continuance after treatment has stopped. Pregnancy often is the ultimate goal. A logical plan must be employed, because indiscriminate therapy may be useless or actually harmful.

The underlying cause of amenorrhea should be treated. In most instances, correction of the basic disorder will be followed by a return of the menses. Emotional status, dietary management, and adequate rest are all factors to consider in therapy. Treat thyroid hypo- or hyperfunction as indicated. Estrogens provide only psychic benefit (causing withdrawal bleeding) in pituitary or ovarian insufficiency. Mild adrenocorticism or the Stein-Leventhal syndrome may be treated with corticosteroids. Wedge resection of the ovaries also may be used for the Stein-Leventhal syndrome.

When no significant disease can be established in the premenopausal woman, prolonged administration of estrogens or progesterone to cause pituitary suppression may initiate a rebound phenomenon of recurring menstruation after steroid therapy has been discontinued.

Low voltage roentgen therapy to the pituitary or ovaries has proved beneficial in nonspecific, secondary amenorrheas of less than 6-12 months' duration. Animal derived gonadotropin therapy has been disappointing. Human pituitary gonadotropin is not yet available commercially. Clomiphene citrate (Clomid®), 50 mg daily orally for 5 days, may induce ovulation.

Prognosis.

Success in reestablishing menstruation in the nonpregnant woman is inversely proportionate to the duration of amenorrhea and the seriousness of the underlying disorder.

26...
The Menopause & Climacteric

Physiologic menopause, the gradual decline and, finally, cessation of menstruation, is an endocrine deficiency state which marks the termination of reproductive function in women. Natural or physiologic menopause due to ovarian aging occurs between the ages of 46-52 years, the mean age being 49 years in the USA. This represents an increase of about 5 years of reproductive life in the past century. Where health and nutritional standards are poor, the menopause or "change of life" may occur 5-10 years earlier. The time of onset and the termination of manifestations of natural menopause are unpredictable.

Artificial menopause may occur at any age after the menarche as the result of pituitary or ovarian destruction or ablation or devastating pelvic disease (e.g., tuberculosis).

The **climacteric** is the period following menopause, normally after middle age, when marked involution or deterioration (aging) due to sex hormone hypo- or dysfunction occurs. Actually the climacteric is evidence that anabolism and repair have not kept pace with catabolism.

Some authors use the terms menopause and climacteric synonymously. Others believe that the menopause is that period during the climacteric when ovarian function diminishes gradually, menstruation ceases, and the body undergoes marked involution. Although noticeable involution begins at about age 35 (e.g., stiffness of joints, skin wrinkles), these findings are only coincidentally related to menstrual function and certainly are not to be considered menopausal. Hence, it is this author's belief that the terms "menopause" and "climacteric" should be distinguished as defined above.

Although it is true that diminished ovarian function causes physical symptoms, cessation of menstruation does not itself impair physical capacity. Nevertheless, the menopause is emotionally disturbing and may cause psychosomatic complications. Fewer than 15% of women require therapy during the menopause, but many eventually seek medical treatment for disorders pertaining to the climacteric.

PHYSIOLOGIC MENOPAUSE

As a result of gonadal failure, the normal reciprocal relationship between the production of ovarian estrogens and progesterone and secretion of FSH changes at the menopause. Anovulation is common after age 40; therefore, no progesterone is produced. The declining estrogen titer releases the "brake" on the hypophysis; FSH then rises from the usual normal level of 5-50 mouse units to as high as 200 mouse units after the menopause.

Estrogen depletion is the most significant factor in the production of menopausal symptoms. Depletion generally occurs gradually following cessation of periodic ovulation in the mid-40's. Symptoms are most severe when the decline or elimination of estrogen occurs rapidly.

There is only a rough correlation between the alteration of normal plasma or urinary estrogen and FSH levels and the degree of discomfort reported by the patient. However, estrogen deprivation is undoubtedly the primary cause of such disorders as atrophic vaginitis and cystitis. Vasomotor symptoms generally are more severe in women with preexisting vasomotor instability. They are due to estrogen decline or increased circulating FSH (or both).

Women who are emotionally unstable before the menopause are prone to suffer more during this time than well-adjusted individuals. Prominent psychic factors may include the following: (1) Fear of loss of libido. Physiologic hormonal variation does not influence sexual desire in women; libido is emotionally determined. (2) Fear of obesity and unattractiveness. Weight gain in middle age is due to overeating and reduced physical activity, not to glandular aberrations. (3) Fear of being useless. Loss of reproductive function does not convert a woman into an "empty shell." Encourage her to seek absorbing, worthwhile diversions. (4) Fear of pregnancy associated with one or more missed menstrual periods may cause profound anxiety.

Clinical Findings.

The diagnosis of menopause cannot be made solely on the basis of menstrual aberration, "nervousness," and vasomotor symptoms; ovarian deficiency must be established by inspection and laboratory tests.
- A. Menopausal Symptoms and Signs: This discussion will include also those complaints commonly but inappropriately attributed to hormonal changes during this period of life.
    1. Alteration in menstrual flow - Irregular and occasionally profuse menstrual periods are common after age 40; they can generally be related to anovulatory cycles. Biopsy and curettage will rule out cancer and benign

tumors. Dysmenorrhea previously associated with ovulation stops.

2. Cessation of menses - Menstrual periods usually become irregular, with wider intervals, scanty flow, and episodes of amenorrhea (oligomenorrhea). Symptoms are apt to be more severe if the periods cease abruptly than when oligomenorrhea precedes cessation of menses.

3. Vasomotor flushes and flashes - These are the most distressing complaints immediately following the menopause. The patient describes a sensation of heat felt first in the epigastrium or over the chest, spreading suddenly over the entire body and accompanied by a facial flush or blush. These unpleasant sensations may occur many times an hour. Concomitant tachycardia and subsequent perspiration are frequent. Vasomotor disturbances occur at short intervals and are most disturbing at night and during periods of fatigue, illness, or emotional tension.

   With appropriate therapy, flushes can be reduced to an occasional mild sensation of warmth. Even with no treatment they usually cease after 1-2 years. However, in some women these symptoms persist until age 65-68. Recording the number of hot flushes experienced during a day permits an appraisal of the degree of disability or success of therapy.

4. Emotional instability - Signs and symptoms of emotional stress are most often due to preexisting psychiatric difficulties; they are not due to cessation of menstruation or estrogen lack and do not disappear when estrogen therapy is given. Fear of insanity is a major concern of some women during the menopause, but there is no physiologic basis for this fear.

5. Gastrointestinal symptoms - Bloating, flatulence, and constipation are commonly attributed to the menopause but are actually due to dietary or allergic factors or to gastrointestinal disease. Aerophagia may accompany anxiety.

6. Headaches - Tension headaches are common during this period but are not related to menopausal alterations. Refractive errors, sinusitis, and hypertension must be considered.

7. Palpitation, dyspnea, and vertigo are usually of emotional origin; hyperventilation may be the immediate cause. Rule out cardiorespiratory and intracranial disorders.

8. Atrophic vulvar and vaginal changes - Contracture of the introitus and thinning of the vulvovaginal tissues occur about 6 months after the menses cease. Irritation, vaginal dryness, and dyspareunia will promptly improve following appropriate estrogen therapy.

9. Local manifestations of depressed ovarian function - These include contracture of the vaginal introitus, pallor and thinning of the mucosa, atrophy of the rugae, loss of elasticity of the vagina, involution of the cervix, diminution of vaginal mucus, and reduced size of the uterus and ovaries.

B. Postmenopausal Symptoms and Signs: Estrogen lack is responsible for disorders which may not occur until one year or more after menstruation ceases.

1. Atrophic (senile) vaginitis - Diminished estrogen levels cause target organs to show variable atrophic changes: shrinkage of the labia and narrowing of the introitus (kraurosis), loss of rugae, blanching of the mucosa, and fissure formation and dryness of the vaginal canal.

2. Atrophic (senile) cystitis - The bladder and urethral mucosa are also responsive to estrogen; atrophy may occur in the lower urinary tract during the climacteric. Cystourethritis causes frequency, nocturia, and urgency—sometimes to the point of incontinence. Bacterial infections must also be considered.

3. Osteoporosis - Demineralization of the skeleton, particularly the vertebrae and long bones, occurs 3-5 years after cessation of menses. Decline in production of steroid sex hormones causes some rarefaction of bone, with the result that pathologic fractures may occur following trivial accidents, cough, or sudden rising to an erect posture. The lumbar vertebrae are most susceptible; fracture of the rarefied head or neck of the femur is also common. Inactivity and inadequate intake of protein and vitamin C are contributing factors.

The clinical symptoms of osteoporosis are back pain and disability upon movement. Backache (in the absence of fractures) may be due to contracture of the periarticular structures; compression of the cartilaginous intervertebral disks contributes to pain.

In advanced osteoporosis, x-ray studies reveal decreased density of bone due to demineralization of trabeculae, particularly in the vertebrae. The cortex may appear dense by comparison. Pathologic fractures of the vertebral bodies (due to compression) are identifiable radiologically.

The diagnosis of osteoporosis is supported by the Sulkowitch test for hypercalciuria.

The differential diagnosis must include radiculitis and osteoarthritis. Decalcification of bone also occurs in Cushing's syndrome, hyperthyroidism, hyperparathyroidism, multiple myeloma, metastatic carcinoma, and osteoporosis of disuse.

4. Arteriosclerosis and coronary heart disease - Degenerative vascular disorders develop when estrogen is

depleted. Coronary heart disease is rare in women prior to the menopause. It is less common in the climacteric in women who have received estrogen therapy.
 5. Skin and hair changes - The aging process after the menopause causes progressive wrinkling and thinning of the skin, loss of skin pigmentation, and hyperkeratosis. Slight generalized alopecia may be noted.
 6. Mental and emotional deterioration cannot properly be attributed to the climacteric.
C. Laboratory Findings: (Indicative of ovarian deficiency.)
 1. Vaginal cytology - Scanty mucus, fewer than 5% cornified cells, numerous basal cells and leukocytes (in the absence of specific infection).
 2. Pituitary gonadotropin (FSH) excretion of more than 100 mouse units per 24 hours.
 3. Endometrial biopsy revealing atrophic endometrium.

Differential Diagnosis.

Amenorrhea and depressed gonadal function may result from severe metabolic and psychic disorders such as adenohypophysial or adrenocortical insufficiency, anorexia nervosa, and myxedema. The incidence is low, but such patients are seriously ill and may present many medical problems.

Prevention of Senile Atrophic Changes.

The increasing longevity of women (American women lived an average of 47 years in 1900; 67 years in 1958) has placed greater importance on the need for continued prophylactic, cyclic sex steroid hormone therapy in the postmenopausal years. The aging changes that characterize this period of female life include the following: (1) Progressive attenuation of the genitalia and pelvic floor structures. (2) Osteoporosis (normal calcification but little bone). (3) Slowly developing kyphosis ("dowager's hump") due to muscle weakness, poor posture, and an attitude of "peering" due to failing vision. (4) Increased atherosclerosis and increased incidence of ischemic heart disease. (5) Keratodermia climactericum, seborrheic keratosis, and neurodermatitis.

Early and adequate steroid sex hormone therapy will usually reduce the extent of mucosal, muscular, fascial, osseous, and, frequently, vascular degenerative changes, but such therapy can only rarely prevent or reverse them. Women receiving sex hormone therapy in the postmenopausal years should receive periodic examinations of the thyroid gland, the breasts, and the female genital organs because endocrine administration may accelerate the growth of dormant malignancies in these anatomic areas.

Treatment.

Amelioration of discomfort and prevention of future disability must be achieved with a minimum of medication. Therapy should be governed by symptomatic responses, not by laboratory tests.

A. General Measures:
 1. Education - Explain the menopause and climacteric and allay unrealistic apprehensions. Reassure the patient that her enjoyment of life will continue as before.
 2. Sedation - Mild vasomotor symptoms can be controlled with phenobarbital, 15-30 mg (1/4-1/2 gr) 2-4 times daily. More severe discomfort is relieved by sedatives combined with antispasmodics. If barbiturates are contraindicated, prescribe glutethimide (Doriden®) or methylparafynol (Dormison®), 0.5 gm at bedtime for sleep. Tranquilizers will control anxiety, e.g., perphenazine (Trilafon®), 2-4 mg 3-4 times daily. Avoid giving dangerous amounts of tranquilizers and sedatives to depressed patients.
 3. Stimulants - The amphetamines relieve depression and increase energy. Give dextro amphetamine sulfate (Dexedrine®), 5 mg twice daily between meals.

B. Specific Measures: Estrogens and androgens both afford relief of menopausal symptoms due to hormonal imbalance, and both have a protein anabolic effect. The estrogens reduce vaginal irritation, contracture, and dryness. The androgens increase libido and have less tendency than estrogens to cause mastalgia and uterine bleeding. Neither hormone is carcinogenic, but estrogen-responsive malignant foci in the breast and endometrium may be stimulated by estrogens.
 1. Estrogens should be prescribed first. Administer the smallest oral cyclic dose which gives relief. Mastopathy and endometrial hyperplasia are thus avoided.

   An unusually sensitive endometrium may be induced to bleed after even minute doses of estrogen. If so, interrupt therapy for 3 months to see if bleeding continues and investigate the possibility of uterine cancer, polyps, or other local causes of bleeding.

   Because a postmenopausal woman will become a physiologic castrate without treatment, the physician should restore and maintain adequate hormone levels by endocrine therapy indefinitely unless contraindicated.

   Experimental studies suggest that protection against vascular deterioration is far more effective with natural conjugated estrogens than with individual natural or synthetic hormones. Nevertheless, all of these products will relieve other symptomatology in appropriate doses. Natural conjugated estrogens (Premarin®, Menagen®) should be given in a dosage of 0.625-1.25 mg orally every other day without a break, or the same dosage daily for 3 weeks each month followed by a rest period of one week. (A dosage of 1.25 mg of natural conjugated estrogens is comparable to diethylstilbestrol, 0.5 mg, or ethinyl estradiol, 0.05 mg.) Cumulative effects and signs of overdosage are uncommon.

Overdosage may be harmful. Parenteral estrogen is indicated only when the patient is in great distress and must have immediate relief, or when oral administration is not feasible. In such cases, prescribe depot estrogen such as estradiol valerate (Delestrogen®), 1 ml (10 mg) in lieu of the first 7 days of oral estrogen. A preliminary examination of the breasts and pelvis for tumors is required. Uterine bleeding is more likely to occur after depot estrogen because of the large initial dose and occasional rapid assimilation.

2. Androgens may be beneficial if estrogens cause mastalgia or uterine bleeding; if uterine fibroids, pelvic endometriosis, or cachexia is present; or if an increase in libido is considered desirable. Prescribe cautiously, because masculinization may occur. Methyltestosterone (buccal), 10 mg, approximates the efficacy of diethylstilbestrol, 0.5 mg, in the immediate postmenopausal years; however, individual variation in response cannot be predicted.
3. Combined estrogen-androgen therapy controls symptomatology and minimizes the undesirable effects of both hormones. Commercial preparations containing half the usual individual dose of each may be obtained.
4. Local sex steroid therapy should be given for vulvovaginal or urinary disorders secondary to ovarian deficiency. Regional application of small doses of sex steroids will relieve pelvic symptoms without the undesirable effects of larger oral or parenteral doses.
   a. Local estrogens are available as diethylstilbestrol in suppositories, 0.1 and 0.5 mg; and diethylstilbestrol creams, 0.25 and 0.5 mg per gm.

   Atrophic vaginal and bladder symptoms will improve in about one month after regular nightly insertion of one vaginal suppository or application of 1 gm of cream for 3 weeks. A less expensive treatment is one diethylstilbestrol suppository, 0.5 mg, inserted every 5th day for 4 doses each month. The best suppositories are made of bases containing a minimum of petrolatum.
   b. Local androgens are available as linguets or buccalets of methyltestosterone, 5 or 10 mg. These highly compressed, slowly disintegrating tablets may be inserted vaginally with excellent results. (Estrogen-androgen equivalents determine the dosage.) Large doses and prolonged treatment must be avoided because of the general systemic effects.

618 Artificial Menopause

Satisfactory symptomatic and metabolic adjustments may be difficult to achieve, and sex steroid hormone therapy may have to be continued indefinitely—regardless of hormone contribution by the adrenal cortex. Be alert to the hazards of hormone deprivation in the aging woman.

C. Treatment of Osteoporosis:
1. General measures - Provide analgesics, e.g., codeine, 30 mg, or aspirin, 0.6 gm, every 4 hours as necessary, and braces or back supports for pain and fractures. Do not keep the patient in bed for protracted periods; further demineralization may ensue. A high protein, high vitamin diet is required. Additional calcium and phosphorus actually may be harmful because they predispose to nephrolithiasis.
2. Steroid therapy - Backache due to osteoporosis in the climacteric is ameliorated in 2-3 weeks after beginning estrogen or androgen therapy. Fractures naturally prolong discomfort. Although marked improvement usually follows therapy, x-ray films will not demonstrate increased bone density until later. Prolonged treatment is required. Interruption of treatment is often followed by recurrence of pain and further skeletal damage is likely.

Prognosis.

The prognosis for an uncomplicated, only mildly disturbing menopause and climacteric is excellent for the well-adjusted, informed woman. Neurotic patients or those who are intolerant of therapy (or for whom medication is contraindicated) may have to endure considerable distress before they "settle down" to a relatively more agreeable old age.

ARTIFICIAL MENOPAUSE

Oophorectomy or intense irradiation therapy to the pelvic viscera causes prompt onset of the menopause. The signs and symptoms of the climacteric develop premature (1-2 months after surgery or radiotherapy). Endocrine therapy must be instituted to prevent metabolic failures such as osteoporosis and coronary heart disease. The treatment of artificial menopause and its sequels is similar to that given for natural cessation of ovarian function. However, endocrine administration is contraindicated if endometriosis or carcinoma of the breast were the reasons for ovarian excision or irradiation.

The benefits of continued ovarian function far outweigh the alleged advantages of routine removal of ovaries after the age of 40 for surgical convenience or to avoid ovarian carcinoma.

27...
Infertility & Contraception

INFERTILITY

A couple is said to be infertile (1) if pregnancy does not result after one year of normal marital relations without contraceptives; (2) if the woman conceives but aborts repeatedly; or (3) if the woman bears one child but aborts repeatedly or fails to conceive thereafter.

Ten to 15% of marriages are childless. In about 40% of cases this is attributable to the male partner. Reproduction may occur when one individual with poor reproductive capacity marries another of greater than usual fertility; but when both partners are grossly infertile, reproduction is not likely to occur. Treatment may correct infertility but not sterility, which is the absolute inability to reproduce.

Infertility in the Female.

Ovulation and conception may occur at any time from the menarche to the menopause. Conception is most likely to occur during the period of reasonably regular ovulation, which begins after adolescence and usually terminates about 5-8 years before the menopause. Normal pregnancy and delivery of a viable fetus depend upon the following sequence of events: (1) A fertile ovum is extruded from the ovary. (2) The ovum finds its way into the fallopian tube within a few hours. (3) Insemination occurs and the spermatozoa migrate to the tube. (4) Fertilization of the ovum occurs in the outer portion of the tube. (5) The fertilized, segmenting ovum implants and develops in a favorable site in the endometrium. (6) Maturation proceeds normally at least until viability.

Female infertility may be due to the following causes:

A. Nutritional: Hypovitaminosis, protein deficiency, and iron deficiency anemia may cause infertility.

B. Endocrine:
   1. Pituitary - Ovulation and pregnancy depend upon the normal production of thyrotropin, adrenocorticotropin, and the gonadotropins (FSH, LH, LTH). Secondary ovarian failure occurs when pituitary function is decreased or increased. Hypopituitarism may be due to circulatory collapse due to hemorrhage and pituitary necrosis (Sheehan's syndrome), granulomas, cysts

and tumors, starvation, and anemia. Pituitary cachexia (Simmonds' disease) is quite rare. Hyperpituitarism is most often due to benign adenoma.
   2. Thyroid - Hypothyroidism results in anovulation, infertility, and abortion. Hyperthyroidism causes infertility when it is severe enough to result in amenorrhea.
   3. Adrenal - Adrenocortical overactivity (Cushing's syndrome) reduces the occurrence of ovulation. Adrenal failure (Addison's disease) causes gonadal atrophy. Hypo- or hyperfunction of the adrenal medulla does not affect fertility.
C. Vaginal: Congenital vaginal anomalies (absence of vagina, gynatresia, imperforate or cribriform hymen, stenosis, septate vagina) prevent intromission and insemination. Vaginitis due to Hemophilus vaginalis, Trichomonas, or Candida infections causes leukorrhea, which reduces the viability of the spermatozoa.
D. Cervical:
   1. Developmental abnormalities ("pin-hole" or double cervix, incompetent cervical os) may prevent sperm migration or cervical containment of an established pregnancy.
   2. Cervical tumors (polyps, myomas) may partially occlude the passage of spermatozoa or cause a discharge which is inimical to spermatozoa.
   3. Cervicitis produces acid, viscid, sometimes purulent secretions which are noxious to spermatozoa. Staphylococci, streptococci, gonococci, Trichomonas, and mixed infections are the most common types.
E. Uterine:
   1. Congenital uterine anomalies (hypoplasia, bicornuate or septate uterus) prevent normal maturation to viability by reducing the capacity of the uterus.
   2. Uterine tumors (polyps, myomas) thin the endometrium, cause bleeding and discharge, alter the blood supply, and distort or reduce the capacity of the uterus.
   3. Endometrial disorders such as polyps, endometritis, or refractoriness to hormonal stimuli prevent nidation or development of pregnancy.
F. Tubal: Closure of the tubal lumen usually is due to infection. Congenital atresia and false passages also occur.
G. Ovarian:
   1. Congenital abnormalities (e.g., ovarian agenesis) cause primary ovarian failure.
   2. Infections of the ovaries cause infertility by extending the preovulatory phase and shortening or eliminating the secretory phase of the cycle. Thickening of the tunica ovarii caused by prolonged chronic infection prevents release of the ovum.
   3. Ovarian tumors may disrupt function or replace or destroy the ovary.

4. Endometriosis disorganizes and scars the ovary, impairing all ovarian function.
H. Psychic: Anorexia nervosa, apprehension or schizophrenia often causes anovulation and amenorrhea.
I. Coital: Douches, lubricants, or deodorant antiseptics may dilute, inactivate, or destroy spermatozoa.

Infertility in the Male.

Male reproductive ability begins at about age 16. After approximately age 45, fertility decreases, although men over 80 have fathered children.

Male infertility may be due to the following causes:
A. Coital: Incomplete vaginal penetration is caused by chordee, epispadias, hypospadias, or extreme obesity.
B. Spermatozoal Abnormalities: The normal values of spermatic fluid are as follows:

> Volume: 2.5-5 ml
> pH: 7.4
> Viscosity: Moderately thin after 30 minutes.
> Motility (at 75° F; 26.5 C): More than 70% motile at ejaculation; 60% at 2 hours; 25-40% at 6 hours; a few still active after 24 hours.
> Count: 50-120 million/ml
> Morphology: Fewer than 30% abnormal spermatozoal heads.

The fresh ejaculate is a whitish, semi-gelatinous fluid containing small opalescent flecks which contain most of the spermatazoa. The first portion of the ejaculate contains the largest number of spermatozoa per volume and the fewest abnormal forms. After 30 minutes, the specimen becomes homogeneous, translucent, and liquified. The presence of blood or pigment is an abnormal finding.

Spermatozoa survive longest in alkaline cervical secretions and are destroyed quickly if they remain in the acid vaginal fluid. The optimal pH for maintenance of spermatozoa is 8.5-9.0. Motility is arrested at pH 6.0, and motility does not return after spermatozoa have been exposed to a pH below 4.0.

Spermatozoa travel at a rate of about 1 cm/hour by their own propulsion. Proper direction is obtained by their tendency to swim against fluid currents and toward the alkaline, glycogenic medium of the upper genital tract. The spermatozoa enter the cervix, traverse the uterus, and are drawn toward the ovum by the ciliary activity of the tubal epithelium, which beat in the direction of the fimbria.

High fertility is assumed to exist when the spermatozoa count approaches 185 million/ml; low fertility is assumed to exist when there are fewer than 50 million active spermatozoa per ml. No definite minimum can be given, although conception is usually possible when the spermatozoa count is below 35 million/ml.

C. Testicular:
   1. Developmental deficiency - Agenesis of the testes is extraordinarily rare; small testes are present in Klinefelter's syndrome. Absence of the testes from the scrotum is usually due to cryptorchism, but migratory testes or physiologic ectopy must be considered. In 2% of postpuberal boys, both testes are cryptorchid, and these individuals are usually sterile at maturity. Unilateral cryptorchism does not affect fertility.
   2. Endocrine - Hypopituitarism, Cushing's disease, and pituitary basophilism cause infertility. Hypothyroidism is associated with infertility, but the reason is not known. Atrophy of the testes occurs in Addison's disease. In Klinefelter's syndrome infertility is due to failure of development of the seminiferous tubules. Cushing's syndrome causes suppression of spermatogenesis. Anemia and poorly controlled diabetes mellitus result in infertility for unexplained reasons.
   3. Infections - Fertility is reduced during and shortly after high fever. Mumps in prepuberal boys only rarely involves the testes; after puberty, mumps is complicated by orchitis in 20% of cases. If orchitis is bilateral, sterility usually results. Chronic debilitating infections (e.g., malaria, tuberculosis, brucellosis) cause temporary infertility.
   4. Physical injury - Irradiation, direct trauma to the testes, and reduced circulation following complicated herniorrhaphy or varicocele repair reduce or destroy testicular function.

D. Penis and Urethra: Congenital malformations or scarring may interfere with erection and intromission. Urethral stricture may prevent ejaculation.

E. Prostate and Seminal Vesicles: These organs produce the liquid vehicle for the spermatazoa; only 5% of the ejaculate is semen. Prostatic fluid contains fibrinogen and fibrinolysin, which cause initial coagulation in the ejaculate and its subsequent liquefaction. Infections of the prostate and seminal vesicles are determined by digital rectal examination and microscopic examination of the fluid expressed.

F. Epididymides and Vasa Deferentia: These structure are spermatozoa conduits from the testes to the seminal vesicles and provide nutritional or maturational spermatozoal factors. Most instances of mechanical obstruction (congenital, inflammatory, or traumatic) occur here. Varicocele and hydrocele may increase scrotal temperature and thus impair spermatozoal maturation.

Diagnostic Survey.

Successful treatment of infertility is possible only if an early and accurate diagnosis can be established. This requires an energetic and systematic approach by the clinician and the cooperation of both partners. Over a period of at least 3 months, with 4 office visits for the wife and 2-3 for the husband, both partners usually can be evaluated and the cause of infertility determined (see Table 27-1). Obscure or multiple causes of infertility may require more time and special technics of investigation.

Table 27-1. Suggested four-visit routine for evaluation of infertility.

	Wife	Husband
First visit	Joint discussion of problem of infertility.	
	Medical history. Explanation. Taking and recording of BBT.	Medical history. Explanation regarding semen collection and analysis.
Second visit (2-4 weeks later) at mid-cycle	Physical examination. Routine and indicated laboratory tests. Preliminary evaluation of BBT chart.	Physical examination. Routine and indicated Laboratory tests. Semen analysis discussed.
Third visit (4 weeks later)	Tubal insufflation (Rubin's test). Evaluation of BBT chart.	Repeat semen analysis if first was deficient.
Fourth visit (4 weeks later)	Spinnbarkeit and fern test. Sims-Huhner test. Repeat Rubin's test if first was unsuccessful.	
Later tests and procedures as indicated	Sex chromatin analysis. Hysterosalpingography when 2 Rubin tests indicate occlusion. Vaginal smear series. Endometrial biopsy. Culdoscopy. Laparotomy.	Testicular biopsy if indicated. Cystoscopy. Definitive genitourinary surgery. Thyroid tests. 17-Ketosteroid and FSH determinations.

624 Infertility

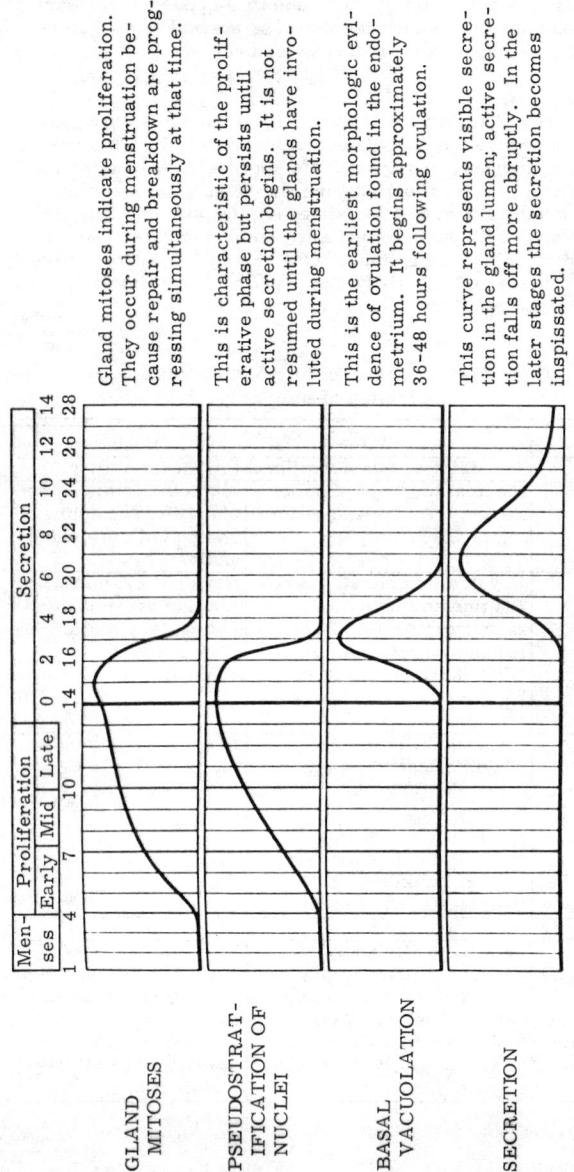

GLAND MITOSES — Gland mitoses indicate proliferation. They occur during menstruation because repair and breakdown are progressing simultaneously at that time.

PSEUDOSTRATIFICATION OF NUCLEI — This is characteristic of the proliferative phase but persists until active secretion begins. It is not resumed until the glands have involuted during menstruation.

BASAL VACUOLATION — This is the earliest morphologic evidence of ovulation found in the endometrium. It begins approximately 36-48 hours following ovulation.

SECRETION — This curve represents visible secretion in the gland lumen; active secretion falls off more abruptly. In the later stages the secretion becomes inspissated.

Fig 27-1. Dating the endometrium. (Approximate relationship of useful morphologic factors.) (Modified slightly after J. P. A. Latour and reproduced, with permission, from Noyes, Hertig, and Rock: Dating the **endometrial biopsy.** Fertil & Steril 1:3-25, 1950.)

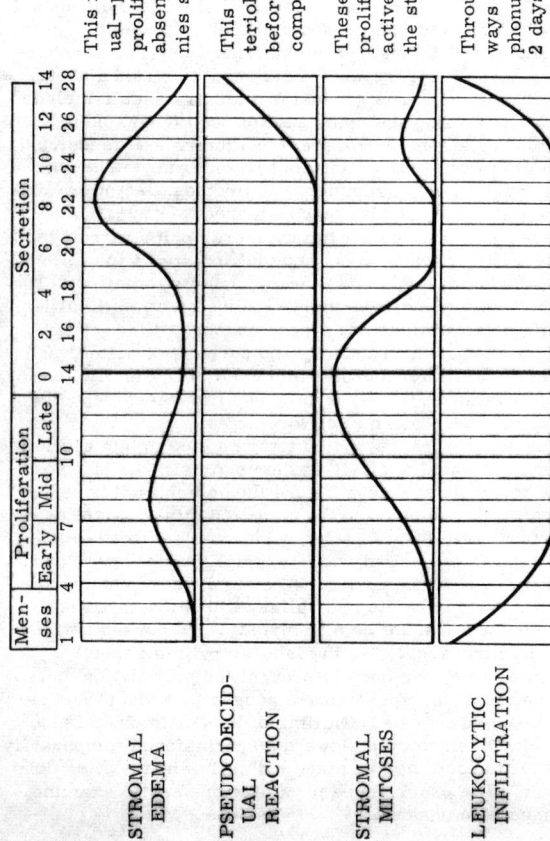

Infertility 625

		Description
STROMAL EDEMA		This factor varies with the individual—particularly the rise during proliferation, which may be almost absent. The edema which accompanies secretion is more constant.
PSEUDODECIDUAL REACTION		This is evident first around the arterioles and progresses until just before menstruation a superficial compact layer is formed.
STROMAL MITOSES		These are most abundant during the proliferative phase, absent during active secretion but reappear during the stage of predecidual formation.
LEUKOCYTIC INFILTRATION		Throughout the cycle there are always a few lymphocytes. Polymorphonuclear infiltration begins about 2 days before the onset of flow.

Fig 27-1. Dating the endometrium (cont'd.).
(Approximate relationship of useful morphologic factors.)

A. First Visit: (Wife and husband.) In a joint interview, the physician explains the problem of infertility and its causes to the husband and wife. Separate private consultations are then conducted, allowing appraisal of marital adjustments without embarrassment or criticism. Pertinent details (e.g., venereal disease or prior illegitimate pregnancies) must be obtained concerning marital, premarital, and extramarital sexual activities. A routine history should be taken. The couple's general health, temperament, diet, and habits should be evaluated, with special inquiry about endocrine problems and hormone therapy. The husband should be questioned regarding mumps; both patients should be asked about chronic infections, venereal diseases, anemia, and medical therapy for these. Past surgical procedures should be discussed. The wife should be asked about abdominal, pelvic, genital, and general surgery; the husband about herniorrhaphy and varicocele correction. Both should be asked about genital injuries. The gynecologic history should include queries regarding the menstrual pattern (e.g., pain, metrorrhagia, and leukorrhea) and the type of menstrual protection worn, either internal or external. The number of pregnancies, abortions, deliveries, lactation, and complications must also be considered. Occupational stresses and hazards of both partners, prior marriages and fertility, pregnancies, and previous tests for infertility, including tests and therapy, must be elicited. The present history includes marital adjustment, difficulties, use of contraceptives and types, douches, libido, sex technics, orgasm, frequency and success of coitus, and correlation of intercourse with ovulation. Family history includes familial traits, liabilities, illnesses, repeated abortions, and abnormal children.

The husband is instructed to bring a complete ejaculate for spermatozoal analysis at the next visit. Sexual abstinence for at least 4 days before the semen is obtained is emphasized. Semen may be collected either by coitus or masturbation. A clean, dry, wide-mouthed bottle for collection is preferred, but a vaginal (Doyle) spoon can be used. Condoms should not be employed, because residual rubber solvents and sulfur, which are noxious to spermatozoa, cannot be eliminated. The corked bottle should be transported to the laboratory in a paper bag held away from the body to prevent the stimulation and dissipation of the spermatozoa caused by warmth and reduced oxygen tension. Chilling of the bottle should also be avoided, since cold slows the spermatozoa temporarily.

Semen should be examined within 1-2 hours after collection. The experienced physician prefers to examine the specimen personally.

B. **Second Visit:** (Wife and husband; 2-4 weeks after first visit.) Abnormal findings are explained briefly but identification of one or the other partner as being responsible for lack of progeny must be avoided, for blame is invariably followed by guilt feelings and resentment. Both the husband and wife will often be found deficient in one or more details relating to infertility.

The woman receives a complete physical and pelvic examination. One must not overlook irritations, discharges, tenderness, maldevelopments, and masses. The rectovaginal examination must be meticulous. The husband's general physical examination, with emphasis on the genital and rectal examination, is done next. Penile, urethral, testicular, epididymal, and prostatic abnormalities are sought. The results of the spermatozoal analysis are explained to the couple without undue optimism or pessimism. Laboratory studies for both husband and wife include urinalysis, complete blood count (including Hct determination), and STS. Thyroid function should be determined.

C. **Third Visit:** (Wife; one month after second visit. The husband is not required to return for a third visit if his physical examination and initial semen analysis are normal.)

Tubal insufflation (Rubin test): Uterotubal insufflation in infertile patients has both diagnostic and therapeutic value. The test is a safe office procedure in properly selected patients if CO_2 is employed and if the pressure is kept below 200 mm Hg. Tubal insufflation at or about the time of ovulation is most likely to be revealing and successful. Pneumoperitoneum (and shoulder pain) is proof of tubal patency. Auscultation over the lower abdomen during insufflation may disclose the whistle of gas passing through one tubal ostium or the other. It is most helpful to secure a kymographic record of insufflation; tubal peristalsis, patency, leakage in the system, tubal spasm, partial obstruction, or release of tubal obstruction may be revealed in this way.

Tubal insufflation is indicated in the investigation of: (1) primary or secondary infertility (after male and other contributing factors have been ruled out), particularly in women who have recently had myomectomy, abortion, operation for ectopic pregnancy, salpingoplasty, appendectomy, and other disorders which may be complicated by tubal obstruction; and as a means of nonoperative tubolysis well after subsidence of salpingitis, appendicitis, etc. **Contraindications** are pregnancy, concurrent or recent genital tract infection, uterine bleeding due to any cause, recent dilatation and curettage, or other uterine surgery, and serious cardiopulmonary or neuropsychiatric disease.

628 Infertility

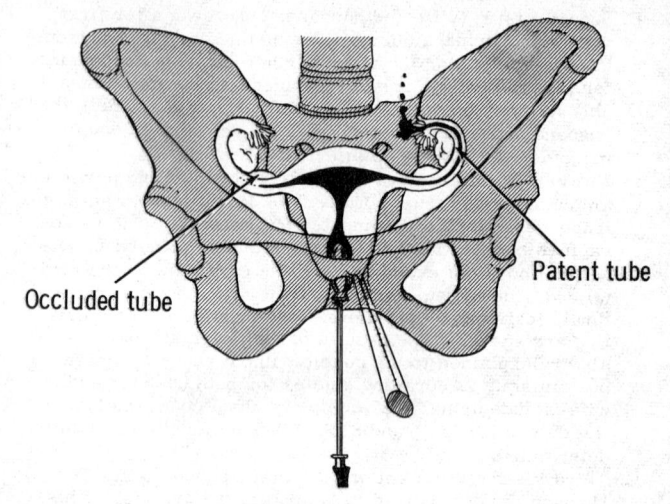

Fig 27-2. Tubal insufflation (Rubin test).

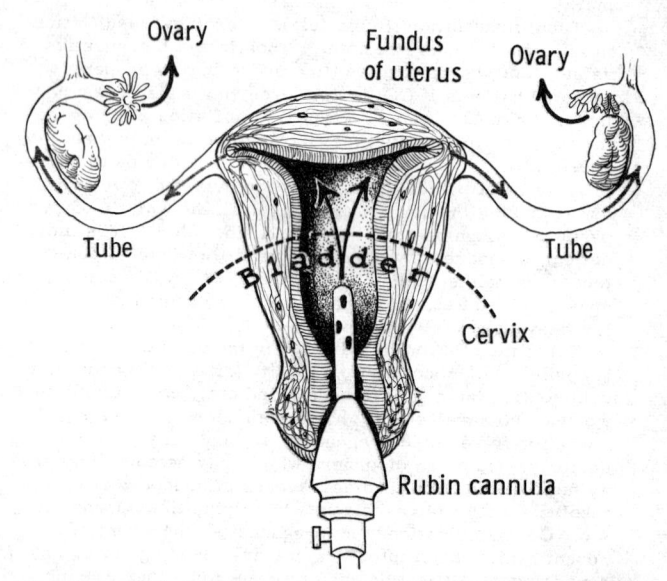

Fig 27-2. Tubal insufflation (Rubin test) (cont'd.). Front view showing dilatation of fallopian tubes.

Infertility 629

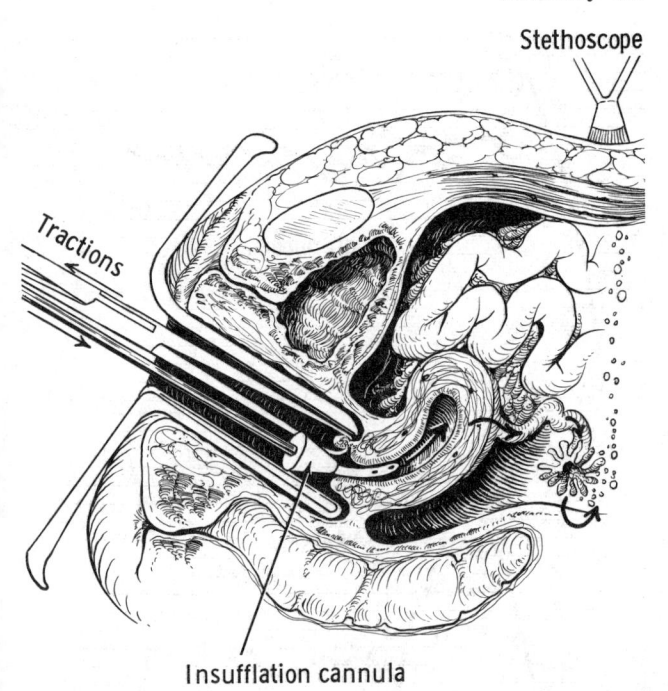

Fig 27-2. Tubal insufflation (Rubin test) (cont'd.).

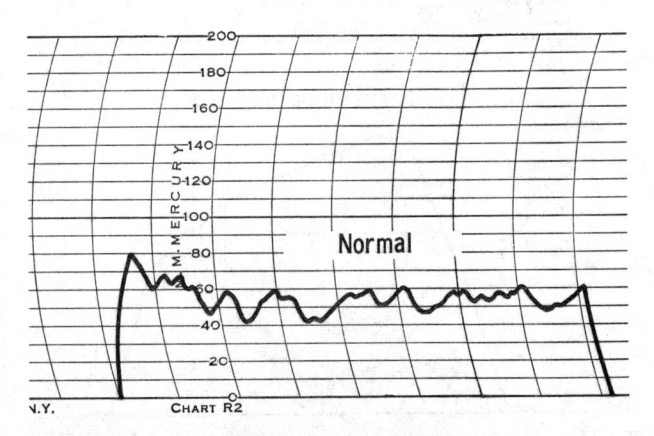

Fig 27-3. Normal kymographic record of insufflation.

630 Infertility

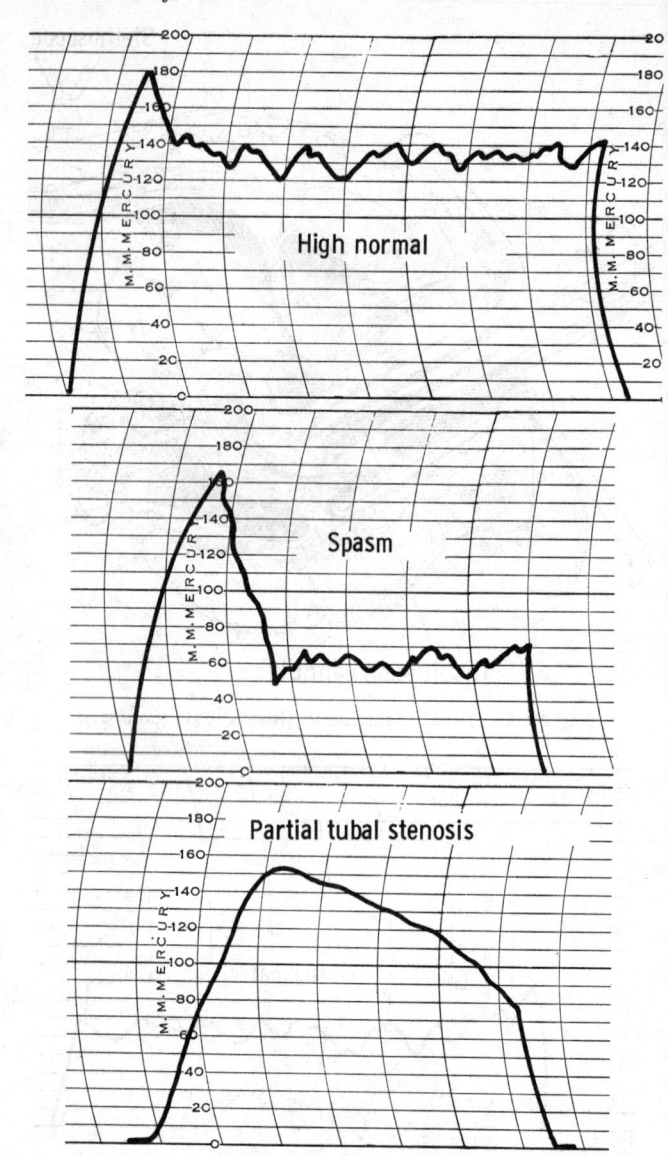

Fig 27-4. High normal and 2 abnormal records of insufflation.

Complications such as gas embolism, upper genital tract infection, tubal rupture, and hematoperitoneum may occur. Early pregnancy may be interrupted. Endometriosis may follow retrograde bleeding and ectopic implantation of endometrium. Peritoneal tuberculosis may occur as a result of spread of contamination from subclinical tuberculous salpingitis.

Repeated, successful tubal insufflation is known to enhance the likelihood of pregnancy.

Spermatozoal analysis is repeated on the third visit if the previous study was abnormal.

D. Fourth Visit: (Wife; one month following the third visit.) The patient returns just prior to ovulation within 6 hours after coitus. The cervical mucus should be thin, clear, and alkaline. Spinnbarkeit or elasticity is an expression of the viscosity of mucus. When a drop of cervical fluid is placed between 2 fingers, for example, the mucus will stretch into a thin strand when the fingers are separated slowly. The mucus is more viscid before and after ovulation. At the time of ovulation, the mucus can often be stretched 10 cm or more. Infection and bleeding also reduce spinnbarkeit. A good spinnbarkeit (stretching to a fine thread 4 cm or more in length) is desirable. A small drop of cervical mucus should be obtained, using a Knight or Kerner forceps, for the fern test and the Sims-Huhner test. The presence or absence of active sperms is noted. The presence in the cervical mucus of 10-15 active sperms per high power field constitutes a satisfactory Sims-Huhner test. The fern test should show clear arborizations: frond-like crystal patterns in the dried mucus. If no motile spermatazoa are found, the Sims-Huhner test should be repeated (assuming that active spermatozoa were present in the semen analysis).

E. Later Tests: (As indicated.) Testicular biopsy is indicated if azoospermia or oligospermia is present. A vaginal smear and an endometrial biopsy may be required to determine if ovulation is occurring. If tests of tubal patency were unsatisfactory, hysterosalpingography is done. Culdoscopy may be required if tubal adhesions or endometriosis are suspected. Laparotomy will be necessary for salpingostomy, lysis of adhesions, and removal of ovarian abnormalities. Sterility on the basis of disorders of the sex chromosomes should be ruled out by examination for "drumsticks" and sex chromatin analysis of desquamated buccal or vaginal cells.

Cystoscopy and catheterization of ejaculatory duct orifices, using a fluid x-ray contrast medium, may be required to demonstrate duct stenosis. Vasography by direct injection of the vas near its origin may demonstrate an occlusion. Needle aspiration of the upper pole of the

632 Infertility

epididymis (globus major) suggests inflammatory closure of the tract if no spermatozoa are recovered.

Treatment.

Treatment in all cases depends upon correction of the underlying disorder or disorders suspected of causing infertility.

A. Infertility in the Female:
1. Infertility due to nutritional deficiencies is frequently corrected by adequate well balanced diets and nutritional supplements.
2. Fertility may be restored by proper treatment in many patients with endocrine imbalance, particularly of hypo- or hyperthyroidism. Stimulation of ovulation by hormonal therapy in women with pituitary or ovarian failure has been most disappointing.
3. Psychotherapy may be of value in women who are fearful of pregnancy and when infertility is related to deep-seated psychiatric problems.
4. Surgical correction of congenital or acquired abnormalities (including tumors) of the lower genital tract or uterus may frequently restore fertility.
5. The alleviation of cervicitis is of value in the restoration of fertility.
6. Surgical excision of ovarian tumors or ovarian foci of endometriosis frequently restores fertility.
7. No treatment is effective for infertility due to marked uterine hypoplasia.
8. Surgical relief of tubal obstruction due to salpingitis will restore fertility in less than 20% of cases.
9. Congenital deficiency or absence of the ovaries is a hopeless sterility problem.
10. Perioophoritis defies medical and surgical treatment.

B. Infertility in the Male:
1. Surgical correction of congenital or acquired abnormalities of the penis and urethra may permit successful vaginal penetration and normal insemination.
2. Testicular hypofunction secondary to hypothyroidism or diabetes mellitus is often corrected by appropriate treatment.
3. Surgical correction of varicocele and hydrocele may restore fertility.
4. Mumps orchitis requires prompt testicular decompression by surgical excision of the tunica albuginea to preserve fertility.
5. Agenesis or dysgenesis of the testes resists all treatment.
6. Infertility due to prostatitis, seminal vesiculitis, and obstructions in the sperm conduit system rarely responds to treatment.

Contraception 633

Prognosis.
The prognosis for conception and normal pregnancy is good if minor (even multiple) disorders can be identified and treated early; poor if the causes of infertility are severe, untreatable, or of prolonged duration. If treatment is not successful within one year, the physician must consider whether he should recommend adoption.

CONTRACEPTION
(Birth Control)

The voluntary and temporary prevention of pregnancy may be indicated or desirable for any of the following reasons: Socioeconomic (spacing children to raise the standard of living and prevent overgrowth of population); medical (improving maternal health during the treatment for diseases such as tuberculosis, renal disease, diabetes); eugenic (avoiding the perpetuation of undesirable traits, e.g., hereditary diseases such as amaurotic familial idiocy); and personal (couples who do not wish children).

In the USA, the prescription, demonstration, and sale of contraceptives is illegal in Massachusetts and Connecticut. In many states, on the other hand, contraception clinics are a part of the public health program. In certain European countries, such as those in Scandinavia, contraceptive materials are sold openly; in Italy and Spain stringent laws prevent the dissemination of contraceptive information and materials. The Planned Parenthood Federation, originally organized by Mrs. Margaret Sanger, is active in many areas of the world to aid interested couples in family planning.

All faiths accept the principle of family planning; the Roman Catholic Church alone requires that this be accomplished by total abstinence or by abstinence during the ovulatory phase of the cycle ("rhythm method"). Protestants and Jews believe that fertility and contraception are providential powers to be used at man's discretion and that pregnancy should not be left to accident; they therefore recognize the couple's right to practice contraception with mechanical devices or in any other way that seems most acceptable to them.

The ideal contraceptive method is simple, acceptable, effective, safe, and economical. No one method has yet been devised which satisfies all of these criteria.

The following types of contraceptives are in current use:

(1) Biologic: Abstinence, including the "rhythm method"; coitus interruptus (onanism); hormonal suppression of ovulation; and tubal or ductal sterilization.

(2) Mechanical: Condoms and sheaths; cervical or intrauterine occlusion, e.g., pessaries, diaphragms, intrauterine devices.

634 Contraception

Table 27-2. Methods of Contraception

0 = none; 1 = poor; 2 = fair; 3 = good; 4 = excellent

Method	By	Acceptance	Effectiveness	Advantages	Disadvantages
Complete abstinence	F & M	0-1	4	No preparation. Accepted by Roman Catholic Church.	Unphysiologic, impractical.
"Rhythm" method Calendar BBT	F & M F & M	3 2	2-3 3-4	Accepted by Roman Catholic Church.	Precise instructions required. Couple must be intelligent, cooperative. Useless postpartum and when cycle is irregular.
Coitus interruptus	M	1	1	No preparation	Unphysiologic, frustrating, risky.
Estrogens	F	3-4	4	Oral tablets	Moderate to high cost. Precise dosage necessary. Steroids potentially dangerous to endocrine balance. Occasional hypermenorrhea and metrorrhagia.
Estrogen-progesterone comb. Enovid-E® C-Quens® Oracon®	F or M	3-4	4	Oral tablets	
Condom or membrane sheath	M	2	3-4	Simple. Prevents venereal disease.	Moderate cost. Impairs gratification.

Cervical cap pessary	F	2-3	3-4	Cap worn 2-3 weeks per month.	Fitting charge. Not applicable to women with rigid hymen, narrow vagina, or deformed cervix.
Diaphragm (only)	F	3	3	Simple, easy application.	Fitting charge. Less satisfactory with large cystocele, rectocele, descensus uteri.
Intrauterine devices	F	3	3-4	Device worn for years	Fitting charge. Cramping and menometrorrhagia. Acute or chronic endometritis and salpingitis in a few users.
Vaginal jelly, gel, cream, suppository (low surface-tension base)	F	3	3-4	Easy application	Moderate cost. May be too lubricating or irritating.
Vaginal foam	F	3	3-4	Simple, inexpensive	May be unaesthetic or irritating.
Douche	F	2	1	Inexpensive	Inconvenient. May be irritating.
Diaphragm and cream or jelly (high surface-tension base)	F	3	3-4	Combines 2 good methods	Fitting charge. Moderate cost.

636 Contraception

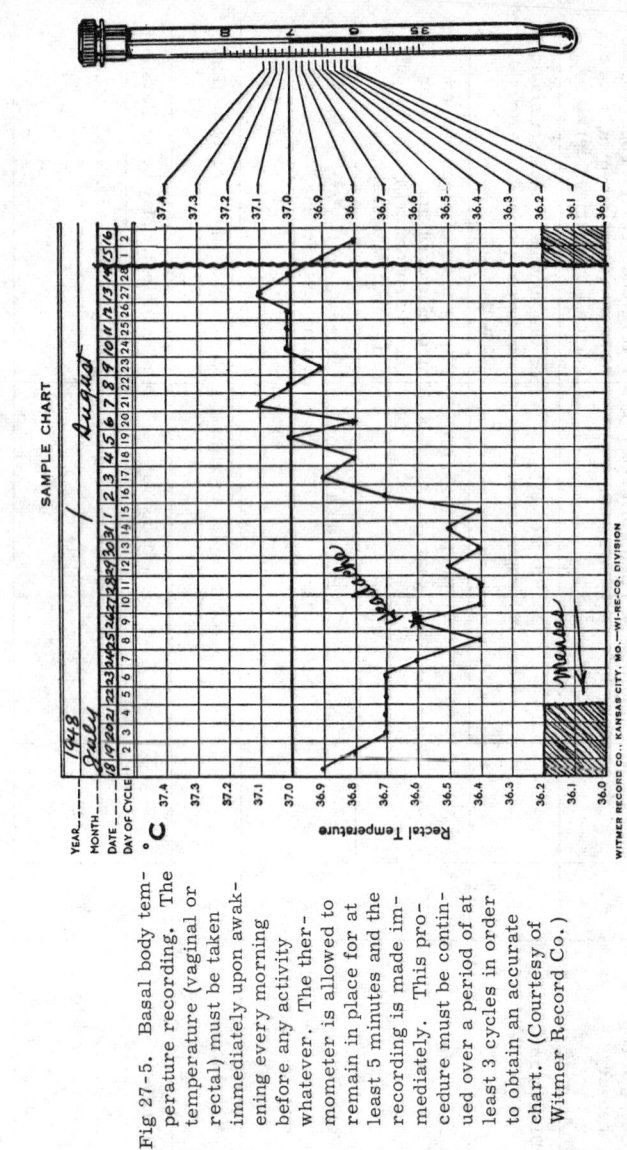

Fig 27-5. Basal body temperature recording. The temperature (vaginal or rectal) must be taken immediately upon awakening every morning before any activity whatever. The thermometer is allowed to remain in place for at least 5 minutes and the recording is made immediately. This procedure must be continued over a period of at least 3 cycles in order to obtain an accurate chart. (Courtesy of Witmer Record Co.)

(3) Chemical: Spermicidal jellies, gels, creams, and suppositories.

(4) Mechanical and chemical: Foam, powder and sponge, douches, diaphragm and cream or jelly.

(5) Immunologic methods are still investigational.

The acceptability, reliability, advantages, and disadvantages of the various types are summarized in Table 27-2.

Complete Abstinence.

If faithfully practiced, this is completely effective as a birth control method. However, it is unphysiologic and generally is unacceptable and impractical for most couples.

"Rhythm Method."

Ovulation occurs approximately 14 days before the onset of the next menstrual period regardless of the length of time between periods; when the cycle is regular, the time of ovulation (the "unsafe" period) can be anticipated.

The ovum and the sperms are probably fertile for about 24 hours. Coitus on the day of ovulation is most likely to result in pregnancy. If one allows 2 days of abstinence before ovulation to make certain that viable sperms will not be in the tube when the ovum descends, and 2 days afterward to make certain that a fertile ovum will not be in the tube when the sperms are deposited, the "unsafe" period may be considered to extend from the 12th through the 16th days of a 28-day cycle. The "safe" periods are from the 1st-11th and the 17th-28th days. However, because ovulation may occur at virtually any time before the 14th day and is delayed in long cycles, and because these calculations are of no value in women recently delivered and when the cycle is irregular, the "calendar" method of determining the time of ovulation is often unreliable. The time of ovulation can be noted more certainly by the use of the BBT record (see Fig 27-5). The vaginal or rectal temperature must be taken immediately upon awakening before any activity whatever. A drop in temperature occurs 24-36 hours after ovulation; a rise of about $0.7°F$ occurs 1-2 days after ovulation and continues throughout the remainder of the cycle. The third day after the rise marks the end of the fertile period. This method requires a great deal of effort and interest on the part of the patient to be sure a true basal temperature chart is being recorded.

Coitus Interruptus.

This method of contraception is rarely acceptable, and its effectiveness is low because of the small but active sperm content of the preejaculate secretion. The Roman Catholic Church considers this method unacceptable.

ESTRINDEX® TEST FOR OVULATION TIME

The sodium chloride content of cervical mucus, which is responsible for crystallization of a dried spread, varies during the menstrual cycle and peaks at ovulation when ferning is also most marked.

A magenta tinted test paper has been developed for the gross color quantitation of chlorides in cervical mucus. The test paper loses color in proportion to the salinity of fluid applied. During the early proliferative phase, the sodium chloride content of the cervical mucus is usually 0.3-0.5%. The mucus will cause only slight fading of the colored test paper. At ovulation, 0.7-0.9% sodium chloride may be present—sufficient to blanch the test sheet.

Utilizing this color change principle, the Estrindex® kit, containing 20 sterile swabs (each packaged in a carton or tube), a chemically treated colored test sheet ruled in numbered squares representing the days of the month, and an explanatory booklet, permits the patient without vaginitis and with no abnormal bleeding to estimate her fertile period. This self-test is reasonably accurate and helpful both as a contraceptive measure and in cases of infertility when it is desirable to know when ovulation is occurring.

Hormones.

The oral contraceptives (see Table 27-3) contain a progesterone-like compound and an estrogen. The patient takes one tablet daily from the 5th through the 24th day of the cycle. Unpleasant reactions, mostly mild and transitory, are reported in about a third of women. Acne and chloasma (the latter particularly prominent in areas exposed to the sun) may be troublesome. Nausea is reported in about 2-5% of women, but vomiting rarely occurs; nausea is usually worse in the first cycle and diminishes with subsequent doses and with subsequent cycles of therapy. "Break-through" uterine bleeding is an annoying symptom in about 10% of patients, usually during the first several months of therapy, it can be readily eliminated by increasing the dose by one-half the daily prescription, continuing through the last day of the treatment cycle. Fluid retention is clinically significant in 15-20% of patients; it may become severe despite reasonable limitation of sodium ion. Thrombophlebitis, usually of the superficial type and sometimes involving the superficial saphenous venous system, is rare; no specific coagulation defect or alteration has been noted in these patients, and discontinuance of hormonal intake and symptomatic therapy are usually sufficient.

The oral contraceptives are not carcinogenic. In theory at least, they should prevent neoplasia from developing in the endometrium because of periodic secretory type of endometrium with regular periods of slough which they produce.

Table 27-3. The oral contraceptives.

Trade Name	Progesterone-Like	Estrogen
Enovid-E	Norethynodrel, 2.5 mg	Mestranol, 0.1 mg
C-Quens*	Chlormadinone acetate, 2 mg	Mestranol, 80 mcg
Oracon†	Dimethisterone, 25 mg	Ethinyl estradiol, 0.1 mg

*Folder contains 15 tablets of mestranol and 5 containing both components.
†Vial contains 16 tablets of ethinyl estradiol and 5 containing both components.

Precipitation or aggravation of diabetes mellitus may occur.

The oral contraceptives should not be given to nursing mothers, women with a history of thromboembolism, or girls who have not attained full growth.

Ovulation may also be prevented by the administration of diethylstilbestrol, 1 mg orally daily, from the third through the 12th days of the cycle. Hypermenorrhea and nausea are complications. If the patient misses even a few sequential doses, ovulation is likely to occur.

Spermatogenesis may be suppressed with oral contraceptives, but nausea, mastalgia, reduced potency, and extended reduction of the normal sperm population have made this method of contraception unacceptable to men.

The potential effect of long-term hormonal medication upon the endocrine balance has not yet been appraised fully.

Condom or Animal Membrane Sheath.

These devices give good to excellent protection. The failures are mainly due to mechanical faults or errors of procedures such as applying the condom after initial intromission. Sheaths have the additional advantage of giving protection against venereal disease, but have the disadvantage of impairing sensation and gratification.

Cervical Cap Pessary.

The use of a plastic or metal cap which fits snugly over the cervix between periods is a successful method of contraception if the cap is fitted accurately and applied properly. Multiparas are more likely to be able to utilize this device because their vaginal canals are wide enough for them to apply the cap themselves after proper direction.

Vaginal Diaphragm.

The diaphragm is almost as reliable as the condom or cap, but it is necessary to teach the patient how to insert it and it must be employed in advance of coitus. The diaphragm should be left in 6-12 hours after copulation. Vaginal or pelvic relaxation may interfere with accurate fitting.

Intrauterine Contraceptive Devices (IUCD). (See Figs 27-6 and 27-7.)

The intrauterine contraceptive device (IUCD) is a plastic or metal coil, spiral, or ring which is inserted transcervically to prevent conception or implantation. It is an excellent method of contraception as long as the device is retained. Apparently, fertilization may occur but the IUCD increases tubal motility so that the endometrium is unprepared for implantation.

The IUCD affords semipermanent, reversible, inexpensive protection without the necessity for personal attention to insertion, as with the vaginal diaphragm. It is best suited for multiparous women, particularly those in the lower socio-economic classes.

The plastic Lippes loop, Margulies spiral, and the Ota rings require no cervical dilatation. They are effective in that order. The Hall-Stone stainless steel ring, one of the most successful IUCD's, requires dilatation of the cervix (usually under anesthesia) for insertion and removal.

Fitting is easiest immediately after a menstrual period; the device can be extracted at any time. Difficulty in insertion (especially in nulliparas), initial cramping, menometrorrhagia, extrusion (10-20% during the first 3 months), and upper genital tract infections (rare) are the disadvantages. IUCD's are contraindicated in young nulligravidas, patients with acute cervicitis, acute or recurrent salpingitis, abnormal bleeding (persistent anovulation with menometrorrhagia, myomas, blood dyscrasias), and in patients whose religion precludes their use.

Vaginal Jellies, Gels, Creams, Suppositories.

These chemical substances, often containing spermatocidal drugs such as phenylmercuric nitrate in a low surface-tension cream base, are easily applied to the upper vaginal canal and are as effective as the best of the mechanical and biologic methods. Their expense, the undesirable lubricating effects, and possible irritating quality are disadvantages. Gels and creams interfere with gratification because they are often considered "slick" or "greasy."

Foam.

This is a combined mechanical and chemical method. A small sponge is moistened, saturated with the powder, and inserted into the vaginal vault. Acid carbon dioxide foam is produced. A new aerosol foam is now available for use within the vagina. It is inserted by means of an applicator, and no sponge is needed. This simple, effective method may be unaesthetic to some women, and the foam may be irritating.

Douche.

Douching with vinegar solution or proprietary acid douches after coitus is not an effective method of contraception because

Contraception 641

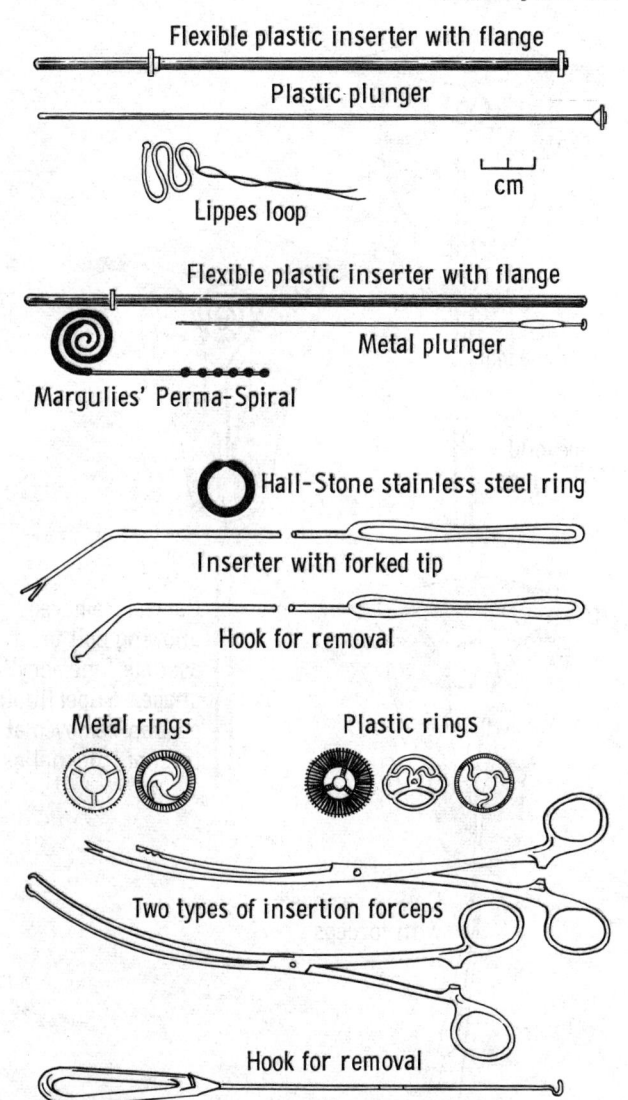

Fig 27-6. Some IUCD's and instruments for insertion and removal.

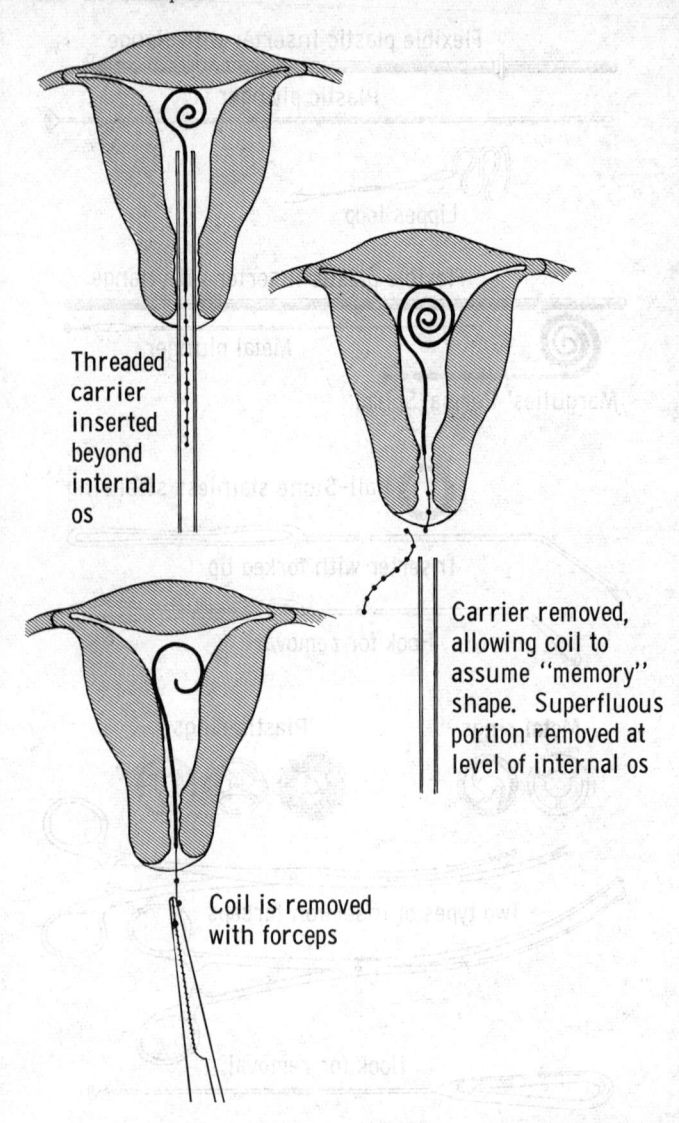

Fig 27-7. Schematic representation of one of the plastic devices (Margulies' Perma-Spiral®) with configurational recall.

it is not true that the sperm specimen can be either washed out of the cervix and vagina or destroyed by the medication. Actual aspiration of the sperm into the cervix occurs immediately after ejaculation, and the semen is often beyond the reach even of potent germicides under high pressure. Furthermore, even if douching were effective, it would be too troublesome for many women.

Diaphragm and Vaginal Cream or Jelly.

This logical combination of 2 good methods of contraception is utilized widely with good to excellent results.

General Procedure.

A bride-to-be or married woman seeking contraceptive advice should be examined and thoroughly indoctrinated into the kinds, advantages, disadvantages, and use of all methods of contraception. In addition, she should be given simple written or printed instructions to follow.

On physical examination all abnormalities should be determined, especially those requiring treatment and those which might contraindicate certain contraceptive devices or methods. A tight, annular hymen, a large cystocele, or marked cervico-uterine descensus may prevent the successful fitting of a vaginal diaphragm.

The ovulatory menstrual cycle and optimal time for conception should be explained, with emphasis on "safe" and "unsafe" periods. It is important to ascertain whether the husband is in accord with delaying the family or whether the woman is there just at her spouse's urging. When in doubt, the final recommendation should be delayed until the husband can be consulted. If the patient is Catholic or if she has agreed to abide by the precepts of the Catholic Church, the "rhythm" method should be described. If this is not pertinent, the discussion should be extended to the pros and cons of several other methods of contraception. Both husband and wife should be satisfied in the choice of contraceptive, as this is a matter of individualization. It may be expedient to favor an oral contraceptive for patients with a snug introitus who might have difficulty with a diaphragm or when one or both parties have aversions to vaginal medication or devices; a diaphragm and cream may be acceptable to other couples. If a mechanical or chemical means of contraception is chosen, the patient should be taught how to use the method and the diaphragm inserted and removed properly under supervision in the examining room. She should be shown how to inspect the diaphragm for damage and made aware that a new one must be fitted after colporrhaphy or vaginal delivery at term. She should be instructed regarding the measurement of doses of vaginal cream, foam, etc., and where to obtain refills. Any other questions she might have should be discussed.

28...
Psychosomatic Gynecologic Problems & Gynecologic Backache

PSYCHOGENIC PELVIC PAIN

Psychogenic (functional) pelvic pain, usually a chronic or recurrent condition, is caused by unresolved emotional conflicts. It may be due to (1) the unperceived presence of disturbing subliminal impulses or (2) the precognition of sensations without conscious awareness. Neurotic women 25-45 years of age are most susceptible. It is far more common in western than eastern society because of European attitudes stressing affect. The incidence in the USA varies from 5-25% of gynecologic patients, depending upon the interests and skills of the physician.

Psychogenic pelvic pain is genuine pain which occurs as a manifestation of unhappiness and serves as a warning of a potentially serious emotional disorder. It represents an abnormal need for solicitude or gratification in the masochistic woman; resentment in the frustrated woman; anxiety in the hypochondriacal woman; guilt in the strict, introspective woman; and a psychic defense mechanism in the borderline schizophrenic woman. The type and degree of pain and the circumstances in which it appears or intensifies vary in accordance with the woman's age and temperament and the culture in which she lives.

Pain which cannot be attributed to physical causes may result when normal physiologic impulses are exaggerated by ignorance, fear, and tension, or when the perceptual threshold to disturbing stimuli is lowered. When pain occurs, it becomes associated in the patient's mind with past or present environmental factors, and repetition of the painful sensation augments and solidifies these associations, so that sensory conditioning "teaches" the woman to feel pain. In her anxiety she may fix her complaints on one anatomic area or organ system.

Patients with psychogenic pelvic pain are often hysterical personality types. All degrees of intelligence are represented. The principal emotional and personality characteristics of these women are as follows: They are egotistic, self-indulgent, and vain; demanding and independent; emotionally immature and shallow; prone to dramatize, exaggerate, and seek attention; excitable, deficient in emotional control, inconsistent in emotional reaction; and coquettish and sexually provocative but sexually fearful and often relatively frigid. Most of these patients have unhappy family histories. Their parents and husbands are frequently described as shown in the table below:

Table 28-1. Typical personality characteristics in mother, father, and husband of women with psychogenic pelvic pain.

Mother	Father	Husband
Domineering, critical	Inadequate, repeatedly unemployed	A passive, friendly "nice guy"
Unaffectionate, cruel	Alcoholic, epileptic, brutal	Hard-working, dependable
Old-fashioned, prudish	Too serious, unaffectionate toward daughter	Less than normally demanding of coitus
A religious fanatic	A faithless woman-chaser	Subject to premature ejaculation
Complaining, chronically ill, tense	Frequently like mother	Uncomplaining, stoical, long-suffering

There is often a history of long-standing conflict between the patient and her mother, who has failed to give the necessary love and support. The resentment and guilt thus created in the patient are repressed, and the result is a masochistic personality with hysterical tendencies. The patient has never been able to confront her mother; her father is frequently unacceptable and therefore is rejected. Women with such a background are invariably led to believe that sex is "dirty" and best avoided.

The girl often marries young to escape the situation at home, and her marriage is usually a dismal, loveless one, even though these girls may marry kindly men unlike their fathers (but not dominant, virile males). Adult life and its responsibilities thus prove unsatisfying, and the patient's sex attitudes are dominated by fear of coitus and aversion to pregnancy.

Clinical Findings.
A. Symptoms and Signs: Complaints are almost invariably multiple. In addition to pelvic pain, which is often in the right lower quadrant and is worse before and during menses, most patients also report frigidity, dyspareunia, leukorrhea, dysmenorrhea, abnormal menses, urinary and bowel dysfunction, headache and backache, "nervousness," agitation, and depression. The signs are usually those of "pelvic congestion": persistent vaginal and pel-

646 Psychogenic Pelvic Pain

vic hyperemia, excessive cervical mucus in the absence of infection, and generalized pelvic tenderness and sensitivity to even gentle palpation of the pelvic viscera. There may be numerous abdominal scars as a result of operations.

Although the patient insists she is in great pain, in about 25% of cases no physical abnormality can be found; in the remainder, insignificant physical variations or minimal lesions are found. The other extreme of a pain spectrum is illustrated by the patient who reports only slight distress despite gross demonstrable organic disease. This may be a psychologically diminished reaction to somatic pain.

B. Special Examinations:
1. Psychologic testing (Cornell Medical Inventory, Taylor Anxiety Score, Saslow Anxiety Quotient, etc) may reveal definite abnormal traits.
2. Psychiatric evaluation - Clues to the diagnosis of psychoneurosis may include unusual attitudes and appearance (seductive dress and mannerisms, heavy make-up, etc), agitation, and rapid breathing ("acting-out" of the problem). Wearing dark glasses indoors may identify a woman sensitive to minor annoyances. Personification of organs or blaming certain viscera may be revealing. ("My right ovary is diseased." "My uterus has given me trouble all my life.") Psychosis may be suggested by crude, illogical, or incongruous remarks or behavior.

Complications.

Surgery does not relieve the underlying emotional distress but may intensify the psychic disorder and lead to medical and surgical complications. Psychoneurosis may progress to psychosis. The patient may commit suicide in a despondent mood.

Differential Diagnosis.

The differentiation of functional versus organic disease can be made by elimination or by recognition of psychoneurosis or psychosis while investigating organic pathology. The latter is preferred since most patients with psychogenic pelvic pain present many characteristic features which make possible a direct diagnosis without extensive studies.

It is curious that popular lay concepts as causes of pelvic pain may be prominent in the physician's mind but rarely occur to the patient as such. "Chronic appendicitis," adhesions, a "painful ovary," or "tipped uterus" are often suspected by physicians as possible causes of pain. Appendicitis is invariably an acute disorder, and pelvic adhesions themselves rarely cause pain. Ovarian cysts without adherence or torsion are almost never painful, and an adherent ovary is sensitive only in the second phase of the cycle. Uterine retropositions may cause specific, periodic pain (dyspareunia, dysmenorrhea).

Chronic salpingitis, chronic urinary tract infection, spastic and other types of colitis, and endometriosis must be ruled out.

The following comparison of organic and psychogenic pelvic pain may be helpful in diagnosis:

Table 28-2. Differentiation of organic and psychogenic pain.

	Organic	Psychogenic
Type	Sharp, cramping, intermittent	Dull, continuous
Time of onset	Any time. May awaken patient	Usually begins well after waking, when social obligations are pressing
Radiation	Follows definite neural pathways	Bizarre patterns or does not radiate
Localization	Localizes with typical point tenderness	Variable, shifting, generalized
Progress	Soon becomes either better or worse	Remains the same for weeks, months, years
Provocative tests	Often reproduced or augmented by tests or manipulation, not by mood	Not triggered or accentuated by examination but by interpersonal relationships

Prevention.

Sex education, marriage counseling, and the early recognition and treatment of emotional illness are the only feasible preventive measures for any psychic disorder. Physicians should cooperate with local mental health facilities and should press for greater emphasis on this aspect of total medical care.

Treatment.

The patient should be admitted to the hospital for examination, observation, and treatment. Reassurance and simple symptomatic therapy are indicated. A complete history should be taken and a thorough physical examination performed. The physician must be a sympathetic, unhurried, "good listener."

Once the diagnosis is established, the disorder is explained to the patient and her husband in direct, convincing terms. The patient should be provided with an acceptable "escape" from her predicament, explaining that, "Our nerves often play tricks on us," "Emotions tie us in knots,"

"The mind governs the body," etc. The physician must gain the patient's cooperation in a basic, perhaps lengthy reorientation and reeducation program.

Narcotics must be avoided, since patients with emotional problems are easily addicted; sedatives should not be given, since these patients are bad suicidal risks; tranquilizers are contraindicated because the patient must adjust to her circumstances and solve her problem without therapeutic crutches. Psychotherapy should be instituted or the patient referred to a psychiatrist for treatment.

Upon discharge to office care, it is well to require numerous visits to maintain contact and ensure the continuity of therapy. Every effort must be made to assist the patient to adjust socially.

Occasional warm douches, external heat (or cold), diathermy, massage, and similar physical measures may be salutary.

Surgery is contraindicated unless psychogenic pain can be excluded. Hysterectomy and other types of sterilizing surgery should be done only on honest indications other than pain.

Prognosis.

Patients with psychogenic pelvic pain are medical "shoppers" or "drifters." Refusal of therapy, interruption of treatment, and the unwillingness to abandon invalidism as a way of life make their medical future discouraging.

About three-fourths of patients with functional pelvic pain will improve temporarily with reassurance and symptomatic therapy, but only a few will derive lasting benefit. Over one-half of psychoneurotic patients will improve markedly, and many can be cured by psychotherapy. The prognosis in psychotic women depends upon the type and severity of the disorder.

GYNECOLOGIC BACKACHE

Backache of gynecologic origin is generally due to a well-defined pelvic disorder. It is rare before puberty and uncommon after the menopause but is frequently reported during adult life. Multiparas are more often afflicted than nulliparas. About 25% of gynecologic patients who complain of backache will be found to have significant genital disease but no orthopedic or other causes of discomfort; 15% of the total will have no gynecologic problem.

Gynecologic backache is frequently associated with orthopedic, urologic, or neurologic difficulties. It may be due to any of the following causes: (1) Traction or pulsion on the peritoneum or the supportive structures of the generative organs or pelvic floor (tumors, ascites, uterine prolapse); (2)

Gynecologic Backache

inflammation of the pelvic contents: bacterial (e.g., peritonitis or salpingitis) or chemical (e.g., due to iodides used in salpingography or fluid from a ruptured dermoid cyst); (3) invasion of pelvic tissues or bone by tumor or endometriosis; (4) obstruction to the genital tract (cervical stenosis); (5) torsion or constriction of the pelvic viscera (ovary enmeshed in adhesions, twisted ovarian cyst); (6) congestion of internal genitalia (turgescence of the retroposed uterus, backache during menstruation); (7) psychic tension (anxiety, apprehension). (See Psychogenic Pelvic Pain, p. 644.)

Most cases of gynecologic backache represent referred pain, but carcinomatous extension to the spine causes direct pain. Irritation of the afferent nerves from the organ involved or abnormal nerve impulses from the site of the disorder to the back via the sympathetic nervous system are responsible. Lumbar, lumbosacral, sacral, sacrococcygeal, or coccygeal distribution of pain depends upon the site, type, and extent of the problem. An infected, distended, or obstructed viscus may cause referred backache. Backache may also be caused by cervicitis associated with lymphangitis and neuritis which may involve the uterosacral ligaments.

Pelvic tumors may cause pain depending upon their size and type. Tumors produce pressure, vascular engorgement, and nerve involvement. Small tumors rarely cause backache. Moderately large tumors, such as ovarian cysts 8-12 cm in diameter, or even the uterus itself in advanced pregnancy, may cause backache by exerting traction on the pelvic ligaments. Very large tumors often do not cause back pain because they tend to be immobile and may even rest upon the bones of the pelvis.

Clinical Findings.

A. Symptoms and Signs: Gynecologic backache is almost invariably associated with other major signs and symptoms of pelvic disease. Fairly constant lumbosacral or sacral backache is often described with salpingitis, pelvic abscess, or twisted ovarian cyst. Discomfort is usually more pronounced on the involved side. Back pain due to endometriosis of the cul-de-sac is referred to the coccygeal region or rectum. Backache due to ovarian, renal, and ureteral lesions commonly radiates toward the inguinal region. Backache due to orthopedic and neurologic disease often radiates down into the buttocks or along the distribution of the sciatic nerve. Tests may reveal faulty posture, bony deformity, muscle spasm, and spinal cord or other back injury.

Hypesthesia, reduced reflex responses, and regional lumbar tenderness are noted on neurologic evaluation in cases of herniated intervertebral disk.

Uterine bleeding, vaginal discharge, pelvic tumor

formation, prolapse of the uterus or ovaries, marked retroposition of the fundus, and similar findings may be observed.
B. Laboratory Findings: Leukocytosis and an elevated sedimentation rate may be indicative of infection. Vaginal cytology may reveal neoplastic cells. Bacteriuria, pyuria, or hematuria suggests urinary tract disease as a possible cause of backache when a catheterized or a clean-catch specimen is examined.
C. X-Ray Findings: AP and lateral films of the spine often disclose a postural, degenerative, neoplastic, or other orthopedic cause of backache. Myelograms may be required to demonstrate a herniated intervertebral disk.

Prevention.
Many cases of gynecologic backache can be prevented by avoiding trauma in labor and delivery, repairing cervical and other obstetric lacerations immediately, treating cervicitis and pelvic infections promptly and adequately, and by examining women periodically so that tumors, hernias, and similar lesions can be treated early.

Treatment.
A. Specific Measures: The underlying problem should be treated definitively. With improvement, backache will be relieved in most instances.
B. Supportive Measures: The patient is placed at bed rest in the most comfortable position on a firm mattress. Heat is applied to the back as necessary for pain and warm water douches given twice daily.

Acetylsalicylic acid with or without codeine should be given every 4 hours as required. Phenothiazines such as prochlorperazine (Compazine®), 5-10 mg 3 times daily, may be given to reduce emotional tension.
C. Local Measures: Cervicitis may respond to topical therapy (see p. 476).
D. Surgical Measures: Tumors, malpositions of the uterus, pelvic hernias, etc may require surgery.

Prognosis.
Multiple causes of backache cloud the prognosis. If the backache is of gynecologic origin, successful treatment of the pelvic problem will almost always eliminate the problem.

DYSPAREUNIA

Dyspareunia (painful coitus) may be functional or organic, or may be due to a combination of organic and emotional causes. Either type may occur early (primary) or late (secondary) in marriage. The location of discomfort may be external (at the introitus) or internal (deep within the genital canal or beyond), and some women describe both types of pain. Early external dyspareunia, either functional or organic, is common among newly married women. Functional dyspareunia is the most frequent type and is more difficult to treat.

Functional dyspareunia may be caused by female psychosexual problems, especially fear of genital damage, venereal disease, or pregnancy. These factors may cause vaginismus, an involuntary spasm of the muscles around the introitus and levators when the thighs are adducted. It is an indication of extreme anxiety. A woman may consider intercourse to be threatening to her ego and security, and she thus becomes hostile and frigid. The husband may be poorly informed regarding sex technics, inept, selfish, and unsympathetic. Marital disharmony and coitus interruptus may also lead to emotionally induced vaginismus and dyspareunia.

Organic dyspareunia, congenital or acquired, is of 2 types: external or internal. External dyspareunia may be due to an occlusive or rigid hymen and postoperative or postpartal vaginal contracture. Inflammatory disorders of the vulva, vagina, urethra, or anus will cause pain upon intromission. Traumatic or infectious processes are often seen in younger patients. Atrophic vulvovaginitis is seen in postmenopausal women.

Organic causes of internal dyspareunia include hourglass contracture of the vagina and septate vagina, severe cervicitis, marked fundal retroposition, uterine prolapse or neoplasia, tubo-ovarian disease, pelvic endometriosis, and severe disorders of the lower urinary tract or large bowel.

Genital infections, a snug hymen, vaginal scarring or other causes of vaginal contracture, pelvic tumors, extreme malposition of the uterus, and similar lesions may cause internal or external organic dyspareunia.

Functional and organic problems are often related. (See Psychogenic Pelvic Pain, p. 644.) A disorder may begin on a functional basis, but organic disease may develop as a consequence. The converse is also possible. Rigidity of the hymen may be a less important cause of dyspareunia than emotionally induced tautness of the introital and pelvic musculature. In contrast, dyspareunia as a result of senile vaginal atrophy may disturb the patient more physically than emotionally.

When vaginismus occurs, further attempts at coitus usually intensify the spasm, and pain develops. Unless the patient's basic problem is resolved or corrected, subsequent coitus often initiates a conditioned reflex: because pain is anticipated, earlier and more severe muscle spasm may result.

Clinical Findings.

A. Symptoms and Signs: The physician should accept the patient's statement that coitus is painful and then differentiate between functional, primary, external dyspareunia and the less common types. In functional dyspareunia there are usually no pertinent physical abnormalities. Serious emotional problems will be notable, however.

Many women with dyspareunia are too embarrassed to complain of painful coitus but will consult their physicians about secondary or related complaints. Many of these complaints are also of psychosomatic origin: dysmenorrhea, pelvic pain, menometrorrhagia, etc. Tactful inquiry about worries, fear of pregnancy, and degree of satisfaction in the sex relationship may encourage a frank and useful discussion of the problem.

Pelvic examination often reveals marked contraction of the perineal and levator musculature with adduction of the muscles of the thighs, even when the patient is "relaxed," and such specific signs as the following: genital hypoplasia, virtually complete or rigid hymen, septate vagina, urethral caruncle, urethral or subvesical tenderness, postpartal or postoperative scarring or contracture of the vagina, vulvovaginitis, kraurosis vulvae, prolapse of the cervix and uterus, uterine retroposition or tumor, tubo-ovarian inflammation or neoplasm, pelvic endometriosis, and rectal or vesical abnormalities.

B. Special Examinations: Psychiatric evaluation is indicated if complex psychosexual problems seem to be present. Specialized technics of physical examination, e.g., cystoscopy, may be required.

Complications.

If not corrected, dyspareunia frequently leads to marital discord, infidelity, and divorce. Psychoneuroses often develop or become intensified, both in the wife and husband. The woman may experience menstrual difficulties and bladder and bowel dysfunction. The husband may suffer from premature ejaculation, impotence, or other sexual problems if his wife's difficulties are not resolved.

Prevention.

Preventive measures consist of premarital sex education of adolescent girls and boys at home, in the schools, and by religious organizations. Personal counseling, courses in "preparation for marriage," scientific films emphasizing pelvic anatomy and genital function, and premarital examination by qualified physicians also are of aid.

Treatment.

A. Specific Measures: Functional dyspareunia can be treated

by marriage counseling. Contraceptive advice for both parties is often helpful. Psychotherapy may be required if the psychosexual problem is deep-seated; both partners should be interviewed. The treatment of organic dyspareunia depends upon the underlying cause.

B. General Measures: In both types of dyspareunia it is helpful to explain the problem to both partners in a tactful and patient manner and to assure them that treatment will probably cure the disorder if their full cooperation is obtained. Mild sedation with phenobarbital, 15 mg ($1/4$ gr.) orally 3 times daily, or a tranquilizer such as prochlorperazine (Compazine®), 5-10 mg orally 3 times daily, may be advisable in cases of extreme emotional tension.

C. Local Measures: For functional dyspareunia the physician may suggest hymenal-vaginal dilatations by the patient with a conical metal (Kelly) dilator or test tubes of gradually increasing size if surgery is not imperative. Local anesthetic ointment may be applied to the introitus before coitus, but this measure is often disappointing and does not correct the problem. Organic dyspareunia due to vaginal dryness may be treated with a simple, nongreasy lubricant. Estrogen therapy is valuable for senile vulvovaginitis.

D. Surgical Measures: Hymenotomy, perineotomy, and other plastic surgical procedures should be done only when obvious gynatresia is present. A hymen that is not completely imperforate but is too small to allow coitus is often found during premarital examination. In most instances the hymen is thin, and the patient's daily dilatation with her fingers over a period of 2-4 weeks will achieve adequate size. If the need for introital enlargement is more urgent, an incision at 6 o'clock, using local anesthesia, is easily performed; bleeding is not serious, and adhesion of the incised surface can be prevented by a lightly placed vaseline gauze pack. If time is not a factor and dilatation is hindered by an inordinate amount of fibrous tissue, the stretching can be facilitated by a series of 1-2 mm nicks at the edge of the hymen. This procedure is relatively painless if the area is numbed by the "pressure anesthesia" of preliminary stretching, especially if a local anesthetic ointment is used and if the knife edge is exceedingly sharp.

Obstructive lesions of the vagina and chronic cervicitis should be treated surgically by appropriate means. The uterus is suspended only when convincing improvement follows fundal replacement and pessary support or when adherent retroversion (and prolapse of the adnexa) are the apparent causes of dyspareunia.

Myomectomy, resection of ovarian cysts, excision of areas of endometriosis, and similar procedures should be done only if these lesions can definitely be shown to be causing painful intercourse.

Prognosis.

The successful treatment of functional dyspareunia requires great delicacy, patience, and sagacity. Few patients are quickly or easily cured. Even when dyspareunia is based upon fear of pregnancy, improvement occurs only gradually as confidence in the contraceptive method develops. Organic dyspareunia yields promptly, often dramatically, to the elimination of the cause of pain.

FRIGIDITY

Failure on the woman's part to achieve normal emotional release or orgasm may be due to temporary situational problems, but more often is evidence of deep-seated, unresolved psychosexual conflicts. Various degrees of relative frigidity occur commonly, but absolute frigidity is rare. In so-called facultative frigidity the patient is responsive to one partner but not to another.

Fear of pregnancy is an important factor in the reduction of sexual responsiveness. Marital disharmony due to ineptitude in sex technics, impotence of the husband (including premature ejaculation), or dyspareunia may be important factors. Vaginismus and, in extreme cases, vaginal hypesthesia may occur.

Frigidity may develop as a result of environmental difficulties such as living in a crowded household or with in-laws. Overwork, discouragement, or unhappiness may provoke or aggravate the problem.

Basically, frigidity is the result of arrested or distorted emotional development. Some patients exhibit homosexual tendencies, infantile fixations, asceticism, or hostility toward men. Social or religious taboos or prejudices may underlie the problem. Critical situations involving rape, perversion, venereal infection, or incest are occasionally described. Nymphomania is a type of frigidity characterized by a constant quest for sexual gratification, always without success.

Out of reluctance to admit that the problem exists, few women consult even the gynecologist with a complaint of frigidity. Most frigid women seeking medical advice describe other symptoms (often dyspareunia) as a subterfuge.

In most instances, frigidity is a far more intricate problem than the rather superficial causes often recorded would indicate. The background of the patient's sexual difficulty must be explored cautiously but carefully. Simple discussion may often be useful in correcting misconceptions and allaying fears, and the physician can sometimes give advice about sex practices that will be of value to both partners. Environmental factors should be manipulated favorably whenever possible. If prompt improvement does not occur, however, an attempt should be made to refer the patient for psychiatric care.

Androgens and aphrodisiac drugs are absolutely worthless in the treatment of frigidity and may be harmful.

The prophylaxis of frigidity consists of the establishment of good mental health.

The prognosis in long-standing, marked frigidity is extremely poor.

MANAGEMENT OF THE TERMINAL CANCER PATIENT

Cancer is a fearsome diagnosis which evokes fears of pain, invalidism, mutilation, social exile, and death. The physician should be sensitive to these implications and must be prepared to extend his personal and professional resources to help the patient live even while she is dying. Management must be individualized. Patients who have family and financial obligations usually should be told of their malignancy. Others should be told as much as they wish to know about their diagnosis and prognosis despite family opinions to the contrary. The exceptions usually are aged or pediatric gynecologic patients who are emotionally unstable or who cannot reason. Unfortunately, severe illness and hospitalization are often interpreted by these patients as punishment for wrongdoing, and this false view must be corrected.

Hope must be kept high. Spontaneous regression of tumors does occur, and new methods of treatment constantly are being developed. Nevertheless, patients must be kept from impoverishing their families in a futile search for nonexistent cures. Much can be done for the patient's comfort and peace of mind. She should know that everything will be done to prevent suffering. Depression must not be permitted to go unnoticed or untreated. The thought of suicide to avoid terminal agony or helplessness or to save the expense of prolonged hospitalization probably occurs to most patients who know they have cancer, but only a few patients with malignancy actually attempt suicide. About 2% of successful suicides have cancer; only 5% of suicides have other types of chronic incurable illness.

The consolation of religion is the greatest source of strength and comfort for many patients in the face of suffering and impending death. The physician should be prepared to cooperate with the patient's religious adviser so that she will derive the greatest possible benefit from her spiritual beliefs.

The management of terminal illness requires emphasis on daily experience. The patient should not be allowed to look back with regret or forward with fear. Insofar as possible, drugs are used which do not impair the mental faculties so that reading, visiting, and entertainment still can be enjoyed.

When the end is near, heroic measures to preserve life for brief periods are seldom justified. The patient should be permitted to expire with dignity.

PRIMARY DYSMENORRHEA
(Essential or Functional Dysmenorrhea)

Primary dysmenorrhea, in contrast to secondary dysmenorrhea (due to organic causes), refers to pain with menstruation for which no organic basis is evident. It accounts for 80% of cases of painful menses. Although primary dysmenorrhea is particularly common during adolescence, it may occur at any time from the menarche to the menopause. The pain is invariably secondary to an emotional problem. Dysmenorrhea and general menstrual discomfort often are described together as "menorrhalgia."

Primary dysmenorrhea is the most common manifestation of neurosis in women. Psychosexual problems and other unresolved emotional conflicts are present in many of these patients, who resent their female status. Many patients are introspective, basically unhappy, and psychologically immature.

Certain physical abnormalities are also described. Diffuse congestion of the pelvic viscera may be noted, but gynecologic examination usually will disclose essentially normal findings in primary dysmenorrhea. Menorrhalgic symptoms usually occur in patients who ovulate. It may be that highly vascularized myometrium and endometrium shed the lining tissue with difficulty during the secretory stage, causing uterine pain. Uterine contractions in primary dysmenorrhea often are hypertonic and dysrhythmic (uterine dyskinesia). Painful contractions are induced with less fluid distention of the uterus than in the asymptomatic woman.

The dynamics of primary dysmenorrhea include the following: (1) Dysmenorrhea due to negative conditioning. Misinformation, taboos, and old wives' tales convince the patient that menstruation and sickness are identical. A neurotic, dysmenorrheic mother or close friend who retreats into invalidism each month personifies this problem. (2) Dysmenorrhea due to childish dependence. Girls of overindulgent mothers frequently have strong oral passive-dependent needs. They crave attention, sympathy, and protection, which often are provided dutifully by a lenient and misguided parent at the time of the menses. (3) Dysmenorrhea due to resentment, hostility, and disappointment toward life situations. The most common cases are sexual arousal without satisfaction, e.g., in petting or restraint because of fear of pregnancy; hatred implicitly expressed, e.g., by the wife in an unhappy marriage; and frustration, e.g., of the infertile wife in an otherwise happy marriage. (4) Dysmenorrhea due to repudiation of the feminine role. The parents push the girl into masculine attitudes and pursuits because of their desire for a boy instead of a girl. (5) Dysmenorrhea due to "castration anxiety." The fantasy of genital trauma is acted out each month. Menstrual flow is the bloody proof of deficiency, inferiority, and suffering to some women. With menstruation, feelings of hostility and resentment are released. (6) Dysmenorrhea due to psychosomatic defense against psychosis. These patients, usually subclinical schizophrenics, project their hatred into organ systems which are psychodynamically significant. Such women may use crude terms such as "rotten uterus" or "an ovary full of pus."

Clinical Findings.

Agitation, abdominal bloating, breast engorgement, and pelvic heaviness often precede dysmenorrhea. Intermittent aching progressing to cramplike discomfort in the lower midline usually accompanies the onset of bleeding. Circulatory engorgement of the vagina and cervix, slight patulousness of the os, and bogginess of the uterus are frequently recorded before and during bleeding. Uterine, parametrial, and adnexal tenderness often are described as well.

Associated symptoms (dysmenorrhea equivalents) such as periodic headache, diarrhea, tenseness, and urinary frequency and urgency indicate monthly dysfunction of other organ systems.

Differential Diagnosis.

A trial of estrogen or estrogen-progestogen therapy may be helpful in diagnosis. Anovulatory periods usually are painless in the absence of cervical obstruction or other genital disorders. Suppression of ovulation usually prevents dysmenorrhea during that month. The patient should be required to keep a basal body temperature chart to document an ovulation.

Primary dysmenorrhea is almost always comenstrual and begins with the bleeding; it is brief (24-48 hours), the flow is rarely profuse, and pre- and postmenstrual spotting do not occur commonly. Clots and hypermenorrhea are not common with essential dysmenorrhea, although shreds of tissue or even an endometrial cast (membranous dysmenorrhea) may be passed by a patient with no known pelvic disease.

Menstrual cramps which develop more than 5 years after the menarche are usually due to organic causes and may include generalized abdominal pain or particularly well localized right- or left-sided pelvic pain. Typical patterns of pain also suggest secondary dysmenorrhea, which often precedes the bleeding, continues during the flow, and may persist even after bleeding has stopped.

Complications.

Patients who experience severe functional dysmenorrhea are emotionally inadequate for marriage, pregnancy, childbirth, and parenthood. Many of these women are relatively frigid. They need psychotherapy, reorientation, and reeducation. If these are not provided and increased stress or further psychosexual conflicts develop, the danger of psychosis or other severe psychiatric conditions cannot be disregarded.

Treatment.
- A. Immediate Measures: Analgesics such as aspirin, 0.6 gm (10 gr), with codeine, 0.03 gm ($1/2$ gr), orally are warranted occasionally until the diagnosis of primary dysmenorrhea is established. Continued use of narcotics should be strictly avoided for fear of addiction.
- B. General Measures:
  1. Warm douches may afford temporary relief.
  2. The patient should be encouraged to be normally active during menstruation. Sports and calisthenics are helpful.
  3. Estrogen therapy - Give diethylstilbestrol, 0.5 mg orally daily for 14 days, beginning with the first day of the period, to suppress ovulation. This course of treatment may be repeated several times. Confidence in the physician will be enhanced if pain is relieved, but hormone therapy for an extended time is not advisable.
  4. Estrogen-progestogen combination (Enovid®, etc.).
  5. Androgen therapy - Give methyltestosterone, 5 mg orally 3 times daily from the 5th through the 10th days after the onset of the period, and continue in this way for 2-3 months. Ovulation is not prevented with androgen therapy, but pain almost always is lessened.
- C. Specific Measures:
  1. Psychiatric - The only treatment which offers a hope of permanent cure is psychiatric. The physician can in most cases undertake this himself if his relationship with his patient is sound enough to permit her to express her fears and conflicts and participate in frank discussions of "personal matters." If the underlying psychodynamics of the patient's emotional problem can be identified, the physician may be able to guide her in the direction of more suitable responses. If his own efforts fail, psychiatric consultation must be recommended.

All superfluous medications should be discontinued. Prolonged use of drugs confuses the issue and permits the patient to take refuge in the assumption that the physician would not prescribe medications unless there were something organically wrong with her. The patient needs encouragement to face facts, accept implied challenges, and strive to overcome her problem.

Individualized treatment of dysmenorrhea can often be based on an understanding of the underlying psychodynamic mechanism: (1) Dysmenorrhea due to negative conditioning is best treated by reeducation. (2) Dysmenorrhea due to childish dependence often requires the severance of identification with the mother figure and establishment of confidence and trust in the physician. The doctor must be kindly and understanding. If reassociation is not successful, relapses will occur or a new psychosomatic disorder, e.g., asthma, irritable colon, or urinary urgency, may be substituted. (3) Dysmenorrhea due to resentment and hostility toward life situations can be relieved by an adequate social and marital adjustment. (4) Dysmenorrhea due to repudiation of the feminine role requires psychotherapy. It is wise to avoid repressive therapy such as surgery (presacral neurectomy), since this intensifies the patient's subconscious conviction that she is seriously ill. (5) Dysmenorrhea due to "castration anxiety" often is improved by hypnosis and dynamic psychotherapy. Surgery should not be suggested unless it is urgently required, for patients may experience a resurgence of anxiety postoperatively. (6) Dysmenorrhea associated with psychosomatic defense against psychosis should be treated by a psychiatrist. If the patient refuses psychiatric assistance, psychotherapy on a superficial level by the personal physician is required. The patient should be allowed to vent her feelings. Emphasis should be placed on symptoms and their treatment, with change of medication when indicated. Explanations and interpretations of "organ language" are to be avoided, but the husband should be informed regarding the problem.

2. Surgical - A paracervical block should be performed in an attempt to evaluate the potential effectiveness of a Doyle paracervical neurectomy, or a Cotte-type presacral neurectomy in the patient unresponsive to other methods of treatment. Hysterectomy is never indicated in the treatment of primary dysmenorrhea.

Prognosis.

In women with satisfactory psychobiologic integration, the prognosis is good. Little can be done for women who use menstrual symptoms as a monthly refuge from responsibility.

29...
Medical Genetics

Many physical abnormalities, metabolic disorders, and instances of infertility, anomalous sex differentiation, Mongolian idiocy, and mental retardation can be explained genetically. Awareness that the clinical characteristics of a specific disorder may be attributable to hereditary factors is basic to proper diagnosis and treatment. Moreover, recognition of hereditary carrier states is important to prevent incompatible matings and to provide dietary advice, specific medical therapy, and environmental control to afflicted individuals.

Basic Concepts.

The nucleus of all cells is made up of a mass of chromatin material which becomes organized into small, discrete rods or strands (**chromosomes**) prior to division of the cell. Chromosomes, which determine the biologic heritage of the individual, are composed of thousands of code-bearing **genes** arranged in linear fashion. It is postulated that the genes are made up of even smaller units, the **cistrons**, each of which may control an enzyme or other metabolic process.

The normal human cell contains 23 pairs of chromosomes. In accordance with the Denver classification, the first 22 are similar in appearance and are called autosomes. The 23rd pair are the sex chromosomes. If the individual is a female, 2 specific X chromosomes are present; if a male, the 23rd pair consists of an X and a Y chromosome.

The genes determine the bodily characteristics and are arranged in pairs of similar (homozygous) or dissimilar (heterozygous) type. If dissimilar, the **dominant** gene determines the trait and the other gene is unexpressed or **recessive**.

Genes also maintain cell activities. They consist of deoxyribonucleic acid (DNA). In the cytoplasm, structures called the ribosomes, containing ribonucleic acid (RNA), have the ability to produce protein. Communications are transmitted between the chromosomes and the ribosomes by means of a transfer of modified or "messenger" RNA.

The reassortment of chromosomes at fertilization is purely a chance distribution. Hence, either chromosome of a pair from one parent has an equal opportunity to combine with either chromosome of the same pair from the other parent.

Normal characteristics and genetically induced diseases may be inherited as autosomal dominant, autosomal recessive, or sex-linked characteristics.

The hereditary constitution or combination of genes characterizing an individual or a group of genetically identical organisms is called the **genotype**. Significantly, the genotype may not be clinically apparent. In contrast, recognizable morphologic or functional expressions of a genetic trait are referred to as the **phenotype**.

Alteration of a gene may occur with or without discernible cause. Moreover, the manifestations of such a transformation are often sudden and dramatic. The new gene occupies the same site (locus) on the original chromosome and is allelic (a partner) to its normal associate. Irradiation, marked temperature change, or certain drugs may cause genetic mutations which manifest new characteristics. The recognition of these alterations is usually easier when they are associated with pathologic changes. Transmission of mutations occurs as a dominant, recessive, or sex-linked hereditary trait.

When 2 gametes (spermatozoon and ovum) join in fertilization, the resultant zygote will normally contain 46 (diploid) chromosome complements. This implies one of each pair of chromosomes from both parents.

A haploid (half or unpaired) number is achieved by meiosis, the reductional division of chromosomes in germ cells. In contrast, mitosis is the division of somatic cells which ordinarily maintains the same number of chromosomes in the daughter cells. The union of the germ cell with a haploid number of chromosomes restores the diploid number of chromosomes.

A **karyotype** is a schematic presentation of photomicrographs or camera lucida drawings of the chromosomes of a single cell. Magnification of 300 times or more is generally required.

An **idiogram** is a diagrammatic representation of chromosomes as determined by chromosomal detail and measurement, usually of numerous cells of the same or different individuals. Generally, only one chromosome of a homologous pair is illustrated, the exception being the sex chromosome when both are depicted.

Alteration in the number of chromosomes is the most easily diagnosed genetic abnormality. Other changes such as elimination of portions of one or more chromosomes have also been identified. Because of the minuteness of the chromosome, only gross genetic abnormalities have been reported thus far. It is known that many genes are lost by **deletion**, which may result in severe phenotypical effects or even death of the individual, especially when autosomes are involved.

When a fragment or even an entire chromosome is relocated or abnormally fixed to another chromosome, the alteration is termed **translocation** or **mosaicism**. Translocation may produce striking developmental and functional anomalies such as Mongolian idiocy.

Generally speaking, both autosomal and sex-linked traits are inherited as either dominant or recessive characteristics. Inheritance of a dominant trait may occur by either the homozygous (DD) or heterozygous (Dd) state. By and large, dominant traits of one of the parents are transmitted to half of the offspring. A vertical transmission from one generation to another is to be expected, and the likelihood of recurrence in subsequent siblings is 50%.

When recessive traits are inherited through homozygous patterns, each parent may be clinically normal but a genetic carrier. Each parent may contribute the same gene to an offspring who may already have 2 such genes. The clinical appearance of the trait in question in the offspring is then assured. The chance of appearance of the trait in another sibling is 25%.

Children of matings by close relatives are more likely to be homozygous for specific genes than offspring of unrelated parents. They are thus more liable to inherit liabilities (as well as assets).

Classification of Genetic Disorders.

A. Chromosomal (Cytogenetic) Abnormalities: Unusual number of chromosomes.
   1. Autosomal trisomy syndromes (e.g., trisomy-21 or Down's syndrome; trisomy "13-15" or "16-18" syndromes).
   2. Sex chromosome abnormalities (e.g., Turner's syndrome, Klinefelter's syndrome).
B. Autosomal dominant hereditary disorders (e.g., osteogenesis imperfecta, retinoblastoma).
C. Autosomal recessive hereditary disorders (e.g., phenylketonuria, galactosemia).
D. X-linked dominant (sex-linked) hereditary disorders (e.g., vitamin D-resistant rickets).
E. X-linked recessive hereditary disorders (e.g., hemophilia).
F. Incompletely understood disorders with possible genetic basis (e.g., hypertension, atherosclerosis, neoplasms).

Diagnosis of Genetic Disorders.

Clinical manifestations which should suggest a possibility of genetic abnormalities to the obstetrician and gynecologist include the following: multiple congenital abnormalities, unusual body size and configuration, abnormal development of the sexual characteristics, delayed menarche, infertility, glycosuria, anemia, and other significant metabolic disturbances.

Proof of a genetic defect may depend upon a careful clinical evaluation, followed by complicated chromosomal or biochemical studies. One must distinguish between acquired congenital defects (e.g., infection or drug toxicity during pregnancy) and hereditary disorders. A complete pedigree should be obtained together with data relative to consanguinity and the occurrence of specific defects in family members. Obviously, such a record may be difficult to obtain because of ignorance, misunderstanding, and shame on the part of the patient or her family. Be prepared to evaluate the genetic constitution of certain of the patient's relatives also to learn whether they are similarly affected, carriers, or normal. Ordinarily, a carrier can be identified only by laboratory studies.

Chromosomal Abnormalities.

It is now possible to determine the number, shape, and even certain structural differences in the autosomes and sex chromosomes by utilizing recently developed cytologic technics such as tissue culture, special staining methods, ultramicroscopy, and photomicrography.

The presence of an abnormal number of autosomes may be compatible with life, but physical or mental abnormalities are likely to occur.

A loss or gain of one or more chromosomes (45, 47, 48, etc) in abnormal developmental states is called **aneuploidy**. Unequal distribution of chromosomes during cell division or in the production of gametes results in abnormalities of chromosome number (**nondisjunction**).

Abnormal daughter cells, one having an extra chromosome and the other lacking a chromosome, occur in nondisjunction when a pair of chromosomes or **chromatids** (half-chromosomes) fails to separate and both halves go to the same pole. Extra autosomes or sex chromosomes may result from this abnormal process.

Trisomy is the aneuploid condition in which one chromosome is represented 3 times instead of twice. Such disorders are identified by the number of the chromosome involved, e.g., trisomy-18. In **tetraploidy**, 4 rather than 2 chromosomes are present.

Mongolian idiocy (Down's syndrome) is the result of trisomy of chromosome 21. It is more likely to occur in children of women who become pregnant late in reproductive life. Mongolism may also occur when a fragmented chromosome 21 becomes attached to another chromosome by translocation.

Severe mental retardation and multiple physical congenital anomalies occur with extra autosomes in the 13-15 chromosome categories or in the other 16-18 chromosomes.

No person lacking an autosome has been described as yet. If and when such an observation is authenticated, the condition will be termed **monosomy** (one body), referring to the presence of but one of a pair of somatic chromosomes.

X-Linked (Sex-Linked) Hereditary Disorders and X Chromosome Abnormalities.

The identical sex chromosomes of the female are called X chromosomes. One such X chromosome together with an entirely different, smaller Y chromosome identifies the male. The sex chromosomes of the female are referred to as XX and those of the male as XY. Many genes of the X chromosome are unopposed by a gene of the Y chromosome. In fact, abnormalities of the X chromosome genes cause disease in the male, whereas in the female the abnormal recessive gene of the sex chromosome is neutralized by the normal allele. For this reason, most of the so-called sex-linked abnormalities cause disease only in males; in contrast, the disease is merely passed through the female. A male and his maternal grandfather are affected and the intervening female serves as a carrier. Sex-linked hereditary disorders may be dominant (e.g., vitamin D-resistant rickets) or recessive (e.g., hemophilia).

The X chromosome of the female carries numerous genes in addition to those determining sex, but the Y chromosome seemingly incorporates only maleness. The term X- (or sex-) linked genes applies to those carried by the X chromosome alone.

A woman receives an X chromosome from each of her parents. She must pass on one or the other of these chromosomes to every child, regardless of sex. The father contributes a Y to a son but another X to a daughter; therefore, in any X-linked recessive disorder (e.g., pseudohypertrophic muscular dystrophy) the mother is a carrier of the disease although she is not clinically afflicted. The chances are that one-half of her daughters will be carriers and one-half of her sons will be affected.

When an X or Y sex chromosome is absent, the individual is described as an XO, the O referring to the missing chromosome. Abnormal males may also have additional X (or Y) chromosomes, i.e., XXY (diplo-X, Y), XXXY (triplo-X, Y), XXYY (diplo-X and diplo-Y).

A well defined hyperchromatic mass in the periphery of the nucleus of 40-60% of mature female cells (Barr body) has been identified as X chromosome substance; females are thus described as "chromatin-positive." However, the normal male has no grossly detectable sex chromatin and is said to be "chromatin-negative." A pathologist needs only a cytologic spread of cells gently scraped from the buccal or vaginal mucosa, fixed in 1:1 ether-alcohol, and stained by the Papanicolaou technic, to determine the number of X chromosomes. Significantly, the number of chromatin bodies is one less than the number of X chromosomes (see Table 29-1).

The presence of a nuclear appendage (the "drumstick") in mature neutrophils in stained peripheral blood smears also probably represents sex chromatin. It is present in 1-3% of normal females, but is absent in normal males.

Autosomal Dominant Hereditary Disorders.

Males and females alike may be affected by an abnormal dominant gene which causes a particular disorder, despite the normality of its paired gene (allele). Afflicted individuals have a 50% likelihood of transmitting the abnormal gene (and the disorder) to each of their children—even when mated with a person genotypically normal. An autosomal dominant type of inheritance is probable if direct transmission of the specific trait over 3 or more generations can be established.

Autosomal dominant inheritance accounts for many serious although uncommon diseases, including chondrodystrophy, Huntington's chorea, Marfan's syndrome, juvenile glaucoma, and Charcot-Marie-Tooth disease. A low incidence of these disorders in the general population is explained by natural selection. Nevertheless, certain disorders, such as Huntington's chorea, have a late onset, and reproduction may have already occurred.

Autosomal Recessive Hereditary Disorders.

For abnormal recessive genes to produce a clinical abnormality, they must be coupled (duplex state). A normal dominant gene makes an abnormal coupled gene recessive. To bring out the trait in an offspring, one abnormal recessive gene must be contributed by each parent who is genotypically affected but phenotypically (clinically) normal.

Autosomal recessive inheritance of a specific disease is difficult to prove. However, certain criteria are used to establish presumptive evidence of this type of transmission: (1) Diagnosis of the identical disease in collateral branches of the same family. (2) Detection of the disease in approximately 25% of siblings in a large family. (3) Consanguinity of individuals within a family increases the likelihood of a duplex status of the affected but recessive genes. The disorder will therefore become more common within that family but less frequent in the general population. (4) Metabolic aberrations similar to those observed in an individual suffering from a clinical disease may be discovered in apparently normal relatives by biochemical studies.

A large number of autosomal recessive diseases have been identified. Enzyme deficiencies, altered plasma proteins, and disorders of the metabolism of specific amino acids can now be determined to identify persons with minimal or no clinical evidence of an autosomal recessive inheritance. More than 300 hereditary metabolic disorders are now recognized, including cystic fibrosis, cystinuria, diabetes mellitus, galactosemia, glycogen storage disease, hepatolenticular degeneration, phenylketonuria, sickle cell disease, peculiar ocular disorders, and instances of mental retardation.

Table 29-1. Sex chromosome abnormalities.* (Modified after Barnes.)

Number of Chromatin Bodies	Number of Chromosomes	Sex Chromosomes (Karyotype)	Physical Appearance (Phenotype)	Diagnosis
None	45	XO (or X)	Female, no significant secondary female sex characteristics.	Turner's syndrome
	46	XY	Female, secondary female sex characteristics; normal external female genitalia.	Testicular feminization; gonads are testes; sterility and amenorrhea.
	46	XY	Male	Normal male
	47	XYY	Male	"Normal" male with mentally defective offspring.
± Barr bodies	46	Xx (partial)	Female, no secondary sex characteristics.	Streak gonads, amenorrhea
One	46	XX	Female	Normal female
	47	XXY	Male	Klinefelter's syndrome
Two	47	XXX	Female	Mental retardation, sterility, abnormal menses.
One	48	XXYY	Male	Klinefelter's syndrome with severe mental retardation.
Two	48	XXXY	Male	
Three	49	XXXYY	Male	
	49	XXXXY	Male	
Four	49	XXXXX	Female	Mental retardation, mongolism.

*Normal male and female included for comparison.

Ill-Defined Genetic Disorders.

Undoubtedly, genetic factors which are still incompletely understood are present in many disorders. It seems likely that hereditary influences play a significant role in idiopathic hypertension, epilepsy, atherosclerosis, schizophrenia, allergic illnesses, and cancer. Unfortunately, it is often impossible to appraise the relative influence of heredity and environment in these conditions. To make the problem even more difficult, the apparent erratic and incomplete expression of recessive abnormalities, so-called "spontaneous" cases, the effects of environmental irradiation, complex dietary and toxic chemical agents, and the problem of securing accurate large-group data defy appraisal.

Genetic Counseling.

Genetic counseling may be difficult and involved but it is most important for the patient, her family, her children, and society. The physician must thoroughly understand the problem and the family milieu. In general, the major concerns relate to the severity of the genetic abnormality and the statistical probability of its appearance in the offspring. Fortunately, a long and useful life is compatible with many clinically severe genetic disorders. The physician should seek to correct misconceptions and false assumptions. He can often alleviate guilt and shame by an accurate interpretation kindly stated.

The problem is an individual one and must be handled as such, especially when giving advice about marriage and procreation. The physician has the responsibility for discreetly discouraging wedlock by carefully and tactfully explaining to the patient the probable occurrence of a significant dominant genetic disorder in her offspring. He must indicate the undesirability of a union of 2 persons carrying serious recessive genetic traits. Regrettably, many patients refuse to accept such advice because of ignorance, disbelief, recklessness, religious persuasion, love, or a desire for children. However, most states and many foreign countries have laws which forbid the marriage of persons suffering from incapacitating hereditary disorders.

30...
Gynecologic Procedures

CAUTERIZATION (COAGULATION) OF THE CERVIX

Cervical cauterization is indicated in the treatment of chronic cervicitis and ectropion (eversion) of the cervix and to obliterate nabothian cysts. A thermal (Post) or high frequency (Cauterodyn®, Bircher) electrocautery may be used.

Linear coagulation should be employed. Cauterization of remaining areas of inflammation may be done at later visits, usually 2-4 weeks apart, avoiding the time of menses. Too extensive coagulation may result in acute exacerbation of cervicitis or cervical stenosis.

Following extensive coagulation, the cervix should be gently dilated occasionally over the following 2 months to ensure patency of the canal.

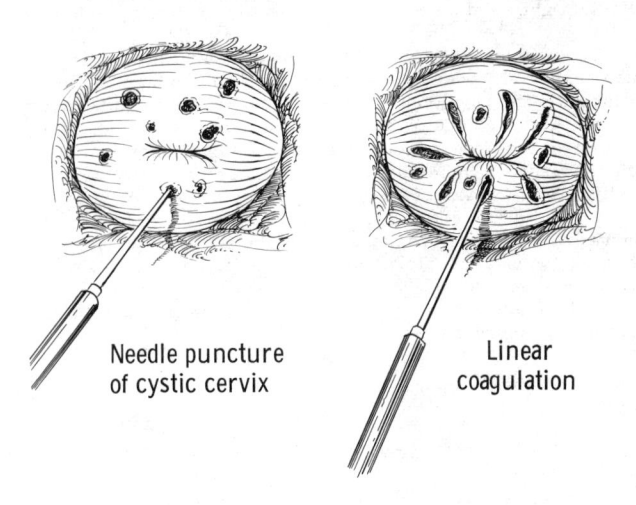

Fig 30-1. Cauterization (coagulation) of the cervix (after Ball).

CERVICAL POLYPECTOMY

Ecto- and endocervical polyps may be removed in a variety of ways. Avulsion of the sessile mass by twisting it on its pedicle, severance of the polyp at its base, and coagulation division at the point of attachment of the polyp are popular methods. Bleeding points should be ligated or sutured rather than cauterized to avoid slough, infection, and spread of possible malignancy. Every polyp should be fixed in 10% formalin or Bouin's solution and evaluated by a pathologist.

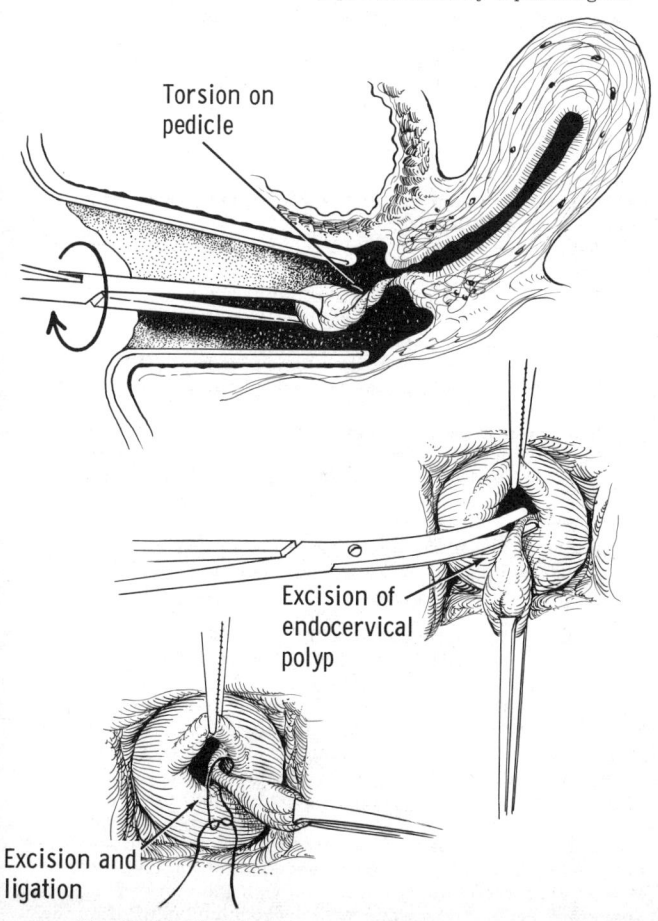

Fig 30-2. Three methods of cervical polypectomy.

ENDOMETRIAL BIOPSY

Endometrial biopsy is a relatively painless office procedure for the study of the uterine lining. It is of value for the following purposes: (1) Appraisal of endocrine effects in infertility (endometrial atrophy, anovulation, inadequate luteal phase, endometritis). (2) Identification of causes of abnormal uterine bleeding and endocrine problems. (3) Evaluation of results of gynecologic hormone therapy. (4) Diagnosis of endometrial cancer, particularly in postmenopausal patients. (In very early cancer, the tissue obtained may be inadequate for diagnosis.)

The procedure is contraindicated in pregnancy and in women with acute pelvic inflammatory disease. Perforation of the uterus, infection, and hemorrhage are rare complications.

Procedure.

Anesthesia is not usually required, but paracervical block can be used if desired.

A. Determine the position of the corpus bimanually to properly direct the curet.
B. Expose the cervix with a suitable speculum.
C. Cleanse the cervical os and portio with antiseptic solution.
D. Gently insert a uterine sound to determine the direction, size, and regularity of the uterine cavity. (If the uterus is large, discontinue the procedure and perform a pregnancy test.)
E. Insert a suction biopsy curet (Novak, Randall), and obtain long individual strips from the anterior, posterior, and right and left lateral walls and the fundus, using slight negative pressure. Fix each specimen in Bouin's solution or 10% formalin.
F. Interpret the histologic picture in relation to the patient's menstrual dates, history, and other findings.

CERVICAL DILATATION & UTERINE CURETTAGE (D & C)

Surgical D & C is a valuable diagnostic and therapeutic procedure. The cause of abnormal uterine bleeding (particularly when cancer is suspected) and obscure incomplete abortion usually are revealed by uterine curettage. Removal of polypoid, often hyperplastic endometrium allows new growth and more normal endometrium in several weeks.

Curettage is most informative when it is timed specifically. For example, irregular shedding of the endometrium is best diagnosed during 6th-8th days of the menstrual period; secretory endometrium cannot be recognized until after the

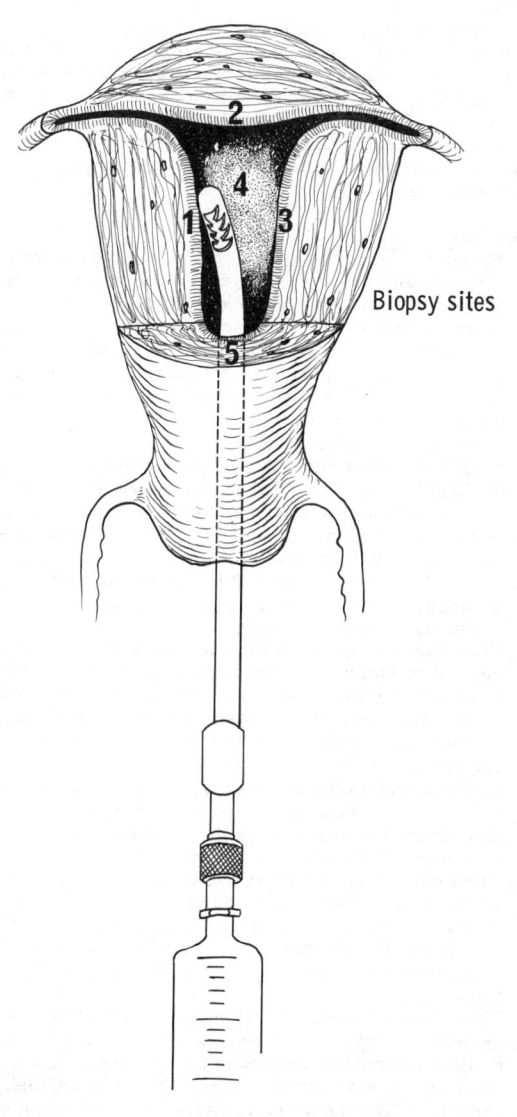

Fig 30-3. Technic of endometrial biopsy.

672 Cervical Dilatation & Uterine Curettage

16th day (assuming ovulation on the 14th day); submucous myomas can be felt best when the endometrium is thinnest—on about the 7th day; endometrial polyps (rarely responsive to hormonal stimulation) are felt more readily when surrounded by soft, secretory endometrium at about 24-26 days.

The **contraindications** include normal intrauterine pregnancy and acute cervicitis, endometritis, or pelvic inflammatory disease.

Procedure.

A. Paracervical, spinal, or general anesthesia may be used.
B. Prepare and drape the patient as for vaginal surgery.
C. Catheterize the bladder to simplify the examination and to permit subsequent replacement of the uterus if it is retroposed and nonadherent. Record the size, shape, position, consistency, and mobility of the fundus and cervix. Identify the adnexa and other pelvic structures. Note the presence of fluid and zones of induration or fixation of the organs.
D. Stain the cervix and vaginal vault with Schiller's reagent or Lugol's solution. Take biopsy specimens or cone cancer suspect zones before endocervical instrumentation.
E. Sound the cervical canal and uterine cavity to note their dimensions and contour.
F. Dilate the cervix to No. 20 Hanks (preferred, perforated dilators) or No. 8 Hegar—a size adequate for insertion of curets of standard size.
G. Curet the endocervix with a small sharp instrument, being careful to obtain no endometrium (differential curettage). Unless the curet is unusually sharp or undue force is exerted, any firm tissue obtained must be considered suspicious and should be fixed separately in Bouin's or 10% formalin solution and appraised by a pathologist.
H. Insert a uterine forceps (e.g., Overstreet) or a gallbladder stone forceps. Grasp for polyps or small pedunculated myomas. Identify any such tissues obtained and prepare them for section and study.
I. Perform a four-quadrant and vault curettage with a small sharp or serrated curet. Obtain long strips of endometrium from each area. Do not squeeze tissue or permit it to dry. Fix the specimens promptly and label the bottle. If questionable specimens are obtained, identify the site and fix separately.
J. Therapeutic Curettage: Therapeutic curettage requires a systematic, vigorous coverage of the entire cavity, including the fundus and each cornual area. Record irregularities such as tumors, septa, scarred regions, and recesses. Wipe the uterine cavity by inserting an open dry sponge and twisting it as it is removed. This procedure will recover detached tissue fragments and blood clots.

Cervical Dilatation & Uterine Curettage 673

K. Reinsert a uterine polyp forceps and grasp for any pedunculated neoplasm previously missed.
L. Replace the uterus in the forward position following curettage A vaginal pessary may be required for 4-6 weeks to hold the fundus in proper anteposition.

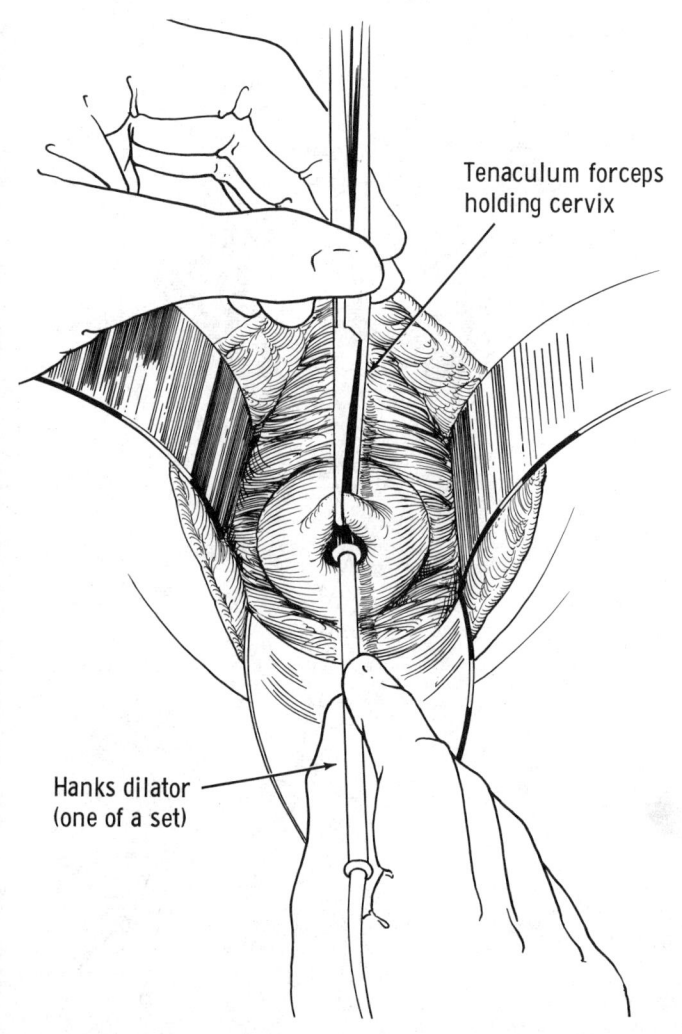

Fig 30-4. Cervical dilatation.

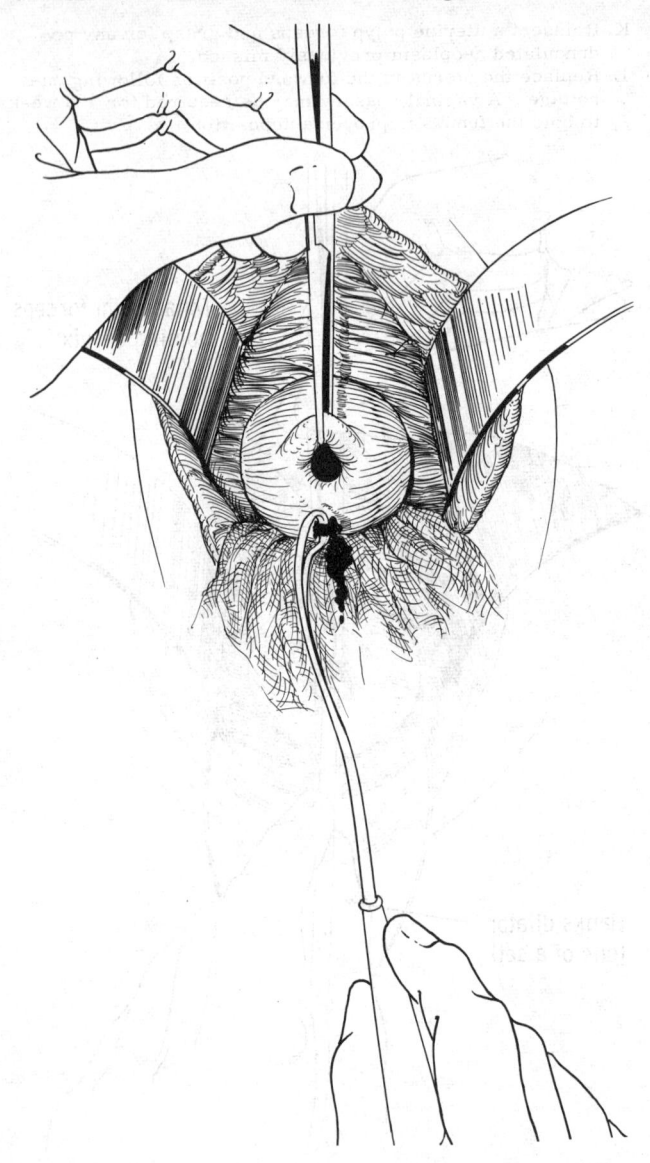

Fig 30-5. Curettage.

Biopsy of the Cervix 675

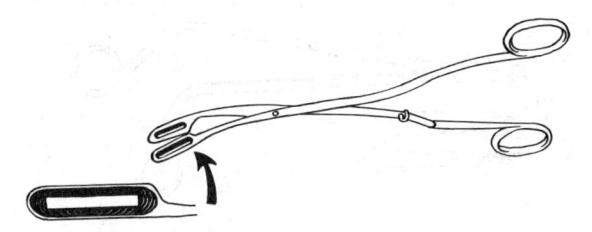

Fig 30-6. Overstreet endometrial polyp forceps.

BIOPSY OF THE CERVIX

Scalpel cervical biopsy is often done, and requires primary suture closure of the defect for control of bleeding. In addition, a variety of biopsy forceps have been developed, and many of these have special advantages. It is important to utilize an instrument that will not crush the tissue and that will remain sharp despite sterilization.

The Tischler biopsy instrument is favored by many because of its simplicity and because its unique construction allows small or generous "bites" with collection of the tissue in a small recess at the tip.

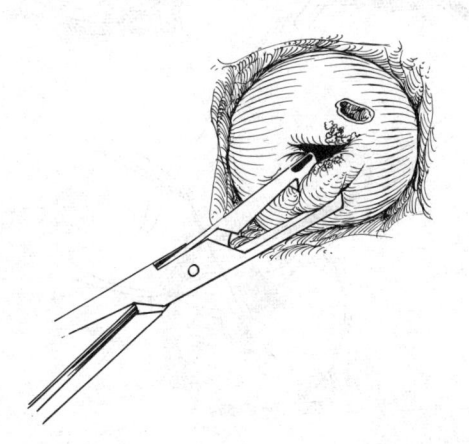

Fig 30-7. Multiple punch biopsy of cervix with Tischler forceps.

676 Biopsy of the Cervix

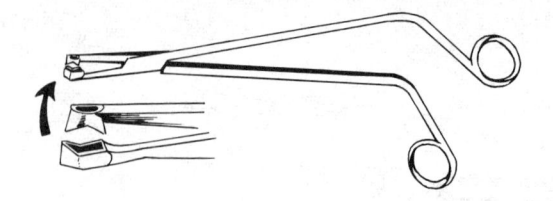

Fig 30-8. Tischler cervical biopsy forceps.

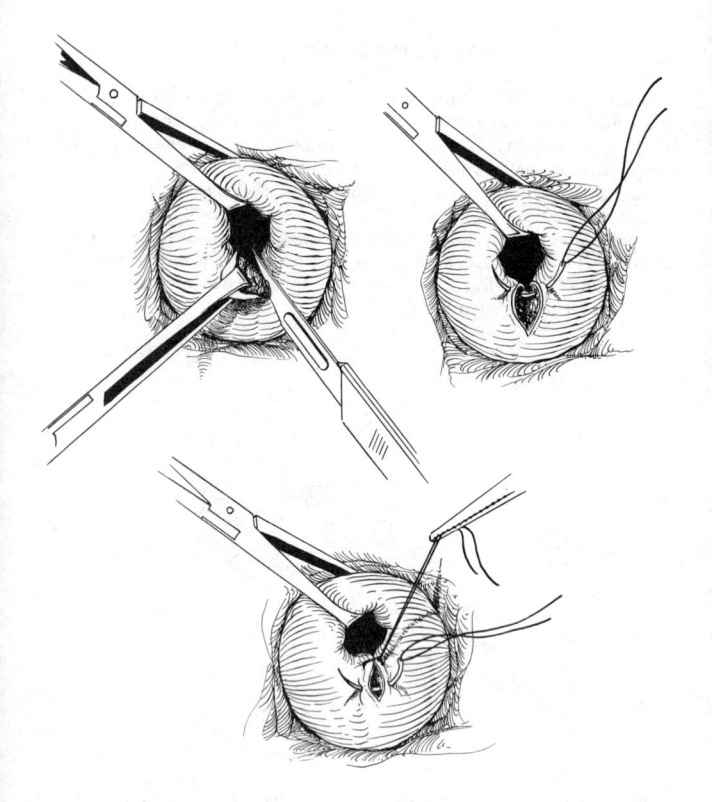

Fig 30-9. Wedge biopsy of the cervix.

CONIZATION OF THE CERVIX

Scalpel or "cold conization" of the cervix, particularly for investigation of early carcinoma, necessitates the removal of a portion of the cervix from the mucosquamous junction to the internal os. For cancer study, the tissue rarely must exceed 0.3 cm in thickness. Preliminary application of Schiller's reagent or Lugol's solution aids in the identification of suspicious areas. The injection of a vasoconstrictor drug (e.g., epinephrine, vasopressin) in normal saline solution reduces bleeding. A uterine sound should be inserted to or just beyond the internal os so that the cervix can be coned without excessive bleeding by directing the tip of the scalpel toward the probe at the internal os. A suture of nonabsorbable material is usually inserted at the top of the cone to aid the pathologist in orienting the tissue for histologic study.

If the cervix is deeply lacerated, segmental excision of tissue may be required to make up a cone. Identification of each of the fragments is required. A diagram and individual numbering with each fragment in a separate bottle of fixative will simplify subsequent pathologic study.

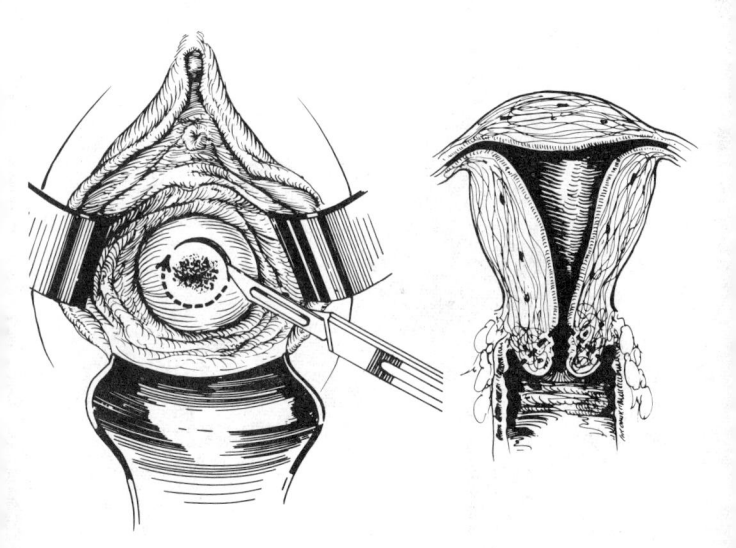

Fig 30-10. Conization of the cervix.

TRACHELORRHAPHY
(Cervical Repair)

Deep, poorly healed cervical lacerations cause gaping of the cervix, eversion of the endocervical lining, excessive cervical mucous discharge, and bleeding. Chronic granulomatous areas within the notched, exposed portions of the cervix are zones of chronic infection. Infertility may develop because of inflammation which hinders sperm migration. Wide exposure of the shortened endocervical canal and cervicitis may predispose to abortion if pregnancy does occur.

Trachelorrhaphy consists of excision of a segment of tissue within the laceration and reconstruction of the cervix utilizing interrupted or mattress type sutures of medium weight (0-1) chromic catgut or nonabsorbable suture material. This is a hospital procedure which requires paracervical or other appropriate anesthesia. The Sänger unilateral and Emmet bilateral trachelorrhaphies are practical corrective procedures. A Sturmdorf trachelorrhaphy may be employed

Denudation of bilateral lacerations

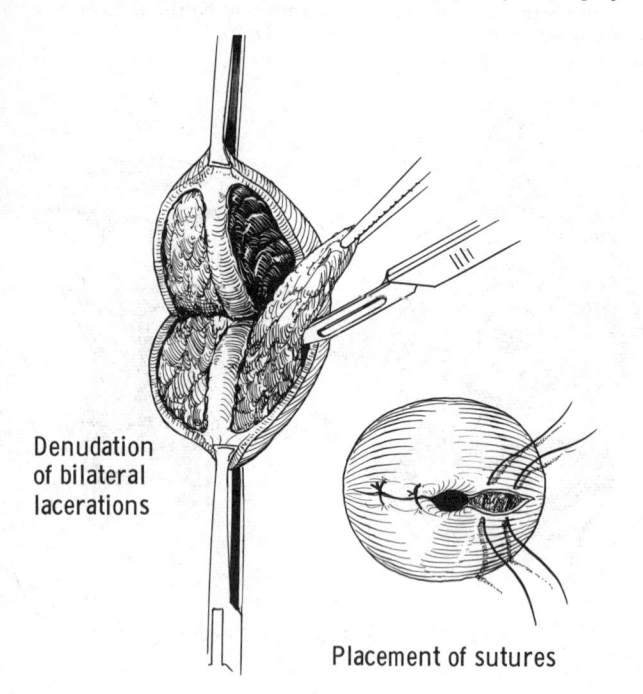

Placement of sutures

Fig 30-11. Emmet's bilateral trachelorrhaphy.

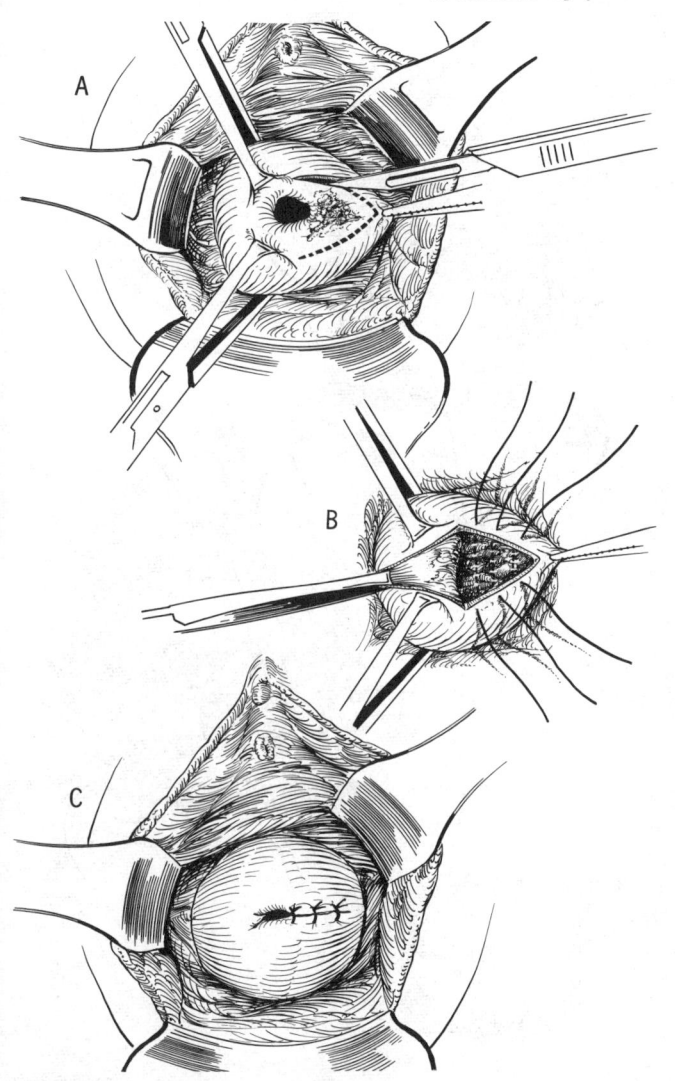

Fig 30-12. Sänger's unilateral trachelorrhaphy. (A) Granulomatous surface in the old lateral laceration undercut and flaps developed. (B) The flap is pulled toward the midline while the deep sutures are introduced. It is then cut off and the sutures tied. (C) Trachelorrhaphy completed.

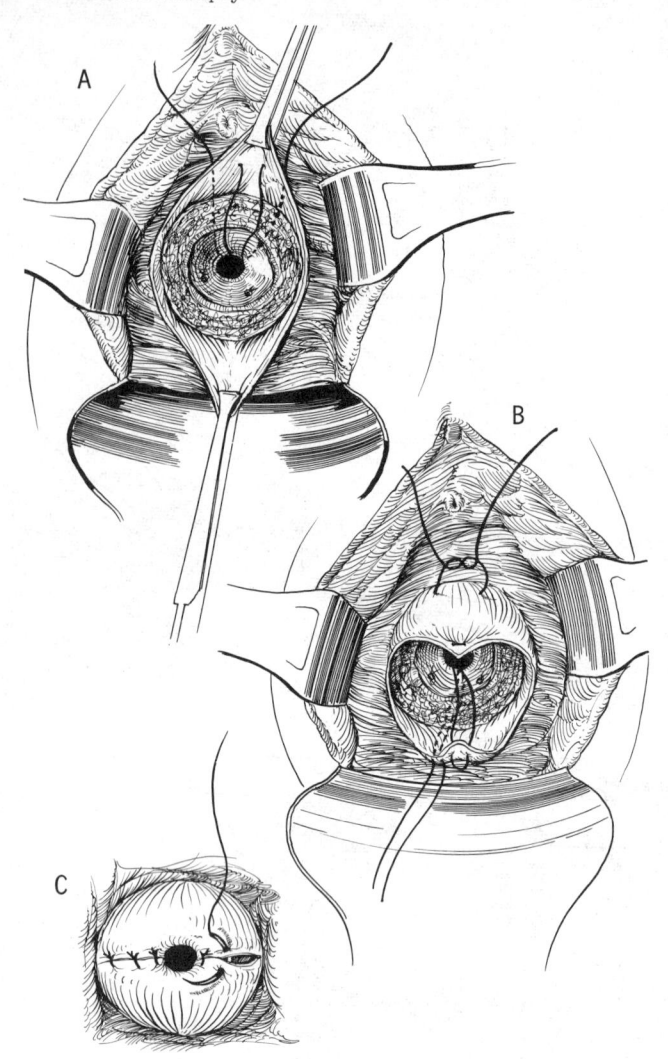

Fig 30-13. Sturmdorf trachelorrhaphy (after Ball). (A, B) Cervix coned (amputated if hypertrophic) and bleeding points controlled by sutures. (C) Interrupted suture closure.

for the repair of a deeply lacerated, hypertrophic, usually chronically infected cervix. This operation requires partial amputation and conization of the cervix with coverage of the denuded area by vaginal mucous membrane, using deep inverting sutures followed by finer superficial sutures for marginal closure.

A Sturmdorf trachelorrhaphy may be employed for the repair of a deeply lacerated, hypertrophic, usually chronically infected cervix. This operation requires partial amputation and conization of the cervix with coverage of the denuded area by vaginal mucous membrane, using deep inverting sutures followed by finer superficial sutures for marginal closure.

CORRECTION OF CERVICAL INCOMPETENCE IN THE NONPREGNANT PATIENT

Cervical incompetence is suggested by a history of repeated midtrimester abortion, usually following a traumatic vaginal delivery, and abnormal patulousness of the cervix (easy passage of dilators to No. 8 Hegar). Occult lacerations in the region of the internal os are a common cause of sequential second trimester miscarriages. It is virtually impossible to locate the precise area of weakness, but excision of a segment of cervix and myometrium, including the area of the internal os, usually will correct the defect and improve function.

An incision is made anteriorly above the cervix and the dissection is continued anteriorly, with displacement of the bladder upward to expose the cervical canal and lower uterine segment. An arrow-shaped portion of tissue is removed with a sharp scalpel and the margins are reapproximated, using interrupted medium weight chromic catgut. Fine catgut sutures are employed for closure of the mucosal layer.

The operation is highly effective in preventing subsequent spontaneous midtrimester abortion.

CERVICAL CERCLAGE
(Shirodkar Operation)

The placement, snug tie, and fixation of a nonabsorbable Mersilene® or comparable strand, ribbon, or band beneath the mucosa and pericervical fascia at the cervicouterine junction may be done during the pregnant or nonpregnant state for correction of cervical incompetence (see Fig 30-15). The physician must then decide whether to release the ligature during labor for vaginal delivery or to perform cesarean section near term.

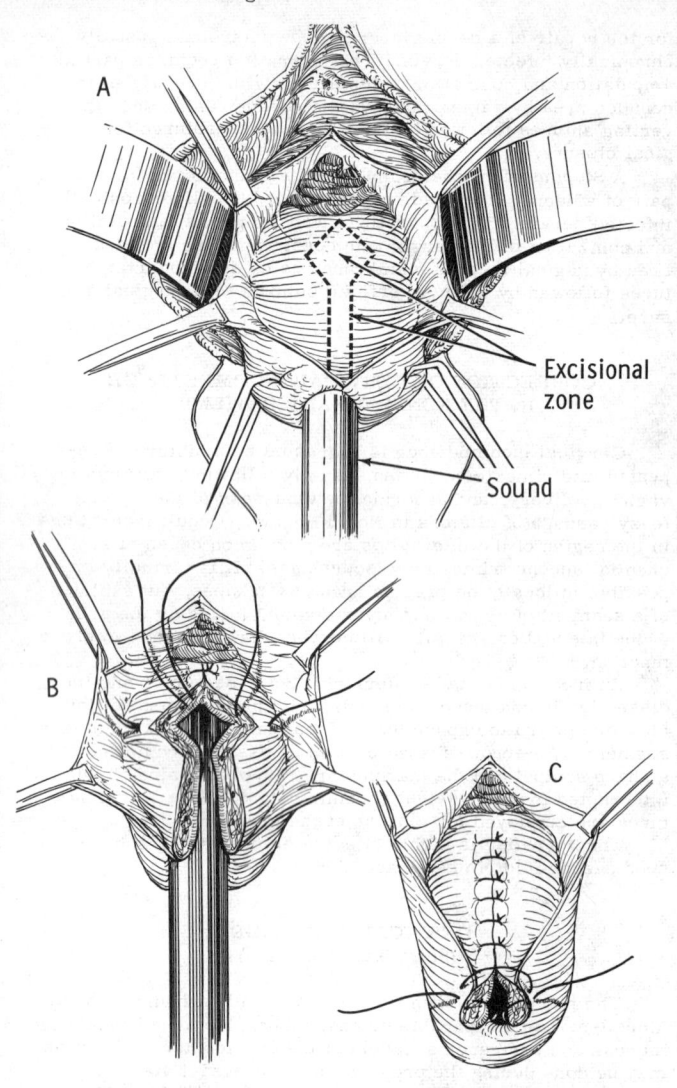

Fig 30-14. Correction of cervical incompetence in the non-pregnant patient (after Ball). (A) Bladder displaced upward, exposing cervicouterine junction. (B) Reapproximation of cervicouterine junction. (C) "Crown suture" mucosal closure.

Cervical Cerclage 683

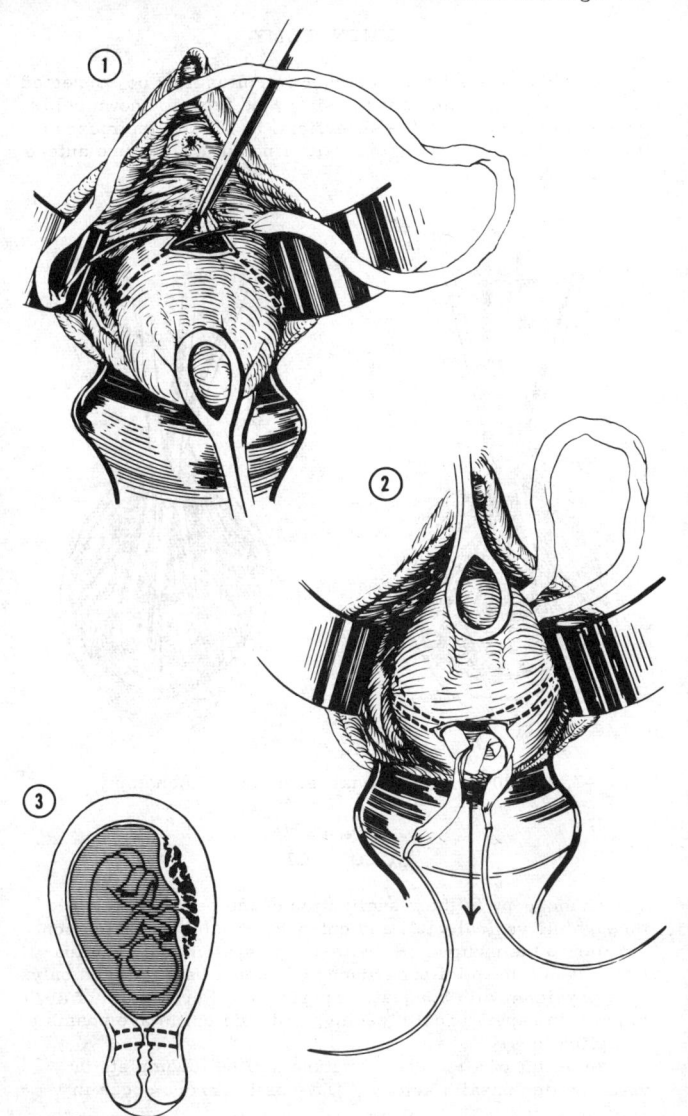

Fig 30-15. Cerclage of the cervix (Shirodkar) with incompetent os in pregnant patient.

HYMENOTOMY

An obstructive hymen or snug introitus may be corrected under local infiltration anesthesia. The technic shown below consists of incision of the superficial tissues to the musculature in the axis of the vagina, with fine suture closure anteroposteriorly.

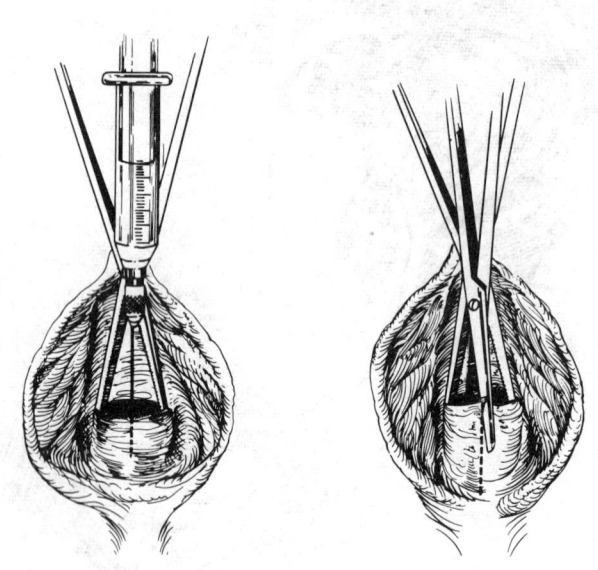

Fig 30-16. Incisional technic of hymenotomy.

CULDOSCOPY

Culdoscopy is the visualization of the pelvic structures through the vaginal vault and cul-de-sac using an instrument similar to the cystoscope, with a lens system and illumination. It is a hospital procedure and should be attempted only by a physician with adequate experience. Perforation of a viscus, intraperitoneal bleeding, and peritonitis are possible complications.

In 5-10% of attempts, puncture will be incomplete or visualization unsatisfactory. Diagnostic errors occur in 1-5% of cases.

Procedure.

A. Administer a hypnotic such as meperidine (Demerol®),

Vault of vagina

Cervix grasped with vulsellum and drawn downward

Culdoscope in cul-de-sac

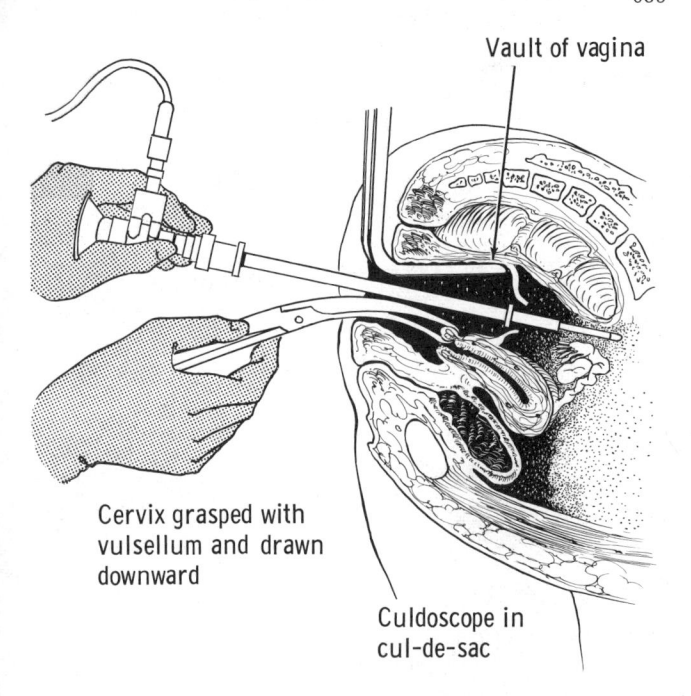

Fig 30-17. Culdoscopy.

   100 mg I. M.
B. With the patient in the knee-chest position and a Sims retractor elevating the perineum, grasp the posterior lip of the cervix with a tenaculum to expose the posterior fornix. Apply an antiseptic solution and then inject 1-2 ml of 1% procaine solution (or equivalent) into the central portion of the fornix. A few minutes later, thrust the sterile culdoscope trocar through the vaginal wall and the peritoneum with one quick movement.
C. Remove the trocar and substitute the sterile culdoscope. Systematically examine the peritoneum, tubes, ovaries, etc.
D. After the examination is completed, remove the culdoscope and expel as much air as possible from the peritoneal cavity through the cannula by exerting pressure on the abdomen.
E. Remove the instrument. It is not necessary to suture the trocar wound; healing will occur within several days.

Appendix

SHOCK

Shock is a state of profound, refractory hypotension which is the general response of the body to an acute reduction in cardiac output, either primary or secondary. There are 3 basic etiologic categories: central vascular, systemic vascular, and peripheral microcirculatory vascular disorders. Very young, very old, or pregnant patients and persons suffering from severe systemic or debilitating diseases are most susceptible. Without early treatment, shock is very frequently fatal.

Pathogenesis of Shock.

Shock is a manifestation of cardiovascular insufficiency which follows a critical decrease in effective circulating blood volume. Causes include the following:
  A. Central Vascular Disorders: Congestive heart failure, myocardial infarction, arrhythmias, and cardiac tamponade which depress cardiac function.
  B. Systemic Vascular Disorders: Hemorrhage or dehydration upsets the balance between the circulating blood volume and the physical capacity of the vascular bed.
  C. Peripheral Vascular Disorders: Severe sepsis, vasotoxic drugs, deep anesthesia, and acute hepatic and renal insufficiency disturb the function and the integrity of the minute vessels in the terminal vascular bed.

There are many factors which perpetuate or sustain shock, including bacterial toxins, reticuloendothelial depression, intense peripheral vascular resistance, inadequate visceral circulation, adrenocortical insufficiency, and electrolyte imbalance.

Microcirculatory insufficiency, or inadequate tissue perfusion, is common to all patients in shock irrespective of the immediate cause. Every system of the body is progressively impaired by circulatory and tissue failure. In time, the microvascular tissue failure becomes self-perpetuating even though the initial problem is eliminated, and shock then becomes irreversible and fatal.

Etiology & Pathologic Physiology of Shock in Obstetrics & Gynecology.

Although shock is an involved symptom complex, for practical purposes patients in shock fall into 2 basic categories: (1) those whose major abnormality is inadequate circulating blood volume, and (2) those in heart failure. One problem may compound the other.

Shock in obstetric or gynecologic patients is often attributable to one or more of the following causes: (1) Hemorrhage, dehydration, and electrolyte imbalance: The volume of circulating blood is depleted. (2) Bacteremia: Sequestration or pooling of blood leading to hypovolemia is a serious feature. (3) Fainting and the collapse following spinal anesthesia or uterine inversion are a result of neurogenic mechanisms. Sudden loss of vascular tone pools blood in the splanchnic and peripheral areas and limits venous return to the heart. (4) Anaphylaxis or idiosyncrasy to drugs: Hypersensitivity results in vascular collapse and reduction in blood returned to the heart. (5) Supine hypotension in obstetric patients, due to amniotic, air, or pulmonary embolism which obstructs afferent cardiac circulation. (6) Arrhythmias, myocardial insufficiency, or other cardiac disorders: Heart failure reduces its pumping efficiency.

In hypovolemia, there is a loss of considerable blood from the vascular space as a result of bleeding or escape of plasma into an injured area. Normally, blood volume represents about 7.5% of the body weight. Rapid loss of 15-20% of the blood volume will result in mild shock; 40% reduction causes severe shock; and a loss of over 50% in a short time is usually fatal.

Very young, very old, and chronically ill individuals—especially those who have sustained severe injuries or who have been given deep general anesthesia or major surgery—are most susceptible to shock. Women with hypoadrenocorticism or those who have received regular therapeutic doses of corticoids (e.g., for asthma or a collagen disease) may develop intractable shock because of reduced adrenocortical reserve unless they receive one of the cortisones as a supportive measure. Pregnant women (particularly those with toxemia) have poor vascular tone and do not resist shock well. During pregnancy, endotoxin released in septic shock may provoke a generalized Shwartzman reaction without previous sensitization.

Hypovolemia in shock is responsible for numerous problems in addition to inadequate cardiac output and reduced capillary circulation. Hypoxic tissues undergo anaerobic metabolism in shock; normal oxidation of lactate and pyruvate to CO_2 and water, for example, fails to occur. Residual acid catabolites accumulate, and acidosis develops. Reduced plasma pH causes an adrenergic release of catecholamines, and vasoconstriction ensues. This protective mechanism may become deleterious when overcompensation occurs because arteriovenous shunts develop to further aggravate cellular oxygen lack and metabolic stagnation. For a time, the blood pressure is supported at the expense of tissue oxygenation. Eventually, vascular collapse results, circulation virtually ceases, tissue becomes devitalized, and death ensues.

In addition to the above, stress causes initial hyperglycemia; but glycogen stores soon become depleted and hypoglycemia results. Catabolism is responsible for azotemia and hyperkalemia; hyponatremia follows fluid shifts. Impaired lung perfusion during hypoventilation, physical exhaustion, or airway obstruction leads to superimposed respiratory acidosis.

The pathologic consequences of shock depend upon its type, degree, and duration. Internal vascular spasm occurs early; vasodilatation occurs later. Tissue degeneration as a result of hypoxia and retention of metabolites is particularly notable in the abdominal viscera. Lower nephron nephrosis or cortical necrosis and hemorrhage into the adrenals or other organs often develop in severe cases. Increased viscosity of the blood and intravascular coagulation may occur. Paradoxically, in rare instances the blood fails to clot.

Clinical Findings.
- A. Impending Shock: A variable period of intense sympathetic activity generally precedes hypotension. Weakness, pallor, cool, moist skin, and tachycardia develop. (**Caution:** Do not confuse with simple fainting.) Fever and shaking chills precede collapse in septic shock. Marked orthopnea, arrhythmia, and severe chest pain are warning signs of cardiogenic shock.
- B. Established Shock: Hypotension (systolic pressure < 100 mm Hg) is superimposed on the above early signs, and tachycardia (> 100) usually develops. (In hypertensive patients, shock may be present when the systolic pressure is > 100 mm Hg.) Thirst, air hunger, severe prostration, and dulling of the sensorium are advanced signs. Coma, cardiac arrest, and death are imminent at this point.
- C. Septic Shock: Chills, high fever, anorexia, and occasional nausea and vomiting are often preceded by a history of criminal abortion, traumatic delivery, or recurrent pyelonephritis. Flushed facies and tachycardia accompany the fever. With bacteremia, initial neutrophilic leukopenia gives way to marked leukocytosis.

    Between 3-9 hours after the first shaking chill, a precipitous drop in body temperature to subnormal levels often heralds disorientation and hypotension, oliguria, and shock.

Treatment.

Because multiple deficits develop, there is no simple and reliable physiologic pattern of patient response to shock. Survival depends upon intensive diagnostic efforts, monitoring of essential parameters, and a flexible plan of therapy based upon vital signs and laboratory data.

Act quickly. Shock is an acute emergency which takes precedence over all other problems except acute hemorrhage, cardiac arrest, and respiratory failure.

Tentatively determine the primary cause of shock promptly. A brief history (if available) and the gross physical findings will permit the identification of hemorrhagic, cardiogenic, septic, or allergic shock in most cases. Except in neurogenic shock due to fainting—a self-limiting condition which can be treated by placing the patient in the recumbent position and administering stimulants—proceed with antishock measures utilizing additional therapy as required for specific problems.

A. Place the patient in the recumbent or head-down (Trendelenburg) position. Disturb her as little as possible.

B. Establish an adequate airway and ensure pulmonary ventilation. Administer oxygen by mask, especially when dyspnea or cyanosis is present.

C. Keep the patient comfortably warm but do not apply excessive external heat because this will cause peripheral vasodilatation.

D. Control pain and relieve apprehension. Shocked patients often have very little discomfort. Choose a sedative such as pentobarbital sodium, 0.13 gm (2 gr) I.V., or, if imperative, morphine sulfate, 10-15 mg ($1/6$-$1/4$ gr), diluted, I.V. (**Caution:** Narcotics are contraindicated for patients in coma, those with head injuries or respiratory depression, and in pregnant women who are likely to deliver within 1-2 hours.)

E. Parenteral Fluids: Restore adequate blood volume immediately. The most effective replacement fluid is whole blood. However, replacement of whole blood for all blood lost in complicated shock states is often harmful. Moreover, acid-base deficits or dehydration may require correction, and protective solutions such as mannitol are usually necessary. Until whole blood can be given, consider I.V. administration of low molecular weight dextran (Rheomacrodex®), 1-1.5 gm/kg in 10% solution in normal saline. Repeat in 8 hours if urine output is good unless bleeding is continuing. This plasma expander reduces blood viscosity, prevents intravascular clotting, and increases capillary circulation. Plasma, plasma products, regular dextran, 5% dextrose, and normal saline are also of value in that order.

Obtain blood for grouping, cross-matching, hematocrit, coagulation time, white blood count, and blood chemistry prior to infusion. If superficial veins have collapsed, puncture a large vein such as the femoral vein for temporary infusion prior to cut-down or percutaneous canalization of a major vessel such as the subclavian vein for central venous pressure determination.

Central venous pressure monitoring should be instituted to measure the hemodynamics and to serve as a guide to treatment. This procedure also serves as a more direct route for therapy to the heart in cases of extreme blood loss, septic shock, serious fluid and electrolyte imbalance, or when the functional capacity of the heart to withstand heroic restorative measures, anesthesia, surgery, or delivery is questionable.

The normal central venous pressure (CVP) is 8-13 cm H_2O. If CVP equals 6-8 cm H_2O, additional fluid replacement is essential and very large amounts of blood or other fluids may be required, as judged by the initial estimate based on the patient's size. If blood volume replacement establishes normal cardiac function and adequate urine production (20-30 ml/hour) with a CVP of 10 cm H_2O, the problem probably was hypovolemia (corrected) regardless of cause. If shock, low arterial pressure, and poor circulation persist despite a CVP of 10-13 cm H_2O, suspect deficient cardiac function, perhaps due to myocardial insufficiency.

1. Whole blood must be correctly grouped and cross-matched for replacement. In dire emergencies, group O, Rh-negative blood may be used without cross-matching. Treatment in cases of shock may require 4-5 liters delivered under pressure in 30 minutes to restore CVP to 10-13 cm H_2O. Use large needles and multiple venipuncture if transfusion is urgently needed. Intra-arterial transfusion is useful when there is marked depression of cardiac action or when citrated blood without calcium is to be used. This will avoid pulmonary vasoconstriction and myocardial depression.
2. Plasma, serum albumin, and Plasmanate® (a reconstituted blood product) may be stored for emergency use and are particularly valuable for the treatment of plasma loss, as in hemoconcentration complicating peritonitis. Homologous serum jaundice is a calculated risk (20%) in patients receiving pooled plasma.
3. Plasma expanders - Dextran 40 (Rheomacrodex®) is a low molecular weight dextran which is superior to others because it reduces the viscosity of the blood and maintains microcirculation much better than regular dextran (see p. 690). Dextran (Expandex®,

Gentran®, Plavolex®) is a water-soluble biosynthetic polysaccharide, 6% in isotonic saline solution. Administer 500-1000 ml I.V. at a rate of 20-40 ml/minute, but do not give more than required to sustain the blood pressure at 90 mm Hg. (**Caution:** Patients with cardiac or renal insufficiency may develop pulmonary edema.) Obtain blood samples before administering dextran because this substance may confuse blood grouping or cross-matching.

4. Saline, dextrose, mannitol solutions - Normal saline or 5% dextrose in saline (500-1000 ml I.V.) will expand blood volume for 1-2 hours until whole blood or blood products can be administered. Mannitol, 10% in normal saline solution, 200-300 ml I.V., reduces renal vascular resistance, causes diuresis, and prevents lower nephron nephrosis. Saline is used as a diluent to avoid hyponatremia.

5. Correction of bicarbonate deficit - Sodium lactate in a $1/6$ molar concentration is approximately isotonic. It is useful in the treatment of acidosis. However, it must be metabolized to bicarbonate before it becomes effective as an alkalinizing agent. In urgent shock therapy, severe acidosis, or when hepatic function is reduced, sodium bicarbonate solution is preferred. This is available in vials containing 3.75 gm (45 mEq) in 50 ml. This is to be added to 5% dextrose in water in the amount required to provide the proper correction of acidosis as indicated by such tests as plasma pH (< 7.35) or CO_2 content (< 26 mEq/liter).

6. Adjustment of acid-base balance - Restore serum sodium, calcium, chlorides, etc. to normal values, using periodic blood chemistry determinations as a guide.

7. Vasoconstrictor drugs - Lack of appreciation of the factors involved in shock leads to the temptation to reverse the most apparent sign, hypotension, and administer vasopressors. However, these agents may further embarrass the already inadequate tissue perfusion. The dose of a vasoconstrictor drug is empiric. With excessive amounts, there will be a redistribution of blood flow from the viscera to other areas. As a result, cellular necrosis may occur. It is far better to augment the blood volume and give corticosteroids than to constrict the vascular space. These drugs may be of temporary value initially to sustain blood pressure before blood or plasma is available. Angiotensin amide (Hypertensin®), 15 mg/500 ml of 5% dextrose in water, is the least deleterious

of the vasoconstrictors in shock therapy. In unusual cases of advanced shock, vasopressors may be necessary to maintain blood pressure and renal function despite apparently adequate blood or plasma.
8. Corticosteroids are not vasoconstrictors but are beneficial in shock because these drugs support the patient in a serious stress state, aid in the transfer of fluids from intra- to extracellular compartments, and, in septic shock, block intense sympathomimetic effects of endotoxin and restore vascular tone. In addition, these drugs have a beneficial antiallergic effect.

F. Treat cardiogenic shock definitively. Convert arrhythmias. Digitalize for myocardial insufficiency. Relieve cardiac tamponade.

G. Combat Anaphylactic Shock:
1. Epinephrine, 1:1000 solution, 0.1-0.4 ml in 10 ml of normal saline slowly I.V.
2. Diphenhydramine hydrochloride (Benadryl®) or tripelennamine hydrochloride (Pyribenzamine®), 10-20 mg I.V., if response to epinephrine is not prompt and sustained.
3. Hydrocortisone sodium succinate (Solu-Cortef®), 100-250 mg I.V. over a period of 30 seconds, as adjunct to epinephrine and diphenhydramine. Dosage depends upon the severity of the condition. The drug may be repeated at increasing intervals (1, 3, 6, 10 hours, etc.) as indicated by the clinical condition.
4. Aminophylline injection, 0.25-0.5 gm ($3^{3/4}$-$7^{1/2}$ gr) in 10-20 ml of normal saline I.V. slowly for severe bronchial spasm. Duration of action 1-3 hours. May repeat in 3-4 hours.

H. Treat hypovolemic shock by monitored blood and fluid and electrolyte replacement (see above).

J. Bacteremic Shock Therapy: In addition to initial general shock therapy, give specific septic shock treatment as follows:
1. Determine CVP and rapidly inject a trial volume expander such as 5% Rheomacrodex® or plasma into a catheter in the vena cava to treat hypovolemia and test cardiac reserve.
2. Treat sepsis -
    a. Give a "push" of diluted chloramphenicol, 1 gm, penicillin G, 10 million units, and streptomycin, 0.5 gm, rapidly into the vena cava.
    b. Start an I.V. infusion of normal saline containing chloramphenicol, 1 gm, penicillin G, 10 million units, and mannitol, 12.5 gm.
    Administer in 24 hours a total of: chloramphenicol, 4-6 gm I.V.; penicillin G, 30 million units I.V.; and streptomycin, 1-2 gm I.M.

c. Administer hydrocortisone hemisuccinate, 1 gm
      I.V., or dexamethasone, 40 mg I.M., per 24 hours.
   d. Give vasopressor drug to avoid extreme hypotension
      and anuria, if necessary.
3. Evaluate cardiac efficiency - Replace Hgb and blood
   loss. Digitalize the patient if heart failure seems
   likely.
4. Correct electrolyte imbalance (usually metabolic
   acidosis).
5. Treat underlying or predisposing medical problems
   vigorously (septic abortion, peritonitis, pyelonephritis, diabetes, etc.).

Evaluation of Antishock Therapy.
   Observe the patient continuously for clinical and labora-
tory responses to therapy. Tachycardia subsides and the
skin becomes warm and dry as blood pressure rises above
100 mm Hg.
   A. Take and record blood pressure, pulse, and respirations
      every 15 minutes.
   B. Maintain a fluid intake and output chart, noting time and
      amount of replacement fluid given and measuring urine
      output every 30 minutes. Acute renal failure often is a
      sequel to deep, unresponsive, or prolonged shock.
   C. Monitor CVP response, especially to initial rapid infusion
      or transfusion, as a guide both to diagnosis (hypovolemic
      versus cardiac shock) and to subsequent treatment. Try
      to rapidly achieve and maintain a normal CVP (8-13 cm
      H_2O). Avoid under- or overreplacement of fluids.
   D. Auscultate the chest periodically for arrhythmia, muffled
      tones (cardiac tamponade), or murmurs. Note the appear-
      ance of rales at lung bases (indicative of congestive fail-
      ure). Obtain an EKG and appropriate medical consulta-
      tion in severe cases.
   E. Determine CO_2 combining power, blood pH, Na^+, K^+,
      Hct, and blood counts at intervals and compare with
      original values. Blood volume determinations (if avail-
      able) may confirm the accuracy of estimates of fluid re-
      placement needed. Nevertheless, these studies often
      are confusing because of regional blood pooling and fluid
      transfer between the intra- and extravascular spaces.

Persistent or Recurrent Shock.
   When intensive therapy does not improve or correct
shock in 30-60 minutes, or when the disorder recurs, consider the following causes:
   A. Incompletely Corrected Blood Volume:
      1. Insufficient blood replacement - Very large transfusions
         rapidly administered are required in severe hemorrhage
         or trauma.

2. Electrolyte imbalance.
   3. Persistent or recurrent bleeding (often concealed).
   4. Inadequate corticosteroid or antibiotic therapy in resistant or septic shock.
 B. Associated Diseases:
   1. Cardiac insufficiency (myocardial failure, etc.).
   2. Cerebral damage (hypoxia, thrombosis).
 C. Irreversible shock.

Anesthesia for the Shocked Patient.

The choice of anesthesia for a major surgical or obstetric procedure for the patient in shock requires a specific knowledge of the pharmacology and physiology involved. Ideally, the patient should be responsive to antishock therapy before operation. If the problem is critical, a calculated risk must be assumed. The following anesthetic methods are justified if the cause of shock has been accurately identified.

 A. Hypovolemic Shock: Inhalation anesthesia with maximum oxygen concentration is preferable. Nitrous oxide and ethylene cause no electrolyte or metabolic impairment. Retention of CO_2 may occur with inadequate pulmonary ventilation using cyclopropane, halothane, or fluroxene. Halothane often causes uterine relaxation, and further bleeding may occur. Regional anesthetic block may result in severe, uncontrollable hypotension. In vascular (caval) obstruction by the pregnant uterus, spinal or caudal anesthesia may further complicate the supine hypotensive syndrome. If this occurs, elevate the uterus; turn the patient to the semilateral position; place a support beneath the right hip to tilt the uterus to the left; and proceed with therapy.
 B. Cardiogenic Shock: Local infiltration with the patient in Fowler's position is recommended.
 C. Bacteremic Shock: Cyclopropane probably is the best anesthetic considering that vascular collapse, renal failure, and fever are present. Nitrous oxide and halothane in low concentration or minimal amounts of succinylcholine (the only muscle relaxant which is well hydrolyzed) is the second choice. (However, succinylmonocholine, produced during oliguria or anuria, may accumulate and retard dissipation of succinylcholine.)
 D. Anaphylactic Shock: Rarely do these patients require surgery until improved. Oxygen, vasopressors, and corticosteroids are of value. For bronchial spasm, give epinephrine by injection or inhalation (spray).
 E. Neurogenic Shock: For replacement of uterine inversion (for example), any anesthetic with a rapid induction time such as cyclopropane is the agent of choice. If considerable relaxation of the lower uterine segment is required, halothane may be used.

EFFECTS OF MATERNAL MEDICATIONS ON THE FETUS AND NEWBORN INFANT

Maternal Medication	Fetal or Neonatal Effect

Sex hormones
  Androgens
  Estrogens
  Progestogens
	Masculinization and advanced bone age

Corticosteroids	Anomalies; cleft palate (?)

Thyroid medications
  Methimazole (Tapazole®)
  Potassium iodide
  Propylthiouracil
	Goiter; mental retardation (?)

Antidiabetes drugs Sulfonylurea derivatives (Orinase®, Diabinese®)	Anomalies (?)
Insulin (shock or hypoglycemia)	Fetal death
Phenformin (DBI®)	Lactic acidosis (?)

Antineoplastic agents
  Amethopterin (methotrexate)
  Aminopterin
  Chlorambucil
	Anomalies and abortion

Anticoagulant drugs
  Bishydroxycoumarin (Dicumarol®)
  Ethyl biscoumacetate (Tromexan®)
  Warfarin (Coumadin®)
	Fetal death, hemorrhage

Vitamin K preparations (excessive)	Hyperbilirubinemia
Cardiovascular drugs Ammonium chloride	Acidosis
Hexamethonium	Neonatal ileus
Reserpine	Nasal congestion and drowsiness
Thiazide diuretics	Thrombocytopenia
Intravenous electrolyte solutions (excessive)	Fluid and electrolyte abnormalities
Antihistamines	Anomalies (?)

EFFECTS OF MATERNAL MEDICATIONS ON THE FETUS AND NEWBORN INFANT (Cont'd.)

Maternal Medication	Fetal or Neonatal Effect
Sedative, hypnotic, and tranquilizing drugs Meprobamate (Miltown®, Equanil®)	Retarded development
Phenobarbital (excessive)	Neonatal bleeding
Phenothiazines (e.g., chlorpromazine)	Hyperbilirubinemia (?)
Thalidomide	Phocomelia, hearing loss, fetal death
Analgesic and narcotic drugs Heroin Morphine	Neonatal death, convulsions, tremors
Salicylates (excessive)	Neonatal bleeding
Tobacco smoking	Undersized babies
Anti-infective drugs Chloramphenicol (Chloromycetin®)	Fetal death ("gray" syndrome)
Chloroquine (Aralen®)	Retinal damage or death (?)
Erythromycin (Ilosone®)	Hepatic injury (?)
Nitrofurantoin (Furadantin®)	Hemolytic reactions
Novobiocin (Albamycin®)	Hyperbilirubinemia
Quinine	Thrombocytopenia, abortion
Streptomycin	Acoustic nerve deafness (?)
Sulfonamides	Kernicterus
Tetracyclines	Hemolysis, inhibition of bone growth, discoloration of teeth
Smallpox vaccination	Fetal vaccinia

Conversion of Metric Weights (gm) to Approximate Avoirdupois Weights (lb and oz)

Metric	Avoirdupois	Metric	Avoirdupois
2000 gm	4 lb 7 oz	3550 gm	7 lb 13 1/2 oz
2050	4 lb 8 oz	3600	7 lb 15 oz
2100	4 lb 10 oz	3650	8 lb 1 oz
2150	4 lb 12 oz	3700	8 lb 3 oz
2200	4 lb 14 oz	3750	8 lb 4 1/2 oz
2250	4 lb 15 1/2 oz	3800	8 lb 6 oz
2300	5 lb 1 1/2 oz	3850	8 lb 8 oz
2350	5 lb 3 oz	3900	8 lb 10 oz
2400	5 lb 5 oz	3950	8 lb 11 1/2 oz
2450	5 lb 7 1/2 oz	4000	8 lb 13 oz
2500	5 lb 8 oz	4050	8 lb 15 oz
2550	5 lb 10 oz	4100	9 lb 1 oz
2600	5 lb 12 oz	4150	9 lb 3 oz
2650	5 lb 14 oz	4200	9 lb 4 oz
2700	5 lb 15 1/2 oz	4250	9 lb 6 oz
2750	6 lb 1 oz	4300	9 lb 8 oz
2800	6 lb 3 oz	4350	9 lb 10 oz
2850	6 lb 5 oz	4400	9 lb 11 oz
2900	6 lb 6 1/2 oz	4450	9 lb 13 oz
2950	6 lb 8 oz	4500	9 lb 15 oz
3000	6 lb 10 oz	4550	10 lb
3050	6 lb 12 oz	4600	10 lb 2 1/2 oz
3100	6 lb 13 1/2 oz	4650	10 lb 4 oz
3150	6 lb 15 oz	4700	10 lb 6 oz
3200	7 lb 1 oz	4750	10 lb 8 oz
3250	7 lb 3 oz	4800	10 lb 10 oz
3300	7 lb 4 1/2 oz	4850	10 lb 11 oz
3350	7 lb 6 oz	4900	10 lb 13 oz
3400	7 lb 8 oz	4950	10 lb 15 oz
3450	7 lb 10 oz	5000	11 lb
3500	7 lb 11 1/2 oz		

Index

-A-

Ablatio placentae, 227
Abnormal uterine bleeding, 599
ABO incompatibility, 170
Abortion, 245, 246
　therapeutic, 400
Abruptio placentae, 227
Abscesses, tubo-ovarian, 548, 552
Accidental hemorrhage, 227
Acetazolamide, 278
Adeno-acanthoma of endometrium, 528
Adenocarcinoma, 466
　of cervix, 483
　of endometrium, 526, 528
　of fallopian tubes, 555
Adenofibroma of ovary, 557
Adenomyoma, 538
Adenomyosis, 538
Adnexa, uterine, palpation of, 440
Aftercoming head, 391
Agglutination inhibition test for pregnancy, 44
Ambulation, early, 192
Amenorrhea, 36, 608
Amicar, 232
Amnesia, obstetric, 142
Amniocentesis in erythroblastosis fetalis, 173
Amnion, 61
Amniotic fluid, 61
Amniotomy, 153
Ampullary pregnancy, 217
Analgesia, obstetric, 142
Anatomy of female reproductive system, 1
Android pelvis, 335, 339
Anemia, iron deficiency, 294
　Mediterranean, 297
　megaloblastic, 295
　pernicious, 295
　refractory, 296
　sickle cell, 296
Anesthesia, caudal, 148
　general, 142, 144
　obstetric, 142
　paracervical, 145
　perineal, 145
　pudendal, 145
　spinal, 149
Aneuploidy, 663

Angiomas, spider, 283
Ankle swelling, 90
Anovulatory bleeding, 599, 602
　cycles, 33
Anteflexion of uterus, 507
Antepartal care, 74
　complications in multiple pregnancy, 212
Anterior pituitary luteinizing hormone, 25
Anthropoid pelvis, 335, 339
Apgar score of newborn infant, 157
Aphthous ulcers, 458
Appendicitis during pregnancy, 300
Arrhenoblastoma, 562
Arthritis during pregnancy, rheumatoid, 306
Arthropathy, pelvic, of pregnancy, 305
Aschheim-Zondek test, 44
Asphyxia neonatorum, 156
Aspiration, vaginal, 495
Atrophic changes, senile, 615
　cystitis, 614
　vaginitis, 455, 614
Autosomal hereditary disorders, 665
　dominant, 662, 665
　recessive, 662, 665
　trisomy syndromes, 662
Axis traction forceps, 366
　handles, 357

-B-

Backache, 85, 648
Ballottement, 43
Bandl's ring, 347
Barr body, 664
Barrier, placental, 63
Bartholin's duct(s), 6
　cyst, 462
　glands, 6
Barton forceps, 358
Basal body temperature, 45, 636
　cell carcinoma, 466
Baths in puerperium, 194
Battledore placenta, 59, 60
Baudelocque's measurement, 81
BBT, 636
BI, 81
Biischial diameter, 79

700 Index

Bimanual examination of pelvis, 440
Bipartite placenta, 58, 60
Birth control, 633
Bladder care in puerperium, 193
  fistula, 592
Blastocyst, 53
Bleeding, abnormal uterine, 191, 602
  anovulatory, 602
  nonplacental, 225
  placental, 225
  postmenopausal, in pelvic cancer, 604
    vaginal, 604
  third trimester, 224
  uterine, abnormal, 599
    hematologic causes of, 601
Block, paracervical, 146
  perineal, 145
  pudendal, 145
Bloody show, 105
Botryoid sarcoma, 480
Bougie, 154
Bowel complications, 582
  cramping, 94
  function in puerperium, 193
Bowen's disease, 467
Bracht's method in breech delivery, 384
Brandt's technic of recovery of placenta, 134
Braxton Hicks contractions, 62, 220
  sign, 41
  version, 243, 378
Breast, carcinoma of, during pregnancy, 304
  examination of, 435
  feeding, 203
  soreness, 90
Breech, complete, 380
  delivery, 383, 384, 386, 388
  extraction, 389
    partial, 385
  frank, 380
  hydrocephalic, 391
  incomplete, 380
  presentations, 110, 112, 115, 379
Breisky pelvimeter, 81
Brenner tumor of the ovary, 572
Bruit, 41
Brunkow urethral advancement, 587

–C–

Call-Exner bodies, 574
Canal of Nuck, 24
Cancer of the cervix, 482
  of the fallopian tubes, 555

Cancer, Cont'd.
  fundal, 526
  of the ovaries, 557
  terminal, management of, 655
  of the uterus, 526
  vulvar, 464
Candeptin, 455
Candicidin, 455
Candida albicans, 442, 452, 457
  vaginitis, 455
Candidiasis, 452, 455, 459
Caput succedaneum, 163
Carcinoma(s), of breast during pregnancy, 304
  of the cervix, 482
  of endometrium of uterus, 527, 528
  epidermoid, of the cervix, 482
  of the fallopian tubes, 555
  of the uterus, 526
  of the vagina, 471
  of the vulva, 464
Carcinosarcoma of the uterus, 536
Cardiac arrest, 288, 289-94
Caruncle, urethral, 587
Caudal anesthesia, 148
CD, 81
Cephalometry, x-ray, fetal, 337
Cerebrovascular accidents during pregnancy, 312
Cervical cancer, 482
  irradiation therapy, 489
  radical total hysterectomy, 493
  staging of, 484
  cap pessary, 639
  dilatation and uterine curettage, 670, 673, 674
  incompetence, correction of, 681, 682, 683
  laceration, repair of, 180
  mucus, changes in, 32
  polyps, 479, 669
  pregnancy, 217, 219
  repair, 678, 679, 680
  scrapings, 495
Cervicitis, 473
Cervix, 10
  adenocarcinoma of, 483
  biopsy of, 444, 675
  cancer of, 482
  conization of, 677
  dilatation of, 108, 668
    and effacement of, 106
  diseases of, 473
  effacement of, 110
  inspection of, 439
  invasive carcinoma of, 483
  softening of, 40
  wedge biopsy of, 676
Cesarean hysterectomy, 395

Cesarean, Cont'd.
  section, 392
CGT, 65
Chadwick's sign, 38
Chamberlen forceps, 356
Change of life, 34
Childbed fever, 265
Childbirth, natural, 154
Chloasma, 37, 282
Chlordantoin, 455
Cholecystitis during pregnancy, 302
Choledocholithiasis during pregnancy, 302
Chorea gravidarum during pregnancy, 312
Chorio-epithelioma, 250, 253
Chorion, 53, 61
  cystic degeneration of, 250
  frondosum, 55
  laeve, 55
Chorionic gonadotropin, 65
Chromatids, 663
Chromosomal abnormalities, 663
Chromosome(s), 660
  sex, abnormalities of, 666
Cineflurography for stress incontinence, 584
Circulation, fetal, 69, 70
  fetoplacental, 54
  immediate postdelivery, 71
  normal, 71
  predelivery phase of, 69
  uteroplacental, 55
Circumvallate placentas, 59, 60
Cistrons, 660
Clark's test, 531, 606
Classical cesarean section, 393
  forceps, 356
Climacteric, 34, 611
Clitoris, 4
Cloaca, 20
Clomid, 566, 578, 610
Clomiphene, 566, 578, 610
Coitus, painful, 650
Colitis, ulcerative, during pregnancy, 301
Colon carcinoma during pregnancy, 301
Colposcopy, 446
Compound presentations, 111
Compression of uterus, bimanual, 182
Confinement, expected date of, 46
Conization of cervix, 677
Conjugata diagonalis, 81, 332
  vera, 81, 332
Conjugate, diagonal, 81, 332
  true, 81
Constriction ring, 347
Contraception, 202, 619, 633
  immunologic, 637

Contraceptives, oral, 639
Contractions, Braxton Hicks, 62, 220
  uterine, 94
Cord, umbilical, 56, 61
  forelying, 262
  prolapse of, 261
  velamentous insertion of, 59
Corpus cancer, 526
  luteum, 14, 53
    cysts, 566
  of the uterus, 11
Cortical stromal hyperplasia, ovarian, 578
Corticoadrenal tumors, 561
Cotyledons, 55
Counseling, genetic, 667
Cramps, leg, 93
Craniotabes, 163
Cranium, major diameters of, 163
Credé maneuver, 128
Cul-de-sac, 7
Culdoscopy, 221, 445, 684
Cullen's sign, 220
Curettement of uterus, 670
  gauze, 181
Curie technic in cervical cancer, 492
CV, 81
Cycle, menstrual, 27
  typical, 29
Cystadenocarcinoma, 558
Cystadenoma, 558
Cyst(s), Bartholin duct, 462
  corpus luteum, 566
  dermoid, 572
  endometrial, 568
  follicle, 566
  granulosa lutein, 566
  inclusion, 568
  inflammatory, 567
  lutein, 566
  ovarian, 565
  parovarian, 23
  theca lutein, 567
  tubo-ovarian, 567
  vaginal, Gartner's, 23
Cystic degeneration of the chorion, 250
Cystitis, atrophic, 614
  senile, 614
Cystocele, 447
Cytologic study, exfoliative, Papanicolaou smear, 495
Cytology, vaginal, 436
Cytomegalic inclusion disease during pregnancy, 324
Cytotrophoblast, 55, 63

−D−

D & C, 670
Danforth's method, 391
Date of confinement, expected, 46
DC, 81, 332
Decidua basalis, 54
    capsularis, 54
    parietalis, 61
DeLee maneuver, 368
Deletion of genes, 661
Deliria, toxic, 421
Deliver(ies), aids to normal, 136
    of the body, 127
    breech, 383, 386
    emotional aspects of, 415
    of the extremities, 127
    forceps, 359
        floating, 360
        high, 359
        indications for, 359
        low, 359
        trial, 360
    of the head, 122
    in the home, 424
    midforceps, 359
    normal, course and conduct of, 104
    obstetric complications of, 217
    operative, 353
    of the placenta, 129
    of the shoulders, 126
    vertex, 119
Demons-Meigs syndrome, 557
Dental care during pregnancy, 101
Depressive reactions, 420
Dermatitides of female genitalia, 457
Dermatologic complications during pregnancy, 282
Dermoid cysts, 572
Descensus uteri, 512
Diabetes mellitus during pregnancy, 316, 320
Diagnosis of pregnancy, 36
Diagonal conjugate, 81, 332
Diameter, biischial, 79, 81
    intertuberous, 79, 330
    posterior sagittal, 81
    'tuberischial, 81
Diaphragm, pelvic, 20
    vaginal, 639
Diet, 95
Dietary allowances, recommended daily, 100
Dilatation of the cervix, 108
Distention, 94
Diverticulum of urethra, 590
Dominant gene, 660
Double ovum twin, 209
Down's syndrome, 662
Drinking during pregnancy, 102
Drugs, effect on fetus, 696
Duct(s), Bartholin's, 6
    cyst, 462
    Müllerian, 22
Duncan mechanism, 129
Duration of pregnancy, 36, 46
Dysfunction, uterine, 346
Dysgerminoma, 571
Dyskinesia, uterine, 656
Dysmenorrhea, functional, 656
    membranous, 31
    primary, 656
Dyspareunia, 650
    functional, 652
    organic, 651
Dystocia, 330
    of fetal origin, 350
    inlet, 333
    midpelvis, 334
    outlet, 335
    pelvic, 330
    due to uterine dysfunction, 344

−E−

EACA, 232
Eclampsia, 268
Eclamptogenic toxemia, 268
Ectopic endometrium, 541
    pregnancy, 217
Eczema, 457
EDC, 46
Edrophonium, 313
Elliott forceps, 356
Embryology, 20
Embryonic growth, 66
Emotional aspects of delivery, 415
    of labor, 415
    of the postpartal period, 416
    of pregnancy, 413, 414
Employment in pregnancy, 103
Endocrine diseases during pregnancy, 314
Endometrial biopsy, 670, 671
    carcinoma, 530
    cysts, 568
    implants, 541
    sarcoma of endometrium, 528
Endometrioma, 568
Endometriosis, 541
Endometrium of uterus, adeno-acanthoma of, 528
    adenocarcinoma of, 526, 528
    carcinoma of, 526
    carcinosarcoma of, 528
    dating of, 624
    ectopic, 542
    sarcoma of, 528
    squamous cell carcinoma of, 528
    stages of carcinomas of, 528

Endosalpingosis, 224
Endosalpinx, 12
Enterobiasis, 459
Enterocele, 447
Epidermoid carcinoma of cervix, 482
Epilepsy during pregnancy, 311
Episiotomy, 136
  incisions, care of, 194
  repair of, 138, 140
  timing of, 140
  types of, 136, 137
Epsilon-aminocaproic acid, 232
Epulis, 38
Erysipelas, 461
Erythema palmare, 283
Erythroblastosis fetalis, 170
Estrogen(s), 25
  natural conjugated, 616
Estrogen-progesterone test for pregnancy, 44
Examination(s), breast, 435
  gynecologic, 432
  pelvic, 436
  postpartal, 201
  rectovaginal, 441
  speculum, 437
  vaginal, 436
Exanthematous diseases during pregnancy, 323
Excretory apparatus, development of, 21
Exercises, Kegel, 586
  postpartal, 195 ff.
Exfoliative cytologic study, Papanicolaou smear, 495
Expected date of confinement, 46
Extraction, breech, 389
Extractor, vacuum, 370
Extraperitoneal cesarean section, 394
Extrauterine pregnancy, 217
Extremities, delivery of, 127
Extrindex test, 638

-F-

Face application of forceps, 363
  presentations, 111, 116, 117
Faintness, 85
Fallopian tubes, 10, 12
  adenocarcinoma of, 555
  anomalies of, 546
  carcinoma of, 555
  diseases of, 546
False pregnancy, 423
Fascia, endopelvic, 20
Fascial planes of the pelvis, 18
Fatigue, 95
Female infertility, 619
  reproductive system, anatomy of, 1

Female reproductive system, Cont'd.
  physiology of, 1
Fern test, 631
Fertilization, 53
Fetal cephalometry, x-ray, 337
  circulation, 69, 70
  dystocia, 350
  growth, 66
  membranes, 61
  nutrition, 68
  weight, Johnson's calculation of, 49
Fetoplacental circulation, 54
Fetus, 53
Fibrinolysins, 232
Fibroid tumor, 521
Fibromas of ovary, 557
Fibromyoma, 521
Fistula(s), bladder, 592
  ureteroenteric, 591
  ureteroperitoneal, 591
  ureterovaginal, 591
  ureterovesical, 591
  ureterovesicovaginal, 596
  urethrovaginal, 591
  urinary, 590
  vesicocervical, 591
  vesicoperitoneal, 595
  vesicouterine, 591
  vesicovaginal, 591
Flatulence, 94
Floating forceps delivery, 360
Flushes, vasomotor, 613
Follicle cysts, 566
Follicle-stimulating hormone, 25
Folliculoma, 574
Forceps application, 360
  face, 363
  axis traction of, 366
  Bailey-Williamson, 355
  Barton, 357, 358
  cephalic application of, 363
  Chamberlen, 356
  classical, 356
  deliveries, 359
  Elliott, 355, 356
  Kielland, 355, 358
  Mann, 356, 358
  McLean-Tucker, 355
  obstetric, 356
  operations, 353
  outlet, 141
  Piper, 355, 358, 390
  rotation, 365
  Simpson, 353, 355, 356
  Tarnier, 356, 357
  types of, 355, 356
  Willett placenta previa, 243
Forelying cord, 262
Fornices of vagina, 7
Fossa navicularis, 7
Fourchet, 7

704 Index

Fourth stage of labor, complications of. See Third stage of labor, 175
Frank breech, 380
Friedman-Hoffman test, 44
Frigidity, 654
FSH, 25
Full-term infant, 155, 162
Functional classification of heart disease, 284
 dysmenorrhea, 654
 dyspareunia, 652
Fundus of the uterus, 10
 cancer of, 527
Fungal dermatitis, 460
Funis, 56, 61
Furunculosis, 461

-G-

Gamete, 661
Gartner's vaginal cysts, 23
Gastrointestinal disorders during pregnancy, 298
Gauze curettement of uterus, 181
Gellhorn pessary, 515
Gene(s), 660
 deletion of, 661
 dominant, 660
 recessive, 660
Generative ducts, embryology of, 22
Genetic(s) counseling, 667
 disorders, 662
 medical, 660
Genitalia, external, 1
 embryology of, 24
 internal, 7
Genital tubercle, 24
Genotype, 661
German measles during pregnancy, 323
Glands, Bartholin's, 6
 para-urethral, 5
 paravaginal, 6
 Skene's, 5
 vulvovaginal, 6
Glomerulonephritis during pregnancy, 309
Gonadal failure, 612
Gonads, origin of, 23
Gonococcal salpingitis, 547
Gonorrheal vaginitis, treatment of, 456
 vulvovaginitis, 452
Gout during pregnancy, 308
Graafian follicles, 14
Granulosa cell tumor, 574
 lutein cysts, 566
Gravindex test for pregnancy, 44
Grawitz tumor, 569

Gynandroblastomas, 561
Gynecoid pelvis, 335, 337
Gynecologic backache, 648
 examination, 432, 435
 history, 432
 problems, psychosomatic, 644
 procedures, 435

-H-

Habitual abortion, 245
Headache(s), 90
 during pregnancy, 310
Head, aftercoming, 391
 delivery of, 122
 extractor, Muirless, 357
Heart disease during pregnancy, 283
Heart-lung resuscitation, 289-94
Hegar's sign, 38, 41
Hemagglutination inhibition test for pregnancy, 44
Hemantigen testing, 172
Hematologic causes of uterine bleeding, 601
 disorders during pregnancy, 294
Hematoma, 178
Hematopoiesis, 68
Hematotrophic transfer, 68
Hemolytic disease of the newborn, 170
Hemophilus vaginalis vaginitis, 455
Hemorrhage, accidental, 227
 postpartal, 175
Hemorrhagic disorders during pregnancy, 297
Hemorrhoids, 89
Hepatitis, viral, during pregnancy, 303
Hereditary disorders, autosomal dominant, 665
 recessive, 662
 sex-linked, 662, 664
Hernia(s), abdominal, 304
 pelvic floor, 512
 pudendal, 512
 vaginal, 447
Herniated intervertebral disk during pregnancy, 313
Herpes gestationis, 282
 progenitalis, 458
 zoster, 458
Hiatus hernia during pregnancy, 298
Hicks's sign, 41
Hidradenitis, 461
Hindgut, 21
History, gynecologic, 432
 obstetric, 74
Histotrophic transfer, 68
Home delivery, 424

Hormonal changes during pregnancy, 34
Hormone, anterior pituitary
 luteinizing, 25
 follicle-stimulating, 25
 luteotropic, 25
 treatment in menopause, 616
Hydatidiform mole, 250, 251
Hydrocephalic breech, 391
Hydropic mole, 250
Hygiene, vaginal, 101
Hymen, 6
Hymenotomy, 653, 684
Hyperemesis gravidarum, 257
Hypermenorrhea, 599
Hypernephroid tumor(s), 561
 ovarian, 569
Hypernephroma, 569
Hyperplasia, ovarian cortical stromal, 578
Hyperthecosis, ovarian, 579
Hypothyroidism in pregnancy, 315
Hysterectomy, cesarean, 395
 radical total in cervical cancer, 493
Hysterography, 252
 in salpingitis, 551
 in uterine malposition, 505
Hysterosalpingography, 221, 556

-I-

Idiogram, 661
Ileus during pregnancy, adynamic, 299
 dynamic, 299
 paralytic, 299
Impetigo, 460
Implantation, 53
Implants, endometrial, 541
Incision(s), episiotomy, care of, 194
 of intestine, 597
Inclusion cysts, 568
Incompatibility, Rh or ABO, 170
Incontinence, cinefluorography for stress, 584
 paradoxic, 586
 urinary stress, 582
Induction of labor, 151
Infant, full term, 162
 immediate care of, 127
 premature, 169
Infectious diseases during pregnancy, 322
Infertility, 619, 625
Inflammatory cysts, 567
Infundibular pregnancy, 217
Injuries, intestinal, 597
 urinary tract, 590
Inlet dystocia, 333

Intercourse in pregnancy, 101
Interstitial pregnancy, 217
Intertuberous diameter, 79, 330
Intervertebral disk, herniated, during pregnancy, 313
Intestinal injuries, 597
Intestine, crushing of, 597
 incision of, 597
 laceration of, 597
Intrauterine contraceptive devices, 633, 640, 641, 642
 pessary, 640
Inversion of the uterus, 186
Involution, uterine, 190
"Iowa trumpet," 146
Isthmic pregnancy, 217
IUCD, 633, 640, 641, 642

-J-

Jacquemier's sign, 38
Jellies, vaginal, 640
Johnson's calculation of fetal weight, 49

-K-

Karyotype, 661
Kegel exercises, 586
Kelly operation, 586
Kidney, primordial, 21
Kielland forceps, 355, 356
Klinefelter's syndrome, 662
Krukenberg tumor, 564
Küstner's sign, 573

-L-

Labia majora, 3
 minora, 4
Labor, complications of, 175
 emotional aspects of, 415
 false, 104
 induction of, 151
 management of first stage, 108
  of second stage, 119
  of third stage, 128
 mechanisms of, 120
 normal, 104, 105
 obstetric complications of, 217
 stages of, 105
 true, 104
Laceration(s), 140
 of intestine, 597
 obstetric, 136
Lactation, 202
 stimulation of, 205
 suppression of, 205
Lacunar system, 55
Ladin's sign, 38, 40
Langhans' stria, 53

706 Index

Last menstrual period, 46, 75
Leg cramps, 93
Leiomyosarcoma of uterus, 536
Leopold's maneuvers, 107, 381
Leukemia during pregnancy, 298
Leukoplakic vulvitis, 464, 465, 466
Leukorrhea, 38, 87, 451
Levamine, 308
LH, 25
Lichen rubor planus, 457
Ligaments, cardinal, 11
  Mackenrodt's, 11
  transverse cervical, 11
  uterosacral, 20
Ligamentum teres, 11
Linea nigra, 37
Listeriosis during pregnancy, 329
Lithopedion, 223
Liver function test values in pregnancy, 304
LMP, 46, 75
Lobes, succenturiate, 60
Locked twins, 213
Lock, English, 354
  French, 354
  German, 354
  Kielland, 354
LTH, 25
Lupus erythematosus, systemic, during pregnancy, 306
Lutein cysts, 566, 567
Luteinizing hormone, anterior pituitary, 25
Luteinomas, 560
Luteoblastomas, 560
Luteomas, 560
Luteotropic hormone, 25
Luteum cysts, corpus, 566
Lymphoma during pregnancy, 298

-M-

Malaria during pregnancy, 328
Malposition(s), hysterography in uterine, 505
  of the uterus, 504
  vaginal pessary for uterine, 508
Manchester-Fothergill operation, 516
Manchester technic in cervical cancer, 491
Manic-depressive psychosis, 419
Manic reactions, 420
Mann forceps, 358
Marginal placenta, 59
Marshall-Marchetti-Krantz operation, 587
Martin pelvimeter, 81
Masculinovoblastomas, 561
Mask of pregnancy, 37
Massage, uterine, 191

Mauriceau's method, 389
McDonald's rule, 48
  sign, 38
Measurement(s), Baudelocque's, 81
  pelvic, 79, 82, 330, 332
Medical complications during pregnancy, 282
  genetics, 660
Medication(s), maternal, effect on fetus, 102, 696
  in pregnancy, 102, 696
Megaloblastic anemia of pregnancy, 295
Meigs's syndrome, 558, 559
Membranes, fetal, 61
Menagen, 616
Menarche, 25, 33
Menge pessary, 515
Menopausal symptoms, treatment of, 615
Menopause, 25, 34, 611
  artificial, 611, 618
  hormone treatment in, 616
  physiologic, 612
  vaginal cytology in, 615
Menorrhagia, 599
Menses, cessation of, 613
Menstrual cycle, 27, 29
  period, last, 46, 75
  previous, 75
Menstruation, 24
  abnormalities of, 599
  anovulatory, 25
  autonomic factors in, 28
  endometrial changes in, 28, 30
  enzymatic factors in, 29
  hormonal factors in, 25
  ovulatory, 25
  phases of, 30, 31
  temperature changes in, 32
  vascular factors in, 28
Mental illness and pregnancy, 418
Mesenchymal tumors of uterus, 536
Mesonephroma, 561
Mesosalpinx, 12
Mesovarium, 13
Metabolic diseases during pregnancy, 314
Metanephros, 21
Metrorrhagia, 599
Midforceps delivery, 359
Midpelvis dystocia, 334
Midwives, 424
Milk production, 204
Minor discomforts of normal pregnancy, 85
Mittelschmerz, 599
Molding, 163
Mole, hydatidiform, 250, 251
  malignant, 253

Molluscum contagiosum, 458
Mongolian idiocy, 663
Monilia, 442
Monosomy, 663
Mons pubis, 1
  veneris, 1
Montgomery's tubercles, 38
Morning sickness, 86
Mosaicism, 662
Mucus, cervical, changes in, 32
Müllerian ducts, 22
Multiple pregnancy, 207
    antepartal complications in, 212
    presentation in, 212
    sclerosis during pregnancy, 312
Myasthenia gravis during pregnancy, 312
Mycotic infections of the female genital tract, 459
Myomas of the uterus, 522
Myomectomy, 526

-N-

Nägele's rule, 46
Natural childbirth, 154
Nausea of pregnancy, 36
Neonatal care, 320
Neoplasms, secondary ovarian, 564
Neurologic diseases during pregnancy, 310, 313
Newborn, hemolytic disease of, 170
  immediate care of, 127
  nursery care of, 155
  resuscitation of, 158
  skull of, 164, 165
Norethindrone test for pregnancy, 44
Norethynodrel test for pregnancy, 44
Nuck, canal of, 24
Nursery care of the newborn, 155
Nursing, 102
Nutrition, fetal, 68

-O-

Obstetric(s), complications of delivery, 217
    of labor, 217
  forceps, 356
    technic of use of, 363
  history, 74
  physical examination, 74
  postcesarean, 398
Obstruction(s), ureteral, 592
  urinary, 590
Occlusion, urethral, 592
Oligohydramnios, 62, 65
Oophoritis, 580

Operation(s), forceps, 353
  Kelly, 586
  Marshall-Marchetti-Krantz, 587
  Wertheim, 535
Ossification centers, fetal, 167
Osteomalacia during pregnancy, 321
Osteoporosis, 614
Outlet dystocia, 335
  forceps, 141
  pelvimeters, Williams, 81
Ovarian cortical stromal hyperplasia, 578
  cysts, 565
  disease, polycystic, 577
  fossa, 13
  hyperthecosis, 579
  neoplasms, secondary, 564
  pregnancy, 217, 219
  seminoma, 571
  tumor, hypernephroid, 569
Ovar(ies), 13
  adenofibroma of, 557
  argentaffin tumors of, 579
  Brenner tumor of, 572
  cancer of, 557
  carcinoid tumors of, 579
  diseases of, 557
  fibromas of, 557
  sarcomas of, 557
  teratoid tumors of, 572
  virilizing tumors of, 537, 560
Ovulation, 31
Oxytocics, postdelivery, 194
  use of, 141

-P-

Packing the uterus, 183, 184
Paget's disease, 465
Pain, abdominal, 94
Pajot's maneuver, 366
Papanicolaou smear, 495
Paracervical anesthesia, 145, 146
Paradoxic incontinence, 586
Parathyroid dysfunction during pregnancy, 322
Paraurethral glands, 5
Paravaginal glands, 6
Parovarian cysts, 23
Pastore technic of recovery of placenta, 134
Pediculosis pubis, 459
Pelves, classification of, 334
Pelvic arthropathy, pregnancy, 305
  cancer in postmenopausal bleeding, 604
  congestion syndrome, 540
  diaphragm, 20
  dystocia, 330
  examination, 436
    bimanual, 39

708 Index

Pelvic, Cont'd.
 floor, 19
  hernia, 512
 inflammatory disease, 546
 joint, relaxation of, during
  pregnancy, 305
 measurements, 79, 81, 330,
  332
 pain, psychogenic, 644
Pelvimeter(s), Breisky, 81
 Martin, 81
 Thoms, 81
 Williams outlet, 81
Pelvimetry, x-ray, 334, 335, 336
Pelvis, android, 335, 339
 anthropoid, 335, 339
 bimanual examination of, 440
 bony, 15
 false, 15
 gynecoid, 335, 337
 platypelloid, 335, 339
 true, 15
Peptic ulcer during pregnancy, 298
Perforation, uterine, 250
Perineal anesthesia, 145
 block, 145
 body, 7
 tears, 139
Perineotomy, 136, 653
Period, last menstrual, 46, 75
 previous menstrual, 75
Peritoneal exclusion cesarean
 section, 395
Peritonitis due to salpingitis, 553
Pernicious anemia of pregnancy,
 295
Personality characteristics in
 psychogenic disease, 645
Pessar(ies), 516
 cervical cap, 639
 Gellhorn, 515
 intrauterine, 640
 Menge, 515
 vaginal, for uterine malposition,
  508
Pfleuger's tubules, 23, 24
Phenotype, 661
Physical examination, obstetric, 74
PID, 546
Pinard's maneuver, 390
Pinocytosis, 64
Pinworm, 459
Piper forceps, 358, 390
Piskacek's sign, 38
Pituitary, anterior, luteinizing
 hormone, 25
Placenta(s), 53
 battledore, 59, 60
 bipartite, 58, 60
 circumvallate, 59, 60
 delivery of, 129

Placenta(s), Cont'd.
 marginal, 59
 mature, 56
 normal, 58
 physiology of, 62
 premature separation of, 227,
  229
 previa, 234, 236
 production of hormones in, 65
 succenturiate, 58
 toxic separation of, 274
Placental barrier, 63
 causes of bleeding, 225
 septa, 55
 transfer, 63
 types, 60
Placentation, 54
Placentography, 239
Planned Parenthood Federation, 633
Plasmotrophoblast, 53, 54, 63
Platypelloid pelvis, 335, 338, 339
Plication of the urethra, 586
PMP, 75
Podalic version, 376
Poliomyelitis during pregnancy,
 325
Polycystic ovarian disease, 577
Polyhydramnios, 62
Polymenorrhea, 599
Polyneuritis of pregnancy, 311
Polyps, cervical, 479, 669
Postcesarean obstetrics, 398
Postdelivery care, 191
 circulation, immediate, 71
Posterior sagittal diameter, 81
Postmenopausal bleeding in pelvic
 cancer, 604
 vaginal, 604
Postpartal care, 195
 examinations, 201
 exercises, 195 ff.
 hemorrhage, 175
Postpartum period, emotional
 aspects of, 416
Postural version, 373
Pouch of Douglas, 7
Prague method, 389
Preeclampsia, 268
Pregnanc(ies), abdominal, 217,
 219
 ampullary, 217
 cervical, 217, 219
 combined, 219
 dental care during, 101
 diagnosis of, 36
  differential, 43
 drinking during, 102
 duration of, 36, 46
 ectopic, 217
 emotional aspects of, 413
 employment in, 103

Pregnanc(ies), Cont'd.
 extrauterine, 217
 false, 423
 history of present, 75
   of previous, 75
 hormonal changes during, 34
 infundibular, 217
 interstitial, 217
 isthmic, 217
 management of normal, 84
 manifestations of, positive, 43
   presumptive, 36
   probable, 39
 mask of, 37
 medications in, 102
 and mental illness, 418
 multiple, 207
 normal, management of, 84
   minor discomforts of, 85
 ovarian, 217, 219
 prolonged, 51
 smoking during, 102
 term, 50
 tests, clinical, 44
   laboratory, 44
 toxemia of, 268
 travel during, 101
 tubal, 217, 219
 vomiting of, 257
Pregnosticon test for pregnancy, 44
Premarin, 616
Premature infant, 169
 separation of the placenta, 227, 229
Prenatal care, 74
Presentation(s), breech, 110, 114, 115, 379
 compound, 111
 face, 111, 116, 117
 in multiple pregnancy, 211
 transverse, 111
 vertex, 110, 112, 113
Primary dysmenorrhea, 656
Primordial kidney, 21
Procedures, gynecologic, 435
Procidentia, 513
Proctodeum, 21
Progesterone, 25
 test for pregnancy, 44
Progestogens, 544
Prolapse of the umbilical cord, 261
 complete, 262
 occult, 262
 of the uterus, 512, 513
Pronephros, 21
Pruritus of pregnancy, 283
 vulvae, 467
Psammoma bodies, 559
Pseudocyesis, 423
Pseudomucinous cystadenoma, 558
Psoriasis, 457

Psychiatric evaluation, 646
Psychogenic disease, personality characteristics in, 645
 pelvic pain, 644
Psychologic testing, 646
Psychosis, manic-depressive, 419
Psychosomatic gynecologic problems, 644
Pudendal anesthesia, 145
 hernia, 512
Puerperal sepsis, 265
Puerperium, 190
 bladder care in, 193
 bowel function in, 193
 first week of, 192
Pyosalpinx, 552

–Q–

Quadruplets, 207
Quickening, 37

–R–

Radioisotope localization in placenta previa, 240
Read, Grantly Dick, 154
Recessive gene, 660
Rectal carcinoma during pregnancy, 301
Rectocele, 447
Rectovaginal examination, 441
Renal diseases during pregnancy, 308
 excretory apparatus, development of, 21
Reproductive system, female, 1
Resuscitation, heart-lung, 289
 of newborn, 156, 158, 159
Rheumatic disorders during pregnancy, 305
Rheumatoid arthritis during pregnancy, 306
Rh incompatibility, 170
Rhythm method in contraception, 637
Ritgen's maneuver, 126
Rubella during pregnancy, 323
Rubin's test, 628, 629, 630
Rupture, uterine, 176, 177

–S–

Sagittal diameter, posterior, 81
 measurements, 79
Salpingitis, 546
 gonococcal, 547
 hysterography in, 551
 peritonitis due to, 552
 pyogenic, 548
 tuberculous, 548

Salpingography, 551
Sarcoma(s), botryoid, 480
  of endometrium, treatment of, 538
  of the ovary, 557
  of the uterus, 536
Scabies, 459
Scanzoni maneuver, 368
Schizophrenia, 421
Schuchardt incision, 137
Schultze mechanism, 129
Seatworm, 459
Semen, examination of, 621
Seminoma, ovarian, 571
Senile atrophic changes, 615
  cystitis, 614
  vaginitis, 614
Sepsis, puerperal, 265
Septa, placental, 55
Serologic test for syphilis, 83
Sex chromosome abnormalities, 666
Sex-linked hereditary disorders, 662, 664
Shock, 687
  anesthesia in, 695
Shoulders, delivery of, 126
Sign, Braxton Hicks, 41
  Chadwick's, 38
  Cullen's, 220
  Hegar's, 38, 41
  Hicks's, 41
  Jacquemier's, 38
  Küstner's, 573
  Ladin's, 38, 40
  McDonald's, 38
  Piskacek's, 38
  Von Fernwald's, 38, 42
Simpson forceps, 356
Sims-Huhner test, 631
Skene's glands, 5
Skull of newborn, 164, 165
Smoking during pregnancy, 102
Souffle, uterine, 41
Speculum examinations, 437
Sperm abnormalities, 621
Spermatic fluid, examination of, 621
Spider(s) angiomas, 283
  vascular, 283
Spinal anesthesia, 149
Spinnbarkeit, 631
Sporostacin, 455
Stations of the fetal head, 110
Stein-Leventhal syndrome, 577
Sterilization, 400, 405
  indications for, 405
  irradiation, 406
  in men, 412
  methods of, in female, 406
Stress incontinence, cinefluorography, 584

Stress incontinence, Cont'd.
  urinary, 582
Stricture, bilateral ureteral, 595
Struma ovarii, 573
STS, 83
Succenturiate lobes, 60
  placenta, 58
Surgery during pregnancy, intra-abdominal, 302
Surgical complications during pregnancy, 282
Syncope during pregnancy, 85, 311
Syntrophoblast, 53, 63
Syphilis during pregnancy, 326
  serologic test for, 83

-T-

Tarnier forceps, axis traction, 357
Tensilon, 313
Teratoid tumors of the ovary, 572
Teratomas, 572
Term pregnancy, 50
Tetany during pregnancy, 322
Tetraploidy, 663
Thalassemia, 297
Theca cell tumor, 569
  lutein cysts, 567
Thecoma, 569
Thiobarbiturates, 145
Third trimester bleeding, 224
Thoms's pelvimeter, 79, 81
  rule, 81
Thyrotoxicosis during pregnancy, 314
TI, 81, 330
"Tipped uterus," 504
Toxemia, eclamptogenic, 268
Toxic deliria, 421
  separation of the placenta, 274
Toxoplasmosis during pregnancy, 329
Trachelorrhaphy, 678, 679, 680
Traction handle, Barton, 357
  Bill, 357
Translocation, 662
Transverse presentations, 111
Travel during pregnancy, 101
Trichomonas vaginalis vaginitis, 442, 452
Trichomoniasis, 459
Trigone test, 584
Triplets, 207
Trisomy, 663
  syndrome, autosomal, 662
Trophoblast, 53
Tubal insufflation, 628, 629, 630
  pregnancy, 217, 219
Tubercles, Montgomery's, 38
Tuberculosis of female genital tract, 461

Index 711

Tuberculosis, Cont'd.
　pulmonary, during pregnancy, 326
Tuberculous salpingitis, 548
Tuberischial diameter, 81
Tubo-ovarian abscesses, 548, 552
　cysts, 567
Tumor(s), corticoadrenal, 561
　granulosa cell, 574
　Grawitz, 569
　hypernephroid, 561
　Krukenberg, 564
　ovarian, Brenner, 572
　　hypernephroid, 569
　　teratoid, 572
　theca cell, 569
　of uterus, mesenchymal, 537
Turner's syndrome, 662
Twin(s), 207
　locked, 213
　ovum, double, 209
　　single, 209

-U-

Ulcerative colitis during pregnancy, 300
Umbilical cord, 56, 61
　forelying, 262
　prolapse of, 261
Ureteral obstruction, 592
　stone during pregnancy, 310
　stricture, bilateral, treatment of, 595
Ureteroenteric fistula, 591
Ureteroperitoneal fistula, 591
Ureterovaginal fistula, 591
Ureterovesical fistula, 591
Ureterovesicovaginal fistulas, 596
Urethral advancement, Brunkow, 587
　caruncle, 587
　diverticulum, 589
　meatus, 5
　occlusion, 591
Urethra, plication of, 586
Urethrocele, 447
Urethrovaginal fistula, 591
Urinary fistulas, 590
　obstructions, 590
　stress incontinence, 582
　symptoms, 87
　tract infection during pregnancy, 308
　injuries, 590
Urogenital fold, 21
　sinus, 21
　tract, embryology of, 20
Urologic complications during pregnancy, 582
Uterine bleeding, abnormal, 599
　hematologic causes of, 601

Uterine, Cont'd.
　contractions, 94
　dysfunction, 346
　　dystocia due to, 344
　dyskinesia, 656
　involution, 190
　malposition, hysterography in, 505
　massage, 191
　perforation, 250
　prolapse, 512
　rupture, 176, 177
Uteroplacental circulation, 55
Uterus, 10
　arcuatus, 503
　bicornis unicollis, 502
　bimanual compression of, 182
　body of, 10
　carcinoma of, 526
　carcinosarcoma of, 537
　complete inversion of, 186
　congenital anomalies of, 500
　corpus of, 11
　didelphys, 502
　diseases of, 500
　duplex bicornis, 502
　fundus of, 10
　inversion of, 186
　inverted, replacement of, 189
　leiomyosarcoma of, 536
　malpositions of, 504
　mesenchymal tumors of, 537
　myomas of, 522
　nonpuerperal inversion of, 186
　packing of, 183, 184
　palpation of, 440
　partial inversion of, 186
　procedure for packing of, 185
　prolapse, 513
　puerperal inversion of, 186
　retrocession of, 506
　retroflexion of, 506
　retroversion of, 507
　septus, 503
　subseptus, 503
　tipped, 504

-V-

Vacuum extractor, 242, 370
Vagina, 7
　carcinoma of, 471
　diseases of, 447
　fornices of, 7
Vaginal aspiration, 495
　bleeding, postmenopausal, 604
　cesarean section, 396
　cysts, Gartner's, 23
　cytology, 436
　　in menopause, 615
　diaphragm, 639
　examinations, 436

712 Index

Vaginal, Cont'd.
   hernias, 447
   hygiene, 101
   jellies, 640
   pessary for uterine mal-
      position, 508
   vault, 7
Vaginismus, 651
Vaginitis, atrophic, 455, 614
   Candida albicans, 455
   gonorrheal, 456
   Hemophilus vaginalis, 455
   senile, 614
   Trichomonas vaginalis, 455
Varicose veins, 91
Vascular spiders, 283
Vasomotor flushes, 613
Veins, varicose, 91
Ventouse, 370
Version, 371
   Braxton Hicks, 243, 378
   combined, 374, 375
   external, 373, 375
      cephalic, 374
   internal, 373, 378
   podalic, 376
   postural, 373
Vertex delivery, 119
   presentations, 110, 112, 113
Vertigo during pregnancy, 311
Vesicocervical fistula, 591
Vesicoperitoneal fistula, 595
Vesicouterine fistula, 591
Vesicovaginal fistula, 591, 595
Vesicular mole, 250
Vestibule, 5
Viral hepatitis during pregnancy, 303

Virilizing hilus cell tumors of the
      ovary, 561
   lipoid cell tumors of the ovary, 560
Vomiting of pregnancy, 36, 257
Von Fernwald's sign, 38, 42
Voorhees bag, 154
Vulva, diseases of, 447
Vulvar cancer, 464
Vulvitis, 452
   leukoplakic, 465, 466
Vulvovaginal glands, 6
   lupus vulgaris, 461
Vulvovaginitis, 452

–W–

Waldeyer's cords, 23
Weight control, 95, 97
   fetal, Johnson's calculation of, 49
Wertheim operation, 535
Wigand's method, 389
Willett placenta previa forceps, 243
Williams' outlet pelvimeters, 81
Wolffian body, 21

–X–

X-ray fetal cephalometry, 337
   pelvimetry, 335, 336

–Z–

Zygote, 53